ENDOSTEAL DENTAL IMPLANTS

Endosteal Dental Implants

Ralph V. McKinney, Jr., D.D.S., Ph.D.
Professor and Chairman
Department of Oral Pathology
School of Dentistry
Professor, School of Graduate Studies
Medical College of Georgia
Augusta, Georgia

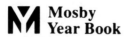 **Mosby Year Book**

St. Louis   Baltimore   Boston   Chicago   London   Philadelphia   Sydney   Toronto

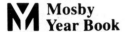

Mosby
Year Book

Dedicated to Publishing Excellence

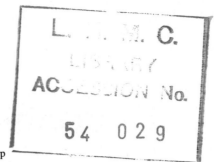

Sponsoring Editor: Robert W. Reinhardt
Associate Managing Editor, Manuscript Services: Deborah Thorp
Production Coordinator: Nancy C. Baker
Proofroom Manager: Barbara Kelly

Copyright © 1991 by Mosby–Year Book, Inc.
A Year Book Medical Publishers imprint of Mosby–Year Book, Inc.

Mosby–Year Book, Inc.
11830 Westline Industrial Drive
St. Louis, MO 63146

1 2 3 4 5 6 7 8 9 0 CL/MV 95 94 93 92 91

Library of Congress Cataloging-in-Publication Data

Endosteal dental implants / [edited by] Ralph V. McKinney, Jr.
     p.   cm.
   Includes bibliographical references.
   Includes index.
   ISBN 0-8151-6044-5
   1. Implant dentures.   I. McKinney, Ralph V.
   [DNLM: 1. Dental Implantation, Endosseous.   WU 640 E56]
RK667.I45E53   1991
617.6'92—dc20   91-13677
DNLM/DLC   CIP
for Library of Congress

This book is affectionately dedicated to Mary, Heather, Holly, Laurel, and Rosemary, my wife and daughters. Their encouragement, love, support, strength, and understanding provided a constant guiding light in the completion of this task.

CONTRIBUTORS

ARTHUR ASHMAN, D.D.S.
New York, New York

CHARLES A. BABBUSH, D.D.S., M.Sc.D.
*Head, Section of Oral and Maxillofacial Implant
    Reconstructive Surgery*
Mount Sinai Medical Center
Cleveland, Ohio

BURTON E. BALKIN, D.M.D.
Implantologist
Narbeth, Pennsylvania

MARTHA WARREN BIDEZ, PH.D.
Assistant Professor
Department of Mechanical Engineering
University of Alabama at Birmingham
Birmingham, Alabama

HARRY C. DAVIS, PH.D.
Consulting Statistician
Office of Research Computing and Statistics
Medical College of Georgia
Augusta, Georgia

THOMAS D. DRISKELL, B.S.
Director, Driskell Bioengineering
Galena, Ohio

L. KIRK GARDNER, D.D.S.
Associate Professor
Department of Prosthodontics
School of Dentistry
Medical College of Georgia
Augusta, Georgia

BARRY M. GOLDMAN, D.D.S., M.S.
Professor, Department of Prosthodontics
School of Dentistry
Medical College of Georgia
Augusta, Georgia

JACK A. HAHN, D.D.S.
*Implantologist, Benmayor and Hahn Dental
    Associates, Incorporated*
Cincinnati, Ohio

WADE B. HAMMER, D.D.S.
*Professor, Department of Oral and Maxillofacial
    Surgery*
School of Dentistry
Professor, Department of Surgery
Medical College of Georgia
Augusta, Georgia

PHILLIP J. HANES, D.D.S., M.S.
Associate Professor
Department of Periodontics
School of Dentistry
Medical College of Georgia
Augusta, Georgia

ANDRAS G. HARIS, D.M.D.
Associate Clinical Professor
School of Dentistry
Louisiana State University
New Orleans, Louisiana

ALFRED L. HELLER, D.D.S., M.S.
Director, The Midwest Implant Institute
Columbus, Ohio

KENNETH W.M. JUDY, D.D.S.
Associate Professor
Department of Prosthodontics
University of Pittsburgh School of Dental Medicine
Pittsburgh, Pennsylvania
Chief of Oral Implants and Implant Prosthodontics
Hollman Hospital Center
New York, New York

ALEX KIRSCH, D.D.S.
Implantologist
Stuttgart, West Germany

DAVID L. KOTH, D.D.S., M.S.
Professor and Chairman
Department of Restorative Dentistry
School of Dentistry
University of Alabama at Birmingham
Birmingham, Alabama

FRANCIS T. LAKE, D.D.S., PH.D.
Associate Professor
Department of Oral Biology/Anatomy
School of Dentistry
Medical College of Georgia
Augusta, Georgia

JACK E. LEMONS, PH.D.
Professor and Chairman
Department of Biomaterials
School of Dentistry
University of Alabama at Birmingham
Birmingham, Alabama

LEONARD I. LINKOW, D.D.S.
Implantologist
New York, New York

W. GREGORY LONG, D.M.D., M.S.
Periodontist
Columbus, Georgia

RALPH V. McKINNEY, JR., D.D.S., PH.D.
Professor and Chairman
Department of Oral Pathology
School of Dentistry
Professor, School of Graduate Studies
Medical College of Georgia
Augusta, Georgia

ROLAND M. MEFFERT, D.D.S.
Professor and Chairman
Department of Periodontics
School of Dentistry
Louisiana State University
New Orleans, Louisiana

GLENN E. MINSLEY, D.M.D.
Associate Professor
Department of Prosthodontics
School of Dentistry
University of North Carolina
Chapel Hill, North Carolina

CARL E. MISCH, D.D.S., M.D.S.
Director, Misch Implant Institute
Dearborn, Michigan
Associate Professor and Director
Oral Implantology Center
Department of Prosthodontics
University of Pittsburgh School of Dental Medicine
Pittsburgh, Pennsylvania

JOSEPH R. NATIELLA, D.D.S.
Professor and Chairman
Department of Stomatology and Interdisciplinary
  Science
School of Dental Medicine
State University of New York at Buffalo
Buffalo, New York

GREGORY R. PARR, D.D.S.
Professor, Department of Prosthodontics
School of Dentistry
Medical College of Georgia
Augusta, Georgia

ANTHONY W. RINALDI, D.M.D.
Prosthodontist
Philadelphia, Pennsylvania

JOEL L. ROSENLICHT, D.M.D.
Oral and Maxillofacial Surgery
Manchester, Connecticut

DAVID W. SHELTON, D.M.D.
Professor, Department of Oral and Maxillofacial
  Surgery
School of Dentistry
Professor, Department of Surgery
Medical College of Georgia
Augusta, Georgia

ALLEN L. SISK, D.D.S.
Associate Professor
Department of Oral and Maxillofacial Surgery
School of Dentistry
Assistant Professor
Department of Surgery
Medical College of Georgia
Augusta, Georgia

DENNIS G. SMILER, D.D.S., M.Sc.D.
Oral and Maxillofacial Surgery
Los Angeles, California

DAVID E. STEFLIK, M.A., ED.D.
Senior Research Scientist
Department of Oral Pathology
School of Dentistry
Medical College of Georgia
Augusta, Georgia

O. HILT TATUM, JR., D.D.S.
Implantologist
St. Petersburg, Florida

MAURICE VALEN
President and Director of Research and
  Development
Impladent Limited
Holliswood, New York

CHARLES M. WEISS, D.D.S.
Implantologist
New York, New York

JACK WIMMER
President, Park Dental Research Corporation
New York, New York

PREFACE

The discipline of dental and oral implantology has suddenly exploded into the practice arena of general and specialized dentistry over the past few years. Yet for the individual interested in learning about the field or examining implant systems available for treatment selection, the dentist has had to rely on promotional literature from the various implant manufacturers or companies. This can not only provide a somewhat limited outlook, but can also fail to present broad general treatment concepts and scientific principles that are important in achieving clinical longevity with dental implants. Previously there was not a comprehensive volume or text available that delineated these general and specific endosteal implant systems for the dentist.

Recognizing this deficiency, this textbook was the direct outgrowth of discussions held between Dr. Frank Paparello (Vice President/Publisher, Mosby-Year Book) and the author. The outcome of these discussions was the decision to develop a textbook on endosteal dental implants that could serve as a reference book for the practicing dentist entering the implant field, and as a textbook for predoctoral and graduate implantology courses and programs. It was decided to assemble a group of authors who were involved directly with a particular implant system, or were recognized clinicians and scientists who could address various aspects of important basic implant biomaterial, biological, and clinical knowledge.

In bringing this work to fruition, I would like to thank all the chapter contributors who happily gave their time and knowledge in providing important material in their chapters. I know that many of them put in extra effort at the late night study lamp. I would like to thank Mr. Richard Wallace of Mosby-Year Book, Inc. for his help, guidance, and, above all, his patience while this book slowly took shape. And finally, an author/editor is only as good as the secretaries who back him up with the heavy task of manuscript production, revisions, more revisions, and telephone contact with multiple authors. Without the sustained superior efforts of Ms. Dora Haines, Ms. Mary Kamaka, and Ms. Angela Williams there simply would not have been a book. To them, my deepest heartfelt thanks for a tremendous task well done.

RALPH V. McKINNEY, JR., D.D.S., PH.D.

CONTENTS

Preface *ix*

PART I: GENERAL *1*

1 / Dental and Oral Implantology: State
of the Art *3*
Ralph V. McKinney, Jr.

2 / History of Implantology *8*
David E. Steflik and Ralph V. McKinney, Jr.

3 / Clinical Considerations
for Implantology *19*
Joseph R. Natiella

4 / Endosteal Implant Biomaterials and
Biomechanics *27*
Jack E. Lemons and Martha Warren Bidez

5 / The Biological Tissue Response to Dental
Implants *37*
*Ralph V. McKinney, Jr., David E. Steflik, and
David L. Koth*

6 / Basic Bone Biology in Implantology *52*
Francis T. Lake

7 / Evaluation and Selection of the Endosteal
Implant Patient *63*
Charles A. Babbush

8 / Basic Surgical Principles
for Implantology *75*
David W. Shelton

9 / Principles of Surgery for Plate/Blade
Implants *88*
Charles M. Weiss

10 / Periodontal Considerations
for Implantology *105*
Roland M. Meffert

PART II: ENDOSTEAL IMPLANT SYSTEMS *117*

11 / The Plate/Blade Oratronics Implant
System *119*
Charles M. Weiss

12 / The Ultimatics Blade-Vent Implant
System *139*
Leonard I. Linkow

13 / The Startanius Implant System *156*
Ralph V. McKinney, Jr., and Jack Wimmer

14 / The Omnii Implant System *163*
O. Hilt Tatum, Jr.

15 / Flexi-Cup Three-Dimensional Blade Implant
Devices *174*
Maurice Valen and Kenneth W.M. Judy

16 / The Stryker Precision Dental Implant System
(Root Form Series) *188*
Thomas D. Driskell

17 / The Stryker Precision Dental Implant System
(Blade Form Series) *203*
Thomas D. Driskell

18 / The Bioceram Implant Systems *215*
*Ralph V. McKinney, Jr., David L. Koth, and David
E. Steflik*

19 / The Titanodont Implant System *231*
Alfred L. Heller

20 / The ITI Implant Systems   *240*
Joel L. Rosenlicht

21 / The Flexiroot Implant System   *255*
Andras G. Haris

22 / The Vent-Plant Osseointegrated Compatible Implant System   *266*
Leonard I. Linkow and Anthony W. Rinaldi

23 / The Nobelpharma Implant System   *293*
Barry M. Goldman and Allen L. Sisk

24 / The Core-Vent Implant System   *315*
Carl E. Misch

25 / The IMZ-Interpore Osseointegrated Implant System   *331*
Charles A. Babbush and Alex Kirsch

26 / The Steri-Oss Implant System   *349*
Jack A. Hahn

27 / The Integral Implant System   *362*
Dennis G. Smiler

PART III: CLINICAL CONSIDERATIONS OF IMPLANT MANAGEMENT   *373*

28 / Practical Implant Prosthodontics   *375*
Glenn E. Minsley and David L. Koth

29 / Clinical Evaluation Tools for Implant Performance   *388*
Ralph V. McKinney, Jr., David L. Koth, and David E. Steflik

30 / Prosthetic Laboratory Relationships for Endosteal Implants   *395*
Gregory R. Parr and L. Kirk Gardner

31 / Oral Hygiene Protocol for Implant Patients   *400*
Philip J. Hanes and W. Gregory Long

32 / Dental Implant Practice Management   *411*
Alfred L. Heller

33 / Clinical Management of Failing Implant Cases   *422*
Burton E. Balkin

34 / Use of Polymeric, Ceramic, and Other Materials as Synthetic Bone in Implantology   *427*
Arthur Ashman

35 / Use of Bone Augmentation or Substitute Material in Implantology   *438*
Wade B. Hammer

36 / The Necessity for Controlled Clinical Implant Trials   *448*
Ralph V. McKinney, Jr.

37 / Implant Clinical Trials: Design and Statistical Management   *452*
David E. Steflik and Harry C. Davis

38 / Future Projections for Implantology   *461*
Ralph V. McKinney, Jr.

Index   *570*

PART I
General

Chapter 1

Dental and Oral Implantology: State of the Art

Ralph V. McKinney, Jr., D.D.S., Ph.D.

OVERVIEW AND PROGRESS

Dental implants have become one of the most exciting and rapidly developing aspects of dental practice in the past decade as dental implants now provide a clear viable treatment alternative to removable dentures. Implants, which are placed into the bone of the jaws and protrude through the mucosal tissues, are used to provide attachment anchorage of replacement artificial teeth for patients. The patient who has lost teeth through dental decay, advanced periodontal disease, or accident can now elect a treatment option that provides for firm anchoring of bridgework or dentures to the bone and tissue. This feature of anchoring provides an alleviation of the fears a patient has about the ability to adequately use removable dentures and to establish the esthetic and social value of their "smile line." As Cervantes wrote in *Don Quixote*, "Every tooth . . . is more valuable . . . than a diamond."

Four scientific breakthroughs in the past 10 years have heralded the rapid development and clinical application of the implant field and are some of the truly significant recent research high-water marks in dentistry. These breakthroughs are (1) the recognition of two basic biomaterials that are nontoxic and respond well to human tissues—titanium, a metal, and single-crystalline aluminum oxide, a dense ceramic substance similar to hard gemstone; (2) the application of computed tomography (CT) to develop

jaw bone models for subperiosteal implants, allowing elimination of one surgical phase; (3) the discovery of the concept of "osseointegration," in which the healing of the jaw bone in direct apposition to the implanted biomaterials provides a stable, predictable structure for bridge attachment; and (4) the discovery, through the use of high-power microscopy, of a "biological" or "transmucosal seal" of the gingival tissues around the implant neck. These last two discoveries allow (1) the firm anchorage of implants in bone, and (2) the development of a "seal" of soft tissue around the implant that prevents the invasion of bacteria and oral debris into the crypt around the implant. These scientific breakthroughs in implantology have direct major health treatment benefits and probably compete with the development of the high-speed drill as research landmarks in dentistry.

BACKGROUND OF THE DISCIPLINE

The concept of dental implants has been around since antiquity. Archeological evidence reveals that Egyptians attempted to implant precious stones and metals into the jaw bone where teeth were lost. Excavation of ancient Mayan civilization ruins has yielded human remains that show the implantation of carved tooth replacements from seashells used as implants into the jaws where teeth were lost (see Chapter 2 for more details).

For the past 100 years or more, scientific approaches to replacement of lost teeth with biological fixed structures has primarily centered on the use of tooth transplants, both autogenic (within the same patient) and allogenic (from one patient to another), and attempts to replant traumatically evulsed (dislodged) teeth. Reinsertion of accident-dislodged teeth and the use of tooth transplants have only been partially successful, the patient often ending up with bone- and tooth-destroying infections and failure of the transplants or replants.

In modern times, dental implants have been utilized in clinical practice since the late 1940s, although only a very small percentage of practitioners used them. In fact, members of the dental profession who used implants were at times severely criticized by other members of the profession because the implants were placed directly into patients without adequate device development or biological investigation of the devices in monitored animal and human clinical trials. But as information began accruing from clinical trials, the dental community began to become aware of the potential for greater use of dental implants. A series of consensus development conference programs co-sponsored by the National Institutes of Health (NIH) in 1978 and 1988 provided an additional impetus for this enhancement of professional interest.[1, 2] The new importance of dental implants was highlighted at the June 1988 NIH Consensus Conference on Dental Implants by the attendance of a large overflow crowd of dentists and dental scientists.

SCIENCE AND DEVELOPING IMPLANTOLOGY

In the past 10 years dramatic technological and biological advances in dental implants have occurred with the end result that a much larger group of Americans can be and are being successfully served by this type of treatment. The advances in successful clinical longevity of dental implants is of great importance for all segments of the population, but especially older Americans because they have suffered the compromising loss of teeth and bone through destructive dental decay and periodontal diseases. The dramatic surge in implant treatment usage is a direct reflection of the impact of science and the investigative technique on a clinical field.

Prior to 1975 dental implantology was practiced by a few dedicated dentists who believed in the viability of this type of treatment. But since almost no basic technological, or experimental animal investigations, or controlled human trials had been performed, the general view of the dental profession was one of skepticism. Most reports by those performing implantology were empiric and retrospective and thus not well received by the profession. This attitude began to change in the late 1970s and early 1980s with the reporting of sound scientific data. It is of note that much of this early research was not supported by governmental funding but instead was sponsored by industrial interests, or was foreign-based research supported by foreign governments. With the reporting of sound implant research the profession suddenly became interested and the field has taken off dramatically as patient demand for services has increased. For the dental patient, dental implants are also a major breakthrough in treatment because, as the patient sees it, they now have the option of conventional removable denture treatment, or implant treatment that will anchor the denture or bridgework to devices implanted in bone. Certainly a new and exciting era of dental practice technology is upon us that is based on sound science. At last a proven successful method for treating dental deformation, accidents, and disease with restoration of esthetics, function, and psychological well-being is at hand.

CURRENT TREATMENT CONCEPTS AND PROGRESS

Dental implants have evolved with two major types of treatment devices in use today. The *subperiosteal implant,* which is a custom-fabricated framework of metal, sits on top of the bone of the jaw but under the oral tissues. Posts (usually four posts) protrude from this framework through the tissue and provide the anchoring foundation for the final bridgework (or denture). The subperiosteal implant is developed by a two-stage surgery procedure. First, an incision is made in the oral tissues and an impression is made of the jaw bone. Then the tissue is closed and the design and fabrication of the implant device framework are carried out on the model of the patient's jaw bone. The prepared framework is then inserted under the oral tissues via a second operation to rest on the jaw bone. Provision is made in the tissue for the protruding posts that will anchor the eventual denture.

One of the very recent significant research advances in the subperiosteal implant treatment modality has been the adaptation of CT to develop a model of the surface of the jaw bone without the use of the first-step surgical procedure.[3] This has worked very well in clinical application, and although expensive, this method is rapidly replacing the two-step surgical technique.

The other basic type of dental implant in use today is the *endosteal implant*. Endosteal or endosseous means "into bone" and this type of implant is placed directly into the bone of the jaw through the oral soft tissue by the preparation of a recipient socket (a process called trephining) using a series of specially prepared drills and tapping burs. The bone and tissue then heal around this implanted biomaterial and once healing is complete, usually after 6 to 10 weeks, the final bridgework can be prepared and attached.

Generally, the *endosteal*-type implants have a configuration of a flat rectangular blade or plate, or a shape somewhat similar to that of a tooth. The blade or plate form is currently the most commonly used type of endosteal implant but it is gradually being replaced by implants shaped like a tooth or cylinder. These latter devices are designed as cylinders, screw forms, tapered cylinders, and cylinders with hollow centers or cutout windows that allow bone to regenerate into the space for stabilization.

One of the dramatic design modifications of the past decade has been the development of the *two-stage endosseous* implant. With the two-stage procedure the root (radicular) portion of the implant is placed in bone and covered up by the soft tissue. Following healing (up to 6 months is recommended by some clinicians) the top of the implant is exposed

through the soft tissue and the top superstructure (coronal) aspect of the implant is attached (via screw, mechanical fit, or cementation) to the buried root portion. This two-stage implant has provided for the rapid development of the concept of osseointegration.[4] The bone is allowed to heal around the implant in an undisturbed state (no biting force load) for approximately 6 months and this provides for a large percentage of *direct bone interface* to the implant. The crown (coronal) portion of the implant is then attached and the functional bridgework completed.

The other significant scientific breakthrough has been the discovery and conceptional understanding of the biological seal around the implant neck.[5] This concept has allowed explanation of the implant viability in the oral cavity and has led to direct alterations in implant design in order to stimulate formation of the biological seal. The seal provides a barrier between the bacteria and plaque-laden oral cavity and the sterile environment of the internal jaw tissues. Knowledge about the seal has also had a direct application to the establishment of oral hygiene protocols for implant maintenance.

RESEARCH INTO BIOLOGICAL AND CLINICAL MECHANISMS OPERATIVE AT THE DENTAL IMPLANT-TISSUE INTERFACE

The implant-tissue interface is "where the action is" and scientific investigations of the past decade have shown that the scientific basis for implant success and clinical effectiveness occurs at this important interface.[6] This is where osseointegration occurs between implant and hard tissue and where the biological seal phenomenon occurs between implant and gingival soft tissue. The role of the body's fibrous tissues are just now being recognized as important in determination of the interface phenomenon.

The investigative studies of this unique interface phenomenon have taken several avenues. Scientists have studied the growth and attachment mechanisms of cells in culture to sheets or plates of implant materials; the materials have been tested for toxicologic and rejection phenomena in animal systems; the surface of implants has been characterized as to type of cell interaction based on smoothness, roughness, and material composition, as well as physical properties and structure; experimental trials have been conducted in animals using implants with and without attached bridgework in which the response of the implant and tissue could be studied by newer technologies, and well-controlled human clinical trials have been conducted wherein clinical data are collected and statistically analyzed by a team of implant investigators. All these studies have shown that stable gingival interfaces (the biological seal) and stable direct bone interfaces (osseointegration) can be achieved. The achievement of these significant research breakthroughs has also shown that strict attention must be paid to several factors. These factors include the use of biologically acceptable materials. The material's performance is a function of its physical, mechanical, chemical, and electrical properties, and its bulk, surface composition, and structure. Of recent interest is the application of additional surface coatings, such as hydroxylapatite crystals and Bioglass (silica-based glass) to enhance healing and anchoring of the device. Further, the diagnosis of quantity and quality of bone and soft tissue at the anatomic site and the use of accurate and atraumatic surgical techniques employing well-cooled, low-speed, incremental bone cutting (vs. overheating bone) and careful aseptic techniques have been revealed as important. Finally, the careful use of one-stage and two-stage implants, the type of bridgework-restorative procedure, and immobilization of the implant during the healing stage are critical steps in achieving a stable implant-tissue interface.

Clinical studies using one- and two-stage implants have demonstrated that the direct bone implant interface (osseointegration) and tissue-implant interface (biological seal) can be *maintained* over the long term, providing successful longitudinal satisfactory service to patients for the support of dental prostheses (bridgework). These clinical results are the outcome of studies revealing the interrelationship between bone remodeling and biomechanics in relation to implant design that occurs when an osseointegrated implant is put into function with attached bridgework. We have learned that the clinical scientist must provide for adequate biodegradation resistance and biomechanics by achieving physiologic force (biting) loads on the bridgework and implant. These important discoveries have come about by employing an interdisciplinary team approach to implants. This approach must be continued.

Biomaterial scientists have made noteworthy contributions to the implant knowledge base by providing rationally designed and theoretically tested implant configurations with the use of biomechanical analyses, usually employing a model called finite stress analysis. Thus new material can be tested and opinions rendered as to whether the device will theoretically be successful before any animal or human clinical trials are undertaken—a noteworthy achievement.

Advances in bone and soft tissue biology and biomechanics have contributed significantly to our understanding of the biology of implantology and its successful application.

IMPLANT DEMOGRAPHICS AND ECONOMICS

Dental implants are the fastest-developing technology in the practice of dentistry today. All facets of the dental profession are interested in this new modern treatment style, general dentists, periodontists, oral surgeons, and prosthodontists being the major groups of practitioners involved in this treatment mode. Some dentists now limit their practices to implantology and others devote a considerable percentage of their time to this treatment option. It is estimated (1987 data) that there are currently 5,900 general dentists (total in the United States, 98,000), 3,800 oral surgeons, and 1,000 periodontists using implants in their daily practices. Estimates for 1987 indicated that 39,500 endosseous implants and 4,500 subperiosteal implants were placed. It is estimated that 300,000 implants will be placed annually by 1992. The endosseous implant (manufacturer's) market alone is estimated to have an economic value of over $40 million.[7] In addition, residency training programs are developing in implantology: four are now active, and three of the current recognized dental specialties require experience in implant treatment in their residency educational programs (periodontics, prosthodontics, and oral surgery).[8] Currently, more implant or implant-related continuing education courses are given than any other type of program in the United States, indicating the heightened educational demand by dentists.

CONCLUSIONS AND SUMMARY

Clearly, dental implants are the most exciting new treatment concept to occur in dentistry in the past decade. The entire dental profession is alive with interest and a desire for knowledge in this field. The fact that two NIH consensus conferences on the subject were held within a 10-year period indicate the high priority this treatment mode has taken in the profession. Three other factors contributing to this phenomenal interest and clinical application have been scientific advancement in implantology, alterations in dental disease patterns, and the socioeconomic status of older Americans. The improvement in dental materials and the biological-mechanistic understanding by dental scientists, the increased interest of scientists in the field, and the conduct of carefully controlled and monitored clinical trials have significantly advanced the scientific basis of dental implants and have helped overcome the bias previously expressed by many dental practitioners. Second, changing disease patterns that have contributed to the surge of interest in implant treatment include the decline of dental caries and the increase in the incidence of periodontal disease. Finally, the increased numbers of middle-aged and older Americans demanding quality dental care, publicity about implant treatment in the lay press, and improvement in third-party (insurance) payments for implant treatment have had a major socioeconomic impact.

In summary, the development of an interdisciplinary dental implant systems approach, clinical applications of the *two-stage implant,* and the discovery of the biomedical phenomena of *osseointegration* and the *biological seal* have provided impetus for this dramatic dental implant treatment change in the 1980s. Dental scientists have now begun to identify the basic biological and material mechanisms that contribute to implant success and are looking further into molecular structure and tissue interactions. However, the application and clinical use of dental implants currently still greatly exceeds the basic knowledge of what makes these devices successful.

REFERENCES

1. Schnitman PA, Schulman LB (eds): *Dental Implants: Benefit and Risk. Proceedings of an NIH-Harvard Consensus Development Conference.* Bethesda, Md, US Department of Health and Human Services publication No (NIH) 81-1531, 1980.
2. National Institutes of Health: *National Institutes of Health Consensus Development Statement: Dental Implants. J Am Dent Assoc* 1988; 117:509–513.
3. McGivney GP, Haughton V, Strandt JA, et al: A comparison of computer-assisted tomography and data-gathering modalities in prosthodontics. *Int J Oral Maxillofac Implants* 1986; 1:55–68.
4. Brånemark PI: Osseointegration and its experimental background. *J Prosthet Dent* 1983, 50:399–410.
5. McKinney RV Jr, Steflik DE, Koth DL: Evidence for a junctional epithelial attachment to ceramic dental implants. A transmission electron microscopic study. *J Periodontal* 1985; 56:579–591.
6. McKinney RV Jr, Steflik DE, Koth DL, et al: The scientific basis for dental implant therapy. *J Dent Educ* 1988; 52:696–705.
7. Worthington P: Current implant usuage. *J Dent Educ* 1988; 52:692–695.
8. Steflik DE, Gowgiel JM, James RA, et al: Oral Implantology instruction in dental schools. *J Oral Implantol* 1989; 15:6–16.

Chapter 2

History of Implantology

David E. Steflik, M.A., Ed.D.
Ralph V. McKinney, Jr., D.D.S., Ph.D.

Since the age of prehistoric man, humanity has suffered from dental pathology and decay. Studies of the teeth of primitive man revealed an extreme form of dental caries and advanced tooth wear due to his abrasive diet.[1, 2]

Tooth decay, and its treatment, can be traced historically to the Babylonians and the god Ea (c. 5000 B.C.). In this period the legend of the tooth-worm developed as the cause of tooth decay and Ea was invoked as the ancient enemy of the tooth-worm.[1, 3] In the fifth century B.C., Herodotus[4] described the practice of medicine in ancient Egypt and wrote, "each physician treats a single disorder and no more . . . some undertaking to cure diseases of the teeth."[1] As Weinberger[1] suggested, Herodotus' reference to such dental specialists reflects a sufficient number of these practitioners during the Old Kingdom in Egypt (c. 3000–525 B.C.) including Hesi-Ra (c. 2600 B.C.) who was recognized as the first dental practitioner and as the "Great One of The Toothers and the Physicians."[1] The art of the dentist was deemed extremely important during this period, and the Code of Hammurabi (c. 1900 B.C.) documented individuals who performed the extraction of teeth.

Therefore, the decay and traumatic loss of teeth have plagued mankind since the dawn of man. Concurrent with these afflictions has been a desire to substitute artificial devices as replacements for the diseased or lost teeth. Congdon in 1915 first defined *implantation* as a term used to "designate the opera-

tion of introducing either a natural or an artificial root into an artificial socket cut into the alveolar process."[5] In this chapter, this definition will be expanded to include the domain of subperiosteal implants. Congdon also suggested that "some of these operations have been attended with success . . . [which] may inspire further experiments in the future. If some cases are successful, why may we not reasonably expect all cases under favorable conditions to succeed?"[5] Congdon's words in 1915 predestined today's desire for reproducibility and guaranteed implant serviceability.

This chapter will highlight the recurring themes not only in dental health care but for oral implantology. "What goes around comes around." We describe six distinct eras of implant dentistry: (1) the ancient era (through A.D. 1000); (2) the medieval period (1000–1799); (3) the foundational period (1800–1910); (4) the premodern era (1910–1930); (5) the dawn of the modern era (1935–1978); and (6) contemporary oral implantology (1978 to the present). Finally, we present the historical origins of implantation protocols and provide a review of the concerns of the dental profession about oral implantology.

THE ANCIENT ERA

The history of dental implants[6–9] is as fascinating as it is ancient. Intraosseous implantation of animal teeth and artificial teeth carved of ivory was performed on court women of the ancient Egyptian dynasties.[7] In fact, lost teeth were considered such a handicap that prior to mummification or preparation for burial, artificial or animal teeth were implanted in the corpse's jaw to assure proper preparation for the afterlife.

Cranin suggests that the earliest recorded dental implant specimen was inserted during the pre-Columbian era.[7] While excavating at the Playa de los Muertos in the Ulua River Valley of Honduras in 1931, Wilson Popenoe discovered a skull with an artificial tooth carved from a dark stone.[3, 10-12] This truly artificial device, not a transplanted natural tooth, was used to replace a lower left second incisor. Dating to A.D. 600, this skull had three tooth-shaped pieces of shell which had been implanted in the sockets of missing lower incisors. Radiographs showed compact bone formation around two of the implants, suggesting that these implants were in situ long enough to permit some type of bone healing. It seems logical, then, that the Mayans practiced the implantation of alloplastic materials in living persons.

In addition to the dental implantations, the Mayans also inlaid precious stones[1, 10-12] and practiced tooth mutilation for esthetic and superstitious reasons. Wooden drill bits would be hand-driven and sand was utilized as an abrasive for these procedures. Prior to these dental treatments, the patient would chew coca and ingest hallucinogenic mushrooms for anesthetic purposes since, presumably, these procedures lasted for hours.

Excavation of pre-Incan South American Indian skulls in Ecuador by Saville suggested that this culture used gold inlays in prepared cavities and performed implantation and replantation of teeth.[1, 11] Saville wrote, "an unusual feat[ure] is found in the right lateral incisor, which does not belong in the jaw, but was implanted to replace the middle incisor."[11] Evidence of inlays was also observed among the Aztecs.[11, 12]

Oral implantology can also trace its history to the Middle East. In 1862 Gaillardot excavated a grave site near the ancient city of Sidon.[1, 3] Here he discovered a prosthodontic appliance dating to 400 B.C., consisting of four natural lower teeth holding between them two carved ivory teeth which served as replacements for two missing incisors, all held together by gold wire.

Dental implant and transplant history can thus be traced to Africa (Egyptians), to the Americas (Mayans, Aztecs, and Incans), and to the Middle East. Also in this earliest historical period, tooth transplants can be traced to the Greeks, the Etruscans, and the Romans.[13, 14] There do not appear to have been any geographical restraints to the desire of early dental practioners to provide replacements for missing or diseased teeth.

THE MEDIEVAL PERIOD

The medieval era of implant dentistry was primarily concerned with the transplantation of teeth. Albucasis (also known as Abul Kasim), an Arab surgeon (936-1013), described transplantation procedures. He also fabricated implants made from ox bone.[1, 6, 15]

In Japan during the 15th and 16th centuries, wooden dental prostheses were designed to function as a dowel crown. The pin of the prosthesis was inserted into the root canal of a nonvital tooth whose crown was missing. This is evidence of an early endodontic implant-supported prosthesis.[3]

Transplantation became fashionable in the European sphere of influence, particularly being performed by the barber-surgeons of the era. A prominant surgeon of the 1500s, Ambroise Paré, emphasized the advantages of transplantation.[1, 6, 15] Morse, in his excellent history of plantation procedures, gave Paré's description in 1530 as follows: "I heard it reported by a credible person that he saw a Lady of prime nobility, who instead of a rotten tooth she drew, made a sound tooth, drawn from one of her waiting maids at the same time, to be substituted and inserted, which . . . grew so firm, as that she could chew upon it as well as any of the rest."[6] Such transplantations grew in popularity for the nobility and for military officers. "If a high ranking officer had a condemned tooth, he had it extracted. Then from the ranks of the soldiers, one would be chosen whose tooth matched the officer's in terms of size and color. The chosen soldier having no chance to object, would lose his tooth."[6]

Tooth transplantation in the 18th century

was supported by such stalwarts as Pierre Fauchard (1678–1761) and John Hunter (1728–1793).[3, 6, 15, 16] During this period, however, transplantation also had its detractors. The satirist Thomas Rowlandson roundly criticized the practice, as did others. Human teeth were expensive and scarce and cadaver teeth were usually repugnant to the patient. We see again the desire for replacements for missing teeth. However, implants made from ivory, shells, and bone, or human teeth used for transplants, were not satisfying the requirements for such replacements. In fact, it was being reported in the 1700s that tooth transplantation could lead to the transfer of disease, and even death. Eventually the procedure diminished in popularity toward the beginning of the 19th century.[14]

THE FOUNDATIONAL PERIOD

Endosseous oral implantology truly began in the 19th century. Maggilio, in 1809, inserted a gold implant into a freshly extracted tooth socket.[6, 7, 9, 17] As Driskell comments,[9] this implant was not truly submerged, but the tissues were allowed to heal passively without a crown. The crown was attached only after the tissues appeared to be healthy. The author of *The Art of the Dentist,* Maggilio also discussed a means for affixing pivot teeth in natural or artificial roots by means of a spring. In 1845 Rogers stated in his *L'encyclopedie du dentiste"* that "the usefulness of the roots for the fixation of artificial teeth seemed so great that the idea of making even [artificial] roots was conceived."[9, 17] Rogers suggested that this procedure was initiated by Maggilio.

The late 1800s saw a resurgence in procedures using implantation of natural teeth. W. J. Younger of San Francisco is credited with introducing the operation in the United States.[5, 17, 18, 19] Congdon wrote that the implantation of teeth "seems to have achieved satisfactory results, though failures were many; two important causes being resorption and exfoliation."[5, 19] Amazingly, these implanted teeth were in situ for up to 11 years, and Younger himself wrote in 1893: "I am happy to state that this operation [implantation] has entered upon its eighth year of life."[19]

Documentation of implanted biomaterials in the

19th century can also be traced to Harris and to Edmunds. Harris[20] reported in *Dental Cosmos* in 1887 that he implanted an artificial porcelain tooth crown on a leaded root in a socket that was artificially formed in the jaw of a Chinese in Grass Valley, California. "The porcelain crown was fixed on a platinum post and around this lead was melted in a mold to resemble a tooth root and was slightly roughened to afford a retaining hold for new tissues in the socket."[20] The operation was said to have originated with Harris.

Even though we can be confident that such implantation procedures can be logically traced to Harris, and even to Maggilio, Edmunds of New York City reported on March 12, 1889, to the First District Dental Society of that city, that he implanted a metallic capsule in the space occupied by the first superior right premolar.[21] The operation itself was probably performed in 1886, or concurrent with the operation of Harris. The metallic capsule comprised platinum foil covered with lead and soldered with pure silver. After injecting 10% hydrochlorate of cocaine as an anesthetic, the socket was formed with spiral knives and reamers and syringed out with a 1:4,000 solution of mercuric bichloride.

It is also interesting that Berry,[22] in 1888, wrote concerning the need to obtain teeth free of danger of communication of disease, a response to the dangers of implantation or replantation of natural teeth. He suggested that possibly porcelain teeth with roots of wood, tin, or silver would be retained if skillfully placed. But, as Berry suggested, since lead is generally tolerated in the body without trouble, it is, no doubt, the best material for roots of teeth for implanting. Berry suggested that the roots of gum teeth be enveloped in beeswax, invested in plaster, boiled to remove the wax, and molten lead poured to fill the spaces. The roots were then filed and reduced in size, as were the sockets to receive them. The roots should also be perfectly round and of equal diameter. So we see in the writings of Berry two interesting considerations: first, the initial proposal for the necessity of immediate congruency of the implant and its tissue encasement; second, the use of a "proven" safe biomaterial—lead. As in the implantology literature today, proven dogmas are indeed subject to future scientific scrutiny.

As we enter the last decade of the 1800s, the use of implanted devices expanded. In 1890, a Massachusetts minister had his lower jaw resected because of a tumor. A unique dental restoration composed of an extensive system of gold crowns soldered together and joined to a hinged device was attached to the remaining dentition as a replacement for the resected mandible.[3] Znamenski,[23] in 1891, reported on the implantation of teeth made of porcelain, guttapercha, and rubber, and Bonwell, in 1895, reported on the implantation of one or two tubes of gold or iridium as a support for individual teeth or crowns.[17] At the National Dental Association meeting in 1898, R. E. Payne gave the first clinic on implantation.[17] In his clinic, "The Implantation of a Silver Capsule," he placed the capsule in the tooth socket with the intent of placing the crown at a later time.

THE PREMODERN ERA

Two innovative clinicians, R. E. Payne and E. J. Greenfield, dominated the first two decades of the 20th century as related to the field of oral implantology. Payne presented his capsule implantation technique at the clinics of the Third International Dental Congress,[24] as reported in *Dental Cosmos* in 1901. Payne wrote of extracting the root, enlarging the socket with a trephine, and the trial-fitting of the capsule. He then placed grooves on both sides of the socket, filled two thirds of the socket with rubber, fitted a crown with a porcelain root into the capsule, and set it with gutta-percha. About the same time, in 1903, Scholl of Reading, Pennsylvania, implanted a porcelain tooth with a corrugated porcelain root.[17]

Greenfield[25-28] was the first to carefully document an original implantation procedure in the scientific literature with accompanying photographs and diagrams. Further, after careful thought, Greenfield considered implant dentistry to be "the missing link of Dentistry."[27] He wrote that "if a surgeon can use metals in the bone, why not dentists? . . . Inspired by this thought I went to work and perfected an artificial root . . . this artificial root embedded in bone is, what I believe, the missing link in Dentistry."[27] Greenfield suggested that "the danger of such an operation may be thought greater than the benefit to be

derived therefrom; but this is not the case if the precaution is taken to have everything sanitary and sterile, a caution every dental surgeon should exercise in performing any operation."[25] Again, history records the sage advice of sterility and cleanliness often overlooked in the middle decades of the 20th century. Negligence led to negative opinions of implantology that we are still disclaiming today. In fact, John Roberts, a noted surgeon of the time, wrote that "when Dr. Greenfield, in describing the operation, says that he cleanses the gum with ether, sterilizes his instruments by boiling, and then fills the cavity with bismuth paste, he is no longer [only] a dentist, he is a surgeon."[29]

Greenfield manufactured an artificial root of 20-gauge iridioplatinum wire soldered with 24-carat gold. Greenfield described his procedure as follows: ". . . when everything is ready, cleanse the gum with alcohol, take out the gum tissue, [use a] cone shaped engine knife to cut the bone tissue; then finish the socket with a reamer. All this consumes about a minute's time."[25] Then, "the root is placed and a splint is cemented. The bands are cemented thus holding the frame firmly until a sufficient deposit of bone cells has filled in between the spaces and the frame becomes embedded in the jaw."[25] Greenfield repeatedly emphasized the importance of the bone being intimately associated with the implant prior to proceeding to the next stage. We see in his writings the first requirements for "osseointegration" and for the concept of submerged implants. Only after there was evidence of embedding of the implant cage in the jaw, usually after 3 months, was the splint removed and the crown placed. Again we see the historical recording of a 3-month period of unloaded healing of the buried implant root.

It should also be noted that Greenfield's clinical case received peer review by an external reviewer. Burton Lee Thorpe wrote: "I have examined a patient of Dr. Greenfield in whose mouth he implanted an artificial root 18 months ago . . . The artificial root is solid in the jawbone and the gum tissue is perfectly healthy around its cervical margin."[25]

Greenfield wrote numerous articles on implantations and constantly emphasized the healing phenomenon of the oral tissues and the lack of mobility of the implant. Greenfield suggested that the patient could be dismissed for 6 to 8 weeks to allow bone tissue to "form through the root" before setting the crown or bridge. Also, "a still further point is the immovability of the root—once implanted, this artificial root is solid; it is stationary. The bony core in the center of the socket assures solidity."[26] Such revelations in 1914 preview the assertions of modern-day hollow basket implants such as the Swiss Hollow Basket and the Core Vent implants, as well as the clinical evaluation criterion of immobility.

The first and second decade of the 20th century also saw the reporting of tooth replantation procedures. The methods of Sebba, Neumann, and Sharp[5] were contrasting procedures, and all seemed at the time to be unsuitable alternatives to implantation. We return to Greenfield who said the clinician should search for a replacement "because of the imperfections of natural tooth implantation."[27]

Leger-Dorez developed one such replacement in the 1920s. This expansible artificial root implant was comparable to a concrete expansion bolt.[6–8] Smollon[8] described the implant as a four-part device, with the shaft buried in bone and its broader, uppermost portion resting near the alveolar crest. The shaft had internal threads to receive a screw, fastening the neck into the shaft. As the screw was inserted into the shaft, the lowermost part of the shaft flared. When the neck was in place, the part bearing the post for the prosthesis was attached. We see here the historical basis for internal screws providing for the retention of prosthetic devices—much like today's submerged implants.

Additional replacements for natural teeth were developed by Tomkins, in 1925, who implanted porcelain teeth, and by Brill, in 1936, who inserted rubber pins in artificially prepared sockets. Adams, in 1937, developed and patented a submerged cylindrical implant in the shape of a screw.[9] The implant had a rounded bottom, a smooth gingival collar, and a healing cap. The ball head was used to retain an overdenture. Driskell[9] correctly remarks the resemblance of such a design to today's implants.

THE DAWN OF THE MODERN ERA

The modern era of implant dentistry most definitely began in the late 1930s with the work of Venable,[30] Strock,[31] Dahl,[32] and Gershkoff and Goldberg.[32] In 1937 Venable developed the cast cobalt-chromium-molybdenum alloy now known as Vitallium. This metallic alloy made possible the innovative implant and prosthodontic procedures of the succeeding decades.

The biomaterials scientist has always worked with the surgeon and the innovator in developing new materials for use in the body, as has been thoroughly documented in the review of Lemons and Natiella[33] of various dental and medical biomaterials. Such was the foundation for the innovators of dental implant devices of contemporary history.

Endosteal Implants: Stage I

An initial use of Venable's Vitallium was the use of a Venable screw-type dental implant by Alvin and Moses Strock beginning in 1939. Strock[31] developed both endodontic and truly endosteal dental implants in the 1940s, with implants providing satisfactory service for up to 17 years. Of equal importance, Strock initiated experimental animal studies to examine the tissue response to such implants placed in dogs. He presented histologic evidence of possible bone congruency to the implants after periods of use. This was our first histologic evidence of osseointegration, or bone apposition.

Subperiosteal Implants

Subperiosteal implant development began with Dahl's 1941 report and his subsequent patent.[7, 32] Gershkoff and Goldberg visited Dahl in Sweden and brought the subperiosteal concept to the United States.[32, 33] The initial subperiosteal implant procedure was performed without direct bone impressions, but rather with an altered standard jaw impression. Isaiah Lew[32] is credited with the development of direct bone impressions and the two-stage subperiosteal procedure in 1951. Berman and Marziani also began experimenting with direct bone impressions for subperiosteal implants.[7, 32] Subperiosteal implant design evolution included Weinberg's unilateral subperiosteal implants, Leonard Linkow's unilateral subperiosteal implants with lingual fingers in 1955, and Bodine's butterfly implant of the 1950s which straddled the bone.[7, 32] Also in the middle 1950s, Salagaray and Sol developed a simple subperiosteal implant with an aerated horizontal bar, and in London Trainin designed subperiosteal implants similar to those in America.

Subperiosteal implant design has evolved rapidly in the past three decades. Weber presented the universal subperiosteal implant in 1968, Mentag introduced the mesio bar concept in 1974, Cranin developed the Brookdale continuous bar in 1978, and D'Alise introduced the O ring.[32] In the late 1970s, James recommended using the buccal surface of both rami for support of the subperiosteal framework. Recently, in fact, James has pioneered the use of computed tomography (CT) scanning as a mechanism to develop mandibular models for subperiosteal implants, thus eliminating an entire surgical procedure for the patient.

Endosteal Implants: Stage II

Additional endosteal implant designs were developed rapidly in the late 1940s, 1950s, and 1960s. Formiggini, in 1947, developed the single helix wire spiral implant made of either stainless steel or tantalum. Zepponi, a colleague and co-worker of Formiggini, described some shortcomings of the Formiggini implant and developed a cast spiral implant. Since all of Formiggini's implants were handmade, the development of a cast implant permitted better treatment planning and reproducibility.[7–9]

Chercheve examined the Formiggini designs and increased the length of the neck and developed a double-helix spiral implant. The increase in neck length is another recurring theme of implants. Since many practitioners believed that implants were probably doomed to failure, primarily due to bone loss at the neck region, implant designers attempted to increase the length of this "fuse" to prolong the "inevitable" (R.A. James, personal communication, 1985).

Chercheve was also credited with the development of a proper surgical armamentarium. Linkow addressed the requirement of a coordinated instrumentation system by saying that Chercheve had a "firm belief that a design cannot be separated from the method of insertion."[9] Smollon also noted that

"Chercheve carefully designed burs and taps to complement the implant."[8]

Other implants developed at this time included Marziani's use of porcelain and acrylic roots to support full dentures[9] and Lee's post design.[8] Lee's central post was narrow with small extensions, which, according to Smollon, "allows blood and bone building elements to encompass the major part of the implant."[8] Also, Scialom developed his tripodial pin design implant in which three thin tantalum pins are inserted and soldered together to support a prosthesis. Benoit and Michelet developed a transosseous implant utilizing a similar pin design.[7]

The period of the 1950s and 1960s was a period of trial and error in the development of implant designs. It was also a period dominated by the work of Linkow. Linkow expanded upon Lew's screw implant, Pasqualini's experiences, and Muratori's hollow implants with screw threads,[9] in developing his vent plant implant. This implant, presented in 1963, had features similar to Greenfield's cage of 1913 and the contemporary core vent and Swiss Hollow Basket. Linkow is probably best noted for the development of the blade implant, an implant that dominated the 1960s, 1970s, and early 1980s. His blade vent design, known as the Linkow blade or Linkow blade vent, was introduced in 1967. Linkow also motivated the development of a professional organization of implant dentists which in 1951 became the American Academy of Implant Dentistry.

During the 1970s implantology grew. Small developed the bone plate and mandibular staple after initial experimental animal studies in 1966 and 1967 and after human clinical trials undertaken between 1968 and 1973. Small and Misiek, in 1986, presented 16-year evaluations of the staple bone plate.[34] In 1974, Bodine reported on evaluations of 27 mandibular subperiosteal implants in situ for 15 to 20 years,[35] and Cranin and co-workers[36] and Linkow[37] reported on endosteal implant trials. Also at this time, Per-Invar Branemark was developing an extraordinary implant study in Sweden (beginning in 1951), Kawahara[38] was developing a ceramic implant in Japan (beginning in 1970), and the ITI group[39] in Switzerland was developing the Swiss Hollow Basket implant. The sphere of oral implantology was indeed expanding.

CONTEMPORARY ORAL IMPLANTOLOGY

Contemporary oral implantology originates with the 1978 conference held at Harvard and co-sponsored by the National Institutes of Health (NIH).[40] The proceedings of the conference, which critically described the benefits and risks inherent to the implant systems then in use, were widely disseminated to the profession at large.[41] This conference for the first time gave the field of oral implantology positive visibility providing awareness of oral implantology via professional respectability.

As the 1980s dawned, three factors[42] continued the growth of oral implantology. These three factors were:

- The results of the 1978 NIH-Harvard consensus conference
- The excitement caused by the results of the Göteborg studies
- The growth of peer-reviewed scientific implant research

The consensus conference has been discussed above. The Göteborg group in Sweden began its experimental studies as early as 1951, but their American colleagues only became fully aware of the importance of their contributions when the research was presented for peer review in 1981 and 1982.[43] Experimental animal studies documented biocompatibility of the implant system which was first known as the Biotes and then as the Nobelpharma implant. In vivo bone rheology studies[44] first documented the degree of possible bone necrosis due to heat generated by drilling, and further studies specifically documented the need for careful and aseptic surgical procedures, a concept first put forth by Greenfield in 1915. The depth of scientific inquiry regarding this specific titanium implant is the major contribution of the Göteborg group led by Branemark and Thomas Albrektsson.[43, 45]

The Göteborg group also presented the results of long-term, large-sample human clinical trials for peer review. Adell and colleagues[46] reported on a sample of 2,768 implants placed into 410 jaws of 371 patients. The size of this patient population was not lost on the North American dental community and a conference on osseointegration in clinical dentistry was held in Toronto, Canada, in 1982.[47] This research, both experimental animal and human clinical evaluations, has been criticized for internal and external validity;[48] however, the composite data presented by the Brånemark and Albrektsson groups represent numbers not previously reported upon in the dental implant literature. It is this factor that helped stimulate the tremendous excitement and interest in dental implants that prevails as we enter the 1990s.

The third factor promoting the enormous contemporary interest in dental implants is the growing amount of dental scientific inquiry concerning both the basic biological response of the oral tissues to implants, and human clinical trials of dental implants. The bridge from theory to practice has always correlated basic and applied science. Contemporary studies, as reported in other sections of this book, document acceptable tissue responses to dental implants. Epithelial attachment has been documented to ceramic,[49, 50] Vitallium,[51] and titanium[52] implants, thus providing a biological seal protection of the apical support systems to implants. Bone has been shown to adequately interface implants, providing structural stability for the implants to serve as abutments for crowns and bridges.[45, 53, 54] Implants can exist within dynamic epithelial and osseous systems.[49, 53, 54] These data have supported the growth of implant dentistry in the 1980s and into the 1990s.

As a result of this increased interest in oral implantology, implant manufacturers began making available numerous implant systems. The ITI Swiss Hollow Basket implant of Sutter and colleagues[39] from the Institute Strauman has been under development since 1974 and follows the design concepts of Greenfield. Kirsch[55] developed the IMZ implant in 1974 and this cylindrical implant has been in clinical use in Germany since 1978. In the early 1970s Kawahara,[38] after positive experimental animal studies in Japan, developed a ceramic cylindrical implant composed of single-crystal alpha aluminum oxide. After clinical experience in Japan, the implant was introduced in North America, first by Johnson and Johnson, and then by the Kyocera Corporation in 1980, where it has undergone extensive experimental animal and clinical investigation.[56] The Stryker-Driskell implant was introduced as late as 1985, but intermediate forms date to the 1970s.

Most cylindrical-type implants were developed following acceptance of the two-stage, cylindrical Branemark implant in the United States in 1981 and 1982. The core vent implant, a modified basket implant made into a two-stage implant, was introduced by Niznick in 1982.[57] Cylindrical implants similar to the Nobelpharma implant, such as the Steri-Oss,[58] Flexiroot, Osseodent, and the Screw-Vent/Swede-Vent were all introduced after 1982. The Integral implant, an implant similar in form to the IMZ but coated with hydroxylapatite, was introduced in 1984. Subsequently, other implant systems offered hydroxylapatite coatings.

PROFESSIONAL STATUS

The cautious attitude of the American Dental Association (ADA) concerning dental implants dates to 1972. The ADA charged Natiella and colleagues with examining the feasibility of dental implants. Their report stated that "there is an obvious limited acceptance of dental implants by the profession and this is a point of international concern."[59] After reviewing the literature, they concluded that "dental implantology has progressed in the past 20 years and has, in many respects, reached a plateau. The scope of dental implantology will be clear only when systematic experimentation and further reporting defines some current conceptions." The research data were nonexistent in 1972.

In 1973, the Council on Dental Materials and Devices co-sponsored with the National Institute of Dental Research (NIDR) a symposium on implants. Based on these reports, including the group report cited above, the ADA in 1974 recommended that "dental endosseous implants be considered as being in the new technique phase and in need of continuing scientific inquiry."[60] The advisors further urged that "endosseous dental implants not be recommended at this time for routine clinical practice."[60] These recommendations emphasized the lack of sufficient information concerning failure and success as well as

the lack of information concerning type of training needed and the qualifications of implantology practitioners.

In 1980 and 1981, the ADA selected criteria for providing provisional acceptance of dental implant devices.[61, 62] This was an expansion of the acceptance program for dental materials, instruments, and equipment to include endosseous implants. At this time, the council's position on endosseous implants remained unchanged, that is, "the council does not currently recommend endosseous implants for routine clinical practice. There is accumulating evidence, although, that when the relative merits of benefit and risk are carefully evaluated and fully discussed with the patient, the endosseous implant may be used. Responsibility for patient selection and information rests with the dentist."[62]

In 1986 only one implant, the Biotes (Nobelpharma), was classified as provisionally acceptable.[63] In the association reports, the Council on Dental Materials, Instruments, and Equipment suggested that after monitoring the scientific review, the organization "still believes there is a need for continued scientific review . . . [and that implants] not be recommended for routine clinical use."[63]

The council did initiate an endosseous implant registry in 1976 to collect data on implants on a nationwide scale.[64] A summary of the data obtained from 93 practitioners concerning 1,885 implants was provided to the council in 1987. Their conclusions suggested that the summary "was in accordance with the position of the Council . . . [that there is] still a need for continued scientific inquiry and longitudinal evaluations."[64] Further, because the registry had served its purpose, it was terminated.

Since 1987, three additional implants have received provisional approval by the Council on Dental Materials and Devices. The Interpore IMZ received provisional approval in 1988, as did the Oratronics blade implant in 1989, and the Core Vent implant in 1989. This number will no doubt increase, possibly until the Food and Drug Administration exercises its control and requires extensive and sophisticated animal and human testing of dental implant devices prior to marketing.[65] This testing was mandated by the second NIH implant consensus conference held in 1988.

SUMMARY

We have examined the extensive history of oral implantology. It became clear that "modern" implantology protocols did indeed evolve from protocols developed by oftentimes forgotten colleagues of times past. The following truism still pertains today—that to see the future we must explore the past.

Implantation procedures indeed can be traced to the ancient Egyptians and to the pre-Columbian South American Indian cultures. Replants and transplants first acted as a substitute for missing or diseased teeth, but were eventually thought of as inadequate or repugnant. As discussed by Greenfield, a new source was needed to restore esthetic and functional dentition. Implants were, and today may be, the "missing link in dentistry."[27] Implant pioneers such as Greenfield, Dahl, Lew, Strock, Linkow, Cranin, James, and Brånemark have attempted to enhance the physical well-being of their patients by developing innovative implantology protocols. Such individuals stand apart from their more avaricious entrepreneurial colleagues. Much of the conservatism of the professional dental organizations and the academic dental community can realistically be traced to the oral implantology environment created by this latter entrepreneurial group.

As we enter the decade of the 1990s, the dental profession and the appropriate governmental agencies are taking a more aggressive stance. Dental implants are entering a new age, an age of sound clinical practice based on basic biological and clinical research—an age in which successful dental rehabilitative treatments will routinely incorporate the multidimensional capabilities of dental implants.

REFERENCES

1. Weinberger BW: *An Introduction to the History of Dentistry.* St Louis, CV Mosby Co, 1948.
2. Keith A: Problems relating to the teeth of the earlier forms of prehistoric man. *Proc R Soc Med [Odont Sect]* 1912–1913; 6:103–124.
3. Ring ME: *Dentistry: An Illustrated History.* St Louis, CV Mosby Co, 1985.
4. Winter GB: *Exodontia: Extraction of Teeth.* St Louis, American Medical Book Co, 1913.
5. Congdon MJ: The plantation of teeth. *Panama-Pacific Dent Congress Trans* 1915; 2:295–305.
6. Morse DR: Plantation procedures: Histology, immunology and clinical considerations. *J Oral Implantol* 1977; 7:176–192.
7. Cranin AN: *Oral Implantology.* Springfield, Ill, Charles C Thomas, Publisher, 1970.
8. Smollon JF: A review and history of endosseous implant dentistry. *Georgetown Dent J* 1979; 43:33–45.
9. Driskell TD: History of implants. *J Calif Dent Assoc* 1987; 15:16–25.
10. Andrews RR: Prehistoric crania from Central America. *Int Dent J* 1893; 3:914.
11. Saville MH: Pre-Columbian decoration of teeth in Ecuador. *Am J Anthropol* 1913; 15:380.
12. Van Rippen B: Pre-Columbian operative dentistry of the Indians of Middle and South America. *Dent Cosmos* 1917; 59:861–873.
13. Reade P: Host reactions to tooth transplants. *Aust Dent J* 1970; (June) 172–178.
14. Kusek JC: A brief history of tooth transplantation. *Dent Students Magazine* 1983; 43:662–670.
15. Costich ER, Haley EW, Hoek RB: Plantation of teeth. *NY State Dent J* 1963; 29(January):3–13.
16. Tompkins HE: Theories and practice of tooth implantation. *Dent Cosmos* 1921; 63:1025–1027.
17. Kirk EC: [Record of implant operations.] *Dent Cosmos* 1913; 55:432–437.
18. Jacobs FO: The question of persistence of vitality in the pericemental membrane. *Dent Cosmos* 1893; 35:446–449.
19. Younger WJ: Some of the latest phases in implantation and other operations. *Dent Cosmos* 1893; 35:102–108.
20. Harris SM: Hints and queries. *Dent Cosmos* 1897; 29:801–802.
21. Edmunds JM: Clinical report in First District Dental Society, State of NY. *Dent Cosmos* 1913; 55:371–372.
22. Berry A. Lead roots of teeth for implantation. *Ohio J Dent Sci* 1888; 8:549.
23. Znamenski NN: The implantation of artificial teeth. *Br J Dent Sci* 1891; 34:314–316.
24. Payne RE: [Report of silver capsule implantation.] *Dent Cosmos* 1901; 12:1401.
25. Greenfield EJ: An artificial root. *Dent Brief* 1910; 15:837–839.
26. Greenfield EJ: Implantation of artificial roots for crown and bridge work. *Dent Rev* 1914; 28:1–7.

27. Greenfield EJ: Implantation of artificial crown and bridge abutments. *Dent Cosmos* 1913; 55:364–369.

28. Greenfield EJ: Implanted artificial roots. *Panama-Pacific Dent Congress Trans* 1915; 2:538–539.

29. Roberts JB: [Discussion concerning Greenfield's paper.] *Dent Cosmos* 1913; 55:431–432.

30. Venable CS, Stuck WG, Beach A: Effects on bone of the presence of metals, based on electrolysis. *Ann Surg* 1937; 105:917.

31. Strock AE: Experimental work on a method for the replacement of missing teeth by direct implantation of a metal support into the alveolus. *Am J Orthodont Oral Surg* 1939; 25:467–472.

32. Linkow LI: Evolutionary design trends in the mandibular subperiosteal implant. *J Oral Implantol* 1984; 11:402–438.

33. Lemons J, Natiella J: Biomaterials, biocompatibility, and peri-implant considerations. Reconstructive implant surgery and implant prosthodontics. *Dent Clin North Am* 1986; 30:3–23.

34. Small IA, Misiek DA: Sixteen-year evaluation of the mandibular staple bone plate. *J Oral Maxillofac Surg* 1986; 44:60–66.

35. Bodine RL: Evaluation of 27 mandibular subperiosteal implant dentures after 15–22 years. *J Prosthet Dent* 1974; 32:188–197.

36. Cranin AN, Rabkin MF, Garfinkel L: A statistical evaluation of 952 endosteal implants in humans. *J Am Dent Assoc* 1977; 94:315–320.

37. Linkow LI: Statistical analysis of 173 implant patients. *J Oral Implantol* 1974; 4:540–566.

38. Kawahara H: Single crystal alumina for dental implants. *J Biomed Mater Res* 1980; 14:597–602.

39. Sutter F, Schroeder A, Straumann F: ITI hollow cylinder system principles and methodology. *J Oral Implantol* 1983; 11:166–196.

40. Schnitman, PA, Schulman LB (eds): *Dental Implants: Benefits and Risks. Proceedings of an NIH-Harvard Consensus Development Conference.* Bethesda, Md, US Department of Health and Human Services publication No (NIH) 81-1531, 1980.

41. Schnitman PA, Schulman LB: Recommendations of the consensus development conference on dental implants. *J Am Dent Assoc* 1979; 98:373–377.

42. Steflik DE: *A Case Study in the Development of Instructional Awareness of Selected Topics in Oral Implantology for Predoctoral Dental Students.* Ann Arbor, Mich, University Microfilms International, Inc., 1987.

43. Branemark P-I: Osseointegration and its experimental background. *J Prosthet Dent* 1983; 50:399–410.

44. Ericksson AR, Albrektsson T: Temperature threshold levels for heat induced bone tissue injury: A vital microscopic study in the rabbit. *J Prosthet Dent* 1983; 50:101–107.

45. Albrektsson T, Branemark P-I, Hansson H-A, et al: Osseointegrated titanium implants. *Acta Orthop Scand* 1981; 52:155–170.

46. Adell R, Lekholm U, Rockler B, et al: A fifteen year study of osseointegrated implants in the treatment of the edentulous jaw. *Int J Oral Surg* 1981; 10:387–416.

47. Zarb GA (ed): *Proceedings of the Toronto Conference on Osseointegration in Clinical Dentistry.* St Louis, CV Mosby Co, 1983.

48. James RA, Altman AF, Clem DC, et al: A critical review of the osseointegrated literature. *Implantologist* 1986; 3:35–41.

49. Steflik DE, McKinney RV, Koth DL: Epithelial attachment to ceramic dental implants. *Ann NY Acad Sci* 1988; 523:4–18.

50. McKinney RV, Steflik DE, Koth DL: Evidence for the junctional epithelial attachment to ceramic dental implants: A transmission electron microscopic study. *J Periodontol* 1985; 56:579–591.

51. James RA, Schultz RL: Hemidesmosomes and the adhesion of junctional epithelial cells to metal implants. *J Oral Implantol* 1974; 4:294–302.

52. Karagienes MT, Westerman RE, Hamilton AI, et al: Investigation of long term performance of porous metal dental implants in non human primates. *J Oral Implantol* 1982; 10:189–207.

53. Steflik DE, McKinney RV, Koth DL: Ultrastructural comparisons of ceramic and titanium implants in vivo: A scanning electron microscopic study. *J Biomed Mater Res* 1989; 23:895–909.

54. Steflik DE, McKinney RV, Koth DL, et al: The biomaterial-tissue interface: A morphological study utilizing conventional and alternative ultrastructural modalities. *Scan Electron Microsc* 1984; 2:547–555.

55. Kirsch A: The two-phase implantation method using IMZ intramobile cylinder implants. *J Oral Implantol* 1983; 11:197–210.

56. Koth DL, McKinney RV, Steflik DE, et al: A clinical and statistical analysis of human clinical trials with the single crystal alumina oxide endosteal dental implant: Five year results. *J Prosthet Dent* 1988; 60:226–234.

57. Niznick GA: The Core-Vent implant system. *J Oral Implantol* 1982; 10:379–418.

58. Hahn JA: Three year clinical evaluation: Steri-Oss

implant system. 1988. Unpublished clinical study, available from Denar Inc, Anaheim, Calif.

59. Natiella J, Armitage J, Greene J, et al: Report on current evaluation of dental implants to Council on Dental Materials and Devices. *J Am Dent Assoc* 1975; 89:1367–1368.

60. Council on Dental Materials and Devices, and Council on Dental Research: Current evaluation of dental endosseous implants. *J Am Dent Assoc* 1974; 88:394–395.

61. Council on Dental Materials, Instruments, and Equipment: Council reevaluates position on dental implants. *J Am Dent Assoc* 1980; 100:247.

62. Association Reports: Expansion of the acceptance program for dental materials, instruments, and equipment: Endosseous implants. *J Am Dent Assoc* 1981; 102:350.

63. Council on Dental Materials, Instruments, and Equipment: Dental endosseous implants. *J Am Dent Assoc* 1986; 113:949–950.

64. Council on Dental Materials, Instruments, and Equipment: Summary of the results of the endosseous implant registry. *J Am Dent Assoc* 1987; 114:672–674.

65. Implantology Research Group and Dental Materials Group of AADR: Safe and effective implants— Criteria for pre-market approval, in SYMPOSIUM VIII, *American Association for Dental Research Annual Meeting, San Francisco, March 18, 1989. J Dent Res* 1989; 68:(special issue):179.

Chapter 3

Clinical Considerations for Implantology

Joseph R. Natiella, D.D.S.

There are many basic response characteristics essential to the clinical success of an endosteal implant. These are complex and include the local and systemic events in healing which begin moments after placement of the implant and the longer-term sequences of repair and regeneration which ensure long duration of use of the implant. Of equal importance are the effects of the host environment on the implant bulk material and surface. A comprehensive understanding of these basic responses is difficult because of the many unique properties of the oral environment and the yet unknown influences of function. The practitioner who plans to utilize the endosteal implant as a treatment modality and who considers the factors that influence success also faces the current dilemma of selecting from a growing list of materials and designs. The criteria for selecting a particular implant are varied and calculation of the benefit-risk ratio must take into account evidence of safety of the material, proof of mucosal adhesion or attachment, and longevity of the optimal intrabony interface. Basically the implantologist strives to achieve a condition of what may be termed "functional biocompatibility." A scheme of this host-implant relationship is illustrated in Figure 3–1. It represents a milieu of responses that integrate host tissue reaction, biological status of the host, properties of the material used, prosthodontic aspects of function, and the influences of handling the implant. This chapter examines some of the factors of the host-implant interrelationship which are associated with important clinical considerations.

HOST TISSUE REACTION

Material Properties

Implant Safety

It is important to determine the safety of all implant materials used in patients on the basis of potential toxicity, hypersensitivity (allergy), and tumor formation. Dentistry has a superb record of assessment of alloy systems and many of the tests developed for determining safety and efficacy of dental alloys apply to endosteal implants.[1-3] Both in vitro and in vivo methods are utilized, the latter often employing the use of small animals, including rats, mice, hamsters, and guinea pigs. Although the American Dental Association recommends 11 tests for evaluating dental implants, some may be modified or combined with others to provide a more selective form of analysis. Autian[4] has differentiated between "safety testing" and "toxicology testing" and he has suggested some methods of evaluation that more appropriately determine the host reaction under conditions simulating use. A number of tests are of considerable importance to discussing the safety of endosteal implants. The hemolysis test allows an evaluation of the effect of particulate forms of the implant material on rabbit blood. Cell culture tests are highly varied and involve the re-

Host vs. Implant

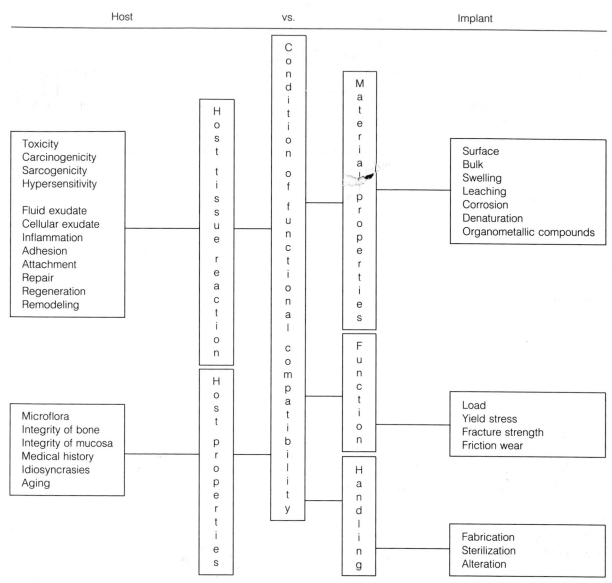

FIG 3–1.
Functional biocompatibility of the host–dental implant relationship.

sponse of tissue growth to the presence of the implant material. The chromium release method is an example of cell culture testing used to evaluate specific alloys used in dentistry.[5] Materials evaluation in cell culture has been extended to the use of ultrastructural analysis[6] and measurement of released radioactive labeled compounds as an index of cytotoxicity.[7] The determination of capsule formation and inflammatory cell re-

sponses form a number of tests which involve the implantation of the material into both the subcutaneous and intramuscular region of rodents.

Special tests for dentistry in a similar category may be used to evaluate materials that penetrate oral mucosa and bone. The bone implant test recommended by the Fédération Dentaire Internationale (ADA/FDI, 211 E. Chicago Ave., Chicago, IL

60611) studies test implants placed for 4 to 20 weeks in the symphyseal region of the rabbit mandible.[3] The tests for systemic toxicity involve administration of material to determine toxic and lethal dose levels and may involve the oral, intravenous, or intraperitoneal route. To study the potential of a material to induce malignant change, the Styles cell transformation and the Ames mutagenicity tests are advocated. The Styles test demonstrates carcinogenic activity of test substances on mammalian cell cultures. The Ames test employs genetically altered bacteria which exhibit a return to the original, normal nutrient requirements when exposed to a carcinogenic test substance.[8]

In 1985 the International Workshop on the Biocompatibility, Toxicity and Hypersensitivity to Alloy Systems Used in Dentistry was held at the University of Michigan.[9] Many tests of importance to consideration of the safety of dental implants were discussed in the proceedings of the workshop. Merritt[10] provided an excellent review of laboratory studies for hypersensitivity reaction to biomaterials. She characterized the type of reaction most commonly seen in biomaterials. This is associated with antigenic recognition involving T cells (lymphocytes) constituting a cell-mediated response. The hypersensitive reaction to a metal is actually to the metal ion–host complex. Reaction to the implant involves wear, corrosion, and ion migration and formation of metallic salts. In vitro tests that explore the potential of hypersensitivity are designed to focus on these products. However, assessing hypersensitivity of reactions to dental implants is difficult. Because the rabbit is used for studies in orthopedics, Merritt and others now recommend the rabbit for other implant studies. It has a dermis that is thick enough for skin testing, repeated blood samples can be drawn, and the rabbit is suitable for such important aspects of testing as migration inhibition factor assays and antibody production.

Generally, dental implants tested with existing protocols and rated on the basis of toxicity hypersensitivity or malignancy appear to be "safe." While there is a paucity of reports that indicate hypersensitivity or allergy to endosteal implants, oral mucosal reactions to crowns, dental alloys, and denture frameworks have been documented.[11–17] These reports include local and distant reaction to nickel, cobalt, chromium, and gold. The reactions range from localized erythema, erosive gingivitis, stomatitis, and oral lichenoid response, to dermatitis, with or without an oral reaction. Patients are suspected of having a sensitivity reaction to an implant material when oral symptoms develop, such as changes in mucosal color and tone, erythematous macular eruption, vesiculation, altered salivary flow, lichenoid mixed keratotic and erythematous lesions, burning mucosa, dysgeusia, and dermatitis. The evaluation of these patients is best done on a team basis by the dermatologist, allergist, and dentist. The patient is frequently skin-tested to a variety of allergens with the patch test method.[18]

The development of malignant disease at the site of dental implants is exceedingly rare.[19] This is reassuring. However, Mjor and Hensten-Pettersen[20] have underscored the fact that carcinogenicity testing is an ever-changing process and that circumstance will modify evaluation protocols for materials used in dentistry. Autian[21] strongly advocates both short- and long-term tests that can adequately illuminate the potential of biomaterial substances, including implants, to stimulate malignant tumor formation in the host. These more comprehensive protocols often extend for a 3-year period and correlate clinical measurements, clinical laboratory testing, and microscopic analysis of organs and tissues in animals that have received implants in various test forms.

There is little evidence available to suggest that the oral environment will act to change implant materials into potential allergens, carcinogens, or organ- or tissue-damaging toxic substances by chemical action. Despite this, leaders in the field of biomaterials have, with increasing frequency, focused on the long-term possibilities of local and distant transfer of substances from the implant to the host. There is concern that current methods of testing may not be sufficient to allow a prediction of long-term effects. In his discussion of the interaction of implants with the body, Black[22] emphasizes that the chronic, low-level release of substances from implants may elicit long-term or delayed effects not detected either in a single-dose test or with repeated doses administered over short test periods. Black urges large-scale epidemiologic studies of implant patients to show the possible development of systemic effects. Particular concern applies to metallic implants, even titanium. Williams[23] has provided an extensive review of the properties of titanium and its biomedical applications. He indicates that although the corrosion rate of titanium is low, it is present in tissues surrounding implants. Further, although titanium is extensively used, and the general consensus is that titanium and titanium alloys are well tolerated, there are actually a small number of reports that comprehensively describe the titanium-host interaction. It is considered important to evolve a more precise understanding of the rate of metal ion release from implants and the mode of chemical activity such as protein binding and the transport phenomena.[24, 25]

Handling the Implant

Enhancement of Initial and Long-Term Response

Knowledge derived from the blood interface–biomaterials field has included the importance of various aspects of fluid adsorption and tissue adherence or attachment (or nonadherence or nonattachment) to the implant surface. The various groups involved in dental implant development and use are increasingly concerned with molecular events occurring at the host-material interface. Norman and others[26] have emphasized the important role of certain cells found in the host fluid exudate at the time of implantation. These investigators have shown the critical and pivotal role played by the monocyte-macrophage cell component thought to involve interaction with adsorbed protein and regulation of fibroblast activity and collagen formation. Further, there is evidence that this "optimum" clot initially formed in the implant crypt may control addition of substances critical to repair and regeneration such as host tissue and macrophage-derived, epidermal, and fibroblast growth factors. The relationship of these molecular events can easily be altered by improper handling of the implant during fabrication or implantation. Studies have shown that adherence of films to implant surfaces may be partially influenced by the surface tension or wettability of the implant. Detailed investigations of the influence of surface properties on the formation of initial "conditioning" films have been conducted by Baier.[27] He has been critical of the tendency in biomaterials research to be mainly concerned with the long-term host response to the device, ignoring the initial events of tissue reaction. It is true that the original surface condition of the implant is often not known and even the accepted methods for finishing implants may be problematic.

Carter and associates[28] studied the conventional finishing and polishing techniques for the preparation of Vitallium subperiosteal implants. The critical surface tension was determined by contact angle measurement providing wettability spectra. They found that organic contamination produced surfaces that were not wetted by water, a condition that could conceivably affect the initial adherence of host fluids and cells. The importance of optimizing and controlling tissue reactions by ensuring the "cleanliness" of the implant surface has also been emphasized by Lemons and Natiella.[29] They stressed maintaining the passivated surface of metal implants and the possible contamination that can occur from faulty steam sterilizers, or from utilization of bead or salt sterilizers as well as the possible addition of harmful substances from trays, packages, and gloves. A number of highly significant biomaterials investigations on dental implant materials have illuminated the almost shocking possibilities of improper handling of the implant prior to insertion. The continuing work of Baier and associates[30, 31] has detailed the common sources and potential surface contaminant derived from faulty implant preparation and sterilization of dental implants, all of which could have a potential role in disturbing the desired host-implant condition. These include low-energy poorly adherent films, detergent residues, organic matter, surfactants, hygroscopic salt particles, corrosion products, metal or alloy constituents, lubricant residues, and other cytotoxic substances.

The long-term response of metallic dental implants is dependant on their corrosion resistance. Metallic implants have an interface chemistry that is determined by the oxide layer that is formed during preparation and sterilization and which persists after insertion. Kasemo[32] has diagrammed the transport and chemical processes that constitute surface oxide and biomolecular interaction. The properties of the oxide zone are dependent on such factors as pressure and speed of machining and sterilization and passivation techniques following alteration of the implant. Departures from recommended methods of handling can be disadvantageous when the issue of corrosion is considered. Van Orden[33] has provided a comprehensive discussion regarding the corrosion of dental implants showing how faulty handling could conceivably compromise the condition of functional biocompatibility. She has described the importance of mechanical factors such as surface abrasion, cracks, and adhesion of films on the potential ionic exchanges from implant to host. Certain endosteal metallic implants may undergo crevice corrosion from dropping, grinding, and other manipulations which destroy the passive oxide film. This critically important film can also be broken, exposing the implant to a hostile environment by bending, which initiates the phenomenon of stress corrosion. Lemons[34] has explained the importance of pre- and postimplantation testing for corrosion inclusive of specimen retrieval analysis. He has continued to advocate scanning electron and optical microscopy for identification of some types of corrosion phenomena and the correlation of these studies with host tissue analysis for biodegradative substances. Lemons has discussed the evolution of in vitro tests for corrosion to more fully simulate the host environment by incorporating proteins and other organic species to test solutions.[34]

HOST VS. IMPLANT: FUNCTIONAL BIOCOMPATIBILITY

Future Testing

Traditional approaches to biocompatibility evaluation usually can be divided into toxicity testing, general biocompatibility testing, and specific usage testing. There is a great overlap between these major forms of implant analysis. The informed practitioner who uses endosteal implants is aware that tests to delineate the host-implant reaction are constantly being developed as new instrumentation and methodologies become available. It is important to understand that many questions remain unanswered. The modern-day approaches to testing are designed to expose the subtle markers of host response and change in the implant material. Such phenomena are characterized by identification of specific enzymes with differential and quantitative counts of peri-implant cell populations. There is a departure from totally descriptive morphologic studies of implant reactions to approaches that incorporate transmission electron microscopy, scanning electron microscopy, and analytical histochemistry.[35] In this way cells important to the long-term success of implants, notably the macrophage, are shown to be influenced by such conditions as implant surface roughness and shape. Tests are now designed to quantitate cellular enzymes important to cell metabolism and provide delicate markers of subtle responses to implants. Implants in animal model sites are graded against their effect on these specific enzymes which include acid and alkaline phosphatase, nonspecific esterase, lactic dehydrogenase, and succinic dehydrogenase.[24] Continued investigation into the properties of the outermost surface layers and coating films now uses sophisticated instrumentation. Surface analysis of trace elements and an indication of the type of bonding and concentration profiles of elements present can be determined within 3,000 to 10,000 Å depths. This is accomplished by techniques using Auger spectroscopy, electron spectroscopy chemical analysis (ESCA), and secondary ion spectroscopy.

This ultramicroscopic and chemical analytical focus is directed toward those cells that may be associated with attachment and those substances on the implant surface that may facilitate and preserve this attachment. These tests often combine animal and human studies. A superb example can be found in the studies of Gould and associates[36, 37] and those of McKinney and his group.[38, 39] These investigations utilized ultrastructural analysis providing characterization of epithelial cell organelle components such as hemidesmosomes, linear electron structures, and basal lamina. This was exciting evidence for the feasibility of the attachment role of mucosal epithelium and was a classic representation of testing which extended from the in vitro mode to usage tests in both animals and humans. Analysis of human implant cases has also helped illuminate the critical area of the microbiology of dental implants. The grading of plaque accumulation and characterization of microbial populations around implants has finally begun on a systematic basis.[40, 41]

Perhaps no single aspect of dental implantology is more developmental than that of understanding the biomechanics and the influence of function on host response. Animal studies by Brunski and Hipp[42] using strain-gauge transducers with hard wiring and telemetric schemes for data collection are innovative and have shown the mechanics of load transmission from implant to fixed bridges. Continued use of finite element analysis and photoelastic models correlated with microscopic analysis is helpful in estimating the effect of forces on host responses.[43] Other studies have been conducted to assess correlations between tissue response and shear strength against displacement of implants.[44, 45] While these studies have been helpful in determining the types of mechanical stress and distribution of force at the implant site, it is probably accurate to say that the optimal design and material for a duplication of tooth function has yet to be developed. The evolution of testing, with the development of newer methods of measurement of forces in animal models and humans, will add to the knowledge base.

DISCUSSION

The selection of an endosteal implant for use in a dental patient requires a comprehensive review of the many factors of the condition of functional compatibility. The questions that must be asked by the practitioner are numerous. What testing has been done on the substances which compose the implant? To what extent does the implant biodegrade and what are the local and distant effects of these products? How is the composition of the implant quality controlled, batch to batch, year to year? Does the manufacturer participate in a retrieval program to identify the possible untoward effects of using the product? Have these tests been done on the specific implant or have results been extrapolated from implants of "similar design or composition?" Does tissue actually attach to the implant? What studies have been done *on that specific implant* to demonstrate attachment over time and under functional conditions that simulate the human condition? What are the precise recommendations for sterilization and handling?

Are these consistent with a good immediate and long-term host-implant response? What studies show this? Are there suggestions derived from longitudinal clinical studies that address the optimal site and condition of loading for the implant system? Are recommendations for periodontal maintenance based on the understanding of the microbiological characterization of the peri-implant tissues? Has the interfacial tissue been described comprehensively by morphometric, histochemical, and ultrastructural analysis? Is the recommendation for a porous or smooth or combined implant surface based on meaningful usage tests?

These questions, which form important clinical considerations, can and should be answered by the existing state of the art of materials testing. There are gaps in our understanding of the host-implant responses that remain. Constant communication between basic scientist, materials scientist, toxicologist, biophysicist, pathologist, dentist, and patient is necessary to evolve an implant system which best duplicates the functional requirements of the dentition.

REFERENCES

1. *ANSI/ADA Document #41 for Recommended Standard Practices for Biological Evaluation of Dental Materials.* Chicago, American National Standards Institute/American Dental Association, 1979.
2. *Methods of Biological Assessment of Dental Materials.* London, British Standards Institute, 1980, BS5828.
3. Fédération Dentaire Internationale: Recommended standard practices for biological evaluation of dental materials, F.D.I. technical report #9. *Int Dent J* 1980; 30:140–149.
4. Autian J: Testing for toxicity, in von Recum AF (ed): *Handbook of Biomaterials Evaluation.* New York, Macmillan Publishing Co, 1986, pp 167–178.
5. Hensten-Pettersen A, Jacobsen N: Biocompatibility of dental base metal alloys as evaluated by subcutaneous implants in rats and by cell culture, in Winter GD, Leray JL, de Groot K (eds): *Evaluation of Biomaterials.* London, John Wiley & Sons, 1980, pp 441–447.
6. Neupert G, Welker D: Morphogenesis of cell-to-substratum adhesion and spreading on Ni-Cr alloys. *Exp Pathol* 1983; 23:121–126.

7. Spangberg L, Langeland K: Biological effects of dental materials. *Oral Surg* 1973; 35:402–414.

8. Lawrence W: Tumor Induction, in von Recum AF (ed): *Handbook of Biomaterials Evaluation.* New York, Macmillan Publishing Co, 1986, pp 188–197.

9. Lang BR, Morris HF, Razzoog ME (eds): *International Workshop on the Biocompatibility, Toxicity and Hypersensitivity to Alloy Systems Used in Dentistry.* Ann Arbor, University of Michigan, 1985.

10. Merritt, K: Biochemistry, hypersensitivity clinical reaction, in Lang BR, Morris HF, Razzoog ME (eds): *International Workshop on the Biocompatibility, Toxicity and Hypersensitivity to Alloy Systems Used in Dentistry.* Ann Arbor, University of Michigan, 1985, sect 5, pp 191–223.

11. Bendlinger D, Tarsitano J: Generalized dermatitis due to sensitivity to a chrome cobalt removable partial denture. *J Am Dent Assoc* 1970; 81:392.

12. Levantine A, Bettley F: Sensitizing to metal dental plate. *Proc R Soc Med* 1974; 67:1007–1012.

13. Young E: Contact hypersensitivity to metallic gold. *Dermatologica* 1974; 149:194–208.

14. Hubler WR: Dermatitis from a chromium dental plate. *Contact Dermatitis* 1983; 9:377–383.

15. Lundstrom JM: Allergy and corrosion of dental materials in patients with oral lichen planus. *Int J Oral Surg* 1984; 13:16–24.

16. Wood JF: Mucosal reaction in chrome cobalt alloy. *Br Dent J* 1974; 136:423–428.

17. Izumi AK: Allergic contact gingivostomatitis due to gold. *Arch Dermatol Res* 1982; 272:3–4, 387–391.

18. Dooms-Goossens A, Ceuterick A, Vanmaele N, et al: Followup study of patients with contact dermatitis caused by chromates, nickel and cobalt. *Dermatologica* 1980; 160:249–260.

19. Friedman K, Vernon S: Squamous cell carcinoma developing in conjunction with a mandibular staple bone plate. *J Oral Maxillofac Surg* 1983; 41:265–269.

20. Mjor A, Hensten-Pettersen A: The biological compatibility of alternative alloys. *Int Dent J* 1983; 33:35–40.

21. Autian J: Carcinogenic potential of metals, in *Workshop on Biocompatibility of Metals in Dentistry. National Institute of Dental Research, National Institutes of Health.* Chicago, American Dental Association, 1984, pp 107–113.

22. Black J: Systemic effect of biomaterials. *Biomaterials* 1984; 5:11–18.

23. Williams DF: Titanium and titanium alloys, in Williams DF (ed): *Biocompatibility of Clinical Implant Materials Vol. I.* Boca Raton, Fla, CRC Press, 1981, pp 9–44.

24. McNamara A, Williams DF: Enzyme histochemistry of the tissue response to pure metal implants. *J Biomed Mater Res* 1984; 18:185–206.

25. Salthouse T: Observations of implanted biomaterials. *J Biomed Mater Res* 1984; 18:395–402.

26. Norman N, Sudilovsky O, Gibbons D: The effects of humoral components on the cellular response to textured and non textured PTFE. *J Biomed Mater Res* 1984; 18:225–241.

27. Baier RE: Conditioning surfaces to suit the biomedical environment. *J Biomech Eng* 1982; 104:257–271.

28. Carter M, Flynn H, Meenaghan M, et al: Organic surface film contamination of Vitallium implants. *J Biomed Mater Res* 1981; 15:843–851.

29. Lemons J, Natiella JR: Biomaterials, biocompatibility and peri-implant considerations, in Guernsey L (ed): Reconstructive implant surgery and implant prosthodontics. I. *Dent Clin North Am* 1986; 30:3–24.

30. Baier RE, Natiella JR, Meyer AE, et al: Importance of implant surface preparation for biomaterials with different intrinsic properties, in Van Steenberghe D (ed): *Tissue Integration In Oral and Maxillofacial Reconstruction.* Amsterdam, Excerpta Medica, 1985, pp 13–40.

31. Baier RE, Meyer AE: Implant surface preparation. *Int J Oral Maxillofac Implant* 1988; 1:9–20.

32. Kasemo B: Biocompatibility of titanium implants. *J Prosthet Dent* 1983; 49:832–837.

33. Van Orden AC: Corrosive response of the interface tissue to 316L stainless steel, titanium-based alloys, and cobalt-based alloys, in McKinney RV Jr, Lemons JE (eds): *The Dental Implant.* Littleton, Mass, PSG Publishing Co Inc, 1985, pp 1–24.

34. Lemons JE: Corrosion and biodegradation, in von Recum AF (ed): *Handbook of Biomaterials Evaluation.* New York, Macmillan Publishing Co, 1986, pp 167–168.

35. Salthouse T: Some aspects of macrophage behavior at the implant interface. *J Biomed Mater Res* 1984; 18:395–401.

36. Gould T, Brunette D, Westbury L: The attachment mechanism of epithelial cells to titanium in vitro. *J Periodont Res* 1981; 16:611–618.

37. Gould T, Westbury L, Brunette D: Ultrastructural study of the attachment of human gingiva to titanium in vivo. *J Prosthet Dent* 1984; 52:418–426.

38. McKinney R, Steflik D, Koth D: Evidence for a

junctional epithelial attachment to ceramic dental implants. A transmission electron microscopic study. *J Periodontol* 1985; 56:579–591.

39. McKinney R, Steflick D, Koth D: Ultrastructural surface topography of the single crystal sapphire endosseous dental implant. *J Oral Implantol* 1984; 11:327–340.

40. Adell R, Lakholm V, Brånemark P: Marginal tissue reactions at osseointegrated titanium fixtures. *Swed Dent J [Suppl]* 1985; 28:175–181.

41. Adell R, Lekholm V, Rockler B: Marginal tissue reactions at osseointegrated titanium fixtures. *Int J Oral Maxillofac Surg* 1986; 15:39–52.

42. Brunski J, Hipp J: In-vivo forces on dental implants. *J Biomech* 1984; 17:855–860.

43. Weinstein A, Klawitter J, Cook S: Finite element analysis as an aid to implant design. *Biomater Med Devices Artif Organs* 1979; 7:169–175.

44. Atkinson P, Seedhom B, Roberts E: The shear strength between bone and porous ceramic root implants in the guinea pig incisor socket. *Biomaterials* 1985; 6:75–81.

45. Cook W, Weinstein A, Klawitter J: Quantitative histologic evaluation of LTI carbon, carbon coated aluminum oxide and uncoated aluminum oxide implants. *J Biomed Mater Res* 1983; 17:519–538.

Chapter 4

Endosteal Implant Biomaterials and Biomechanics

Jack E. Lemons, Ph.D.
Martha Warren Bidez, Ph.D.

OVERVIEW

Dental implant biomaterials and biomechanics represent an area of relatively active research and development over the past two decades. A great deal of basic and applied information has evolved with the overall interpretation and application influencing most clinical practices.[1-3]

This chapter provides a general summary of the various biomaterials used for the construction of endosteal dental implants with emphasis on the bulk and surface properties; the basic biomechanics of the synthetic and biological substances that make up the implant and tissue support regions; and a general evaluation of the biomaterials-to-tissue interface as influenced by the tissue type, force transfer, and the chemical stability of the implant surface.

Roles of Science and Technology

The successful applications of surgical implant devices are multifactorial with many direct and indirect influences supporting the final result. Basic science studies provide the opportunities for new and improved systems; however, these basic concepts must be developed through engineering for optimization prior to application. Technology controls whether the developments will proceed to actual devices and can be a critical limitation.

Science and technology in biomaterials and biomechanics, although directly interrelated, proceed through independent disciplines. As these disciplines are carried forward to clinical devices, they must be merged and extended to the dental practitioner. This requires a complex series of communications which often delays science and technology transfer. As the discipline of implant dentistry continues to develop, the basic textbook and journal publications should shorten the time between invention and application. Because the various steps are all critical, short cuts may result in less-than-optimal clinical devices.

Previous, Current, and Future Trends

Early applications of endosteal dental implants utilized available materials with clinical procedures specifically related to the dentist providing the restoration. Little interaction with other disciplines existed and the success ratios were quite dependent on the device and the individual inventor.[4] Over the following decades of expanded applications, a multidisciplinary approach evolved and several devices became routine modalities of treatment.[5] At present, from device manufacturers to long-term intraoral care, many of the procedures follow rigorous protocols. The basic and applied research programs are extensive and current trends suggest that new biomaterials and systems for transferring force will continue to be introduced.[6] In part, future results and improved opportunities for dental implants will directly depend upon studies of biomaterials and biomechanics.[7]

BIOMATERIALS

Metals and Alloys

Metals and their alloys represent the most common category of biomaterials used for dental implants. These materials, in general, are similar to those used in other surgical disciplines. This class of materials has been studied in depth, and standards on surgical implant devices for bulk and surface properties have been published by the American Society for Testing and Materials Committee F-4 (ASTMF-4).[8] The metallic biomaterials and their related ASTMF-4 standards are summarized in Table 4–1. The standards associated with these metallic biomaterials provide a listing of systems chemical analyses and basic mechanical properties. The general recommended practice for surface finish and preparation is also included in Table 4–1. Although the practice is required for surgical stainless steel, most metallic biomaterials are passivated as one of the final steps of finishing.

Titanium and its alloy are frequently selected for endosteal implants because of the surface oxide that forms spontaneously in air and in physiologic saline.

Insertion techniques can alter the surface layers and this reoxidation (passivation) is recognized as a significant advantage with respect to minimizing biodegradation.

Surgical stainless steel is subject to crevice and pitting corrosion in saline if the chromium-rich oxide layer is removed; therefore, passivation and protection of the oxide layer is critical for this alloy system. Mechanical properties of stainless steel are excellent, as is the case for titanium alloy. Commercially pure (cp) titanium is somewhat weaker, but does exhibit excellent ductility, which is often a significant advantage for some implant devices.[9, 10] The casting alloy of cobalt is often used to make custom dental devices and although cobalt alloy is somewhat less ductile, strengths and surface properties are adequate for long-term implantation. Cobalt alloy is relatively inert in a passivated condition with the complex chromium-oxide surface providing a significant reduction in corrosion phenomena. Where increased strengths are required, mechanically processed (forged or hot isostatically pressed) alloys are selected and tungsten is substituted for molybdenum to permit elevated temperature treatments. Limited applications of other alloys, such as tantalum, also exist, but these are not commonly used for currently available implant devices.

Ceramics and Carbons

The inert biomaterials include aluminum oxide (alumina and sapphire) ceramics, carbon, and carbon silicon compounds. These are summarized in Table 4–2, which also includes the surface-active and biodegradable forms.

Ceramic forms of hydroxyapatite (called *hydroxylapatite* to represent the *ceramic* form) have been introduced as a particulate for bone augmentation and as a surface coating. An extension of this general class of biomaterials includes the partially or totally resorbable tricalcium phosphates (TCPs) or calcium aluminates (ALCAP).[11] A number of other ceramics has been investigated, e.g., zirconia, but very few have been extended to endosseous systems.

Selected silica-based glasses, such as invert soda-lime glass with additions of calcium and phos-

TABLE 4–1.

Dental Implant Metals and Alloys and Associated American Society for Testing and Materials Committee F-4 (ASTMF-4) Standards

Biomaterial	ASTMF-4 Standard
Fe-Cr-Ni (316L SS)	F-138, 139, 621
Ti	F-67
Ta	F-560
Ti-6Al-4V	F-136, 620
Co-Cr-Mo (cast)	F-75
Co-Cr-W-Ni (wrought)	F-90
Co-Ni-Cr-Mo (wrought)	F-562
Co-Cr-Mo-W-Fe (wrought)	F-563
Practice for surface preparation and marking of metallic surgical implants	F-86

TABLE 4–2.

Ceramic and Carbon Biomaterials for Dental Implant Devices

Biomaterial	Standard
Aluminum oxide (Al_2O_3)	
Alumina	F-603
Sapphire	(draft)
Zirconia (ZrO_2)	(draft)
Hydroxylapatite [$Ca_{10}(PO_4)_6(OH)_2$]	(draft)
Tricalcium phosphate [$Ca_3(PO_4)_2$]	(draft)
Silica-based glass (Bioglass)	—
Calcium aluminate (ALCAP)	—
Carbon (glassy or vitreous)	—
Carbon silicon	—

phate (Bioglass or Ceravital), have been investigated for direct bonding to bone. To date, applications as dental implants have been limited.[12] Studies of biodegradation phenomena have shown carbon and carbon silicon compounds to be inert, and these types of biomaterials can be manufactured with elastic properties similar to bone.[13] Significant difficulties with these have included their color, electrical and thermal conductivities, and brittleness. In theory, carbon should be an ideal dental implant biomaterial, both as a structural material and as a coating; however, this substance cannot be connected to stainless steel in saline environments without the possibility of introducing electrochemical breakdown of the stainless steel. Carbon manufacturing and surface coating are technologically dependent, and high-quality products require precise controls.

The general group of ceramics and carbons is different from metallic biomaterials in physical, mechanical, chemical, and electrical properties. Inertness, conductivity, modulus of elasticity, brittleness, and surface reactions for bonding are notable differences. Properties should be carefully evaluated for each endosseous implant system. This is especially critical with regard to handling and sterilization. While metallic biomaterials can be sterilized by most available techniques, the ceramics must normally be processed by dry heat. Extreme care should be taken in sterilization because of well-recognized limitations and possible changes in the basic material and its related biocompatibility.[14]

Polymers and Composites

A wide range of polymeric biomaterials used for other surgical and medical devices have been investigated for use as dental implants and as surface coatings (Table 4–3). In general, these polymers have not found extensive use as major structural components of dental implants owing to their relatively low strengths and high ductilities. Some surface coatings and abutment post applications continue. Primary concerns have been low creep (cold flow) resistances under cyclic loading conditions. Considering the theoretical opportunities afforded by new composite systems, the biomaterials community anticipates an expanding utilization of composites fabricated to suit selected implant requirements. Most notable are the possible cost reductions and the ability to introduce anisotropic properties that are designed to meet the basic recommendations from biomechanical analyses.

Basic and Applied Research

Metallic, ceramic, and polymeric biomaterials provide a wide range of properties for device applications with biomaterials now being designed and manufactured to meet specific property require-

TABLE 4–3.

Polymeric Biomaterials and Composites for Endosseous Dental Implants

Biomaterial	Standard
Ultra-high-molecular-weight polyethylene (UHMW-PE)	F-639, 648
Polyethylene terapthylate (Dacron)	—
Polytetrafluoroethylene (PTFE)	F-754
Polymethylmethacrylate (PMMA)	F-451, 500
Dimethylpolysiloxane (silicone rubber)	F-604
Polysulfone (PS)	F-702
Thermoset epoxy	F-602
Thermoplastic polyurethane	F-624
Polycarbonate resin	F-997
Fiber-reinforced polymers	
Dacron-silicone rubber	—
Carbon-PTFE (Proplast)	—
Alumina-PTFE	—
Polysulfone on alloys	
Carbon-PMMA	—

ments. In former years, metallic and ceramic systems were used because they were available; however, their primary use was other than as a biomaterial. Basic and applied research in both biomaterials and biomechanics should lead to improved surgically implanted devices.[15]

BIOMECHANICS

Physiologic Loads and Force Transfer

An endosteal dental implant serves to accept the physiologic loads or forces imposed on it and subsequently to distribute those forces into the surrounding tissues. The resultant force-per-unit area in the tissues is referred to as stress. Bone is known to remodel in response to applied stress[16]; therefore, the manner in which endosteal implants distribute stress in interfacial tissues is of paramount importance when the stability of the tissue-to-implant interface is considered.

Forces imposed on dental implants may be described by magnitude, direction, mode of loading (static, cyclic, or intermittent), and duration. The range of human bite force capability is quite broad and very dependent on the state of dentition in an individual. The maximum bite force has been shown to decrease with increasing age and the loss of natural teeth.[17] The detailed prosthodontic restorative treatment applied to a dental implant also may alter the character of the load imposed on the device.

Design of a dental implant must accommodate physiologic loads which do not result in failure of the implant or of the surrounding biological tissues. Excessively high, localized stresses that exceed the implant material's yield strength may result in permanent deformation and possible failure. Clinical experience has shown that bone undergoes disuse atrophy in response to excessively low stress levels in the tissue, as well as overuse atrophy as a consequence of excessively high stresses. Quantification of "Wolff's Window," the window of tissue stress levels indicative of physiologic health, has not been definitively described in the published literature and multiple bone-remodeling theories have been proposed.[18]

Many investigators have reported maximal bite strengths in individuals with natural dentition[17, 19–22] in the approximate ranges of 98 to 716 N in the molar region and 9.8 to 431.2 N in the incisor region. Bite force data on patients with reconstructed dental implant systems are relatively scarce and usually refer to only one osteointegrated implant device.[23] The load that is applied to the bridge is not, however, necessarily the load which the implant experiences. Investigations have developed hard-wiring and telemetry methods to measure axial (vertical) components of physiologic forces actually experienced by a dental implant in a dog mandible.[24] Such studies provide more precise load data for use in implant analyses and should be expanded to include various dental implant designs.

Biomaterial and Biological Properties

Mechanical properties of many of the currently available biomaterials used in dental implants are listed in Table 4–4, and those of the human musculoskeletal system are provided in Table 4–5. Trabecular bone, into which endosteal implants are placed, may be described as a structure of variable density and structural rigidity based on the quantity and distribution of the trabeculae within the region.[25] The results of some studies suggest that the microstructural material properties of trabecular and cortical bone are quite similar.[26–28] These findings have led to the development of an empirically derived power relation whereby the compressive strength and modulus of elasticity of trabecular bone are expressed as power functions of the specimen density.[29] Thus, the mechanical properties of any density of trabecular bone may be approximated based on knowledge of the trabecular density and of the mechanical properties of compact (cortical) bone.

When dental implants are designed properly, the mechanical properties of commonly used biomaterials are generally adequate to withstand physiologic loads without failure of the implant; however, the design must necessarily consider both material composition and implant geometry.

Implant Design and Function

Endosteal dental implant designs may be generally categorized as blade or root form. Blade form

TABLE 4–4.
Mechanical Properties of Selected Surgical Implant Biomaterials

Property		Ti (Wrought)	Ti-Al-V (Wrought)	Co-Cr-Mo (Cast)	Co Alloy (Wrought)		Fe-Cr-Ni (316L)		C-Si	Sapphire	Al₂O₃ Alumina	UHMW Polyethylene	PMMA	PTFE
					Annealed	Cold Worked	Annealed	Cold Worked						
Density (g/cc)		4.5	—	8.3	9.2	9.2	7.9	7.9	1.5–2.0	3.99	3.9	0.94	1.2	2.2
Hardness (Vickers)		R$_b$100	—	300	240	450	170–200	300–350	—	—	HV23,000	D65	M60–100	D50–65
Yield strength														
MPa		170–485	795–827	490	450	1050	240–300	700–800						
(ksi)		(25–70)	(115–120)	(71)	(62)	(152)	(35–44)	(102–116)						
Ultimate tensile strength														
MPa		240–550	860–896	690	950	1540	600–700	1000	350–517	480	400	21–44	55–85	14–34
(ksi)		(35–80)	(125–130)	(100)	(138)	(223)	(87–102)	(145)	(51–75)	(70)	(58)	(3.0–6.4)	(8.0–12.3)	(2–5)
Elastic modulus														
GPa		96	105–117	200	230	230	200	200	28–34	414	380	1	2.4–3.3	0.4
(ksi × 10³)		(14)	(15–17)	(29)	(34)	(34)	(29)	(29)	(4.0–4.9)	(60)	(55.1)	(0.145)	(0.348–0.479)	(0.058)
Endurance limit (fatigue)														
MPa		—	170–240	300	—	240–490	300	230–280						
(ksi × 10³)			(24.6–35)	(43)		(35–71)	(43)	(33.3–40.6)						
Elongation (%)		15–24	10–15	8	30–45	9	35–55	7–22	0	0	0	400	2–7	200–400

TABLE 4–5.

Mechanical Properties of Selected Tissues

	Tissue						
Property	Cortical Bone	Dentin	Enamel	Ligament	Hyaline Cartilage	Collagen	Elastin
Ultimate tensile strength							
MPa	140	40	70	0.03	0.03	0.56	0.01
(ksi)	(20.3)	(5.8)	(10.2)	(0.004)	(0.004)	(0.081)	(0.001)
Compressive strength							
MPa	130	145	260	—	—	—	—
(ksi)	(18.9)	(21)	(37.7)				
Modulus of elasticity							
GPa	18	14	50	—	—	0.14	0.61
(ksi $\times 10^3$)	(3)	(2)	(7.25)			(0.02)	(0.09)
Elongation (%)	1	0	0	5–160	1.8	—	—

implants are typically narrow in the buccal-to-lingual dimension and elongated in the distal-to-mesial dimension, whereas root form implants are generally cylindrical. Both implant types have experienced wide clinical use with multiple variations currently available in each category.

The neck design in either implant system is particularly important in the consideration of implant geometry because the physiologic load is transmitted through the neck region to the implant body and the surrounding tissues. As the cross-sectional area of the neck decreases, the stress levels in the neck and surrounding tissues increase (recall: stress = force/area). Such highly localized peak stresses may lead to tissue necrosis or "cratering" in the zone immediately adjacent to the implant neck. One clinical advantage for the implant neck characterized by a reduced cross-sectional area is that the implant head and neck may be deformed or bent to achieve parallelism during prosthodontic reconstruction. Some implant designs have attempted to take advantage of the favorable stress distribution that a larger neck cross-sectional area can produce and still maintain the ability to achieve parallelism through special design modifications. While it is obvious that a dental implant must be restored prosthodontically to achieve the function for which it was designed, the current state of knowledge cannot substantiate the use of one particular method for achieving parallelism over any other.

The implant body must exhibit a macrogeometry suitable for acceptable levels of force transfer to the surrounding tissues as well as for implantation into a bony site of a particular anatomic size. Cylindrical implant geometry has been shown to produce a favorable stress distribution[30]; however, such a design imposes size constraints on the geometry of the implantation site. Blade implants are designed to serve in those bony sites which are too narrow to accommodate root form implants. Whereas the body of blade form implants generally demonstrates a significantly reduced cross-sectional area available to resist axial loads as compared to the root forms, clinical success in excess of 15 years has been documented for these devices.[31] Due to anatomic variability in the dental implant patient population, the use of a single design for all clinical cases encountered does not seem justifiable. Biomechanical studies which evaluate the effect of bone macrogeometry on the stress profiles around different implant geometries are not available in the published literature. Such investigations are necessary to evaluate the biomechanical efficacy of using a root form vs. a blade form implant in a given anatomic site.

Perforations or "vents" in the body of an endosteal dental implant provide a means for bone ingrowth into the device with resultant stabilization of the implant within the tissues. In blade form implants, vents also serve to increase the amount of cross-sectional area available to resist axial loads. No published work is available that provides detailed explanations of the effect of vent design or distribution on the biomechanical performance of dental implants.

Clinical Experience and Biomechanics Research

A multitude of endosteal dental implant devices have been designed and utilized in the patient population. Most of these devices have been designed based on "physical intuition" with respect to the suitability of the implant for a specific clinical case, rather than on rigorous, engineering design criteria.

As advancements have been made in the field of implant dentistry, the long-term success of any dental implant has been recognized as dependent upon the tissue-to-implant interface in situ. The tissue type and stability of such an interface may be due to such parameters as the type and duration of loading, the macrodesign of the implant and any suprastructure devices, the biomechanical and biocompatibility characteristics of the implant biomaterial, and the clinical protocols and techniques utilized in placement and intraoral restoration. A paucity of information exists in the published literature on these and other biomechanical variables.

IMPLANT-TO-TISSUE INTERFACES

Biomaterial and Surface Conditions

Bulk and surface properties of synthetic biomaterials for dental endosteal implants have been continually improving and the concept of mechanically and chemically clean implants has now become a reality for most systems. Tissue interface stability is the final test for these conditions and biomaterials can directly influence the nature of the biological interface. The 316L alloy of surgical stainless steel has shown an adjacent fibrous tissue, while titanium and titanium alloy interfaces have demonstrated a direct association with bone at the optical microscopy evaluation level.[32] This characteristic is dependent upon the surface oxide and the relative chemical analysis of the surface, assuming acceptable force transfer conditions.

The same type of direct bone interface has also been demonstrated for ceramics, carbons, and selected polymers.[33] The basic nature of the contiguous interface and whether the material surfaces have some type of chemical bond is an area of continuing research. On a relative scale, the interfacial bonding seems to be greater in magnitude for Bioglass and hydroxylapatite surfaces, of lower strength for titanium and titanium alloy, and minimal to nonexistent for carbon, aluminum oxide, and most polymers. These considerations are summarized in Table 4–6, which presents the surface, the nature of the surface-to-tissue interaction, whether active or passive, and opinions of whether a bond does or does not exist between the biomaterial and bone.

The various biomaterials can be separated with respect to their interface characteristics with bone. These characteristics directly influence designing, manufacturing, handling, sterilizing, and placing endosteal implants. Since no emphasis has been placed in this chapter on the periodontal soft tissue regions and the biomaterial and biomechancial influences, general summary statements are provided.

Metals and alloys do not appear to offer soft tissue-to-oxide bond strengths of significant magnitudes. Direct contact and some surface interactions have been reported, but most devices have been shown to function through a relatively tight "cuff" region at the implant neck. For this reason, most metallic biomaterials are prepared with a polished surface and with the final polishing marks oriented circumferentially around the neck region. This surface feature is proposed to influence adjacent tissue development and maturation.[34, 35]

Ceramics have been extensively studied along the peri-implant interface with reports of "Sharpies-like" fibers attaching to hydroxylapatite regions. These results need to be confirmed and extended to human retrievals. Smooth surface conditions on aluminum oxide and hydroxylapatite appear to be favorable to soft tissue adaptation.

Polymeric biomaterials in porous and solid conditions have been investigated as a means to stabilize the soft tissue-to-implant interface. Although certainly an excellent idea from a theoretical biomechanical standpoint, no system has been developed for routine clinical use.

Probably one of the critical considerations of

TABLE 4–6.

Biomaterial Summary of Surface and Interface Properties

Biomaterial*	Surface	Active (A) or Passive (P)	Bonded (B) or Not (N) to Bone
Metals			
Fe-Cr-Ni	Cr_xO_y	P	N
Ti and Ti-6Al-4V	TiO_2	A-P	B
Co alloys	Cr_xO_y	P	N
Ceramics and carbons			
Al_2O_3	Al_2O_3	P	N
HA	$Ca_{10}(PO_4)_6(OH)_2$	A	B
TCP and ALCAP	$Ca-PO_4$	A	B
Bioglass or Ceravital	$Ca-PO_4$	A	B
C and C-Si	C or C-Si	P	N
Polymers and composites			
PE	Polymer	P	N
Dacron	Polymer	P	N
PTFE	Polymer	P	N
PMMA	Polymer	P	N
Silicone rubber	Polymer	P	N
PS	Polymer	P	N
Composites	Polymer	P	N

*HA = hydroxylapatite; TCP = tricalcium phosphate; ALCAP = calcium aluminate; PE = polyethylene; PTFE = polytetrafluroethylene; PMMA = polymethylmethacrylate; PS = polysulfone.

implant maintenance is oral hygiene and the ability to clean at the sulcus site. Rough material surfaces are difficult to maintain adequately. Another factor is the position of the subjacent bone and the presence or absence of attached gingiva. Both are influenced by the specific biomaterial and design used for the device.

Chemical and Biochemical Interactions

Consideration of the relationships between the chemical properties of the synthetic biomaterial and the tissue biochemical characteristics is important. Bone and soft tissues have very different properties with respect to structure, rates of reaction, and reaction types.[36, 37] The basic biochemical reactions of tissues are quite different and a single biomaterial surface chemistry should not be expected to optimize tissue interactions. In this regard, the introduction of new polymer-metal, ceramic, ceramic-metal, or polymer-ceramic-metal composites should provide significant advantages for future devices.

Biomechanical Considerations

Two distinctly different interfacial morphologies have been observed in functioning endosteal dental implants: a fibrous tissue-to-implant interface and a direct bone-to-implant interface with a minimal interpositioned fibrous tissue layer. Proponents of the fibrous tissue-to-implant interface argue that such a "peri-implant" zone most closely simulates the natural tooth–periodontal ligament system and is advantageous to implant function by providing a shock absorber capability. Proponents of the bone-to-implant interface argue that long-term stability may only be achieved with direct bone contact without the possibility of an ever-widening fibrous tissue membrane sometimes seen in failed implant systems.

Studies have shown that stress distribution through surrounding interfacial tissues and displacement profiles exhibited by the implant relative to interfacial tissues directly influence the formation of a specific interfacial morphology. A literature base has been developed by a Swedish group on the characterization of direct bone-to-implant interface for titanium dental implants.[38] After leaving implants externally unloaded for over 3 months, the group reported bone to be firmly adherent to the titanium implants. Very little information exists in the scientific literature to describe the precise nature and mechanical behavior of a fibrous tissue-to-implant interface. Some studies have suggested that excessive relative motion between the implant and surrounding tissues may elicit a fibrous tissue-to-implant interface.[39]

Investigators have performed finite element analyses on blade and root form dental implants.[40-44] A soft tissue, interpositional membrane (compared to direct bone-to-implant attachment) was demonstrated to significantly reduce the stress levels in the alveolar bone surrounding the implant. The precise clinical ramifications, if any, are at present unclear.

SUMMARY AND CONCLUSIONS

Biomaterial and biomechanical properties have been shown to directly influence tissue responses and thereby the clinical longevities of dental implant restorative procedures. This chapter has provided an overview of basic biomaterial and biomechanical characteristics for existing dental implant devices and the properties of these devices have been extended to implant-to-tissue interfaces with opinions about optimal combinations of conditions.

A wide range of biomaterials and designs are in current clinical use within implant-dependent restorative treatments. A chemically and mechanically clean implant condition is fundamental to the desired tissue response for each biomaterial selected. Control of force transfer through implant and restorative crown and bridge design, geometry, and material composition is equally fundamental to long-term tissue stabilities. These basic concepts related to materials and mechanics should always be applied to treatments utilizing surgical implants because a blend of clinical experience and engineering analysis is required for device longevity. The study of dental biomaterials and biomechanics must be pursued aggressively in the basic and applied science laboratories and transferred to the clinical realm to enhance future developments in the field of implant dentistry.

REFERENCES

1. Williams DF (ed): *Biocompatibility of Clinical Implant Materials,* vol 1. Boca Raton, Fla, CRC Press, 1981.
2. Smith DC, Williams DF (eds): *Biocompatibility of Dental Materials,* vol 4. Boca Raton, Fla, CRC Press, 1982.
3. McKinney RV Jr, Lemons JE (eds): *The Dental Implant.* Littleton, Mass, PSG Publishing Co Inc, 1985.
4. Cranin AN (ed): *Oral Implantology.* Springfield, Ill, Charles C Thomas, Publisher, 1970.
5. Schnitman PA, Schulman LB (eds): *Dental Implants: Benefit and Risk—Proceedings of an NIH-Harvard Consensus Development Conference.* Bethesda, Md, US DHHS publication No. 81-1531, 1980.
6. English CA: Cylindrical implants. *Calif Dent J* 1988; (Jan):17-38.
7. Lemons JE: Dental implant research. *Calif Dent J* 1987; (Oct):27-35.
8. *Medical Devices. ASTM Standards, 13.01.* Philadelphia, American Society for Testing and Materials, 1987.
9. Lemons JE: Surface conditions for surgical implants biocompatibility. *J Oral Implantol* 1977; 7:362-374.
10. Lemons JE: General characteristics and classifications of implant materials, in Lin O, Chao E (eds): *Perspectives in Biomaterials.* Amsterdam, Elsevier, 1986, pp 1-15.
11. Ricci JL, Berkman A, Bajpai PK, et al: Development of a fast-setting ceramic-based grout material for filling bone defects. *Soc Biomater Trans* 1986; 9:132.
12. Hench LL, Ethridge EC (eds): *Biomaterials,* vol 4. New York, Academic Press, 1982.
13. Meffert RM, Block MS, Kent JN: What is osseointegration. *Int J Periodont Restor Dent* 1987; 4:9-23.
14. Lemons JE: Surface evaluations of materials. *J Oral Implantol* 1986; 12:396-406.
15. Ducheyne P, Lemons JE (eds): *Bioceramics: Material Characteristics Versus In Vivo Behavior,* vol 523. New York, Academy of Science, 1988.
16. Wolff J: *Pas Destez der Transformation der Knochen.* Berlin, Hirschwald, 1892.
17. Helkimo E, Carsson GE, Helkimo M: Bite force and state of dentition. *Acta Odontol Scand* 1977; 35:297-303.
18. Huiskes R, Weinans H, Grootenboer HJ, et al: Adaptive bone-remodeling theory applied to prosthetic-design analysis. *J Biomech* 1987; 20:1135-1150.
19. Gibbs CH, Mahan PE, Mauderli A, et al: Limits of

human bite force. *J Prosthet Dent* 1986; 56:226–229.

20. Mansour RM, Reynik RJ: In vivo occlusal forces and moments, I: Forces measured in terminal hinge position and associated moments. *J Dent Res* 1975; 54:114–120.

21. Mansour RM, Reynik RJ: In vivo occlusal forces and moments, II: Mathematical analysis and recommendations for instrumentation specifications. *J Dent Res* 1975; 54:121–124.

22. Pruim GJ: Asymmetries of bilateral static bite forces in different locations on the human mandible. *J Dent Res* 1979; 58:1685–1687.

23. Haraldson T, Carlsson GE, Ingervall B: Functional state, bite force and postural muscle activity in patients with osseointegrated oral implant bridges. *Acta Odontol Scand* 1979; 37:195–206.

24. Brunski JB, Hipp JA: In vivo forces on dental implants: Hard wiring and telemetry methods. *J Biomech* 1984; 17:855–860.

25. Galante J, Rostoker W, Ray RD: Physical properties of trabecular bone. *Calcif Tissue Res* 1970; 5:236–246.

26. Martin RB: The effects of geometric feedback in the development of osteoporosis. *J Biomech* 1972; 5:447–455.

27. Pugh JW, Rose RM, Radin EL: Elastic and viscoelastic properties of trabecular bone: Dependence on structure. *J Biomech* 1973; 6:475–485.

28. Townsend PR, Rose RM, Radin EL: Buckling studies of single human trabeculae. *J Biomech* 1975; 8:199–201.

29. Carter DR, Hayes WC: The compressive behavior of bone as a two-phase porous structure. *J Bone Surg* 1977; 59A:954–962.

30. Atmaram GH, Mohammed H, Schoen FT: Stress analysis of single-tooth implants I. Effect of elastic parameters and geometry of implant. *Biomater Med Devices Artif Organs* 1979; 7:99–104.

31. Kapur K, Deupree R, Frechette A, et al: VA cooperative study on dental implants, part 4 (abstract 55, IADR). *J Dent Res* 1987; 66(special issue):113.

32. Albrektsson T: The response of bone to titanium implants. *Crit Rev Biocompatibility* 1985; 1:53–84.

33. Baier RE: Surface preparation. *J Oral Implantol* 1986; 12:389–396.

34. Ten Cate AR: *The Gingival Junction, Tissue Integrated Prostheses*. Chicago, Quintessence, 1985, pp 145–155.

35. Lemons JE, Natiella JR: Biomaterials, biocompatibility and peri-implant considerations. *Dent Clin North Am* 1986; 30:3–23.

36. Lucas LC, Bearden LF, Lemons JE: Ultrastructural examinations of in vitro and in vivo cells exposed to solutions of 316L stainless steel, in Fraker A, Griffin C (eds): *ASTM STP 859*. Philadelphia, American Society for Testing and Materials, 1985, pp 208–221.

37. Macon N, Lucas L, Lemons J, et al: Tissue response to Ti-6Al-4V/Co-Cr-Mo implants. *Biomed Eng* 1985; 4:11–18.

38. Hansson HA, Albrektsson T, Brånemark PI: Structural aspects of the interface between tissue and titanium implants. *J Prosthet Dent* 1983; 50:108–112.

39. Brunski JB, Moccia A, Pollack SR, et al: The influence of functional use of endosseous dental implants on the tissue-implant interface. I. Histological aspects. *J Dent Res* 1979; 58:1953–1969.

40. Privitzer E, Widera GE, Tesk JA: Some factors affecting dental implant design. *J Biomed Mater Res Symp* 1975; 6:251–255.

41. Buch JD, Crose JG, Bechtol CO: Biomechanical and biomaterial considerations of natural teeth, tooth replacements, and skeletal fixation. *Biomater Med Devices Artif Organs* 1974; 2:171–186.

42. Widera GE, Tesk JA, Privitzer, E: Interaction effects among cortical bone, cancellous bone, and periodontal membrane of natural teeth and implants. *J Biomed Mater Res Symp* 1976; 7:613–623.

43. Cook SD, Weinstein AM, Klawitter JJ: Parameters affecting the stress distribution around LTI carbon and aluminum oxide dental implants. *J Biomed Mater Res* 1982; 16:875–885.

44. Bidez MW: *Stress Distributions Within Endosseous Blade Implant Systems as a Function of Interfacial Boundary Conditions* (dissertation). University of Alabama at Birmingham, 1987.

Chapter 5

The Biological Tissue Response to Dental Implants

Ralph V. McKinney, Jr., D.D.S., Ph.D.
David E. Steflik, M.A., Ed.D.
David L. Koth, D.D.S., M.S.

Dental implantology is a unique field of specialization because it involves the bringing together for treatment the skills of the dental practitioner, the use of inert materials in the human body, the physiologic and masticatory operation of the jaws, and the theoretical design and physical parameter applications of biomaterialists and engineers. Although dentists as a profession are routinely using inert materials for the restoration of teeth, the tooth is a fully developed hard tissue structure that is not going to change or degenerate during interface with restorative materials. The most that occurs in tooth restoration is that the vital pulp dies, and even this can be treated by use of inert materials, i.e., filling the pulp chamber with an endodontic material(s).

The closest speciality area in the dental-medical field that approaches oral implantology is implant use by orthopedists. But important differences exist between implant orthopedics and implant dentistry as is discussed in the section on the biological seal.

THE SPHERE OF BODY-IMPLANT INTERACTIONS

The overall realm of body-implant reactions can be divided into four major areas we call the *four B's of implantology:* biomaterials, biomechanics, biolog-

ical tissues, and body serviceability (Fig 5–1). The spheres of influence reflect the various areas of basic and clinical science that together contribute to the successful longitudinal service of dental implants in the restoration of normal human physiologic function.

Biomaterials is the scientific study of materials that are compatible with living tissues. The physical properties of materials, their potential to corrode in the tissue environment, their surface configuration, tissue induction or lack thereof, and their potential for eliciting inflammation or a "rejection response" are all important factors in this area. Also important are the practical guidelines for handling of the biomaterials by the dentist.

Biomechanics is the scientific study of the load-force relationships of a biomaterial in the oral cavity. Biomechanical questions quickly become apparent when we ask: Can the implant support the projected prosthesis? What is the stress distribution to the jaws? Will bone resorb under adverse stress? These are all scientific questions requiring a scientific basis for successful implantology.

Biological tissues concerns the reaction and response of living cells and tissues to the implanted biomaterial and its supposed prosthesis. Especially important is the healing of these tissues following implant surgery and the long-term results of their in-

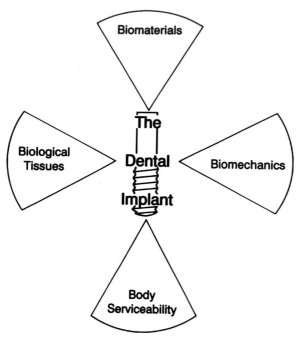

FIG 5–1.
The four B's of dental implantalogy: the spectrum of clinical and basic science knowledge needed that cumulatively contributes to the successful serviceability of dental implants in the treatment of human oral disease and restoration of physiologic function.

timate biomaterial relationship. Comparison studies are a must in this area.

Body serviceability stresses the need for scientifically designed longitudinal clinical implant trials with quantifiable, easily measured evaluation parameters that can be carried out by the dental practitioner.

Dentists have their own basis for implant serviceability. What the practitioner wants to know is: Are the selected implants safe to use? How does this particular implant function biologically and is it successful? How can I select the correct implant to match the patient with certain diagnostic situations? How can I predict the long-term outcome for the implant I have selected? What type of prosthetic technique and design should I utilize for a specific implant? And what type of hygiene maintenance program do I use to maintain these implants for maximum longevity? All these practitioner-oriented

questions must be answered by biological experimentation and adequately controlled clinical trials.

PURPOSE

This chapter reviews and presents theoretical concepts as well as state-of-the-art scientific knowledge as to how the human body and its tissues respond to the invasion of endosteal dental implants. The primary focus will be on the last two implant B's: biological tissues and body serviceability (see Fig 5–1).

BIOLOGICAL TISSUE RESPONSE TO DENTAL IMPLANTS

Data for this section on biological tissue response come primarily from tissue interface scientific studies conducted in the Department of Oral Pathology at the Medical College of Georgia (MCG). Where other scientific work is discussed, appropriate reference citations are given. The MCG studies involved the use of mongrel dogs and the placement of one-stage endosteal dental implants composed of polymethyl methacrylate, cobalt-chromium-molybdenum alloy, single- and polycrystalline aluminum oxide ceramics, and commercially pure (cp) titanium. The implants supported fixed prostheses or were left freestanding in the oral cavity. For investigative methodology concerning animal handling, and surgical, prosthetic, specimen preparation, and microscopic protocols, the reader is referred to selected references.[1–10] During the animal protocols, information was also collected and validated concerning clinical evaluation indices applicable to dental implants (see Chap 29 for more on this subject).

Peri-implant Gingival Response

Of great interest is the peri-implant gingival response, which forms the biological seal between tissue and implant. Figure 5–2 is a scanning electron micrograph of a titanium dental implant in situ in the

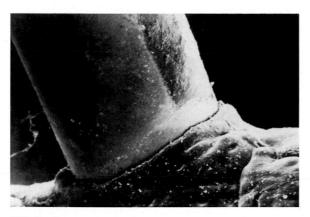

FIG 5–2.
Scanning electron micrograph of a titanium one-stage endosseous dental implant in a dog mandible. Note the regenerated attached gingiva around the implant transmucosal post and the formation of a free gingival margin. Plaque can be seen on the implant post that was not visible clinically.

jaw bone of a dog. From this micrograph it is evident that the attached gingiva has regenerated around the implant after surgery and a new free gingival margin has developed around the implant device.

Regeneration of the attached gingival tissues occurs around the implant post and provides a protective barrier between the oral cavity and the internal jaw environment.

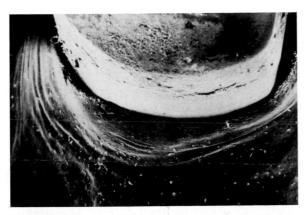

FIG 5–3.
Higher-resolution scanning electron micrograph showing the anatomic structures of the gingival sulcus and free gingival margin which have formed around an implant transmucosal post. The implant was placed in an edentulous section of the jaw.

Oral surgery procedures disrupt the gingival epithelium, both the attached gingiva and the alveolar mucosa, when a flap is used to create the soft tissue opening to bone. The surgically traumatized gingiva heals around the implant transmucosal post, as well as reattaches to bone, and during healing a new anatomically free gingival margin complete with gingival sulcus and free gingival groove is formed. Scanning electron microscopy verifies that the regenerated epithelium has reestablished a stratified squamous epithelial layer and a re-formation of the gingival sulcus (Fig 5–3). The genetic control factors initiating reestab-

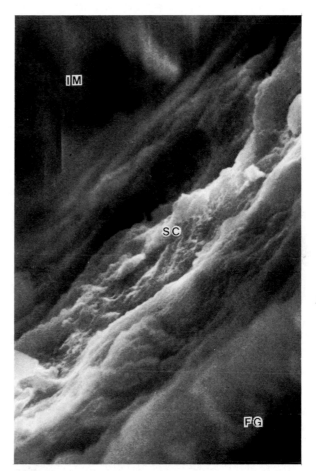

FIG 5–4.
Close examination of the interior of the regenerated gingival epithelium visualizes the surface of the nonkeratinized gingival sulcus cells *(SC)*. The implant surface is indicated at *IM* and the crest of the free gingival margin is *FG*.

lishment of these anatomic structures are unknown, but obviously must reside in the gingival tissues of the oral cavity, since reestablishing a gingival margin occurs in a previously edentulous jaw area.

Using the resolving power of the scanning electron microscope, one can look into the gingival sulcus and see the reestablished sulcular epithelium composed of individual epithelial cells (Fig 5–4). These epithelial cells forming the sulcus are in contact with the implant face at the bottom of the new gingival sulcus; actually, pseudopodia (fingerlike projections) extending from the cells contact the implant face.[6, 7] This reaction and repair around the implant by the gingival cells is very similar to what happens around a natural tooth following periodontal surgery.[11]

The nature of the epithelial cell zone of contact on the implant can be studied by high-resolution transmission electron microscopy.[9, 10] Figure 5–5 is a transmission electron micrograph of the cells found along the implant-crevicular epithelial front. These cells demonstrate the characteristics of junctional epithelial cells with organelles, tonofilaments, vesicles containing dark material, and hemidesmosomes on the fingerlike projections emanating from the cell that is in contact with the implant.

The presence of epithelial hemidesmosomes on gingival cells in contact with implant biomaterial

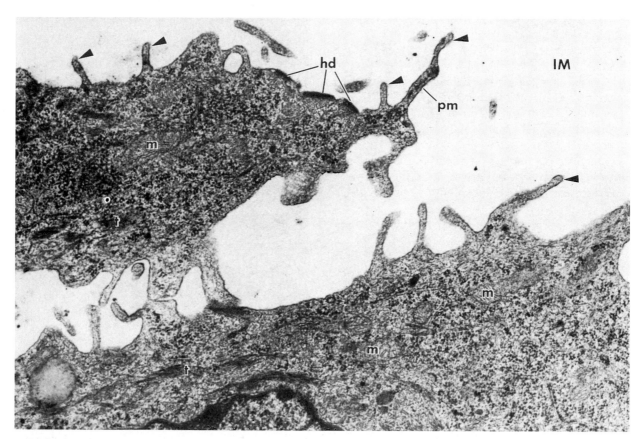

FIG 5–5.
Transmission electron micrograph showing the close-up detail of the gingival epithelial cells at the bottom of the sulcus that contact the implant face. Identified are the cell membrane *(pm)*, mitochondria *(m)*, tonofilaments *(t)*, hemidesmosomes *(hd)*, and fingerlike projections arising from the cells *(arrowheads)*. The implant, which occupied the space at *IM*, was removed prior to final tissue sectioning.

faces was initially described by Listgarten and Lai[12] and by Swope and James.[13] Formation of these epithelial attachment plaques has also been described by investigators using explants of gingival epithelial cells growing on biomaterials in vitro.[14] Obviously, it appears that this organelle is a very necessary component of the attachment phenomenon for epithelial cells to biomaterials.

In our laboratories, we have been able to achieve a complete ultrastructure picture of the implant-tissue contact by junctional epithelial cells utilizing a cryofracture technique (Figs 5–6 and 5–7). Combining cryofracture with a standard electron microscopic protocol, we have been able to observe the entire basal lamina structure against the epithelial plasma membrane.[9, 10, 15] Although the revelation of these interface structures is exciting to the dental scientist, it can look just like a series of black and white lines to the clinical dentist (see Figs 5–6 and 5–7). Thus, to present the concept of structure organization, we have created a diagram portraying the fine structure of the attachment zone (Fig 5–8). When the actual electron micrographs (see Figs 5–6 and 5–7) are compared with the diagram (see Fig 5–8), one can observe the gingival plasma membrane with the hemidesmosome structure and substructure, the component layers of the basal lamina, and the glycocalyx or linear body on the implant face. Comments on how these structures interact with one another are found later in this chapter.

Peri-implant Bone Response

Using in situ block jaw specimens containing implants and employing a laborious technique of plastic embedding, sectioning, and polishing,[4] we have been able to produce thin microscopic sections. Figure 5–9 is a study of the bone adjacent to a ceramic implant in the jaw. Figure 5–10 is from a jaw containing a titanium implant showing bone adaptation. Under higher magnification, mature cortical bone shows the presence of osteon units and the direct interface of bone with the implant face (Fig 5–11).

The regenerative capability of bone is tremendous. Bone regenerates around the ridges and grooves of screw-type implants, into the pores of porous root implants, and through the pores of blades and hollow cylinder–type implants (Fig 5–12). Bone is readily compatible with many dental biomaterials including polymethyl methacrylate, stainless steel, and Vitallium, as well as titanium and ceramic materials.[1, 2, 16]

When bone is in direct apposition to an implant, the phenomenon is often referred to as "osseointegration," or "osteointegration" in current implant ter-

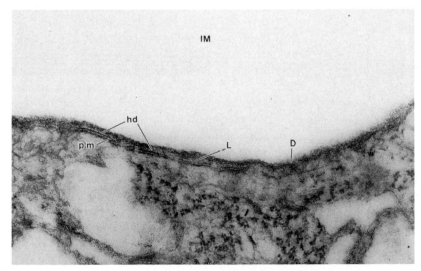

FIG 5–6.
A cryofracture-prepared transmission electron micrograph of an epithelial cell against an implant *(IM)* showing the plasma membrane *(pm)* with hemidesmosomes *(hd)* and the lucent *(L)* and dense *(D)* layers of the basal lamina. Original magnification ×108,200.

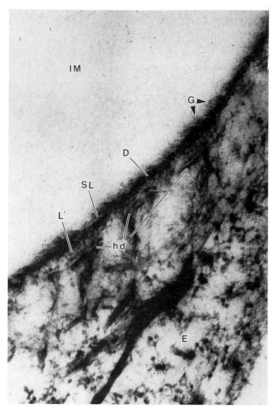

FIG 5–7.
A cryofracture electron micrograph specimen revealing the plasma membrane edge of the gingival epithelial cell *(E)* with hemidesmosomes *(hd)* and the lamina lucida *(L)*, lamina densa *(D)*, and sublamina lucida *(SL)* layers of the basal lamina. The outer layer, which interfaced the implant *(IM)*, reveals some remnants of the glycocalyx *(G)*. Original magnification × 108,200.

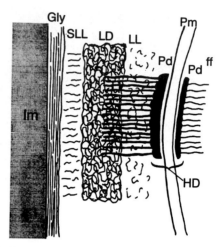

FIG 5–8.
Diagram demonstrating the anatomic structures that form the attachment mechanism between the regenerated junctional epithelium and the implant face. This diagram is oriented to show the epithelial plasma membrane *(Pm)* containing the hemidesmosome *(HD)* with its component parts, the peripheral densities *(Pd)* and fine filaments *(ff)*, that extend into the cytoplasm and the basal lamina. The components of the basal lamina are the lamina lucida *(LL)*, lamina densa *(LD)*, and sublamina lucida *(SLL)*, which contains chains *(wavy lines)* of fibronectin. *Gly* is the glycocalyx, also called the linear body, and is found on the implant face *(IM)*.

minology.[17] Other terms utilized are "rigid support" and "ankylosis," but from a pathologist's viewpoint, this is not ankylosis since the bone is not actually fused to the biomaterial, although proponents of bioactive surface materials might disagree.[18] A much better term would be "direct bone interface," which describes the actual morphologic condition. *Osseointegration* was coined by the Swedish research teams and refers to light microscopic evidence of direct bone implant contact,[19] but is by no means limited to titanium two-stage implants. A direct bone interface or contact can be observed with ceramic, other metal, and one-stage implants.[20]

In addition to a cortical bone interface, trabecu-lar (cancellous) bone also directly contacts implant surfaces (Fig 5–13). The interior of the maxilla or mandible is composed of trabecular bone and so the only place cortical bone is in continuity with the implant passage is at the outer jaw surfaces such as the crest of the ridge. Sections through bone and teeth will reveal a similar bone (cortical or trabecular) relationship to the tooth. In the mandible the apex of the implant radicular portion may extend into the inferior alveolar canal or fibrofatty marrow space.

Radiographically, a cortical bone interface appears as a unified structure around the radicular aspect of an implant device. Figure 5–14 is a radiograph of titanium cylindrical root form implants supporting a fixed prosthesis. This radiograph would warrant the clinical interpretation of "direct bone interface" or "osseointegration." However, we are viewing in two dimensions a three-dimensional object, the jaw and implant, and though radiographically it appears the implant is surrounded totally by cortical bone, in reality this is not the case. A bucco-

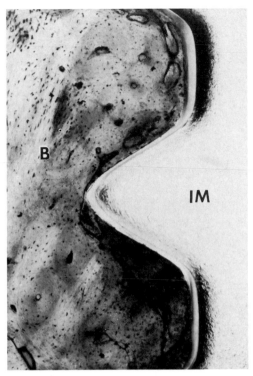

FIG 5–9.
Light photomicrograph demonstrating direct bone *(B)* interface against the radicular portion of a ceramic screw-type endosteal implant *(IM)*.

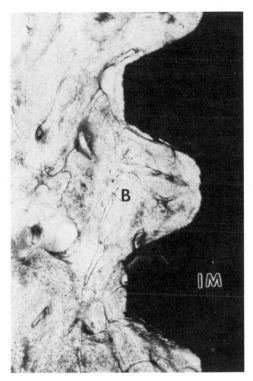

FIG 5–10.
Light photomicrograph demonstrating direct bone *(B)* interface against the radicular portion of a cp titanium one-stage screw-type implant *(IM)*.

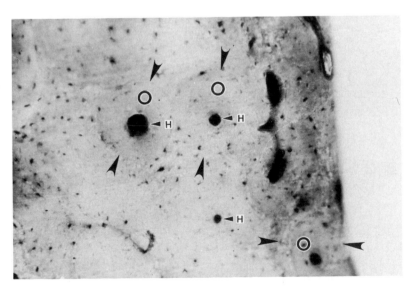

FIG 5–11.
Bone interfacing a ceramic endosseous implant and demonstrating prominent osteon units *(O, between arrows)* and haversian canals *(H)*, hallmarks of normal cortical bone.

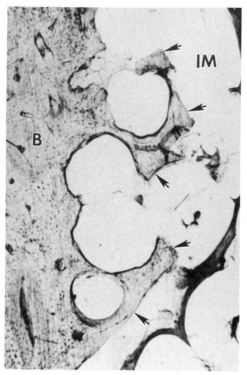

FIG 5–12.
The remarkable regenerative capacity of bone tissue *(B)* is portrayed in this microscopic section revealing bone ingrowth between the polymethyl methacrylate spheres of a porous root implant *(IM)* to the depth indicated by the *arrows.*

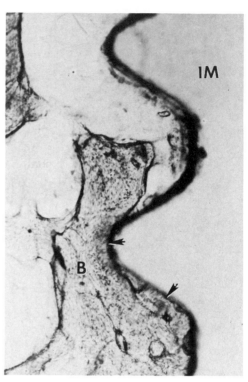

FIG 5–13.
Trabecular (cancellous) bone *(B)* in direct apposition (contact) to the surface of a ceramic implant *(IM).*

FIG 5–14.
Periapical radiograph of two cp titanium one-stage implants supporting a fixed prosthesis in the mandible.

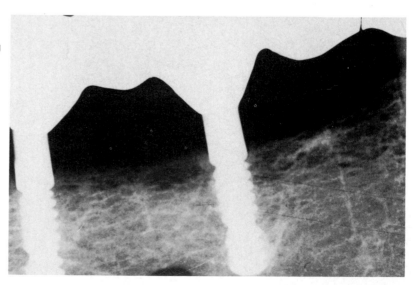

lingual section of an implant in situ reveals that the implant is generally supported by cortical bone only in the upper one third of the implant radicular portion (Fig 5–15). Generally this cortical bone support only extends along one fourth to one half of the occlusal length of the implant root surface. Initial studies from our laboratories suggested that the middle one third of the endosseous implant radicular portion is supported by trabecular bone (see Fig 5–15), and the apex or lower one third of the root portion of an endosseous implant is primarily in contact with fibrofatty marrow space, particularly in the mandible.[21] However, we have recently conducted computer-assisted studies on the bone interface area around screw-type implants and our preliminary results reveal that the maximum bone area contact occurs, as expected, at the occlusal one third of the implant root while the next area of most bone area contact is the *apical third*.[22] This is somewhat of a surprise and may alter our thinking of the amount of bone support needed for an implant. Biomechanical studies suggest that the implant in bone does not have to be very long for appropriate occlusal force distribution.[23]

Another interesting finding from our histologic studies is that implants that are placed and heal with a direct bone interface will demonstrate an active bone-remodeling process after placement of the prosthesis. Implants will be completely surrounded by connective tissue 2 to 4 months after loading, the remodeling process removing bone that directly opposed the implant.[24] This remodeling process proceeds for a period of 5 to 6 months, and the bone may then regenerate with microscopic evidence indicating that basic bone osteogenesis occurs in the connective tissue space between implant and bone.[25] Thus, as the remodeling continues, bone *again* develops direct contact with the now-loaded implant. Following all these biological changes histologically is a laborious process through clinical trials and specimen preparation, but our initial results of the tissue changes after loading are exciting and indicate the pressing need for more biological studies to completely understand the body response to implants.

Peri-implant Connective Tissue Response

A direct bone interface is not always the result of implant placement and often a large area of the implant may be surrounded by connective tissue or collagen following healing.[2] This is often a perplexing issue both to the clinician and the basic scientist. What are the control factors that result in this type of interface? Excessive mobility? Poor surgical placement? Even eliminating these variables, a predominant connective tissue interface still occurs.

Sometimes these collagen bundles run from bone to implant, creating a peri-implant ligament around the implant similar in morphology to that of a periodontal ligament (Fig 5–16). It would be nice to be able to predict reliably whether implants would achieve predominantly a bone or organized ligament interface around the radicular portion. Knowledge

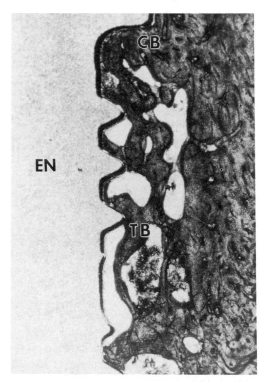

FIG 5–15.
Low-power light photomicrograph showing the variance in bone support around an implant post. Cortical bone *(CB)* interfaces the occlusal region of the intraosseous cylinder *(EN)*. In the middle portion of the intraosseous cylinder, trabecular bone *(TB)* is the predominant tissue type.

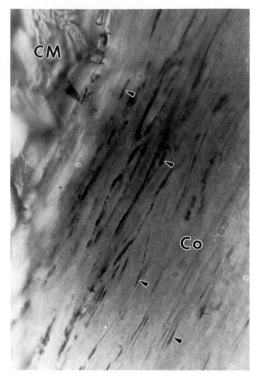

FIG 5–16.
Connective tissue response around a ceramic implant *(CM)* showing parallel collagen fiber *(Co)* organization present between the implant face and trabecular bone (out of figure at lower right). The nuclei of the fibroblasts are evident *(arrowheads)* among the collagen fibers.

about a soft tissue interface and the remodeling that occurs after occlusal loading strongly suggests that two-stage implants which heal with a direct bone interface may be converted to a connective tissue interface after prosthetic loading. This important biological activity cannot be overlooked by the clinician. Weiss considers the presence of the peri-implant ligament response an important concept for maintenance of root form and blade form endosteal implants.[26, 27] He calls this tissue response interface the "fibro-osseous integration" concept and assigns it a shock-absorbing role similar to a periodontal ligament.

When a radiograph reveals an endosteal implant with a thin radiolucent line around the implant device, and yet clinically this implant is successful, it suggests that an organized connective tissue interface between bone and implant can be a successful result, just as much as a direct bone interface.[27] We need to know what role collagen fibers actually play in serving as anchoring, nonrotational, or limiting structures in stabilization of the implant. Does a collagen interface actually have shock absorber or suspensory ligament roles, as theorized?[27, 28]

ROLE OF THE TISSUE-IMPLANT BIOLOGICAL SEAL

Dental implants provide a unique treatment modality because an inert material inserted into the tissues and bone of the jaws serves as an anchoring attachment for fixed prostheses. Dentist and dental scientists have long dreamed of such a treatment in order to assist patients in the firm anchorage of prosthetic appliances to the jaws, particularly for those patients who experience problems in adjusting to removable dentures or have compromised bone because of trauma or disease.

Approximately 30 years ago implantologists began to recognize that for a dental implant to be successful and survive for an extended period of time in the jaws, there had to be an important biological acceptability between the implant biomaterial and the jaw tissues. It became obvious that the role of the gingival epithelium and its interface with the implant post was of singular importance because this is the area where initial peri-implant tissue breakdown would begin with the onset of inflammatory reaction and destructive disease processes. Thus, Lavelle postulated the concept of the "mucosal seal" around the dental implant.[29] Lavelle and others pointed out the necessity for the attached gingiva to adapt appropriately to the implant and provide a barrier to the movement of bacteria and oral toxins into the space between the implant post and biological tissues.[30] Others have called this area the zone of the "transmucosal seal."[31] Although implantologists began to recognize that this was an important area they were frustrated at their attempts to effectively prevent the development of inflammation and bacterial ingress around this critical attached gingival zone. Much of this frustration developed because of the lack of scientific data and the inability to recognize the joint role of biomaterial surface and biological tissue response.

James and Schultz were the first to begin a systematic scientific study to investigate this seal phenomenon.[32] Using a combination of light and electron microscopy they were able to show that the gingival epithelium following surgery regenerated a series of epithelial cells around the implant that were consistently similar to those seen around the natural tooth. They showed the presence of hemidesmosomes associated with crevicular epithelial cells and the presence of an Oricin-positive deposition on the implant face that suggested the presence of a dental cuticle-like structure that would assist in creating a positive attachment between gingival epithelium and implant.[32] In addition, they showed the presence of connective tissue fibers below this epithelial interface and the role of these fibers in supporting the surface epithelium.[33] These types of studies were carried out in further detail by McKinney and co-workers who positively identified the regeneration of the attached gingiva and its ability to form a gingival sulcus lined by crevicular (sulcular) epithelium.[2, 6, 34] Thus, the presence of a gingival attachment apparatus with epithelial components similar to that seen around natural teeth was firmly established.[9, 16]

The philosophy of the gingival epithelial role in forming the *biological seal* is one of great importance in implant dentistry. All implants, whether they be endosteal forms, and that can include root, cylindrical, spiral, screw, and basket shapes, or one- or two-stage procedure implants, must have a superstructure or coronal portion that must pass through the submucosa (lamina propria) and the covering stratified squamous epithelium into the oral cavity. This transmucosal passage then creates the "weak link" between prosthetic attachment and predicted bony support of the implant. This transmucosal zone is the potential area where initial tissue breakdown may result in eventual tissue necrosis and destruction around the implant.

Subperiosteal implants, although not inserted into the bone of the jaw, rest upon the surface of the jaw bone and the framework is placed below the fibrous connective tissue stroma (lamina propria and periosteum) underneath the gingival epithelium. But even though the concept of bony support for this implant modality is totally different from the endosteal dental implant, it has posts arising from the subperiosteal framework that serve as the coronal portion to support the prosthetic restoration. Thus the subperiosteal implant has the exact same features—a *transmucosal passage* through connective tissue and epithelium to exit into the oral cavity. Thus, both types of major implant modalities in use today, the endosteal and subperiosteal implant, are faced with the need to create an *effective* biological seal.

The biological seal thus becomes a pivotal factor in endosteal or subperiosteal implant longevity. The seal must be effective enough to prevent the ingress of bacterial toxins, plaque, oral debris, and other deleterious substances taken into the oral cavity such as food, alcohol, and tobacco. All these agents are known initiators of tissue and cell injury and must be prevented from gaining access from the external environment of the oral cavity into the internal environment of the jaw bone. The biological seal is a physiologic barrier that must be developed by the recipient host tissues around the dental implant device in order to prevent the encroachment of toxic and destructive agents into the area of implant support.[31] No matter how carefully we perform the surgery with low-speed non–heat generating techniques, no matter what the design of the implant and its surface physical characteristics, and no matter how well we achieve direct bony adaptation to biomaterial (osseointegration), all these carefully planned and controlled and resultant treatment features are for nought if the biological seal adaptation phenomenon does not work. The biological seal zone must form a sufficient physiologic barrier to prevent the movement of destructive agents into the internal environment of the jaws. Once destructive agents gain access to the interior environment they will establish inflammatory processes, either acute or chronic, that will eventually lead to destruction of the collagenous stroma beneath the epithelium and of the alveolar bone supporting and surrounding the implant device.

The mechanisms of bone destruction are at first inflammation and osteoclastic activity causing reabsorption of bone in direct contact with the implant. With loss of direct bone support, the implant becomes mobile and allows a percolation or pumping action of oral bacterial toxins and degenerative agents into the internal environment of the implant crypt. Finally, sufficient destruction occurs that potentially gives rise to acute suppurative inflammation, or acute inflammation with pain, particularly upon mastication, or extensive mobility that renders support of the fixed prosthesis impractical.[20] In any case, these features are treated by only one route, that is, removal of the implant and debridement of the tissue area to clear up the inflammation and infection and allow the tissues to heal. Of course, if sufficient bone is lost during this disease process, then the possibility of the patient's jaws supporting another implant is severely compromised.

Current information developed from our investigative studies indicates the biological formation of this *transmucosal seal* following implant surgery. As described in detail in the section on peri-implant gingival response, the tissue forms an epithelial "cuff" (free gingival margin). Even though the area has been edentulous, in some cases for long periods of time, the regenerating epithelium regenerates the free gingival margin complete with free gingival groove and a gingival sulcus. Gingival epithelium regenerates and lines this sulcus with nonkeratinized sulcular (crevicular) epithelium and a zone of epithelial cells at the base of the sulcus that interface the implant surface. These epithelial cells at the base produce attachment structures that are recognized as normal components of cell biology. The attachment structure includes formation of a basal lamina composed predominantly of type IV collagen, hemidesmosomes, which are the attachment plaques holding epithelial cells to the basal lamina, a glycocalyx (also called a *linear body*), and an enzyme called *laminin* which serves as a molecular bonding agent between the epithelial cells and the layers of the basal lamina.

Although collagenous components of the linear body cannot physiologically adhere or embed into the implant biomaterial as they do in the living cementum of the tooth, the high content of glycosaminoglycans (mucopolysaccharides) in the linear body which coats the dental implant has sufficient "stickiness" or gluelike properties to form a biologically active and trauma-resistant attachment interface at the gingival sulcus. A summary of the research evidence supporting an implant-tissue biological seal is presented in Table 5–1. The longevity of this regenerated structure can be demonstrated by the measuring and probing of the re-created gingival sulcus in long-term implant trials and the successful longevity of many different types of implants that have been placed and followed by critical clinical analysis for many years.[35–39]

Thus, the biological seal around dental implants is a definitive biological entity that must be present to prevent the external toxins and agents of the oral cavity from moving into the internal environment of the jaw. The biological seal serves as an effective

TABLE 5–1.

Summary of Research Evidence Supporting an Implant-Tissue Biological Seal

Light microscopy
    Verification of the regeneration of crevicular epithelium
    Juxtaposition of a junctional epithelial structure next to the implant
    Presence of gingival sulcus
Scanning electron microscopy
    Observation of epithelial cells involved in regeneration of the free gingival margin, sulcus, and junctional epithelium
    Normal gingival epithelial maturation patterns
    Interface of junctional epithelial pseudopodia and the implant
Transmission electron microscopy
    Presence of cell organelles, basal lamina, and other structures constituting an attachment complex
    Presence of a glycosaminoglycan molecular coat on the implant face
    Development of a cell attachment apparatus consistent with current cell biology knowledge

barrier to maintain these two distinct environments separate in the peri-implant environment. It is up to the clinical dentist to employ good dental prophylaxis procedures and instruct the patient in adequate home care maintenance to keep the biological seal viable and healthy, and preserve the structural integrity of this biological area between oral cavity and internal jaw environment.

THE IMPLANT-TISSUE ATTACHMENT COMPLEX

Combining our knowledge from light microscopy, and scanning and transmission electron microscopy, we are now able to show conclusively that the various components of the unique gingival tissue attachment to teeth also exist in the regenerated epithelial tissue interfacing dental implant posts. This research evidence is summarized in Table 5–1. Using current concepts of cell biology, it is possible to theorize how the attachment complex of the biological seal forms. Figure 5–17 serves as a guide to the descriptive series of events that follow. During the regeneration of the attached gingiva and the formation of the free gingival margin, fibroblasts produce glycosaminoglycans that coat the implant face. Fibroblasts as well as new capillary sprouts in the heal-

ing area produce fibronectin, a tissue component necessary for adhesion of the basal lamina to other tissue structures. The regenerating crevicular epithelial cells produce the basal lamina with hemidesmosomes as they regenerate around the implant, and in the process they also produce laminin. The laminin and hemidesmosomes tack the basal lamina to the epithelial cells. The fibronectin produced by the fibroblasts and capillaries serves as the "final glue" or molecular adhesion material between the glycosaminoglycan coat on the implant and the basal lamina.[16] In this manner the biological seal is completed.

CONCLUSIONS

Dental implantology is an exciting treatment concept that relies on surgical, prosthetic, periodontal, and restorative skills, and scientific understanding by the practitioner of today. We are now seeing the widespread acceptance of implant treatment because a sound scientific basis for this treatment mode is emerging. We now understand the necessity for controlled surgical procedures that provide a good environment for healing of the gingiva and bone tissues around the implant post. From scientific investigations, we have gained an understanding of how the tissue heals around the implant post and how a

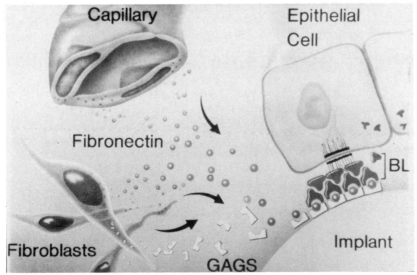

FIG 5–17.
Artist's illustration of the development of the attachment complex and the implant *biological seal.* The epithelial cell regenerating around the implant post produces the basal lamina *(BL)* and hemidesmosomes. Fibroblasts in the healing environment produce glycosaminoglycans *(GAGS)* which coat the implant surface as the glycocalyx (linear body) *(white u blocks).* Fibroblasts, plus the new capillary sprouts, produce fibronectin *(spherules)* which serves as the adhesive enzyme in the sublamina lucida space. See text for further details and compare with diagram in Figure 5–8.

biological seal forms that can prevent the ingress of bacteria and oral debris into the peri-implant tissues supporting the implant. However, there are still many areas of concern and much that is unknown about the biological reactions of human tissues to dental implants. All of these areas require in-depth scientific inquiry by both clinician and basic scientist.

REFERENCES

1. Koth DL, McKinney RV Jr: The single crystal sapphire endosteal dental implant, in Hardin JF (ed): *Clark's Clinical Dentistry*. Philadelphia, JB Lippincott Co, 1981, chap 53.

2. McKinney RV Jr, Koth DL: The single crystal endosteal dental implant: Material characteristics and 18-month experimental animal trials. *J Prosthet Dent* 1982; 47:69–84.

3. McKinncy RV Jr, Koth DL, Steflik DE: The single crystal sapphire endosseous dental implant. II. Two year results of clinical animal trials. *J Oral Implantol* 1983; 10:619–638.

4. Steflik DE, McKinney RV Jr, Mobley GL, et al: Simultaneous histological preparation of bone, soft tissue and implanted biomaterials for light microscopic observations. *Stain Technol* 1982; 57:91–98.

5. McKinney RV Jr, Koth DL, Steflik DE: The single crystal sapphire endosseous dental implant. I. Material characteristics and placement techniques. *J Oral Implantol* 1982; 10:487–503.

6. McKinney RV Jr, Steflik DE, Koth DL: The biologic response to the single-crystal sapphire endosteal dental implant: Scanning electron microscopic observations. *J Prosthet Dent* 1984; 51:372–379.

7. McKinney RV Jr, Steflik DE, Koth DL: Ultrastructural surface topography of the single crystal sapphire endosseous dental implant. *J Oral Implantol* 1984; 11:327–340.

8. Steflik DE, McKinney RV Jr, Koth DL: Scanning electron microscopy of plasma etched implant specimens. *Stain Technol* 1984; 59:71–77.

9. McKinney RV Jr, Steflik DE, Koth DL: Evidence for a junctional epithelial attachment to ceramic dental implants. A transmission electron microscopic study. *J Periodontol* 1985; 56:579–591.

10. Steflik DE, McKinney RV Jr, Koth DL: Epithelial attachment to ceramic dental implants. *Ann NY Acad Sci* 1988; 523:4–18.

11. Listgarten MA: Electron microscopic study of the junction between surgically denuded root surfaces and regenerated periodontal tissues. *J Periodont Res* 1972; 7:68–90.

12. Listgarten MA, Lai CH: Ultrastructure of the intact interface between an endosseous epoxy resin dental implant and the host tissues. *J Biol Buccale* 1975; 3:13–28.

13. Swope EM, James RA: A longitudinal study on hemidesmosome formation at the dental implant-tissue interface. *J Oral Implantol* 1981; 9:412–422.

14. Gould TR, Westbury L, Burnette DM: Ultrastructural study of the attachment of human gingiva to titanium in vivo. *J Prosthet Dent* 1984; 52:418–420.

15. McKinney RV Jr, Steflik DE, Koth DL: The epithelium dental implant interface. *J Oral Implantol* 1988; 13:622–641.

16. Steflik DE, McKinney RV, Jr, Koth DL: Ultrastructural comparisons of ceramic and titanium dental implants *in vivo:* A scanning electron microscopic study. *J Biomed Mater Res* 1989; 23:895–909.

17. Branemark PI, Hansson BO, Adell R, et al: Osseointegrated implants in the treatment of the edentulous jaw. Experience from a 10-year period. *Scand J Plast Reconstr Surg [Suppl]* 1977; 16.

18. Gross U, Strunz V: The interface of various glasses and glass ceramics with a bony implantation bed. *J Biomed Mater Res* 1985; 19:251–271.

19. Brånemark PI: Osseointegration and its experimental background. *J Prosthet Dent* 1983; 50:399–410.

20. McKinney RV Jr, Steflik DE, Koth DL, et al: The scientific basis for dental implant therapy. *J Dent Educ* 1988; 52:696–705.

21. McKinney RV Jr, Steflik DE, Koth DL, et al: Histomorphometry of endosteal implant-tissue interfaces. *J Dent Res* 1985; 64(special issue):299.

22. Cason L, McKinney RV Jr, Larke V, et al: Histomorphometric analysis of endosteal bone implant interfaces. *J Dent Res* 1990; 69(special issue): 347.

23. Skalak R: Stress transfer at the implant surface. *J Oral Implantol* 1988; 13:581–593.

24. McKinney RV Jr, Steflik DE, Koth DL, et al: Histological results from a comparative endosteal dental implant study. *J Dent Res* 1987; 66(special issue):186.

25. Steflik DE, McKinney RV Jr, Koth DL: Light and scanning electron microscopic characterizations of the apical support system to endosteal dental implants. *Trans Soc Biomater* 1989; 12:62.

26. Weiss CM: Tissue integration dental endosseous implants: Description and comparative analysis of the

fibro-osseous integration and osseous integration systems. *J Oral Implantol* 1986; 12:169–214.

27. Weiss CM: A comparative analysis of fibro-osteal and osteal integration and other variables that affect long-term bone maintenance around dental implants. *J Oral Implantol* 1987; 13:467–487.

28. James RA: Connective tissue-dental implant interface. *J Oral Implantol* 1988; 13:607–621.

29. Lavelle CLB: Mucosal seal around endosseous dental implants. *J Oral Implantol* 1981; 9:357–371.

30. James RA: Tissue response to dental implant devices, in Hardin JF (ed): *Clark's Clinical Dentistry*. Philadelphia, JB Lippincott Co, 1986, chap 48.

31. McKinney RV Jr, Steflik DE, Koth DL: Per, peri, or trans? A concept for improved dental implant terminology. *J Prosthet Dent* 1984; 52:267–269.

32. James RA, Schultz RL: Hemidesmosomes and the adhesion of junctional epithelial cells to metal implants. A preliminary report. *J Oral Implantol* 1974; 4:294–302.

33. James RA: Tissue behavior in the environment produced by permucosal dental devices, in McKinney RV Jr, Lemons JE (eds): *The Dental Implant. Clinical and Biological Response of Oral Tissues*. Littleton, Mass, PSG Publishing Co Inc, 1985, chap 9.

34. Steflik DE, McKinney RV Jr, Koth DL, et al: The biomaterial-tissue interface: A morphological study utilizing conventional and alternative ultrastructural modalities. *Scan Electron Microsc* 1984; 11:547–555.

35. Koth DL, McKinney RV Jr, Steflik DE, et al: Clinical and statistical analyses of human clinical trials with the single crystal alumina oxide endosteal dental implant: Five-year results. *J Prosthet Dent* 1988; 60:226–234.

36. Schnitman P, Rubenstein J, Jeffcoat M, et al: Three-year survival results: Blade implant vs. cantilever clinical trials. *J Dent Res* 1988; 67(special issue):347.

37. Kapur K, Deupree R, Frechette A, et al: VA cooperative study on dental implants. Part IV: Comparisons between RPD and FPD. *J Dent Res* 1987; 66(special issue):113.

38. Smithloff M, Fritz ME: The use of blade implants in a selected population of partially edentulous adults. A 15-year report. *J Periodontol* 1987; 58:589–593.

39. Albrektsson T, Dahl E, Enbom L, et al: Osseointegrated oral implants. A Swedish multicenter study of 8,139 consecutively inserted Nobelpharma implants. *J Periodontol* 1988; 59:287–296.

Chapter 6

Basic Bone Biology in Implantology

Francis T. Lake, D.D.S., Ph.D.

Bone is a vital tissue that is constantly undergoing change. Throughout the life of bone the normal sequence of events includes the continuous replacement of preexistent bone with new bone. In addition, injured bone has the ability to regenerate itself which leads to complete anatomic and physiologic repair. Bone is one of the few organs of the body that has this regenerative capacity. One of the factors that determines the success of an endosseous implant is the healing of the bone into which the implant is placed. This chapter presents current concepts concerning basic bone anatomy and physiology related to endosseous implant preparation, insertion, and function.

BONE TISSUE

Bone is unique in the body in that it exists both as a tissue and as an organ. An example of the organ bone would be the mandible or the maxilla. Each of the bony organs that we collectively call the *skeleton* is composed primarily of a tissue that is also called *bone*. Therefore, the bony skeleton is constructed from the same basic building material, which is called *bone tissue*. In the following discussion we concern ourselves with bone tissue, since it is the common denominator for all the bones of the body.

EMBRYOLOGIC DEVELOPMENT OF THE JAWS

From an embryologic perspective each bone is given one of two names that reflects the method by which the bone was developed within the embryo. The upper and lower jaws are *intramembranous* or *membrane bones,* which means that they developed within a membrane. This type of bone begins its development as a nidus of osteogenic cells in the embryonic connective tissue. This nidus of cells produces the initial osteoid matrix, which rapidly mineralizes to form bone (see next section). This contrasts with the long bones, such as the femur and humerus, which are *endochondral* or *cartilage bones.* This type of bone develops within a previously laid-down cartilage model. The bone is formed upon remnants of cartilage that are present in the area, and the formative process does not imply that cartilage turns into bone. Early in development there is cartilage associated with the lower jaw. This cartilage is called *Meckel's cartilage* and develops prior to any bone formation. As such it is called *primary cartilage* to differentiate it from *secondary cartilage,* which appears after bone formation begins. Meckel's cartilage does not give rise to the bone of the mandible, and very few remnants of Meckel's cartilage remain in the postnatal human. Most of the bone of the mandible and maxilla is formed by intramembranous mechanisms, but a secondary cartilage does develop in the mandible which eventually gives rise to a portion of the ramus that includes the condylar process.

The bone associated with the secondary cartilage develops by endochondral mechanisms.

BONE FORMATION

There are many types of bone tissue present in the human body. A few of the common terms used to describe different types of bone are mature bone, immature bone, fine-fibered bone, coarse bundle bone, compact bone, and trabecular bone. In addition, each of these terms has synonyms, which makes it even more confusing for the uninitiated! Each of these terms describes bone tissue from either a gross or microscopic anatomic level. To simplify the situation consider the fact that regardless of the type of bone tissue that is being described, it is produced in the same manner as any of the other types of bone. It is important, then, to understand this basic mechanism by which bone tissue is formed. The process of bone formation is called *osteogenesis* or *ossification*.

There are within the body certain cells that are programmed (predetermined) to become the bone-forming cells *(osteoblasts)*. These predetermined cells are called *osteoprogenitor cells* or *osteogenic cells*. The osteoprogenitor cells originate from more primitive cells which are called *mesenchymal cells*. The mesenchymal cell is thought to be able to differentiate into many different cell types depending upon the signal that it receives or its microenvironment, or both. When bone is needed the osteoprogenitor cells differentiate into osteoblasts. The osteoblasts produce bone. Following the proper signal, but prior to bone formation, the osteoblasts send out cytoplasmic processes which contact cell processes from other osteoblasts. A network of cells connected by long, thin cell processes is thereby formed (see Fig 6–1,A and B). As will be discussed later, the contact of cell processes of different osteoblasts is quite important for the future vitality and function of the osteoblasts.

Between the osteoblasts and their processes are large spaces. Collectively the spaces constitute what is known as the *intercellular space*. Initially the osteoblasts produce and secrete *organic components* into the intercellular space (see Fig 6–1,B). The organic secretions of the osteoblasts can be classified

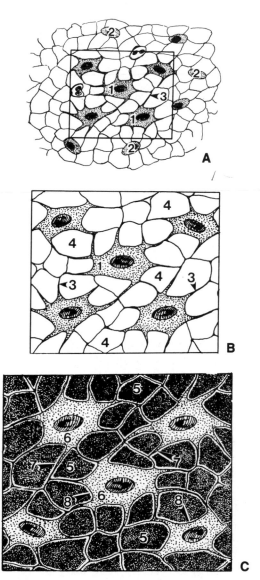

FIG 6–1.
This figure shows the steps that occur during bone formation. **A** and **B** show a network of osteoblasts *(1)* which have differentiated from osteoprogenitor cells *(2)*. Cell processes *(3)* from one osteoblast join with those of other osteoblasts. The osteoblasts secrete collagen and amorphous ground substance into the intercellular matrix *(4)* to produce osteoid. **C** depicts fully formed bone which is produced by the mineralization of the matrix. The matrix *(5)* is now calcified. Nutrients reach the cells, which are now called osteocytes *(6)*, through canaliculi *(7)*. The spaces around the osteocytes are called lacunae *(8)*. All types of bone tissue are formed in a similar way, i.e., osteoblasts produce osteoid which undergoes mineralization to form mature bone tissue.

into a *fibrous component* and an *amorphous component*. The fibrous component is primarily collagen (type I), while the amorphous component consists of proteoglycans, noncollagenous proteins, and glycoproteins. *Osteonectin* and *osteocalcin* are two components of the amorphous component of the matrix. Osteonectin is a protein found only in bone. Its function is to cement the collagen fibers in the matrix to the bone mineral. Osteocalcin is a calcium-binding protein which is thought to be involved in the mineralization of the matrix. The organic components and water which fill the intercellular space are called the *organic matrix*. The organic matrix produced by the osteoblasts is called *prebone* or *osteoid*. Osteoid or prebone has not yet undergone mineralization.

Once the osteoid is formed it undergoes a process called *mineralization* or *calcification* (see Fig 6–1,C). During this phase of bone formation, calcium and phosphate ions are deposited into the organic matrix. The calcium-phosphate complexes that precipitate into the organic matrix are known chemically as *hydroxyapatite* crystals. The exact mechanism of control of the mineralization process is unknown at this time, but many investigators believe that it is under the control of the osteoblasts.

Therefore, the formation of bone tissue takes place in two distinct phases: the initial phase of organic matrix production *(osteoid formation phase)*, followed by the mineralization of the matrix by hydroxyapatite crystals *(mineralization phase)*. Bone formation is schematized in Figure 6–2.

After the matrix mineralizes, the cells (former osteoblasts), which are now surrounded by the mineralized matrix, are called *osteocytes* (see Fig 6–1,C). Since the osteocytes are enclosed by a mineralized matrix, they cannot receive nourishment or get rid of waste products by diffusion through the matrix as they did prior to mineralization. Therefore, another mechanism must be provided to meet the metabolic demands of the osteocytes. Following mineralization, nutrients reach the osteocytes by traveling in the space between the cell processes and the mineralized matrix. Not only is there a space between the cell processes and the mineralized matrix but there is a similar space between the cell body of the osteocyte and the mineralized matrix. These spaces are filled with tissue fluid and provide the necessary conduit for the passage of substances to and from the embedded cells. The space in which the cell body of the osteocyte resides is called a *lacuna,* while the tunnel which encloses the cell process is called a *canaliculus* (see Fig 6–1,C). Eventually the tissue spaces surrounding the cell body and the cell processes communicate with a blood supply located within the medullary spaces of the bone, in the periosteum covering the bone, or in a structure called a *haversian canal,* which is located within the substance of the bone.

Osteocytes were at one time osteoblasts that eventually became trapped within the mineralized matrix. Not all osteoblasts, however, become osteocytes since some of them migrate as the organic matrix is produced. In this case the osteoblasts remain on the surface of the newly developed bone. They become a component of the membranes that cover the surfaces of all bones. These membranes are called the *periosteum* and the *endosteum* (see Figs 6–3 and 6–4).

Another cell type, the *osteoclast,* is also found on the surfaces of bone. These cells are responsible for *osteoclasia,* which is the removal of bone tissue (see Fig 6–4,B). Osteoclasts are derived from cells of the monocyte-phagocyte system, which arises from monocytes that have migrated into extravascular spaces from circulating blood. Osteocytes are also thought to be able to remove bone from the walls of their lacunae. This process of bone removal is called *osteolysis.*

THE MEMBRANES OF BONE

Most of the surfaces of a bone are covered with a membrane. Outer bone surfaces are covered with

---

> **Undifferentiated mesenchymal cell → Osteoprogenitor cell →**
> **Osteoblasts → Organic matrix → Mineralization of the matrix → "The tissue bone"**

FIG 6–2.
Steps in the formation of bone tissue.

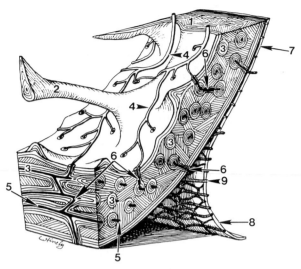

FIG 6–3.
This is a higher magnification of the area labeled *6* at the bottom of Figure 6–5,B. Note the cortical bone *(1)*, a trabeculum *(2)*, haversian systems or osteons *(3)*, and blood vessels within the marrow spaces *(4)*, and within the haversian canals *(5)*. Also note the connecting Volkmann canals *(6)*. The bone tissue seen in this figure is of the mature or lamellar type. The periosteum is seen attached at *7* and lifted from the surface of the bone at *8*. The fibrous portion of the periosteum has been lifted from the surface of the bone, while the majority of the cellular layer remains on the bone surface. The periosteum is quite vascular as demonstrated by the numerous vessels within the periosteum *(9)*. The periosteal vessels connect with the haversian vessels via Volkmann's canals *(6)*

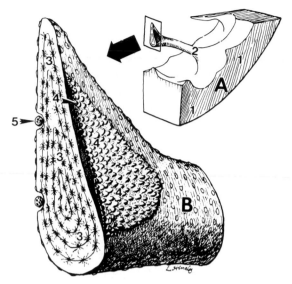

FIG 6–4.
A shows a portion of a mandible which contains cortical bone *(1)* and trabecular bone *(2)*. **B** is a high magnification of a portion of the trabeculum *(2)* seen in **A.** Note that the trabeculum is composed of lamellar bone *(3)*. The surface of the trabeculum is covered with endosteum which consists mainly of osteoblasts and osteoprogenitor cells *(4)*. Osteoclasts *(5)* are also seen on the surface which indicates that bone resorption is taking place. All of the internal surfaces of bone, including the haversian canals, are covered or lined with endosteum. The endosteum is an excellent source of osteoprogenitor cells.

the *periosteum,* while the inner surfaces, including the haversian canals, are covered or lined with the *endosteum* (see Figs 6–3 and 6–4).

The periosteum consists of two distinct layers: an inner *cellular layer,* which is adjacent to the bone, and an outer *fibrous layer*. The cellular layer consists of osteoprogenitor cells, osteoblasts, and osteoclasts. The cellular layer can vary in thickness depending on its location on the bone, the activity of the cells, and the age of the individual. With age and decreased cellular activity, the cellular layer of the periosteum becomes thinner. The cells become attenuated, and the number of layers of cells in the cellular layer is reduced. The cellular layer contains nerve fibers and an abundant blood supply. The outer fibrous layer consists mainly of dense collagenous fibers produced by fibroblasts within the fibrous layer.

The fibrous layer gives a toughness to the periosteum. Periosteum is not seen on articulating surfaces, or at sites of tendon and ligament attachment.

The endosteum differs from the periosteum in that it consists of only one layer of cells. This single layer of cells is similar to the cellular layer of the periosteum in that it contains osteoprogenitor cells, osteoblasts, and osteoclasts. In either case, the cells of the cellular layer of the periosteum and endosteum can produce new bone if properly stimulated. Therefore, both the periosteum and the endosteum are sources of cells that can repair damaged bone.

TYPES OF BONE TISSUE

Morphologic Classification.—When viewed grossly, i.e., with the unaided eye, bone tissue can be classified into two types: *compact bone* and *trabecular bone* (see Figs 6–5 and 6–6). The type of bone that makes up the outer surfaces of most bones of the skeleton is quite dense and has very few spaces within the bony tissue. This type of bone is called *compact, cortical,* or *dense bone.* The other type of bone seen grossly has considerable space within the bony tissue. This type of bone is called *trabecular, spongy,* or *cancellous bone.* The spaces among the bony trabeculae in this type of bone constitute that portion of the organ bone called the *medullary cavity.* The interior of most bones consists of marrow, which fills the medullary cavities. Some bone marrow is actively producing blood cells, in which case it is called *red marrow.* In most human bones, the red marrow is converted into a fat storage site and is then called *yellow marrow.* In mature human jaws the marrow spaces are filled with fat. Yellow marrow can revert to red marrow if the demands of the body require additional blood elements.

Histologic Classification.—When a bone is viewed with the light microscope, two general categories of bone can be identified. They are *immature bone* and *mature bone.* These two types of bone can be distinguished by the number of osteocytes present within a given area of bone, the size of the osteocyte lacunae, and by the arrangement of the osteocytes within the matrix.

Immature bone is formed earlier and more rapidly than mature bone and is the type of bone that forms during the initial phase of bone repair. With time immature bone is usually replaced by mature bone. There are two subclassifications of immature bone. They are *woven bone* (also called *repair bone*) and *bundle bone.* In woven bone the collagen fibers within the matrix run in various directions giving the bone a woven appearance when viewed microscopically with polarized light. In bundle bone the collagen is arranged in large bundles which run parallel to one another with the osteocytes located between the bundles of collagen. This is the type of bone which attaches the periodontal ligament to the bone of the alveolus.

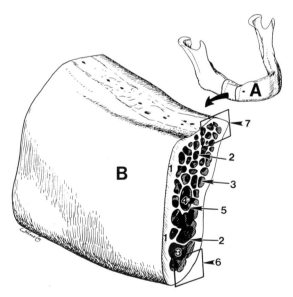

FIG 6–5.
An edentulous human mandible is seen in **A.** The residual ridges show moderate resorption. This mandible would be able to accept an appropriate endosseous implant. A portion of the bicuspid molar region is enlarged in **B.** Note the cortical bone *(1),* the trabecular bone *(2),* the marrow spaces *(3),* and the neurovascular bundle *(4)* within the mandibular canal *(5).* Blocks labeled 6 and 7 are discussed in Figures 6–3 and 6–6, respectively.

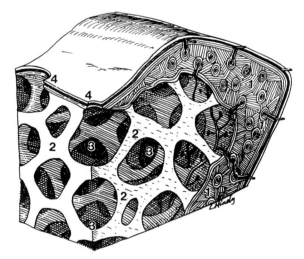

FIG 6–6.
This represents a high magnification of the area labeled 7 at the top of Figure 6–5,B. Cortical bone *(1)* and trabecular bone *(2)* are seen. Marrow spaces are seen at *3.* Marrow spaces in adults are usually filled with fat tissue. Note that the cortical bone becomes quite thin or nonexistent at the crest of the residual ridge *(4).* In these areas the residual ridge consists of trabecular (cancellous) bone that is covered by the oral mucosa.

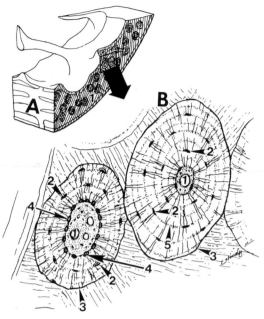

FIG 6–7.
A shows a portion of bone from the mandible. **B** is a high magnification of the box outlined in **A. B** shows two osteons which have been cut in cross section. Note the haversian vessels *(1)*, osteocytes *(2)*, and the cement line *(3)*. The endosteum, composed of osteoblasts and osteoprogenitor cells, is seen at *4*. The osteocytes *(2)* and the resting lines *(5)* which connect them form concentric lamellae.

Mature bone is called *fine-fibered bone* and *lamellar bone* (see Fig 6–4). In this type of bone the matrix is produced in a very ordered manner, and is described as having a layered or lamellar appearance. In general the collagenous fibers within the matrix of one lamella are at right angles to those in adjacent lamellae. *Haversian* or *osteonal bone* is a type of mature bone in which the lamellae are arranged in concentric circles *(concentric lamellae)* around a blood supply (see Fig 6–7). Mature bone replaces immature bone in most instances.

REMODELING OF COMPACT BONE

Compact bone is continually being removed and replaced within the body. The removal of the bone can occur on the surface of the bone by way of osteoclastic activity on the bone surface, or it can oc-

cur within the depths of the bone. In either case, the bone is removed by cells called *osteoclasts*. When bone becomes fatigued or necrotic, osteoclasts aggregate at a bone surface and begin to remove bone. In addition, clusters of osteoclasts can aggregate at the surface of bone or in haversian canals within the bone tissue and eventually create a tunnel within the depths of dense bone. This cluster of osteoclasts is called a *cutting cone* and the tunnel that is produced by the osteoclasts is called an *erosion (resorption) tunnel* (see Fig 6–8). The cutting cone will continue to burrow into the bone until all the necrotic or weakened bone tissue is removed. Following immediately behind the cutting cone, and inserting itself into the bony tunnel, is a blood capillary. Associated with the capillary are osteoprogenitor cells which accompany the capillary as it grows into the erosion tunnel. These ostcoprogenitor cells are located around the periphery of the capillary and are sometimes called *perivascular cells* (see Fig 6–8). Perivascular cells are also found associated with capillaries throughout the bone marrow and periosteum. The osteoprogenitor cells disassociate themselves from the capillary, move away from the capillary, and approximate the bony walls of the erosion tunnel. By this time the cells have differentiated into osteoblasts and begin to lay down osteoid on the tunnel walls. The osteoid mineralizes and bone can once again be seen within a portion of the erosion tunnel (see Fig 6–8). As the bone is laid down, some of the osteoblasts remain behind and become entrapped within the mineralized matrix to become osteocytes. Bone continues to be laid down within the tunnel and eventually the majority of the tunnel is filled with new bone. The blood vessel that originally entered the erosion tunnel is now surrounded by bone. The canal that is produced by this process is called a *haversian canal*. The haversian canal is lined with either ostcoblasts or osteoprogenitor cells. These cells constitute the *endosteal* lining of the haversian canal. The bony structure that forms within the original erosion tunnel is called an *osteon* or a *haversian system*. These osteons are more properly called *secondary osteons* to distinguish them from *primary osteons,* which do not require the presence of an erosion tunnel for their formation. The outermost portion of a secondary osteon can be visualized with

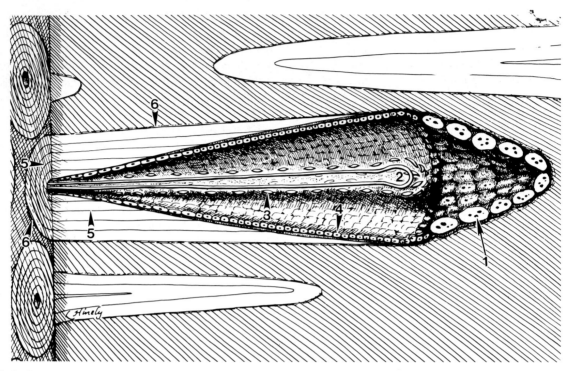

FIG 6–8.
This figure illustrates remodeling of bone and the production of secondary osteons by means of a cutting cone of osteoclasts *(1)*. As the bone is removed, a capillary *(2)* invades the space bringing with it osteoprogenitor cells *(3)*. These cells are sometimes called perivascular cells. The osteoprogenitor cells migrate to the walls of the erosion tunnel, which has been produced by the osteoclasts, and differentiate into osteoblasts *(4)*. The osteoblasts produce bone tissue in the form of concentric lamellae *(5)*. The cement line is seen at 6. When bone formation is completed, a mature secondary osteon or haversian system will have been formed.

the light microscope and is called the *cement line* (see Figs 6–7 and 6–8). It represents the original wall of the erosion tunnel produced by the cutting cone. The osteon is essential in maintaining the vitality of osteocytes which lie deep within compact bone. Osteonal bone makes up a large portion of compact bone in humans. The process of secondary osteon formation is also seen in the repair of damaged bone following the placement of an endosseous dental implant and is discussed in a later section.

BLOOD SUPPLY TO BONE

The circulation of blood within long bones is *centrifugal,* that is, the blood circulates from the medullary region outward through the cortical bone to end in vessels located in the periosteum and other soft tissues associated with the bone. The blood supply to the medullary region is from *nutrient arteries,* which are relatively large vessels that pass through the bone by way of nutrient canals to enter the medullary spaces. Within the marrow the nutrient artery forms a network of vessels called the *endosteal* or *medullary plexus.* Vessels from this plexus enter the cortical bone through *Volkmann's canals* and eventually reach the surface of the bone. While passing through the cortical bone, numerous vessels are given off at right angles to these vessels. These branches become the vessels that are found within the haversian canals of the osteons (see Fig 6–3). Osteonal bone is a major type of bone found in the cortical bone of the jaws. Once the intraosseous vessels reach the outer surface of the bone they anastomose with vessels within the cellular layer of the periosteum or with arteries supplying the soft tissues.

The network of vessels associated with the periosteum is called the *periosteal plexus*. The periosteal plexus in turn communicates with vessels that are supplying arterial blood to muscles and other soft tissues in the area (see Fig 6–3).

The mandible and maxilla are membrane bones and as such do not develop in the same manner as long bones. It is generally agreed, however, that the circulation of blood within the mandible is *centrifugal under normal circulatory conditions*. Centrifugal circulation of blood within the maxilla has not been demonstrated although it may very well exist under normal conditions. As in the long bones, there are endosteal and periosteal plexuses that are interconnected with one another. In addition to these vascular networks, a *periodontal plexus* is found associated with the teeth. When teeth are present, *intraosseous vessels* send branches into the alveolar processes *(intraalveolar arteries)*, to the teeth *(apical arteries)*, and to the periodontal plexus. The intraalveolar arteries and periodontal plexus in turn connect with vessels of the periosteal plexus as well as with vessels within the soft tissues surrounding the bone. Once a tooth is removed its periodontal plexus is lost.

Under abnormal circulatory conditions within the mandible, e.g., occlusion of the nutrient artery, the blood supply to the mandible can reverse so that the direction of flow is from the outside to the inside of the bone. This is called *centripetal circulation*. Angiographic studies by Bradley (see Selected References) of living human subjects of all ages demonstrated blockage of the inferior alveolar artery in almost 80% of all persons studied, and in 33% of the subjects arterial flow was absent. The incidence of blockage of the inferior alveolar artery increased with age. The reduction or absence in flow within the inferior alveolar artery may be associated with tooth extraction. Studies of completely edentulous humans indicated that the inferior alveolar artery degenerated to such an extent as to be negligible in the supply of blood to the mandible. In these cases, the blood supply to the bone and internal structures was dependent upon the connections with the external blood supply located within the periosteum and soft tissues associated with the mandible. Similar blood flow reversal with age has not been reported in the maxilla, but the final comment concerning blood flow in the aged edentulous maxilla awaits further investigation.

All bone cells lie within a distance of 0.1 mm of a blood supply. As mentioned previously, the blood supply is found within the marrow spaces, the periosteum, and within haversian canals. Tissue fluid from the arterial capillaries bathes the osteoblasts and supplies them with the necessary nutrients and oxygen. The osteocytes, which are surrounded by mineralized matrix, are also bathed by tissue fluid which reaches the cell by way of canaliculi. The canaliculi eventually join the lacunae which surround the cell bodies. The void between the cell body and its cellular processes and the lacunar and canalicular walls provides the space in which tissue fluid circulates. Waste products are returned to the bloodstream in the reverse direction.

EFFECTS OF VITAMINS ON BONE FORMATION AND REPAIR

Various vitamins and hormones can affect the formation and repair of bone tissue. It is essential that the dental practitioner understand these effects since the repair and replacement of bone around endosseous dental implants is an essential requirement for the success of the implant.

When bone tissue begins to form, the osteoblasts produce osteoid that consists primarily of type I collagen. The collagen precursors are produced by the osteoblasts and are secreted into the intercellular space where they mature into collagen. The proper production of collagen is dependent upon adequate quantities of vitamin C being available during the assembly of the collagen precursors within the osteoblasts. Inadequate amounts of vitamin C can lead to the disease known as *scurvy*. The repair process in both hard and soft tissues requires adequate amounts of vitamin C.

Once a normal osteoid is produced, the next process in the development of bone tissue is the mineralization of the osteoid. Proper mineralization is dependent upon the availability of proper quantities of calcium and phosphorous. Calcium and phosphorous absorption from the gut is dependent upon adequate supplies of vitamin D. The active metabolite of vitamin D is 1,25-dihydroxyvitamin D [1,25(OH$_2$)D]. Vitamin D is obtained in equal amounts from the diet and from an endogenous reaction within the skin produced by ultraviolet radiation. The vitamin D is converted to its active form [1,25(OH$_2$)D] in the kidneys. The active metabolite increases the absorption of both calcium and phosphorous from the gut. It also promotes osteoclastic resorption of bone which releases calcium and phosphorous and increases the serum levels of these minerals in the blood. Thus, inadequate amounts of vitamin D, or low levels of calcium and phosphorus within the body, can lead to a defective mineralization phase of bone formation. This defect leads to the condition known as *rickets* in the child, or to *osteomalacia* in the adult. In both conditions the amount of osteoid increases in the bone tissue since it continues to be produced, but it does not undergo normal mineralization.

Accordingly, each phase of bone formation is dependent upon critical vitamins and nutrients being available during the formative process. A vitamin C deficiency will not affect the mineralization phase of bone formation, just as a deficiency of vitamin D will not affect the initial organic (osteoid) phase of osteogenesis.

EFFECT OF HORMONES ON BONE FORMATION AND REPAIR

Parathyroid hormone (PTH) is produced by the parathyroid glands and controls the calcium and phosphate levels in the blood. Increased PTH release causes an increase in osteoclastic activity with a resultant rise in blood calcium levels. The parathyroid glands' secretion of PTH is determined by the concentration of calcium in the blood. Low levels of calcium initiate the release of PTH. Increased blood levels of calcium cause the parathyroid glands to cease their production of PTH. Thus, the level of calcium is under the control of PTH as well as vitamin D. Vitamin D works in conjunction with PTH to promote osteoclasia with the resultant release of calcium into the blood. In contrast, calcitonin (CT), also called thyrocalcitonin (TCT), promotes the lowering of calcium in the blood by inhibiting bone matrix resorption by decreasing the number and the activity of osteoclasts.

Other hormones that cause an increase in bone resorption include glucocorticoids and excess levels of thyroid hormone. The glucocorticoids decrease the absorption of calcium from the gut. In adults, excess levels of thyroid hormone (von Recklinghausen's disease) cause an increase in bone resorption by osteoclasts without a concurrent increase in bone formation. This leads to the thinning of trabeculae and increased porosity of the cortical bone which results in a net loss of bone from the skeleton. Fibrous tissue subsequently fills in the bony defects.

Hormones that produce an increase in bone formation include the sex hormones, growth hormone (normal levels), and normal levels of thyroid hormone. Sex hormones generally act to increase the amount of bone formation, although the exact mechanism of their actions is not known. The use of estrogens in the treatment of osteoporosis has become widespread. Apparently, this hormone acts by increasing the amount of calcium absorption in the small intestine. Postmenopausal women also have an increased response to PTH. While estrogen receptors have not been found in association with osteoclasts, it is felt that estrogen inhibits the action of PTH in some manner. Regardless of its mechanism of action, the use of estrogen in the treatment of osteoporosis in postmenopausal women has been clinically successful.

HEALING OF FRACTURED AND DAMAGED BONE

Like any other living cells, the cells of bone require an adequate supply of nutrients and oxygen to remain vital. When a bone is fractured the blood vessels within the fracture site are ruptured. The osteocytes supplied by these vessels are deprived of nourishment and die. Thus, nonvital bone is produced on both sides of the line of fracture. Blood from the vessels fills the tissue spaces and forms a clot.

The injury to the bone signals osteoprogenitor cells present in the periosteum, endosteum, and marrow (perivascular cells) to differentiate into osteoblasts. These cells, as well as other osteoblasts already present within the area, begin the process of new bone formation. The first bone that is formed in the damaged area is immature (woven, repair) bone. The purpose of this bone is to join the damaged bone fragments on either side of the fracture. This repair bone is also called the *callus*.

Simultaneously, osteoclasts that are located in the area, or that migrate into the area, begin the process of removal of necrotic bone. Much of the nonvital bone is removed by osteoclasts forming cutting cones which tunnel into the area of nonvital bone. Following the removal of the bone by the cutting cone, a capillary grows into the erosion tunnel bringing with it osteoprogenitor cells. These cells leave the capillary and move to the surface of the bony tunnel where they differentiate into osteoblasts and begin laying down bone. Eventually, all of the nonvital bone is removed and is replaced with mature bone.

RESPONSE OF BONE TO ENDOSTEAL IMPLANT PLACEMENT

According to Roberts and colleagues (see Selected References), approximately 1 mm of bone adjacent to an endosseous implant dies as a result of the trauma associated with the preparation of the implant site and the subsequent placement of the implant. The majority of the damage is due to inflammation and the interference with the blood supply to the cortical bone in these areas.

Between the bony wall of the surgical site and the surface of the implant a lattice of new bone is laid down rapidly by osteoblasts. This bone is an immature, trabecular type of bone, and as such does not have enough strength to resist masticatory loads. If given enough time prior to loading, the spaces between the lattice of immature bone will fill with mature (lamellar) bone so that most of the area between the original surgical site and the implant will consist of bone tissue. The resulting "compacted" bone (i.e., immature and mature bone with little space between) is quite strong and can resist the forces of mastication. Based on research with rabbits and dogs, Roberts et al. estimate that compaction of the

implant interface bone takes approximately 18 weeks in humans.

While compaction of bone at the surgical site is occurring, the nonvital bone in the area is also being removed. Necrotic bone is removed via osteoclastic activity on the bone surface facing the implant, or within the depths of the damaged bone. To remove the deeply placed necrotic bone, osteoclasts form cutting cones which burrow into the nonvital bone as described previously. The process differs from normal remodeling seen in cortical bone in that the secondary osteons which are produced by the process are oriented at right angles to the long axis of the bone rather than parallel to the long axis. Emanating from the initial erosion tunnels, other channels are formed which are at right angles to the implant interface surface.

Maintenance of the bone-implant interface requires the continuous remodeling of the bone at the interface as well as the surrounding supporting bone. The removal of fatigued bone at these sites is accomplished by osteoclasts using the cutting cone mechanism previously described. This system is quite efficient since osteoclasts tend to remove the most highly mineralized bone. Highly mineralized bone tends to be the oldest bone present in the area and as such is the bone that is most prone to be damaged.

The healing process just described applies only to cortical bone present at the implant site. The effects of implantation on trabecular bone are not well understood, and research is needed.

CONCLUSION

The dentist who places implants should understand the basic concepts of bone biology in order to increase the probability of successful treatment. The implantologist should have a firm understanding of the bone formation process as well as the process of bone repair. The practitioner should be aware of the effects of nutrition, vitamins, and hormones on normal bone development, as well as their effects on the repair process in bone. In addition, the role of the periosteum and endosteum in providing osteoprogenitor cells for the repair of bone at implant sites is essential if one is to consistently obtain successful results with endosseous implants. Finally, an understanding of the blood supply to bone will not only assist the dentist in performing successful implant surgery but will also be useful in understanding the basic techniques used in periodontal and oral surgery. It is hoped that this short review will encourage the dental implant practitioner to become more familiar with that very dynamic tissue we call bone.

Acknowledgments

Special thanks to Lewis Hinley for the medical illustrations, to Vera Larke for her photographic assistance, and to Linda Cullum for her excellent secretarial and editing skills.

SELECTED REFERENCES

Bell WH: Revascularization and bone healing after anterior maxillary osteotomy: A study using adult rhesus monkeys. *J Oral Surg* 1969; 27:249–255.

Bell WH: Biologic basis for maxillary osteotomies. *Am J Phys Anthropol* 1973; 38:279–290.

Bell WH, Levy BM: Revascularization and bone healing after anterior mandibular osteotomy. *J Oral Surg* 1970; 28:196–203.

Bourne GH: *The Biochemistry and Physiology of Bone,* ed 2, vols 1–4. New York, Academic Press, 1972–1976.

Bradley JC: Age changes in the vascular supply of the mandible. *Br Dent J* 1972; 132:142–144.

Bradley JC: A radiological investigation into the age changes of the inferior dental artery. *Br J Oral Surg* 1975; 13:82–90.

Brookes M: *The Blood Supply of Bone.* London, Butterworths & Co Ltd, 1971.

Castelli WA, Nasjleti CE, Diaz-Perez R: Interruption of the arterial inferior alveolar flow and its effects on mandibular collateral circulation and dental tissues. *J Dent Res* 1975; 54:708–715.

Cormack DH: *Ham's Histology.* Philadelphia, JB Lippincott Co, 1987.

DeLuca HF: Metabolism and mechanism of action of Vitamin D—1981, in Peck WA (ed): *Bone and Mineral Research Annual,* vol 1. New York, Elsevier Scientific Publishing, 1983, pp 7–73.

Enlow DH: *Handbook of Facial Growth.* Philadelphia, WB Saunders Co, 1975.

Frost HM: *The Physiology of Cartilagenous, Fibrous, and Bony Tissue,* vol 2. Springfield, Ill, Charles C Thomas, Publisher, 1972.

Hellem S, Ostrup LT: Normal and retrograde blood supply to the body of the mandible in the dog. II. The role played by periosteo-medullary and symphyseal anastomoses. *Int J Oral Surg* 1981; 10:31–42.

Peck WA: *Bone and Mineral Research,* vols 1–4. New York, Elsevier Scientific Publishing, 1983–1986.

Rhinelander FW: Circulation of Bone, in Bourne, GH (ed): *The Biochemistry and Physiology of Bone.* New York, Academic Press, 1972, pp 1–77.

Roberts WE, Smith RK, Zilberman Y, et al: Osseous adaptation of continuous loading of rigid endosseous implants. *Am J Orthod* 1984; 86:95–111.

Roberts WE, Turley PK, Brezniak N, et al: Bone physiology and metabolism. *J Calif Dent Assoc* 1987; 15:54–61.

Ten Cate AR: *Oral Histology: Development, Structure and Function.* St Louis, CV Mosby Co, 1985.

Tonna EA: Electron microscopy of aging skeletal cells III. The periosteum. *Lab Invest* 1975; 31:609–632.

Vaughn J.: *The Physiology of Bone.* Oxford, Clarendon Press, 1981.

Chapter 7

Evaluation and Selection of the Endosteal Implant Patient

Charles A. Babbush, D.D.S., M.Sc.D.

SELECTION OF PATIENT

Many factors are required to carry out and maintain successful long-range implant reconstruction. The implant modality itself must have proven efficacy. The professional team—surgical, restorative, and laboratory technician—must be adequately trained and clinically experienced to achieve success with their choice of implant system. Last, the patient must be appropriately screened and ultimately selected to initiate the entire reconstruction with a high degree of potential long-term success.

Over the past 20 years I have developed and worked with a system to evaluate and select the appropriate implant candidate. This chapter reviews my approach to the implant patient selection process. Basically, the patient is reviewed from both the dental and medical aspects.[1-11]

DENTAL EVALUATION

Various aspects of clinical dentistry must be included in this phase of the evaluation process in order to adequately review the potential candidacy for implant reconstruction.[5-8]

1. Dental history
2. Clinical examination
3. Radiographic review

   a. Periapical
   b. Panoramic
   c. Occlusal
   d. Lateral headplates
   e. Computed tomography (CT) scan
4. Study casts
5. Photographs

DENTAL HISTORY

The dental history of the patient is an extremely important aspect of the selection process. If the patient is totally edentulous the ability to evaluate the etiologic factors which contributed to the loss of dentition is much more difficult. The tooth loss may have been a result of periodontal disease, caries, trauma, tumors, or gross neglect. The decision-making process then becomes more difficult owing to the lack of adequate diagnostic information. The question remains as to whether the patient who has lost the natural dentition as a result of periodontal disease or gross neglect will repeat his or her past lack of care or maintenance and cause the premature loss of the implants. However, if the patient presents with a semiedentulous condition, a more accurate evaluation of the overall oral health status can be made. A comprehensive history of semiedentulous tooth loss must be obtained. The patient must be examined with regard to the total reconstruction—implant,

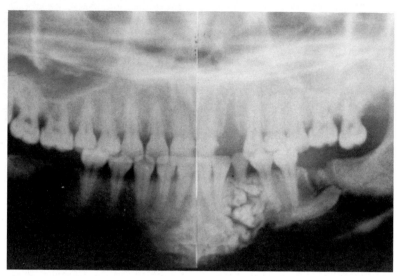

FIG 7–1.
Panoramic radiograph showing a pathologic region which should be eliminated prior to implant placement and reconstruction.

prosthodontic, periodontic—and rehabilitation. All other therapy, endodontic, periodontic, exodontic, oral surgical, and operative procedures, must be completed prior to implant placement.

If the patient presents with a tenuous dental history and oral environment, all preliminary procedures should be carried out and the patient placed in a transitional controlled program of oral hygiene. The patient should be followed for a period of 6 to 12 months. A reevaluation at that time will disclose the patient's ability and understanding related to the maintenance of a potential implant reconstruction. If this transitional period demonstrates a favorable result, a comprehensive treatment plan and reconstruction may then be carried out. On the other hand, if the patient's response or the results are negative, it is evident that implant rehabilitation is contraindicated.[8]

CLINICAL EXAMINATION

A comprehensive examination of the oral structures must be carried out in conjunction with the dental history. This evaluation should be performed

FIG 7–2.
Panoramic radiograph demonstrating the presence of postextraction defects as well as a postoperative pathologic defect. There should be no evidence of this type of defect prior to implant placement.

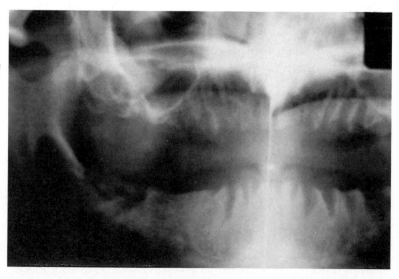

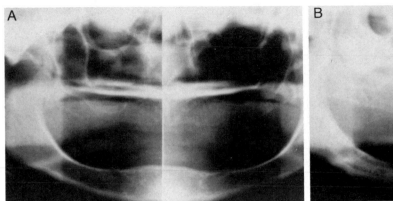
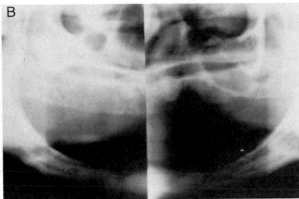

FIG 7–3.
A, panoramic radiograph demonstrating the lack of trabecular patterns. **B,** panoramic radiograph demonstrating a consistent dense trabecular pattern.

in an orderly precise fashion, on a routine basis.

The hard and soft tissue should be evaluated as to both quality and quantity. The radiographs must be evaluated in conjunction with this portion of the clinical examination to ensure the absence of pathologic bony defects (Fig 7–1). The complete healing of postextraction defects should also be verified by the absence of postextraction defects or phantoms on the radiograph (Fig 7–2). The presence of a good trabecular pattern should be verified (Fig 7–3,A and B).

The abscence of tori as related especially to the potential prosthetic reconstruction should be noted and treatment planned for modification or removal (Fig 7–4). The soft tissues, especially in the intended area of implantation, should be evaluated for unfavorable frenum (Fig 7–5) and muscle attachments and for the presence of attached gingiva (Fig 7–6). If there is not sufficient quality or quantity of keratinized tissue at these critical locations, the treatment plan should be modified to include a satisfactory grafting procedure to rectify the situation. With the increased use of two-stage osteointegration procedures the use of soft tissue grafts has increased and is recommended in the treatment at the time of the second-stage implant recovery or reopening session. This consolidates the number of surgical procedures that the patient must undergo and establishes the exact location of the implant at this time, thus avoiding miscalculations.

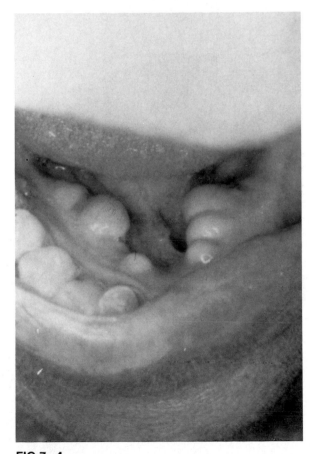

FIG 7–4.
A clinical photograph of bilateral lingual tori which could interfere with implant placement and subsequent prosthetic reconstruction.

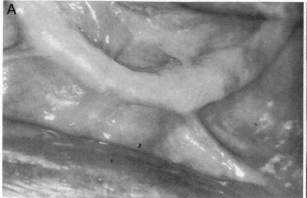

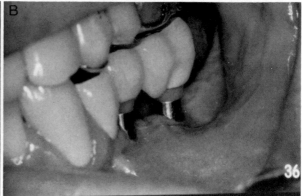

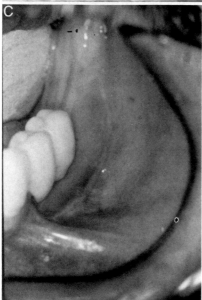

FIG 7–5.
A, clinical photograph demonstrates an unfavorable frenum which must be modified to obtain a favorable long-range prognosis. **B,** mucosal tissue surrounds the implant posts instead of the attached gingiva. **C,** this photograph depicts an unfavorable muscle attachment in the bicuspid area.

FIG 7–6.
Attached or keratinized gingival tissue should be present in the immediate implant abutment area in order to *maintain* a high level of periodontal integrity and health.

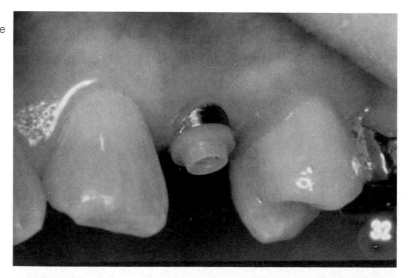

The jaw relationships must be accurately evaluated, especially when severe Class II or III abnormalities are present. Interceptive orthodontics or combined orthodontic-orthognathic surgical correction may be required before implant reconstruction.

The number and health of the opposing and adjacent dentition must be evaluated. A long-range favorable prognosis for these dental units must be determined. In many instances we have found that a dental unit with a guarded prognosis may be a hazard to overall survival of a comprehensive rehabilitation. Therefore, in many instances these compromised teeth are indicated for removal.

Jaw movement in all directions—lateral, protrusive, and vertical—must be evaluated before initating therapy. Restriction of motion may impair surgical as well as prosthetic procedures and the final reconstruction. Parafunctional habits should be diagnosed, treated whenever possible, and the treatment plan developed with these habits in mind. Occlusal compromises or pathologic conditions must be evaluated and corrected prior to final treatment.

Each aspect of the oral and dental clinical examination has its place in diagnosis and treatment. Only with these factors in mind can one hope to achieve a favorable long-range prognosis for implant reconstruction.

RADIOGRAPHS

The radiographic examination remains one of the most valuable of diagnostic tools. The practitioner must identify the adjacent vital structures such as the floor of the nasal cavity, the floor of the maxillary sinus, the mandibular canal, and the mental foramen (Fig 7–7). The use of only periapical radiographs severely limits these findings (Fig 7–8). The panoramic radiograph allows for a more comprehensive view and better interpretation of these anatomic structures. In the totally edentulous patient, especially in the mandible, the lateral mandibular radiograph is very beneficial because it relates to symphyseal angulation, thickness, and true vertical bone height (Fig 7–9). The use of an occlusal film at the region of the symphysis exposed with the periapical radiographic machine may provide an accurate two-dimensional interpretation of this area.

The CT scan (Dentascan, MPDI, Torrence, Calif.) has the ability to go beyond the standard two-dimensional radiographs mentioned above. The production of exact cross-sectional radiographic views (three-dimensional) of the residual bone of the mandible or maxilla is possible with the use of specialized computer algorithms to enhance the standard axial CT examination. The patient is placed in a comfortable supine position, the head immobilized with tape or Velcro, and scanned in the axial plane.

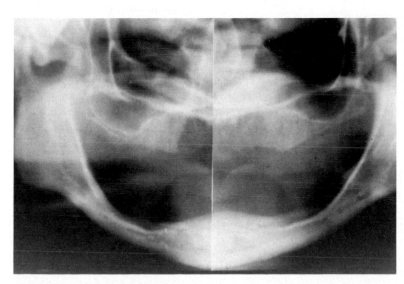

FIG 7–7.
A good panoramic radiograph will enable the surgeon to identify the anatomic boundaries of such vital structures as the maxillary sinus, nasal cavity, inferior alveolar canal, and mental foramen.

FIG 7–8.
Two periapical radiographs were superimposed over the panoramic view demonstrating the loss of anatomic as well as pathologic entities.

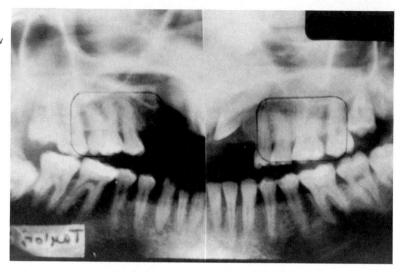

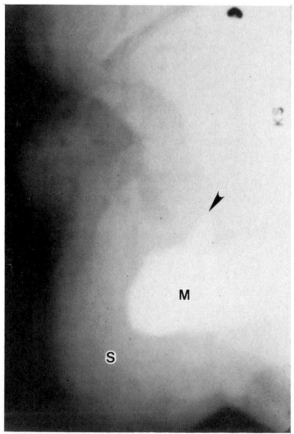

FIG 7–9.
A lateral jaw radiograph allows identification of the height, width, angulation, and even the genial tubercle *(arrowhead)* of the mandible *(M)*. Soft tissues of the face are also visualized *(S)*.

The total examination (patient time) takes less than 30 minutes per jaw. The data can then be rearranged by the computer software program which yields cross-sectional images that are exactly perpendicular to the curvature of the alveolar ridges. When scanning data of this type are used, it is called *multiplanar reformation (CT/MPR)*. This technology allows the surgeon in the presurgical planning to first establish the candidacy of the patient. If sufficient quantities of residual bone are available, then it can provide the necessary knowledge as to the exact three-dimensional size and location of endosseous implants as well as avoid or minimize the risk to adjacent vital structures.

CT/MPR allows visualization of the maxilla or mandible in three views. The axial plane is the plane in which the patient has actually been viewed by the scanner. This is the first view. Two additional projections are then processed by the computer. A series of CT panoramic interpretations, similar to conventional panoramic views, are also displayed (Fig 7–10,A and B).

Radiographic Measurement Template

The use of presurgical measurement splints has been an accurate cost-effective means of determining various bone dimensions. Study casts should be mounted on a semiadjustable articulator. A clear acrylic splint is fabricated to extend over the edentulous areas of the arch where implant placement is an-

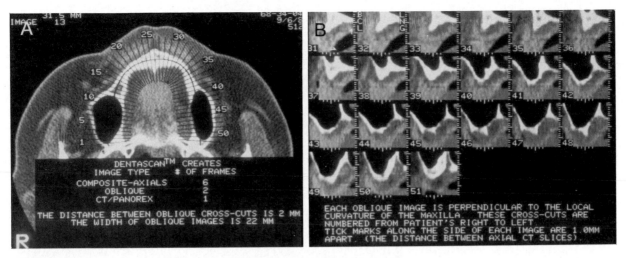

FIG 7–10.
A, an occlusal CT view of the maxilla with a series of oblique cross-sectional lines perpendicular to the curvature of the ridge.
B, cross-sectional CT images are viewed individually.

ticipated. This fabrication can be carried out nicely with an Omni-Vac procedure. The intended implant site should be marked on the cast. A compatible bur is used to create a slight depression in the acrylic splint. A 5-mm precision stainless steel ball bearing* is placed mesial and distal to the intended implant site. The ball bearing is secured with one drop of Super Glue (Fig 7–11). Once the ball bearing is secured, the entire splint is placed in the oral cavity

*Implant Support Systems, Irvine, Calif.

and a panoramic radiograph is obtained (Fig 7–12). The ball bearing image on the radiograph is measured with a millimeter gauge to determine the distortion factor of bone in a vertical fashion. If the 5-mm ball bearing now measures 6 mm on the radiograph, a 20% distortion factor is present. Therefore, for each multiple of 6 mm, or fraction thereof, there is only 5 mm of available bone for placement of an endosseous implant. In a similar fashion the splint can be maintained in the oral cavity and an occlusal film may be exposed to obtain a

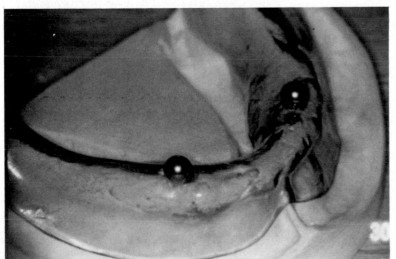

FIG 7–11.
A mandibular template with 5-mm precision stainless steel ball bearings secured in position.

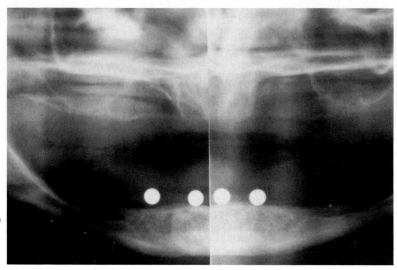

FIG 7–12.
The radiograph is obtained with the 5-mm ball bearings in position. The true vertical dimension of bone is then calculated.

guide as to the buccolingual or the horizontal dimension of bone in the area of the intended implant site. In the totally edentulous mandible a straight lateral radiograph will also provide knowledge of bony dimension at the midsymphyseal area.

The presence of pathologic entities should preclude implant placement. The abnormality should be corrected, excised, or revised, and a sufficient postsurgical period should ensue to allow for healing and a healthy receptor site to be established. These decisions are usually confirmed by posttreatment radiographs which would demonstrate the lack of any further bony defects.

STUDY CASTS

The use of diagnostic study casts has been well documented over the years. All cases, whether they be a single tooth replacement or a full-arch implant prosthetic reconstruction, would benefit by study casts mounted on a semiadjustable articulator (Fig 7–13). Only with this diagnostic and planning tool can the centric relationship, interarch occlusal clearance, occlusal discrepancies, and opposing and adjacent dentition be evaluated. With this method the number and position of required implants can be evaluated, based on diagnostic wax-ups of the potential reconstruction.

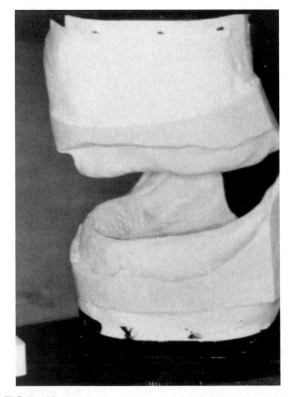

FIG 7–13.
Mounted study casts should be used for presurgical evaluation whether or not the patient is edentulous.

PHOTOGRAPHS

Most practitioners agree that treatment is carried out today in a litigious environment. For this reason alone, pretreatment photographic documentation is an excellent format for increased-risk management practice. Photographic documentation is also of value during the formulation of the treatment plan to allow recall of the anatomy, physical structures, and so forth in the absence of the patient; it is especially valuable in the team approach to implant reconstruction procedures. The surgical and prosthetic restorative team members will have a more realistic concept without the physical presence of the patient during their diagnostic and treatment planning sessions. On numerous occasions over the past 20 years, patients have expressed their needs, wants, and desires of implant reconstruction to be related to the restoration of function, improved chewing and speaking ability, increased retention and security, and the elimination of pain. Unfortunately, many are really seeking rejuvenation, a fact which they either conceal from us, intentionally or otherwise. In most instances a functional success is obtained for patients in general. Unfortunately, this goal does not always match the patient's expectations, and if an esthetically pleasing, cosmetic, "youthful," result is not achieved, a potential patient failure may surface. The presentation at this time of the pretreatment photographs—full face, lateral face, and intraoral views—can in most instances reverse this potentially negative psychological result.

MEDICAL EVALUATION

Since the head, neck, and maxillofacial region are integral parts of the human body, there is no means by which they can be evaluated without a review of the medical aspects of each implant candidate. After all these years, it is still my firm belief that a comprehensive health questionnaire should be the first avenue of review for each potential implant patient. The American Dental Association long-form health questionnaire remains my mainstay.*

*American Dental Association, 211 E. Chicago Ave., Chicago, IL 60611.

Evaluation of the Medical History

Once the health questionnaire is completed by the patient, it should be reviewed by the practitioner as he or she is the person with the training, clinical experience, and final decision making capability as to whether or not the patient is a potential candidate for surgery and subsequent reconstruction. The areas that should receive primary attention are the following[8–11]:

- Cardiovascular system
- Respiratory system
- Gastrointestinal system
- Excretory system
- Nervous system
- Endocrine system
- Vascular system
- Skin and mucous membranes

Diseases of the Cardiovascular System
Patients with a history of cardiac disease, including angina, myocardial infarction, and arrhythmias, are subject to recurrent episodes when placed in a stressful situation. Even placement of a single implant could compromise cardiovascular function.

Many cardiovascular abnormalities, such as coronary artery disease, are amenable to surgical correction. Many of these patients are then susceptible to infections, or complications of the graft site, or both. Rheumatic heart disease, as well as mitral valve prolapse, are categories to which the practitioner must give attention. Careful consideration should be given to the prophylactic use of antibiotics and consultation with the patient's physician. This group of patients is usually indicated for some method of intravenous sedation for tranquilization to allay fears and emotional trauma with the reduction of intraoperative stress.

Diseases of the Respiratory System
Several diseases of the respiratory system interfere with the ability to function in normal daily activities and therefore change the normal physiology of the body. Chronic bronchitis, pulmonary embolism, emphysema, and lung tumors may severely interfere with the normal healing mechanisms of the

body. These pathologic processes may create a potentially high risk for this patient intraoperatively or may entirely contraindicate surgery.

Diseases of the Gastrointestinal (GI) System

Such states as nervous stomach with vomiting, hypersecretions, xerostomia, and hyperacidity all contribute to changes in the pH of the saliva, which will interfere with healing of the mucous membranes.

Various ulcers of the GI tract are sometimes indicative of the patient's life stresses and strains. This may be revealing with regard to the overall treatment, as this patient may manifest his or her emotional states in the form of bruxism, clenching, or various tongue habits which may, in turn, contribute to eccentric forces being applied to the implant that will lead to its failure.

Diarrhea, constipation, and colitis are significant factors in the ability to properly digest food and maintain emotional stability.

The liver has many functions, some of which, when impaired, may influence the normal healing mechanisms. These functions include the storage, filtration, and formation (on demand) of blood cells; carbohydrate metabolism; production of prothrombin and other coagulation factors; synthesis of plasma proteins; and so on.

In recent years eating disorders—anorexia, bulimia, etc.—have been recognized as being detrimental to the oral structures. These patients should be carefully evaluated prior to implant therapy. In addition, consultation with the treating professional staff is strongly recommended.

Diseases of the Kidney and Urinary Tract

The kidneys are responsible for filtering the blood, among other functions. They excrete the waste products of body metabolism. Such disease states as nephritis, glomerulonephritis, chronic urinary tract infections, and tumors of the kidney will all cause disturbances of normal kidney function, and thus a change in the normal composition of the blood. Since kidney transplants are becoming a more common procedure, consultation with the patient's

physician should be sought prior to initiating any implant procedure on an organ transplant patient.

Diseases of the Nervous System

Epileptics are subject to convulsive disorders followed by states of unconsciousness. The forces that can be exerted during these seizures can be traumatic to implants. In addition, many of these patients are treated with phenytoin (Dilantin), an anticonvulsant.

One of the effects of phenytoin is gingival hypertrophy, which occurs only when teeth are present. The epileptic patient who has implants may be subject to gingival hypertrophy around the abutment neck and should be warned of this possibility because subsequent surgical corrections may be necessary.

Other neurologic disorders, such as trigeminal neuralgia, Bell's palsy, glossopharyngeal neuralgias, or existing paresthesia, should be noted on the patient's medical history preoperatively.

Diseases of the Endocrine System

The eight endocrine glands in the body are responsible for numerous functions dealing with growth, sexual development, metabolism, and reproduction.

Such states as gigantism, dwarfism, and acromegaly all demonstrate abnormal growth with subsequent abnormally large or small maxillofacial skeletal size which could influence implant intervention. Myxedema and cretinism are also states which lead to retarded dental development, either in pattern of eruption or with malformation of the structures.

The parathyroid glands are responsible primarily for calcium and phosphorus metabolism. Ninety-nine percent of body calcium is found in the organic matrix of bone and teeth. Calcium is essential for numerous functions in the body. The formation of bone and teeth as well as its role in the coagulation of blood are among the more important actions of calcium. Therefore, any abnormal calcium activity in the body requires complete review before placement of dental implants.

The islands of Langerhans, which lie in the pancreas, secrete insulin. The most common disease associated with the pancreas is diabetes—the inability of the body to metabolize carbohydrates. Diabetics are prone to periodontal disease; they have a decrease in local as well as general resistance to infection. The selection of the diabetic patient to receive implants must be carefully considered. Consultation with the patient's physician should also be sought. Patients should be informed of the potential for complications or failure related to their preexisting disease.

Diseases of the Blood

The patient with anemia should be treated with care, as even an elective surgical procedure can cause a sudden drop in the blood count. A marked increase in leukocytes and hyperplasia of the tissues that form white blood cells is termed *leukemia.* Any form of acute leukemia would contraindicate dental implants. Continuous bleeding with ulcerative stomatitis is a frequent finding. The chronic leukemias are usually not as violent, but the oral symptoms are similar.

Classic hemophilia is found only in males and is characterized by a deficiency of plasma factor VIII. These patients have prolonged bleeding following the most minute trauma or surgical procedure. Usually these patients are not considered for dental implants.

The category of pathologic entities known as purpuras are characterized by hemorrhage into the skin and mucous membranes. These patients will have prolonged or spontaneous bleeding and should not be considered for dental implants.

A group of drugs, anticoagulants, are used to "thin out the blood." Heparin, given only intravenously, will cause an increase in the coagulation time. Warfarin sodium (Coumadin) prolongs the prothrombin time and can be administered orally as well as intravenously. Both of these drugs will cause hemorrhage, and patients taking them are poor implant candidates. If these patients can be regulated to a more normal level for favorable intraoperative and postoperative safety, they may be acceptable candidates. Consultation and teamwork with the attending physician or hematologist are advisable.

Diseases of the Skin and Mucous Membranes (Dermatologic)

Such pathologic states as lichen planus, erythema multiforme, lupus erythematosus, and pemphigus all affect the mucous membranes and skin. This group has also been categorized as collagen or connective tissue defects. Patients with these disorders will often be very ill and will not even present for dental treatment. However, many of these patients will have subacute or mild cases of these diseases and will seek treatment. In general, this category of patients is a poor group for implant restoration, as the physiologic healing mechanism is impaired.

Malignant Disease

Many patients with malignancies are treated by radiation therapy or antimetabolites or both. Patients who have had, or are receiving, radiation therapy to the head and neck region have a change in the normal physiologic processes of the mucous membranes and bone. The vascular supply to regions either primarily or secondarily irradiated has been impaired. When an elective procedure, such as an implant insertion, is carried out, the additional interruption of the tissues may be sufficient to cause further impaired vascular supply with a resultant failure or even radiation osteonecrosis. However, recent reports have demonstrated favorable two-stage osteointegrated reconstruction in selected cases.[12]

Chemotherapeutic agents severely affect the overall physiologic composition of the body, with a resultant decrease in its ability to protect itself against infection. Implant reconstruction is usually contraindicated for patients who have been or are being so treated. However, consultation with the oncologist should be sought to determine the return to a physiologic normal baseline.

Laboratory Tests
Sequential Multiple Analyzer (SMA 12/60, SMA 6/60).—Blood studies are considered to be a good overall screening mechanism and an integral part of the patient's overall evaluation.[1–6, 8]

SUMMARY

Since my writings[8] in the 1970s and early 1980s, many aspects and modalities of implant reconstructive procedures have changed. Instead of being concerned about the proximity of the maxillary sinus, inferior alveolar neurovascular bundle, or the inferior border of the mandible to the implant body or its apical portion, we are now concerned about filling, augmenting, and moving these anatomic structures to allow reconstruction of otherwise impossible cases. However, we must be aware of and knowledgeable about the various anatomic variations, diagnostic tools, and implant modalities that will be most efficacious for our patients.

REFERENCES

1. American Academy of Implant Dentistry (AAID): *Implant Criteria Workshop,* Dearborn, Mich, June 1976.
2. American Dental Association, Council on Dental Materials and Devices and Dental Research: *Workshop on Dental Implants,* Chicago, December 1975.
3. Babbush CA: Medical contra-indications and the implant candidate. Presented at the American Academy of Implant Dentistry Annual Meeting, Washington, DC, November 1974.
4. Babbush CA: Selection of the implant candidate. Lecture presented at the University of Southern California, July 1975.
5. Bicoll NA: Preparation, the keywork for implant dentistry. *J Oral Implantol* 1973; 3:4.
6. Franko JM: Blood scanning in oral implantology patients. *Oral Health* 1976; 66:5,34–36.
7. Dripps RD, Eckenhoff JE, Vandam LD: *Introduction to Anesthesia,* ed 5. Philadelphia, WB Saunders Co, 1977.
8. Babbush CA: *Surgical Atlas of Dental Implant Techniques.* Philadelphia, WB Saunders Co, 1980.
9. Rose LF, Kaye D (eds): *Internal Medicine for Dentistry,* ed 2. St Louis, CV Mosby Co, 1990.
10. Scully C, Causpm RA: *Medical Problems in Dentistry.* Boston, Wright-PSG, 1982.
11. Little JW, Falace DA: *Dental Management of the Medically Compromised Patient.* St Louis, CV Mosby Co, 1984.
12. Esser E, Montag H: Conventional transplant surgery and endosseous implants—A treatment concept for rehabilitation after radical tumor surgery of the mandible. *Dtsch Z Mund Kiefer Gesichtschir* 1987; 11:77–87.

Chapter 8

Basic Surgical Principles for Implantology

David W. Shelton, D.M.D.

In this chapter, some of the principles of surgery are explored. Because dental implantology involves the placement of a foreign body into the bone of the jaws and because this implant must communicate with the oral environment and eventually bear considerable forces, it is clear that these principles are especially basic to dental implantology. Wound healing is briefly reviewed as well as factors which tend to enhance and impede it. Because surgical intervention is required, hemostasis is discussed along with aspects of detecting potential problems with blood clotting. A number of pharmacotherapeutic agents are used in the treatment of the dental implant patient including local anesthetics, sedative agents, antibiotics, and analgesics. Factors that may alter the expected response to a particular drug or a particular dose of a drug in an individual patient are reviewed and discussed. The microbiology of wound infections is reviewed as well as basic considerations operative in managing these infections. The role of surgical incision and drainage, debridement, and antimicrobial chemotherapy is discussed.

WOUND HEALING

Wound healing is one of the most basic considerations in surgery. The day-to-day clinical practice of surgery, whether it be in the operating room or in the office, must be based upon a knowledge of the biochemical and mechanical aspects of the tissue reparative phenomenon. Unquestionably, wound healing is altered in a number of pathologic as well as nonpathologic states. Diabetes mellitus, anemia, uremia, and jaundice are examples of pathologic states, and advanced age is an example of a physiologic state in which wound healing is impaired. Surprisingly, relatively little attention has been accorded the wound healing process, either on a clinical or experimental research level.

Connective tissue repair and the formation of scar tissue are the hallmarks of soft tissue wounds. Granulation tissue forms within the space of the wound. Granulation tissue is a highly vascularized and cellular tissue. It is within this environment that collagen and the components of ground substance are laid down. The quantity of scar tissue laid down is proportional to the quantity of granulation tissue formed.[1]

Healing of soft tissue wounds may occur in two ways. When the edges of an incised wound are approximated and maintained in an appropriate way, i.e., with sutures, primary healing occurs. When tissue is lost or when the wound edges become separated, as with wound dehiscence, secondary wound healing takes place. There is considerably more granulation tissue formation associated with wounds healing in this fashion and, subsequently, greater scarring. The collagen fibrils of the connective tissue and of the ground substance are derived from the granulation tissue. The normal formation and structure of connective tissue is briefly reviewed below as a precursor to wound healing.

Collagen

Collagen is produced within the fibroblast cell.[2] Collagen production begins with the synthesis on the intracellular ribosomes of three polypeptide chains known as alpha chains. The alpha chains contain a high content of the amino acids proline and lysine, which are converted to hydroxyproline and hydroxylysine by enzymatic processes during the ribosomal phase of collagen synthesis.[3] Among other things, the process requires ascorbic acid and oxygen. It has been shown that deficiency of ascorbic acid (vitamin C) and tissue hypoxia (anemia) have adverse effects on wound healing. It should also be mentioned here that measurements of hydroxyproline and the turnover of radioactively labeled proline are indicators of collagen metabolism.

The next step in the collagen synthesis pathway is glycosylation of the collagen which also requires enzymatic processes. It is also dependent upon the hydroxylation of lysine taking place at the ribosomal level. Variations in the proportion of lysine residues which are hydroxylated and the degree of glycosylation accounts for the various types of collagen.

After the final bonding together of the alpha chains, the collagen molecule is extruded from the fibroblast cell. The source of energy enabling the collagen molecule to be extruded from the fibroblast cell is probably adenosine triphosphate.[4] The mature collagen provides the healing wound with mechanical strength.

Ground Substance

Varying amounts of amorphous material between the cells and the fibers is present in virtually all connective tissues. It is a colloid-rich phase in equilibrium with a water-rich phase.[5] This amorphous material contains electrolytes, water, glycoproteins, and compounds called *proteoglycans*. The proteoglycans are comprised of several types of chondroitins, sulfates, and hyaluronic acid. Proteoglycans are synthesized by fibroblasts.[6] The precise

function of these molecules is not known but they are in some way involved in collagen maturation.[7]

The polymorphic glycoprotein fibronectin has been shown to be an important component of connective tissue. It is present in the blood and basement membranes of all vertebrates. The circulating form of fibronectin is called *cold-insoluble globulin*.[8] Fibronectin is synthesized by connective tissue fibroblasts.[9] It appears to have an important role in the cell-to-cell and cell-to-matrix adhesion in tissues.[10] In addition, recent information suggests that fibronectin stimulates platelet-collagen adhesion at sites of endothelial injury.[11]

Another fibrous protein, elastin, also synthesized by fibroblasts, occurs to a limited extent in scar tissue. Apparently, for this reason, the scar tissue of healing wounds is very brittle and inelastic, leading to suggestions that elastic tissue does not regenerate. However, two studies have cast doubt on this conclusion and have indeed shown that elastic fibers do appear in soft tissue healing wounds after approximately 60 days.[12, 13]

Cellular Components of Wound Healing

Healing of soft tissue wounds is generally accepted to occur in three phases. The first phase of soft tissue wound healing consists of inflammation and mobilization of the cells which will produce granulation tissue. In the second phase, granulation tissue appears in the wound and proteoglycans and collagen are formed by the granulation tissue. As a result, the mechanical strength of the wound is increased. In the third phase, there is extensive remodeling and additional increase in the strength of the wound.

The first phase is characterized by an immediate vascular response, i.e., vasoconstriction of vessels in the wound margins which is quickly followed by vasodilation and changes in capillary flow. With slowing of the blood flow, polymorphonuclear neutrophil leukocytes adhere to the walls of the capillaries. There is an increase in capillary permeability.

Studies have shown that polymorphonuclear leukocytes and some lymphocytes are present in the wound within 3 hours, and these cells are surrounded by a network of glycoproteins (including fibronectin) and fibrin.[14] By the fifth day mononuclear macrophages become dominant in the wound and are actively engaged in phagocytosis. Endothelial cell proliferation from capillaries in the wound edges also occurs in the first stage of wound healing. There is some evidence to suggest that the young endothelial cells secrete a plasminogen activator which digests fibrin along the path of the advancing capillaries.[15] Fibroblasts, derived from undifferentiated mesenchymal cells, also appear in the late stages of the first phase of wound repair.[16]

The second phase of soft tissue wound healing is characterized by the appearance of extracellular collagen and proteoglycans synthesized by the fibroblasts and is detectable by the fourth or fifth day.[17] Fibroblasts and endothelium become more prominent and the endothelial cells acquire a lumen and communicate with the capillaries of the wound margin. At the height of the second stage of wound healing, the wound appears filled with vascular granulation tissue encompassing capillaries, fibroblasts, macrophages, and mast cells. By the fifth or sixth day after wounding the collagen within the wound begins to interdigitate with the collagen of the incisional space and these changes in collagen account for the development of the intrinsic mechanical strength of the wound.[18]

The third phase of wound healing is characterized by decreased numbers of fibroblasts, capillaries, and macrophages. Cellularity in the wound becomes progressively less with only a few inflammatory cells and foreign body giant cells or round cells remaining around buried suture material. The final appearance is that of a dense and relatively avascular scar of collagen fibers.

Chemical Mediators

A number of chemical mediators may be involved in wound healing. In the early phase of wound healing, histamine from platelets and tissue mast cells may be the initiators of vasodilation following injury.[19]

There is some evidence to suggest that serotonin, bradykinin, kallidin, and prostaglandins all act as mediators.[20] Leukocyte emigration may be due to several chemotactic agents. Serum complement provides for some chemotactic factors.[21] Several bacterial factors are involved in leukotaxis, and it has been suggested that kallikrein as well as some prostaglandins is a leukocyte emigration mediator.[22]

Bone Healing

With respect to the healing of bone following injury by trauma or surgery, the process of repair is characterized by many of the same events that take place during healing of soft tissue injuries. The wound space is filled with blood and there follows the appearance of polymorphonuclear neutrophil leukocytes, lymphocytes, and a network of glycoproteins, including fibronectin, and fibrin. The site then becomes infiltrated by mononuclear macrophages as the process progresses. Fibroblasts and endothelium become more prominent. The vascular granulation tissue consisting of capillaries, fibroblasts, macrophages, and mast cells, accompanied by osteoblasts and osteoclasts (derived from pluripotential mesenchymal cells, endosteum, and periosteum), give way to a considerable quantity of collagen which spans the defect. This defect-spanning mass of fibroblasts, collagen, osteoblasts, osteoclasts, and contributing ground substance material constitutes the callus. An external callus is characteristic of cartilaginous bone healing and an internal callus is characteristic of membrane bone healing. In the absence of pathologic complications or mechanical interferences, the callus takes up inorganic material and ossifies.

Summary

Thus, in summary, healing of wounds and injuries of soft tissue and bone proceeds in identifiable stages:

1. An immediate vascular response, i.e., vasoconstriction followed by vasodilation with emigration of inflammatory cells into the wound space.
2. The initial contents of the wound space are replaced by macrophages and fibroblasts. Synthesis of collagen becomes apparent during this phase.

3. The wound becomes more acellular during this phase and the collagen undergoes a virtually complete remodeling.

HEMOSTASIS

As with wound healing, hemostasis is basic to surgery. Every surgeon is obligated to be in possession of knowledge, in some depth, of the biologic and mechanical processes involved in hemostasis. The normal and intact mechanisms are more than adequate to promptly seal off bleeding resulting from loss of integrity of the capillaries and small vessels. Bleeding from larger vessels may require additional interventions, i.e., applied pressure, stick tie, clamping and suture ligation, and on occasion ligation of selected regional vessels. When the normal hemostatic mechanism fails, dramatic, even torrential and overwhelming hemorrhage may ensue following seemingly minor trauma.

Hemostasis involves a complex integrated interaction of blood vessels, platelets, and coagulation cascade to form a localized stable mechanical seal that subsequently undergoes slow removal by fibrinolysis.[23]

Blood Vessels and Endothelium

Cellular metabolic exchange takes place as blood flows through the capillaries. All blood vessels are lined by endothelium. In the orderly combination of related and successive events constituting hemostasis, endothelial cells contribute in a number of ways. For example, they represent a barrier to the formed elements of the blood, the synthesis of factor VIII/vWF (von Willebrand factor), fibronectin, and the processes of vascular repair. So long as the endothelium is undisturbed it is nonreactive with the constituents of the circulating blood such as platelets and coagulation factors. Disruption of the endothelium promptly results in vasoconstriction, adhesion of platelets to exposed subendothelial surfaces, the coagulation cascade is initiated, and finally, fibrinolysis is begun by the release of activator substances from the endothelial cells.

Platelets

Platelets circulate in the blood as small, colorless, biconcave disks. They are produced by the megakaryocyte of the bone marrow and are approximately 3 μm in diameter or a little less than half the size of the red blood cell. Under normal conditions there are between 150,000 and 300,000 circulating platelets per microliter. When the platelet count drops below about 60,000/μL there may be excessive bleeding following a surgical procedure that leaves raw surfaces, for example secondary epithelialization vestibuloplasty, or a similar procedure. When the platelet count drops below 20,000/μL the patient develops a serious bleeding tendency which may include a threat of central nervous system bleeding.[24] The normal life span of the platelet is approximately 8 to 10 days. They are then removed by phagocytosis, primarily in the liver. Without adequate numbers of platelets (thrombocytopenia) normal hemostasis is impossible. The primary functions of platelets are maintenance of vascular integrity by sealing over endothelial disruptions, initial plugging of vascular defects, contribution of clotting factors (primarily platelet factor 3) to the coagulation cascade, and promotion of vascular healing.

Coagulation

Blood clotting is initiated either by surface-mediated factors (intrinsically) or by a tissue-derived factor pathway (extrinsically).[25] The two systems converge upon a final common pathway which leads to the insoluble fibrin gel which is formed when thrombin acts on fibrinogen. The coagulation cascade is outlined in Figure 8–1.[26]

The activation of factor VII by tissue thromboplastin (factor III), which becomes exposed when the vessel is disrupted, constitutes the extrinsic system. The activation of factor XII by any one of several means, severance of the vessel with a scalpel being one example, exposing the blood vessel surface with resultant cascading of the other coagulation factors, represents the intrinsic system.

The subsequent conversion of factor X to its active form is the meeting point of the two systems and

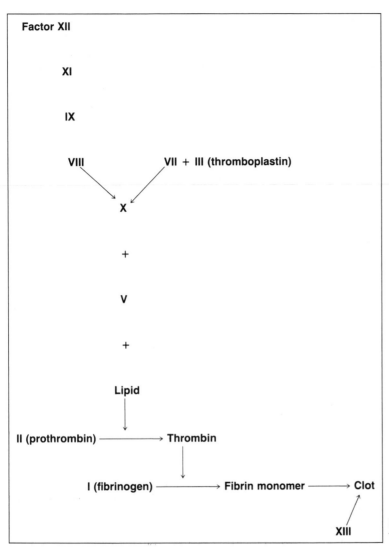

FIG 8–1.
The coagulation cascade.

represents the common pathway. In its active form and in the presence of lipid, factor V then mediates the conversion of prothrombin to thrombin. Thrombin splits the fibrinogen molecule. The resulting fibrin monomer polymerizes to form the clot which is stabilized by factor XIII. All of the coagulation factors (with the probable exception of factors VIII and VIII/vWF) are synthesized in the liver. Thus, conditions effecting the liver may produce a bleeding diathesis. Alcoholic liver cirrhosis is one example.

The implant surgeon should note that there are three important individual coagulation tests which

may document positive findings in the history: the prothrombin time (PT), the partial thromboplastin time (PTT), and the bleeding time.

The PT is the time to clot formation in vitro, normally 10 to 15 seconds. The factors primarily measured by the PT are II, VII, V, and X. It is, thus, essentially a test of the extrinsic system. These four factors are dependent upon vitamin K for their binding properties. At the present time, the most commonly used anticoagulant drug is warfarin sodium (Coumadin). Warfarin acts by depressing synthesis in the liver of factors VII, IX, X, and II. Following oral administration, hypoprothrombinemia is induced in 36 to 72 hours. Its half-life is 2½ days; its effect, however, may persist for 4 to 5 days after stopping the drug. Excessive prothrombinopenia, with or without bleeding, is readily controlled by stopping the drug, and if necessary, the administration of vitamin K_1.

The PTT is the time to clot formation in vitro, normally 25 to 35 seconds. The primary factors evaluated by the PTT are XII, XI, IX, VIII, X, and V; thus, it is a test of the intrinsic system. The congenital abnormalities of coagulation, i.e., the hemophilias, are manifestations of factors of the intrinsic system.

It should be remembered that the function of platelets is to plug small holes in blood vessels and to contribute in a major way to the formation of the clot. Neither the PT nor the PTT provides any information about platelet function. The bleeding time is normally 4.5 minutes and is a reasonable measure of platelet function. It is especially useful when the patient gives a history of bruising or bleeding. A bleeding time of 8 to 10 minutes should be considered borderline and beyond 10 minutes is an indication of a significant bleeding diathesis.

In terms of platelet function, aspirin is of particular clinical interest. Aspirin is a commonly used drug and is contained in a number of compounds which are available without prescription. Platelet ag-

gregation is mediated, in part, by the platelet prostaglandin pathway, summarized in Figure 8–2. Arachidonic acid is released from the platelet membrane during aggregation and is metabolized by the enzyme cyclooxygenase to a variety of prostaglandins, cyclic endoperoxides, and thromboxanes. Thromboxane A_2, produced by this pathway, is a potent stimulus to aggregation. When thromboxane production is blocked by aspirin, which inhibits cyclooxygenase, total aggregation does not occur. The platelet does not recover from the aspirin injury and is permanently impaired. As mentioned above, the normal life span of the platelet is 8 to 10 days.

Patient history is a vital factor in the recognition, diagnosis, and treatment of patients with bleeding disorders. The questions contained in Figure 8–3 are offered as a guide to the bleeding history.[27]

Summary

Hemostasis occurs as a result of an integration of interactions involving blood vessels, endothelium, platelets, and a coagulation cascade of a host of factors and enzymes to first seal off the rent in the vessel and subsequently form a clot. Lastly, through fibrinolysis, the clot is gradually removed. The patient's history should be scrutinized for any information suggesting a problem with bleeding. In this

FIG 8–2.
Prostaglandin metabolism. * = site of aspirin inhibition; † = potent stimulus to aggregation.

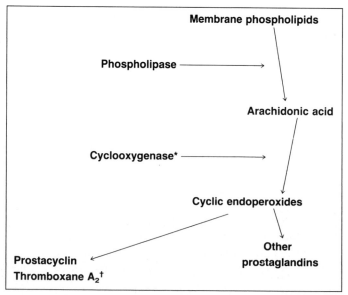

Membrane phospholipids

Phospholipase

Arachidonic acid

Cyclooxygenase*

Cyclic endoperoxides

Other prostaglandins

Prostacyclin
Thromboxane A_2†

Name_____   Age_____

1. Have any of the following members of your family ever had a problem with prolonged or unusual bleeding? Parents, brothers and sisters, children, grandparents, great-grandparents.   Yes_____   No_____

2. a. Have you ever had marked bleeding for up to 24 hours after a surgical procedure, e.g., tooth extraction or tonsillectomy?   Yes_____   No_____

   b. Have you ever required a blood transfusion after surgery?   Yes_____   No_____

   c. (Females) Do you feel that you have abnormal bleeding during menstruation?   Yes_____   No_____

3. Do you get bruises larger than the size of a quarter for which you cannot remember the injury?   Yes_____   No_____

4. Do you experience numerous and severe nosebleeds for up to several hours?   Yes_____   No_____

5. Do your gums often bleed not related to trauma or toothbrushing?   Yes_____   No_____

6. Are you taking any blood thinner (anticoagulant)?   Yes_____   No_____

7. Have you taken any medication, i.e., pills, powders, or liquids, in the past week?   Yes_____   No_____

8. Have you had or do you have any liver disease?   Yes_____   No_____

FIG 8–3.
Sample bleeding history.

event, it is recommended that the patient complete the bleeding history presented in Figure 8–3.

PHARMACOLOGIC CONSIDERATIONS

In the performance of implant surgery the patient may be exposed to a number of therapeutic agents. Local anesthetics, sedatives, analgesics, and antibiotics being some examples. Some of these agents may be administered simultaneously or in an overlapping fashion. Not uncommonly, the patient may be taking one or more drugs at the time treatment is begun and is given medication to be taken after completion of the procedure. While the prudent use of pharmacotherapeutic agents in the uncompromised ambulatory patient is not ordinarily attended by adverse effects, a number of other factors may be responsible for deleterious events following the administration of drugs that ordinarily cause no problem at all. Examples are kidney and liver disease, sex, age, race, weight, and genetic defects.[28] Although compromise of other body organ systems such as the endocrine, cardiovascular, and pulmo-

nary systems is important, in terms of drug effect enhancement, prolongation of action, and increased toxicity, kidney and liver disease are preeminent.[29]

Kidney Disease

The agents affected by the presence of kidney disease that are of interest to the implant surgeon are the aminoglycoside antibiotics streptomycin, gentamicin, tobramycin, kanamycin, and amikacin, agents used in the treatment of soft tissue or bone infections from which certain gram-negative bacilli are cultured; e.g., *Escherichia coli* or *Pseudomonas aeruginosa*. None of these antibiotics are metabolized, and they are excreted primarily by glomerular filtration.[30] In addition, aminoglycoside antibiotics have the potential for ototoxicity, the incidence ranging from 3% to 24% in various studies. In the presence of renal insufficiency, increased levels of aminoglycosides in the serum and perilymph have been demonstrated in both animals and humans.[31] The aminoglycosides also possess the potential for nephrotoxicity, the most commonly encountered toxicity associated with these agents. Binding of drugs to serum albumin is impaired in the presence of chronic renal disease. Among the drugs of interest to the implant surgeon so affected are the barbiturates, salicylates, and certain narcotics, notably morphine.[32] The potential toxicity of these drugs is therefore increased accordingly.

Liver Disease

The biotransformation and metabolism of many drugs occurs in the liver. Of interest to the implant surgeon are the barbiturates and the benzodiazepines. Albumin is produced exclusively by the hepatocyte.[33] Thus, compromised liver function may decrease the serum albumin available for drug binding. Drugs administered at normal dosage levels become more toxic when serum albumin binding is diminished. A number of drug-related problems arise in patients with deficient liver function that are due to delayed drug metabolism. As mentioned earlier, there may also be deficient synthesis of clotting factors. Caution must be exercised when giving any drug to a patient with compromised liver function.

Age

The association of increased drug intolerance and increasing age is well documented.[34] A reduction in the glomerular filtration rate of 30% in persons over 65 years of age and 50% in those 90 years of age has been shown.[35] Clearly, drug doses for the elderly must be determined with care.

Sex

Women have been shown to demonstrate a higher incidence of adverse drug reactions than men in a number of studies. The incidence of allergic skin reactions to commonly used drugs has been reported to be 50% greater in women.[36] In a study from Switzerland it was shown that of 171 hospitalized patients having evidence of adverse drug reactions, approximately two thirds were women.[37]

Weight

If optimum pharmacotherapeutic efficacy is to be achieved not only body mass but also body composition must be taken under consideration in determining drug dosages. Obviously, adjustments may be required for abnormally lean or obese patients. Distribution of the drug in fat, extracellular fluid, and lean body mass must be considered.

Genetic Factors

Genetically transmitted defects may manifest in a broad spectrum of clinical presentations. Diabetes mellitus, the hemophilias, sickle cell anemia, and certain neuromuscular diseases are examples. Two of the genetically mediated entities of interest in relation to drug administration, particularly in the outpatient surgery setting, are glucose-6-phosphate dehydrogenase (G6PD) deficiency and porphyria.

G6PD deficiency is an intrinsic erythrocyte abnormality in which hemolytic anemia is produced by oxidant drugs. This enzyme normally functions by enhancing the intracellular metabolism of glucose when the red blood cell is undergoing stress by oxidant compounds. Thus G6PD facilitates metabolic processes and prevents cell lysis.[38] More than 40 agents capable of inducing hemolysis in the presence of G6PD deficiency have been identified. Prominent among them and of interest to the implant surgeon are antipyretics, including aspirin, and certain analgesics, including phenacetin, commonly present in compounds such as aspirin-phenacetin-caffeine (APC).[39] In a survey of 2,874 patients, 102 instances of G6PD deficiency were found, an overall incidence of 3.6%. Of the 102 patients with documented G6PD deficiency, 72 (71%) were black. Of all black males tested in the survey, 13% were deficient in G6PD activity. The incidence of decreased G6PD activity among white males was 0.9%. Hemolytic crises may also be precipitated by bacterial and viral infections and other metabolic problems, e.g., diabetic ketoacidosis.[40] G6PD deficiency should be suspected in any black male who gives a history of darkening of the urine. If a simple follow-up complete blood count (CBC) shows decreases in hematocrit, hemoglobin, and the red cell count, the patient should be appropriately consulted prior to treatment.

Porphyria, although uncommon, is a usually inherited error in the biosynthesis of the heme portion of the red blood cell. Porphyrins are intermediate pigments in the biosynthesis pathway of heme and are probably synthesized in cells throughout the body but primarily in the bone marrow and in the liver.[41] The various types of porphyrias that become clinically manifest represent overproduction, accumulation, and excretion of the intermediate metabolites (porphyrins) of heme biosynthesis.[42] The most common porphyria is porphyria cutanea tarda of which skin photosensitivity (increased facial pigmentation, fragility of the skin to trauma, erythema, and vesicular and ulcerative lesions) is the only major manifestation.[43] The acute stage of the porphyrias is characterized by episodes of intense colicky abdominal pain, vomiting, hemolytic anemia, neuromuscular weakness or paralysis, and psychiatric manifestations. Drugs of particular interest to the implant surgeon that are known to aggravate or precipitate attacks are listed in Table 8–1.

Summary

The use of drugs and medications associated with implant surgery must be based upon an appreciation of the individual patient. The patient's age, race, sex, weight, and above all, his or her history of factors that may alter drug action must be carefully scrutinized. Liver and kidney disease are preeminent and certain genetically transmitted defects may be critical.

WOUND INFECTIONS

Some of the more difficult problems in surgery are related to infections and their management. This is no less applicable to dental implant surgery since the overwhelming majority of implant devices are inserted in a "contaminated" field, i.e., the oral cavity. In spite of this, infections associated with implant surgery are relatively uncommon, probably owing to the abundant vascularity and the high resistance to infection of the mouth, jaws, and face. The critical aspects of these infections, when they do occur, are twofold. Those that fail to respond to initial therapy have a propensity to become worse in a brief period of time. Additionally, because the anatomic regions into which they spread are in juxtaposition to the

TABLE 8–1.

Drugs That Aggravate or Precipitate Porphyria Attacks

Drugs acting on the central nervous system
  All barbiturates
  Phenytoin (Dilantin)
  Meprobamate (Equanil)
  Chlordiazepoxide (Librium)
Analgesics
  Phenylbutazone (Butazolidin)
  Indomethacin (Indocin)
Antimicrobials
  Sulfonamides
  Griseofulvin (antifungal)
Hormones
  Estrogens (Premarin)
  Progesterone (birth control pills)
Alcohol

airway and to vascular access to the meninges and the brain, very aggressive management may be required, including hospitalization and adequate incision and drainage as well as other supportive measures. It is therefore clear that a brief review of the microbiology of these infections and their antimicrobial management be included in this discussion.

Microbiology

It is well known that the oral cavity and pharynx are colonized by a known spectrum of microorganisms existing in a symbiotic state. When this symbiosis is altered by mechanical, chemical, environmental, physiologic, or nutritional disturbances the result is a pathologic state. Table 8–2 lists the distribution of important groups of indigenous microorganisms in the head and neck region, including the oral cavity and pharynx.

The causative microorganisms of infections associated with implant surgery may be introduced by trauma or by surgery, resulting in entry into the underlying soft tissues. The infection may remain localized if the host defense mechanisms are capable of containing it or if the infection is promptly and adequately treated with appropriate antimicrobial agents. However, if the host defenses are overwhelmed and drug therapy is inadequate or inappropriate, abscess and cellulitis may result as well as osteomyelitis.

TABLE 8–2.

Distribution of Important Groups of Microorganisms of the Head and Neck*†

Organism	Mouth	Oropharynx
Gram-positive facultative cocci		
α-Streptococcus	++++	++++
β-Streptococcus	+	++
Nonhemolytic streptococcus	+++	+++
Pneumococci	+	++
Staphylococcus epidermidis	+++	+
Staphylococcus aureus	+++	+++
Gram-positive anaerobic streptococcus		
Peptostreptococcus	+++	+++
Gram-positive facultative rods		
Diphtheroids	++++	+++
Lactobacillus	+++	0
Actinomyces	+++	+++
Gram-positive anaerobic rods		
Clostridium	+	0
Diphtheroids	+++	+++
Gram-negative facultative cocci		
Neisseriaceae	+++	++++
Gram-negative anaerobic cocci		
Veillonellacea	++++	+++
Gram-negative rods		
Pseudomonas	+	0
Coliform bacteria	+	+
Gram-negative anaerobic rods		
Fusobacterium	+++	+
Bacteroides	+++	+
Spirochetes	+++	+
Yeasts	+++	+++

*Adapted from Schuster GS: The microbiology of oral and maxillofacial infections, in Topazian RG, Goldberg MH: *Oral and Maxillofacial Infections.* Philadelphia, WB Saunders Co, 1987, pp 33–71.
†++++=generally present as major component of cultivatable flora; +++=generally present as a minor component of cultivatable flora; ++=may be present as minor component or transient; +=often present as minor component or transient; and 0=not normally present.

Antimicrobial Therapy

The first and foremost principle of treating infections resulting in abscesses, cellulitis, and osteomyelitis is surgical drainage and removal of the causative agent. It is unfortunate when management of the infectious process entails removal of an implant; however, when it is the source of the infection, it must be removed.

In recent years it has become increasingly apparent that the use of penicillin alone in the treatment of many infections of the cervical-maxillofacial region has become somewhat less than a panacea, even when combined with what ordinarily would be con-

sidered adequate incision and drainage. In two recent studies the failure rate of penicillin in treating acute group A β-hemolytic streptococcal infections was 20% to 25%, while the failure rate of a second course of penicillin therapy was 40% to 80%.[44, 45] One possible explanation for the failure of penicillin to eradicate streptococcal infections is the "protection" that is provided to the organisms by β-lactamase–producing aerobic and anaerobic bacteria which also reside in or accompany these infections.[46]

Ideally, selection of the antimicrobial agent, or agents, should be based upon culture of the material recovered from the infection at the time of incision and drainage combined with antibiotic sensitivity testing. However, in most instances it is necessary to make a selection empirically based upon the clinical presentation of the infection and a knowledge of its usual microbiology. Generally, penicillin is the drug of choice. However, if the infection has progressed to an abscess or to frank cellulitis, it is advisable to initiate antimicrobial therapy so as to provide broad-spectrum coverage. A reasonable choice is penicillin and metronidazole, or in advanced cases, clindamycin. It should be mentioned here that a simple Gram's stain will often provide useful information and can be done quickly. For example, gram-positive and gram-negative cocci and rods can frequently be identified, thus offering some confirmation of the mixed nature of many, if not most, of these infections. Later, after culture and sensitivity information is available, there may be an indication to change the antimicrobial regimen. While any of the groups of microorganisms listed in Table 8–2 may be involved, Table 8–3 summarizes the organisms most commonly cultured from these infections and indicates their sensitivity to selected antibiotics.

Having treated the infection with surgical inci-

sion and drainage and removal of the causative agent and the initiation of antimicrobial therapy, it is then imperative to follow the patient closely in order to monitor the postoperative course of healing or initiate changes in therapy if indicated. Some of the causes of treatment failure include depressed host defense mechanisms; inadequate surgery; difficulties with antimicrobial therapy, e.g., wrong drug, inadequate dosage, and noncompliance on the part of the patient to take outpatient oral medications; misrepresentation or misinterpretation of the culture material; and residual foreign material left in the wound. If the infection does recur, it is probable that the wound will require reexploration, debridement, irrigation, and drainage as well as a repeat course of antimicrobial therapy.

Summary

Management of infections in the oral and maxillofacial region is one of the most important aspects of implant surgery. These infections have a propensity to worsen rapidly and their proximate location to the airway and to vascular access into the meninges

TABLE 8–3.

Average Reported Incidence of Microorganisms Isolated From Infections of the Oral and Contiguous Structures and Antibiotic Sensitivities*

Microorganisms	Percent	Antibiotic of Choice
Streptococci (α- and nonhemolytic)	50	Penicillin
Streptococcus faecalis	13	Ampicillin + gentamicin
Anaerobic streptococci (*Peptostreptococcus* sp)	18	Penicillin
Staphylococci	16	Penicillin or oxacillin (if β-lactamase producer)
Proteus sp	4	Gentamicin
Escherichia coli	4	Gentamicin (if nosocomial) Ampicillin (if urinary)
Diphtheroids	4	Penicillin
Actinomyces sp	4	Penicillin
Neisseria sp	5	Penicillin
Proprionibacterium sp	20	Clindamycin
Bacteroides sp	15	Clindamycin
Fusobacteria	5	Clindamycin
Veillonella sp	29	Clindamycin
Candida albicans	7	Amphotericin B

*Adapted from Schuster GS: The microbiology of oral and maxillofacial infections, and Peterson LJ: Principles of antibiotic therapy, in Topazian, RG, Goldberg MH: *Oral and Maxillofacial Infections.* Philadelphia, WB Saunders Co, 1987, pp 33–71, 122–155.

and brain makes it imperative that the gravity of these infections be recognized. Many, if not most, of these infections are of mixed aerobic and anaerobic microflora. A high percentage of them contain β-lactamase–producing species, and thus broad-spectrum antimicrobial agents are frequently indicated. Adequate surgical incision and drainage is an essential component of treatment, and removal of the causative agent is critical. Close follow-up is required after initial treatment of the infection in order to monitor the patient's progress.

REFERENCES

1. Irvin TT: The healing wound, in Bucknall TE, Ellis H (eds): *Wound Healing for Surgeons*. London, Bailliere Tindall, 1984, p 3.
2. Ross R, Benditt EP: Wound healing and collagen formation. *J Cell Biol* 1965; 27:83.
3. Chvapil M, Hurych J: Hydroxylation of proline in vitro. *Nature* 1959; 184:1145.
4. Rasmussen H: Cell communication, calcium ion, and cyclic adenosine monophosphate. *Science* 1970; 170:404.
5. Goldin EG, Joseph NR: Response of connective tissue ground substance in wound healing. *Arch Surg* 1968; 97:753.
6. Berenson GS, Lumpkin WM, Shipp VG: Study of the time course of production of acid mucopolysaccharides by fibroblasts in synthetic medium. *Anat Rec* 1959; 132:585.
7. Jackson DS: Biosynthesis of collagen fibers. *Clin Sci* 1970; 38:7.
8. Stenman S, Vaheri A: Distribution of a major connective tissue protein fibronectin in normal human tissues. *J Exp Med* 1978; 147:1054.
9. Hahn LHE, Yamada KM: Identification and isolation of a collagen binding fragment of the adhesive glycoprotein fibronectin. *Proc Natl Acad Sci USA,* 1979; 76:1160.
10. Culp LA, Murray BA, Rollins BJ: Fibronectin and proteoglycans as determinants of cell substratum adhesion. *J Supramol Struct* 1979; 11:401.
11. Gordon JL: Mechanisms regulating platelet adhesion, in Curtis ASG, Pitts JD (eds): *Cell Adhesion and Mobility*. Cambridge, Cambridge University Press, 1980, pp 199–233.
12. Williams G: The late phases of wound healing: His-
tological and ultrastructural studies of collagen and elastic tissue formation. *J Pathol* 1970; 102:61.
13. Longacre JJ, Berry HK, Basom CR, et al: The effects of Z-plasty on hypertrophic scars. *Scand J Plast Reconstr Surg* 1976; 10:113.
14. Ross R, Odland G: Human wound repair: Inflammatory cells, epithelial mesenchymal interrelations and fibrogenesis. *J Cell Biol* 1968; 39:152.
15. Lack CH: Some biological and biochemical consequences of inflammation in connective tissue. *Biochem Pharmacol* 1978; (suppl) 197.
16. MacDonald RA: Origin of fibroblasts in experimental healing wounds. *Surgery* 1959; 46:376.
17. Dunphy JE, Udupa KN: Chemical and histochemical sequences in the normal healing of wounds. *N Engl J Med* 1955; 253:847.
18. Gillman T: On some aspects of collagen formation in localized repair and in diffuse fibrotic reactions to injury, in Gould BS (ed): *Treatise on Collagens,* vol 2B. London, Academic Press, 1968, pp 331–407.
19. DiRosa M, Giround JP, Willoughby DA: Studies on the mediators of the acute inflammatory response induced in rats in different sites by carrageenan and turpentine. *J Pathol* 1971; 104:15.
20. Vane JR: Prostaglandins in the inflammatory response, in Lepow IH, Ward PA (eds): *Inflammation: Mechanisms and Control*. New York, Academic Press, 1972, pp 261–279.
21. Ward PA: Natural and synthetic inhibitors of leukotaxis, in Lepow IH, Ward PA (eds): *Inflammation: Mechanisms and Control*. New York, Academic Press, 1972, pp 301–307.
22. Turner SR, Tainer JA, Lynn WS: Biogenesis of chemotactic molecules by the arachidonate lipoxygenase system of platelets. *Nature* 1973; 257:680.
23. Thompson AR, Harker LA: *Manual of Hemostasis and Thrombosis*. Philadelphia, FA Davis Co, 1988.
24. Rapaport SI: *Introduction to Hematology,* Philadelphia, JB Lippincott Co, 1987.
25. Jackson CM, Nemerson Y: Blood coagulation. *Annu Rev Biochem* 1980; 49:765.
26. Waterbury L: *Hematology for the House Officer*. Baltimore, Williams & Wilkins Co, 1986.
27. Tullman MJ, Spencer WR: *Systemic Disease in Dental Treatment*. New York, Appleton-Century-Crofts, 1982.
28. Shelton DW: Review of adverse drug reactions, in Irby WB, Shelton DW (eds): *Current Advances in Oral and Maxillofacial Surgery*. St Louis, CV Mosby Co, 1983, pp 222–246.

29. D'Arcy PF, Griffin JP: Introduction, in D'Arcy PF, Griffin JP (eds): *The Milieu of the Emergency*. Chicago, John Wright & Sons Ltd, 1980, pp 1–16.

30. Kagan BM: *Antimicrobial Therapy*. Philadelphia, WB Saunders Co, 1980.

31. Brummett RE, Bendrick TW, Himes DL, et al: Ototoxicity of tobramycin, gentamicin, amikacin, and sisomicin in the guinea pig. *J Antimicrob Chemother* 1978; (suppl A) 73.

32. Koch-Wesser J, Sellers EM: Binding of drugs to serum albumin. *N Engl J Med* 1976; 294:311,526.

33. Isselbacher KJ, La Mont JT: Diagnostic procedures in liver disease, in Wilson JD, Braunwald EB, Isselbacher KJ, et al (eds): *Harrison's Principles of Internal Medicine*. New York, McGraw-Hill Book Co, 1980, pp 1450–1453.

34. Caranasos GJ, Stewart RB, Cluff LE: Drug induced illness leading to hospitalization. *JAMA* 1974; 228:713–717.

35. Agate J: *The Practice of Geriatrics*. London, William Heinemann Ltd, 1963.

36. Arndt KA, Jick H: Rates of cutaneous reactions to drugs: A report of the Boston Collaborative Drug Surveillance Program. *JAMA* 1976; 235:918.

37. Klein V, Klein M, Strum H, et al: The frequency of adverse drug reactions as dependent upon age, sex, and duration of hospitalization. *Int J Clin Pharmacol* 1976; 13:187.

38. Beutler E, Dern RJ, Flanagan CL, et al: The hemolytic effect of primaquine. VII. Biochemical studies of drug sensitive erythrocytes. *J Lab Clin Med* 1955; 45:286.

39. Rollo IM: Drugs used in the chemotherapy of malaria, in Goodman LS, Gilman A (eds): *The Pharmacologic Basis of Therapeutics*. New York, Macmillan Publishing Co, Inc, 1980.

40. Grant FL, Winks GF: Primaquine sensitive hemolytic anemia complicating diabetic acidosis. *Clin Res* 1961; 9:27.

41. Griffin JP: Some genetic factors underlying drug induced emergencies, in D'Arcy PF, Griffin JP (eds): *Drug Induced Emergencies*. Chicago, John Wright & Sons Ltd, 1980, pp 17–39.

42. Hoffman WS: *The Biochemistry of Clinical Medicine*. Chicago, Year Book Medical Publishers, Inc, 1970.

43. Meyer VA: Porphyrias, in Wilson JD, Braunwald EB, Isselbacher KJ, et al (eds): *Harrison's Principles of Internal Medicine*. New York, McGraw-Hill Book Co, 1980, pp 494–500.

44. Gastanaduy AS, Kaplan EL, Huwe BB: Failure of penicillin to eradicate group A streptococci during an outbreak of pharyngitis. *Lancet* 1980; 2:498–502.

45. Smith TO, Huskins WS, Kim KS: Efficacy of beta-lactamase–resistant penicillin and influence of penicillin tolerance in eradication of streptococci from the pharynx after failure of penicillin therapy for group A streptococcal pharyngitis. *J Pediatr* 1987; 110:777–782.

46. Brook I: The role of beta-lactamase–producing bacteria in the persistence of streptococcal tonsillar infection. *Rev Infect Dis* 1984; 6:601–607.

Chapter 9

Principles of Surgery for Plate/Blade Implants

Charles M. Weiss, D.D.S.

BASIC SURGICAL PRINCIPLES

The basic principles of oral surgery apply to the insertion of endosseous plate or blade form implants. All accepted and correct techniques for maintaining *sterility* are utilized, as for the extraction of an impacted third molar.

Good access is often the difference between optimal and troubled implant insertions. *Direct visualization* of the tissues involved, including landmarks, undercut areas, and the like, is indispensable. *Gentle handling* of tissues is axiomatic: Edema is lessened, healing is hastened, complications are fewer.

A *trained dental assistant* who understands the general requirements of oral surgical procedures, as well as the basics of oral implantology, is an asset. Teaching tapes are available on plate or blade form techniques. They convey all necessary information and procedures.

AVOIDING METAL TRANSFER AND CONTAMINATION

Most endosseous plate or blade form implants are made of titanium. To avoid metal transfer, the implants must be protected from contact with other metals. Prudence dictates that all instruments that contact implants be titanium-tipped, to ensure that the implants are not contaminated during the insertion process. In setting up the instrument tray, the instruments are arranged in the sequence in which they will be used: tissue marker first, then the scalpel, periosteal elevators, trimming and shaping rongeurs, and so on. The titanium-tipped instruments are grouped together and away from others, again to avoid metal transfer contamination. During sterilization, titanium-tipped instruments and implants should not contact aluminum sterilization trays or other instruments. They should be wrapped in gauze, utilizing glass containers or bagging.

THE PREINSERTION VISIT

The One-Stage vs. Two-Stage (Submerged or Semisubmerged) System

The one-stage configuration of plate or blade form endosteal implants is recommended and routinely utilized. Its validated sequencing, which can result in total case completion in 4 to 6 weeks' elapsed time, is usually the method of choice for solo practitioners.

There are circumstances in which two-stage submerged or semisubmerged configurations are the better choice. In the team approach, the practitioner inserting the implant should consider the advantages to the restorative dentist of a completely healed implant. Solo practitioners have control of sequencing; team members often do not. The two-stage approach is also advised in marginal situations, defined as:

1. Cases that have less than optimal bone for implant insertion
2. Cases requiring more than a 15-degree bend between the long axis of the body and the abutment head
3. Cases in which the opposing arch is a natural dentition, a fixed prosthesis, or a combination of both
4. Cases with high vertical dimension
5. The elderly

There are slight variations in insertion for one-stage and two-stage systems. These are discussed later in the chapter at each step of the procedure. Ideal two-stage configurations permit the final abutment head to be placed on the implant body during the insertion procedure. With these abutment heads in position, the implant has the appearance of, and is inserted in the same manner as, a one-stage configuration. After insertion, at the appropriate time, depending on whether the submerged or semisubmerged approach is used, the final abutment head is removed and a healing collar is placed.

Preparing and Temporizing Natural Co-abutments(s) That Will Serve as Support Under the Same Prosthesis as the Implant(s)

When teeth will serve as co-abutments under the same prosthesis as the implants, they are prepared before or at the time of the insertion of the implant(s). Endodontic and periodontal therapy is completed first.

In extended cases, natural abutments are prepared before the time of implant insertion, and temporized. After the implant(s) are inserted, the provisional teeth are extended or completely redone to include the new implant abutments, particularly in areas that are important in terms of esthetics.

In small fixed bridge cases, natural abutments are usually prepared first, at the same visit as the implant insertion. After one-stage implant insertion, the

natural and implant abutments may be included in the provisional prosthesis. Often, the implant abutments remain freestanding and are not included in the provisional prostheses, depending on occlusion, esthetics, and other factors discussed later.

Two-Stage System Variations

When utilizing two-stage submerged or semi-submerged systems, the natural co-abutments are prepared and temporized at or just prior to the visit during which final abutment heads are attached.

SELECTING THE PROPER IMPLANT

To select the proper implant, the amount of available bone must be determined. During clinical examination, the width of the alveolar ridge is palpated and noted. Only intraoral palpation can determine whether or not the width is adequate for the placement of a plate or blade form implant. In the maxilla, because of its excessive and variable tissue thickness, direct visualization after tissue reflection is often necessary to determine width (Fig 9–1). When examining a partially or totally edentulous ridge, it may be noted that the maxilla heals predominantly at the expense of the buccal and labial plates of bone. Resorption occurs superiorly and medially. This results in a ridge crest that is in a relatively lingual position. When selecting and implanting maxillary plate or blade form implants, this effect on placement and abutment head parallelism must be considered.

Plate or blade form implants are placed to bisect the cortical plates of the patient's residual alveolar ridge. Properly placed implants will protrude through attached gingiva into the oral cavity medial to where the central fossae of the natural teeth once were, toward the lingual side of the planned abutment crown. To achieve a favorable result the final prosthesis will require extra contouring toward the buccal and the labial aspect for acceptable occlusion and esthetics. Radiographs determine the length of the ridge, and its depth apically to the roof of the inferior alveolar canal, mental foramen, sinus areas,

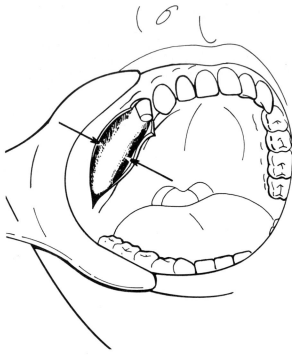

FIG 9–1.
Direct visualization of bone width in the maxilla via use of the surgical flap.

and nasal cavity. A long-cone periapical radiograph will provide the most accurate image of the area of available bone under consideration. The ridge crest, roof of the inferior alveolar canal, mental foramen, adjacent tooth root, sinus floor, and other landmarks can be marked directly on the radiograph with a felt pen to clearly outline the length and depth of available bone.

Use of the Plate/Blade Form Selector for Final Model Selection

Once the amount of available bone has been assessed, a plate or blade form selector, which has life-sized prints of each implant configuration on transparent film, will aid in the selection of the particular implant configuration that most nearly fills the area of available bone. With the plate or blade form selector held over a periapical radiograph, the base of the abutment head is placed at the ridge crest, and the configuration whose body fully utilizes the available bone is selected, leaving a 1- to 2-mm landmark clearance for safety (Fig 9–2).

If palpation reveals that the crest of the ridge is narrow, a narrow blade with a shoulder width of 1.2 mm is selected. In cases that exhibit adequate width, wider blade implants are recommended. When possible, wider implants are chosen to reduce stress transfer to the surrounding tissues.

Panoramic radiographs distort images, the distortions varying depending on the panoramic unit, the area of film being viewed, and patient positioning. Panoramic films reveal excellent relevant diagnostic anatomic information, but cannot be used reliably for implant selection. Long-cone periapical radiographs are the most accurate for implant selection.

The Single- vs. Double-Headed Implant

A key question concerns correct implant placement under the proposed prosthesis. Many implant models are supplied with either one or two abutment heads. These should be positioned to harmonize with the opposing dentition, not where an embrasure should be. The tooth positions for the projected prosthesis are planned in advance, and that implant is selected whose abutment heads project under the proposed teeth, and not into interproximal areas (Fig 9–3). Newer models are supplied with off-center abutment heads. Reversing the mesial and distal automatically repositions the head anteriorly or posteriorly for improved prosthodontic location. In closed bite cases, two-head models are preferred, where possible because they are shorter. Also, two heads offer added cement retention.

Adjusting the Implant to Clear Landmarks

Many implant configurations are available so adjusting the implant to avoid landmarks is rarely required. However, if trimming is required, metal implants, especially titanium, must be repassivated prior to use.

The implant is placed over the area of available bone on the periapical radiograph, and the portion of the implant that impinges on any landmark is determined. A disc or stone is used for trimming. A metal

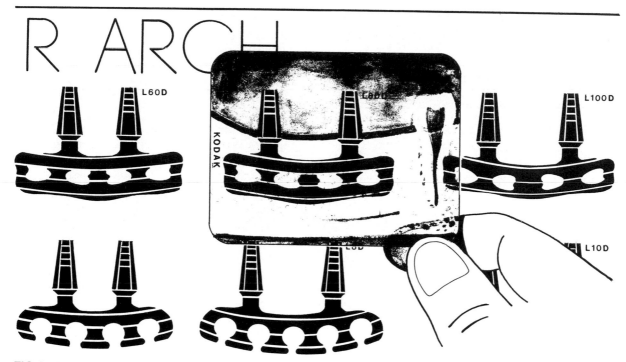

FIG 9–2.
Utilizing the plate or blade form selector to choose the correct implant model.

bur is not used in order to avoid metal transfer contamination.

This is best done after selecting the implant, prior to sterilization at the implant insertion visit.

Adjusting the One-Stage and Two-Stage Abutment Heads for Interocclusal Clearance

Interocclusal clearance of the implant abutment heads is tested and adjusted. In centric occlusion, a minimum of 2-mm clearance from the top of the abutment head to the opposite occlusal surface is required. The abutment head is 7 to 8 mm high. Its base is placed against the ridge crest. In the mandible the gingival thickness is most often 1 mm. In the maxilla it is often thicker. If, for example, the height from the gingival crest to the opposite occlusal surface is 10 mm or more, no adjustments are required. If less, adjustments are required.

The millimeter adjustment lines on the abutment head are used for guidance (Fig 9–4). The abutment head is shortened with stones, discs, diamonds, and wheels. Interocclusal clearance should be checked and readjusted if necessary.

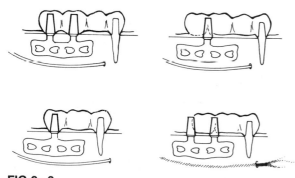

FIG 9–3.
Relating implant abutment head position to final prosthesis.

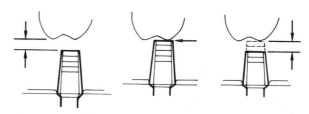

FIG 9–4.
Adjustment of a blade implant for interocclusal clearance.

It is preferable to adjust for occlusal clearance prior to sterilizing the implant at the insertion visit.

THE INSERTION VISIT

Preoperative and Postoperative Medication

Most patients do not require sedation or medication for edema control. Prophylactic antibiotic coverage is usually recommended. Medication to control postoperative discomfort is usually prescribed. An ice pack can be helpful.

Local Anesthesia

Gentle but thorough local anesthesia allows the patient to remain ambulatory and comfortable. During the insertion procedure, if the patient experiences the slightest discomfort, an additional anesthetic should be administered. An adequately anesthetized patient is more relaxed, exhibits less anxiety, is cooperative, and requires little if any sedation. Bupivacaine hydrochloride (Marcaine) will provide long-lasting block anesthesia, and where the use of a minimal vasoconstrictor (1:200,000) is indicated. In the mandible, a double inferior alveolar-lingual block with bupivacaine may be administered. Using lidocaine with epinephrine 1:100,000 to control bleeding, the buccal and labial fold is infiltrated. The injection is made anteriorly and posteriorly to what will be the *pontic areas* of the proposed prosthesis. This avoids edema caused by anesthetic fluid in the planned pontic area should one choose in single implant cases to take master impressions immediately postoperatively. In the maxilla a posterior superior alveolar block (bupivacaine) and infiltrate (lidocaine) are administered along the buccal and labial fold, as well as palatally.

When the anesthesia is effective, the insertion procedure may begin.

The Incision

Every effort should be made to ensure that implant abutment heads protrude into the oral cavity through areas of attached gingiva.

The incision line is marked on or just buccal to the crest of the ridge, in attached gingiva. In order to achieve proper access to the entire receptor site opening on the crest of bone, a mark is made 3 to 5 mm beyond the length of the implant of each end of the proposed incision line. If the incision extends within 5 mm of the next tooth, it is carried directly through the cuff of the natural tooth. The incision line is generally made in the same direction as the blood supply and bleeding is therefore minimal. A right-angle incision is not made because it would cut across the blood supply and cause increased bleeding, edema, and discomfort during the healing process (Fig 9–5).

The scalpel is positioned distally and pressed firmly against the crest of bone. The incision is made through the gingiva *and* the periosteum, and continued anteriorly to the end of the incision line. In approaching the distal surface of the next natural tooth, the scalpel is turned around and pressed against the distal surface cleanly and completely (Fig 9–6).

The incision in an edentulous arch extends from retromolar pad to retromolar pad in the mandible and from tuberosity to tuberosity in the maxilla. The gingival tissue in the maxilla varies in depth. It can be more than 10 mm, though most often it is 2 to 5 mm thick. The incision is extended from distal to the midline on each side, and the incision lines joined carefully, making sure that the incision is made

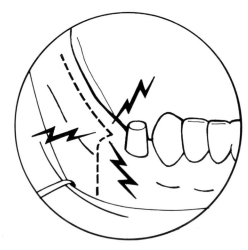

FIG 9–5.
Incisions at right angles to the direction of the blood supply are avoided.

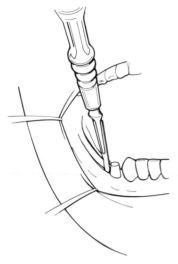

FIG 9–6.
The scalpel is reversed to incise cleanly through the gingival cuff.

through the periosteum down to the bone. This facilitates tissue reflection, reduces trauma, and avoids unnecessary bleeding.

Tissue Reflection

A periosteal elevator is passed *under* the periosteum to reflect the gingival tissue from the bone (Fig 9–7). The periosteum is composed of dense, tough

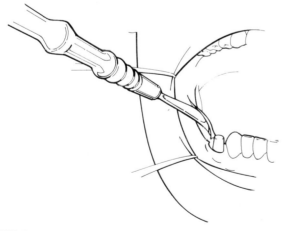

FIG 9–7.
Initial positioning of the periosteal elevator under the periosteum.

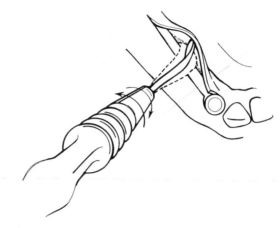

FIG 9–8.
Rotational reflection of tissue.

tissue. If the elevator is passed cleanly between the bone and under the periosteum, problems will not occur. If the periosteum is separated from the connective tissue between it and the gingival crest, increased bleeding and added edema will occur.

The elevator is placed at one point along the incision line, teased 4 to 5 mm between the periosteum and the bone. There are now several options to complete the reflection. One is to rotate the elevator mesially and then distally to lift the flap (Fig 9–8). Another involves moving the elevator bodily along the incision line anteriorly and posteriorly, carefully lifting the tissue away (Fig 9–9). A third option is to place the end of the elevator between the bone and periosteum, and hold it there firmly, raising the handle to reflect the tissue (Fig 9–10). The key to

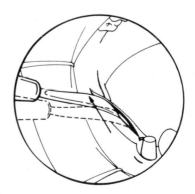

FIG 9–9.
Tissue reflection through anteroposterior bodily movement.

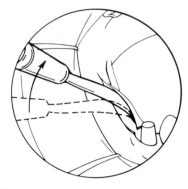

FIG 9–10.
Tissue reflection through elevation.

proper reflection is to maintain the elevator under the periosteum at all times. Generally, 10 to 15 mm of exposed alveolar ridge, as measured from the crest apically, is adequate access. The reflection is extended to that depth.

Reflection of the tissue in the maxilla is done in same way as in the mandible, but a larger or broader periosteal elevator is used. The maxillary mucosa is thicker in the tuberosity and less so anteriorly. Generally it is more difficult to reflect tissue in the maxilla, because maxillary bone is more porous, providing anchorage for tissue tags to fasten the periosteum to the bone.

Once the flaps arc laid back, the exposed alveolar ridge is examined for width, undercuts, imperfections, spines, and residual tissue tags. The available bone is reevaluated to reconfirm its adequacy for the planned procedure.

Trimming the Edges of the Incision

After the periosteum is completely reflected bucally/labially and lingually, and the ridge can be observed directly, the straightness and evenness of the edge of the soft tissue incision line are confirmed. If the edges are jagged or uneven, they are trimmed with tissue scissors. A clean, even incision line helps promote suturing and ensures good primary intention healing.

Cleansing the Ridge Crest

The crest of the ridge is examined for the presence of tissue tags or bony projections. If they are present, a curet is used to scrape off the tissue tags. Bony projections are trimmed with a rongeur. The rongeur requires a bayonet design to allow it to pass over natural teeth and permit orientation of the cutting edge parallel to the crest. A bone file is used to smooth the crest in areas where bone was removed.

The general rule is to touch or alter the bone as little as possible to avoid unnecessary resorption.

Locating the Implant Receptor Site

The implant is placed firmly in an implant carrier with the manufacturer's logo or other distinguishing feature toward either the buccal or lingual aspect of the ridge. Remembering this orientation will ensure proper replacement after correcting adjustments are made to the implant, and it is reintroduced into the oral cavity. The flap is retracted and the implant placed against the crest of the ridge in the area of the planned receptor site (Fig 9–11). Posteriorly, in the mandible, it is important to prepare the receptor site to avoid the mental foramen and roof of the inferior alveolar canal. Most often, the implant is placed 1 to 2 mm distal to the foramen. Receptor sites are prepared 1 to 2 mm longer at each end, to ease implant insertion and afford mesiodistal leeway to promote correct anteroposterior abutment head positioning. The location of the planned receptor site is noted, or the bone marked with a small round bur at several sites.

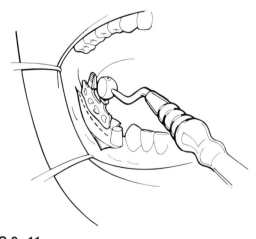

FIG 9–11.
The planned extent of the implant receptor site is verified.

Preparing the Receptor Site

Endosseous plate or blade form implants are always placed within receptor sites that are prepared 1 mm deeper than the depth and slightly narrower than the width of the selected implant (Fig 9–12). This promotes complete seating and good press fit at insertion, and promotes essential implant immobilization during healing. To create the receptor site, appropriate bone burs are applied intermittently, at high or low speed, with a copious external water spray, or internally cooled bone burs where possible, also with an additional external water spray. Coordinated burs are generally slightly narrower than their compatible implants. The manufacturer's suggestions should be followed faithfully.

Before penetrating the cortical plate to start the receptor site, the channeling bur is angled so as to bisect the cortical plates of bone. The receptor site is to be centered within the cancellous bone of the alveolar ridge. Parallelism with other natural or implant abutments is not a consideration at this point. In most cases, the abutment heads will not project into the oral cavity parallel with other abutments. They will be adjusted for parallelism in a subsequent step.

With the correct bone bur a series of penetrations is prepared approximately 3 to 5 mm apart along the crest of the ridge, just through the cortical bone, into the cancellous bone. The angle of the bur is maintained to keep bisecting the cortical plates. The contra-angle may be fitted to supply sterile wa-

ter. A copious external or internal spray provides important cooling and cleansing during the bone removal sequence. When the series of penetrations into cancellous bone have been made, the holes are carefully connected, keeping the proper angulation to bisect the cortical plates at all times. Bone is removed intermittently to join the holes, maintaining a copious flow of water. The receptor site has not yet been prepared to its predetermined depth.

Most receptor sites are not straight, owing to the anatomy of the posterior ridge and the curved anterior and canine areas. In cases exhibiting straight receptor sites, an alternate first step can be the use of compatible channeling saws, with a copious flow of water at low speed (Fig 9–13). Some saws are equipped for internal cooling. The axis of the saw is held so as to bisect the cortical plates of bone and penetrate into the underlying cancellous bone.

After the penetration holes have been connected, a channel curet and depth gauge are passed within the partially prepared receptor site to remove and harvest any bone chips that may remain. The harvested bone is stored in a sterile dappen dish. The implant is placed in its partially prepared receptor site to confirm that the mesiodistal length can accommodate the length of the implant, with an extra 1.5 to 2.0 mm at each end to ensure ease of seating and correct mesiodistal prosthodontic positioning. With this verified, the preparation is completed by bringing the receptor site to its proper depth. To accomplish this, before inserting the correct bone bur, the tip is positioned opposite the base of the abutment head, making sure the implant and bur do not touch. Noting the point on the shank of the bur that

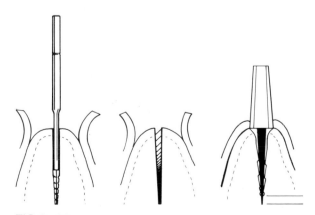

FIG 9–12.
The receptor site is prepared slightly narrower than the implant width, but 1 mm deeper than the implant to be seated.

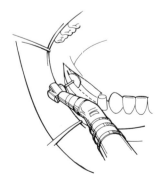

FIG 9–13.
A saw may be utilized for straight receptor sites.

is opposite the base of the implant, 1 mm is added and that point marked on the shank by spinning it against a disc (Fig 9–14). Some bone burs are premarked for depth.

This helpful step determines that point on the bur's shank which must be brought flush with the crest of bone to ensure the proper depth of channel preparation. This will safely and predictably avoid landmarks.

Now the receptor site channel is prepared to its proper depth. Bisecting the cortical plates, a series of holes are made 3 mm apart, brought to their final depth, and connected, while maintaining a copious water flow. With the implant in a carrier, the channel curet and depth gauge are held opposite the implant so that the tip of the depth gauge is at the base of the abutment head, noting the point on the depth gauge that is opposite the bottom of the implant (Fig 9–15).

The proper depth of the channel is now confirmed at every point. The depth gauge is inserted and moved along the channel base. If a portion of the channel is too shallow or uneven, this should be corrected.

In the case of asymmetric implants, such as those indicated for use anteriorly, to the sinus, in the posterior mandible, or in the presence of uneven ridge resorption, the bur shank is marked to indicate the deepest and shallowest insertion depths (Fig 9–16). Each portion of the channel is brought to its final depth by penetrating the bur to the depth mark-

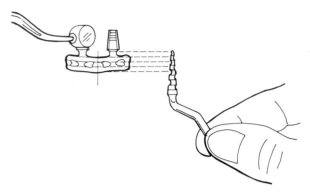

FIG 9–15.
Proper penetration is determined with a depth gauge.

ing that corresponds to the depth of the implant at that point.

In cases where two or more implants are being inserted during the same visit, consideration should be given to preparing the receptor site(s) for the other implant(s) at this time. Then, preliminary seating and final adjustments for parallelism and interocclusal clearance can be made on all implants at the same time, often with greater ease.

Preliminary Bending Adjustments to the Implant Body

Because the dental arches are curved, receptor sites are usually curved. It may be necessary to bend the implant along the shoulder to reflect the bone's natural contour. Previous periodontal conditions and the results of prior surgical intervention may have caused uneven ridge healing. The implant is now adjusted to accommodate this. In ideal configurations, final abutment heads for two-stage systems are attached to the implant body during all bending, adjusting, and insertion procedures. They are removed

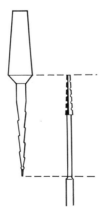

FIG 9–14.
The bone bur is marked for proper depth.

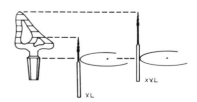

FIG 9–16.
Depth control for asymmetric implants.

after final insertion of the implant, prior to closure, to permit submerging or semisubmerging after placement of healing collars or caps. All bending is now done with the titanium-tipped bending pliers. The implant is wrapped in sterile gauze and held in the bending pliers so that they are parallel and near the shoulder of the implant, which is bent to match the curve of the arch as closely as possible (Fig 9–17). In the canine area, as the implant turns the arch, greater bends may be required. The shoulder and inferior borders of the implant are inspected to determine whether the adjustments are adequate. The implant is inserted passively 1 to 2 mm into the receptor site.

Preliminary Seating of the Implant

With the implant positioned just into the receptor site, a seating instrument is placed over the abutment head(s) (Fig 9–18). The implant is tapped and seated evenly until the base of the abutment head(s) is 2 mm above the ridge crest. The long axis of each seating instrument is held parallel to the long axis of the *body* of the implant so that all tapping forces are in the direction of the central axis of the receptor site (see Fig 9–17). The seating instruments are bayonet-shaped to allow easy access and full visibility. When seating a maxillary implant, the patient's head is placed against the head rest. In the case of the lower arch, the inferior border of the mandible must be supported. In the case of either a single-headed or double-headed implant the mesial may be seated

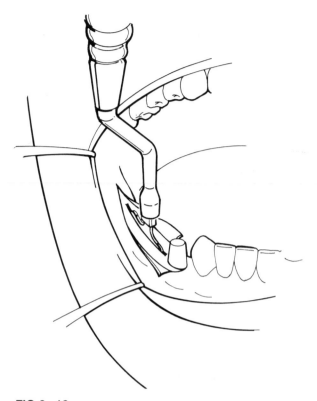

FIG 9–18.
The position of the seating instrument is oriented to the long axis of the implant body.

first, and then the distal, rocking the implant into position. To accomplish this, the shoulder set-point or set-slot seating instrument is used, first on the mesial and then on the distal (Fig 9–19). Another option is to seat the implant evenly with a single- or double-head seating instrument. When preliminary seating is completed the base of the abutment head should be 2 mm from the ridge crest.

Progress films may be taken. They will verify the correctness of the previous adjustments. If too little available bone remains, and adjusting the body cannot solve this problem, a smaller model may be indicated. Practitioners often sterilize implants that are one size larger and one size smaller than their primary selection, for use if needed.

With the implant preliminarily seated, the abutment head(s) is checked to see that it is parallel to the long axis of the crowns of the planned natural abutment teeth, or existing or planned adjacent implant abutment heads. If not, bending is required.

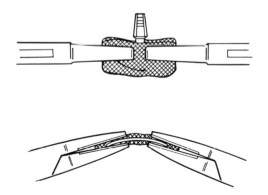

FIG 9–17.
The implant is adjusted to follow the curved receptor site using special titanium-tipped bending pliers.

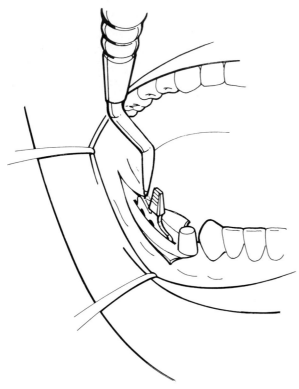

FIG 9–19.
Off-center seating is applied to level the shoulder.

verse with the force applied vertically (Fig 9–20). The receptor site must *not* be widened by luxating the implant buccolingually or labiolingually. To adjust an abutment head for parallelism, the titanium-tipped adjusting pliers are positioned as follows: one pliers over the abutment head or under its base, with its beak end parallel to the base, and the second pliers with its beak end parallel to the first, 2 to 3 mm below it (Fig 9–21). The body of the implant below the abutment head may be wrapped in sterile gauze. The section of the implant between the parallel beak ends is bent across, while viewing the implant in the mesial profile. This angle affords greater control. The head may also be rotated for better line-up as the arch is turned, particularly in the canine area. Heads may also be bent anteroposteriorly to achieve parallelism in that plane. Newer models have abutment heads with greater taper mesially and distally to avoid bending in those directions, and are prebent

The next consideration is whether sufficient interocclusal clearance exists. The distance between the *base* of the abutment head and the crest of the ridge is approximately 2 mm when the implant is preliminarily seated. Thus, when the implant is fully seated, there will be 2 mm *more clearance* when the patient closes into centric occlusion. Preliminary adjustments for interocclusal clearance were made prior to the implant insertion visit. Further abutment head shortening may be necessary now. All of these adjustments are made extraorally.

Bending Adjustments to the Abutment Head

With the implant preliminarily seated, and with the base of the abutment head 2 mm above the ridge crest, the angle of bend (if any) required to achieve parallelism with other abutments is determined. The implant is removed by engaging an implant remover under the base of the abutment head, tapping in re-

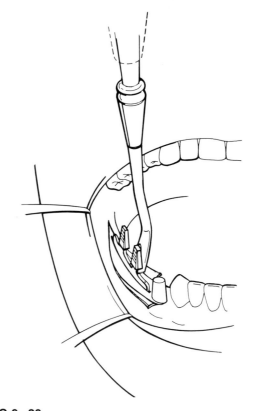

FIG 9–20.
Reversal of the mallet implant remover.

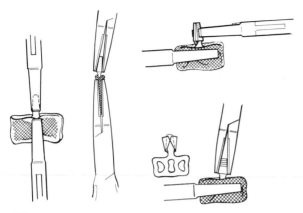

FIG 9–21.
Bending the abutment head for parallelism.

buccolingually. When reversed in the receptor site, parallelism may often be achieved without bending. The implant is reinserted, with the base of the abutment head 2 mm above the ridge crest, and the accuracy of all adjustments is checked. The necessary corrections are made. In the maxilla, achieving parallelism is difficult owing to the significant resorption of the buccal and labial plates in this area. As a result, the abutment heads protrude buccally and labially, and have to be bent lingually to achieve parallelism. Often the magnitude of the bend required is between 20 and 45 degrees; most often it is 15 to 20 degrees.

It is proper to adjust parallelism by bending rather than to grind the head after final seating. Grinding in the mouth may be done if required, after suturing, exercising care that grinding debris and metal chips do not contaminate an open receptor site area.

Ideally, the placement and adjustment of final abutment heads on two-stage implants at the insertion visit *ensure absolute control of parallelism.* After implant insertion, they are removed and set aside. Healing collars or caps are placed until completion of long-term healing.

Adjusting Head Height for Interocclusal Clearance

After paralleling and rotational abutment head bends are made, and the implant is partially seated

with the base of the head 2 mm above the ridge crest, the patient is asked to close into centric occlusion if opposing teeth are present. Any previous pre-insertion head height adjustments are checked. If the patient can close into centric occlusion at this time and not touch the abutment head, there will be at least a 2-mm clearance after final seating. In final seating the implant will seat 2 mm more to engage the abutment head base at the ridge crest. If the abutment head interferes with closure prior to final seating, the implant is removed and sufficient metal is removed to produce adequate clearance. The implant is then reinserted and tested for accuracy.

In the case of two-stage implants, interocclusal clearance adjustments of the final abutment heads may be accomplished with the head(s) on or off the implant body.

Final Seating

Final seating of the implant is done with either a shoulder set-point or shoulder set-slot single- or double-headed seating instrument, depending on the implant configuration and the degree of previous abutment head bending for parallelism. As seating progresses, and the implant vents approach the ridge crest, an anorganic bone mineral granular graft that has been mixed with harvested bone (if any) is prepared and inserted to fill each vent. If the head was bent more than 15 degrees, and the long axes of the head and the body diverge significantly, only a shoulder set-point or shoulder set-slot seating instrument can be used. All seating forces must be directed in the long axis of the implant body when the seating instrument engages the implant during tapping with the mallet. With gentle tapping and full vision, the implant is seated until the base of the abutment head engages the ridge crest. The body of a correctly seated implant must press-fit tightly and securely against cancellous bone. No movement is permissible. Frictional press-fit keeps the implant immobile and promotes proper healing. When there is a significant abutment head bend for parallelism, which is often seen in the maxilla, the base of the abutment head may engage the lingual but not the buccal or labial crest of bone (Fig 9–22). The implant should then be removed, reducing only the lin-

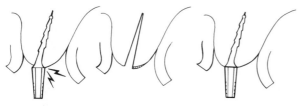

FIG 9–22.
The ridge crest is adjusted to ensure equal engagement of the safety stop.

gual crest of bone in the area of the base of the abutment head. On reseating, the abutment head base will engage both plates of bone. If there is a firm lingual crest and a thin labial crest, the implant can remain seated with the abutment head base engaging only the lingual crest. The abutment head is tapped and a solid ringing sound will indicate that the implant is securely and properly seated.

Occasionally a receptor site is prepared too wide, or is inadvertently widened during repeated preliminary insertions in order to make adjustments. In this case, the body is bent into a gentle curve to establish three-point contact, with the mesial and distal ends snug against the lingual of the receptor site and the middle portion snug against the labial or buccal of the receptor site. This is the last bending adjustment to the implant body prior to final seating. This adjustment is rarely needed, but is essential if required. No adjusting bends of any type should be made to coated plate or blade form implants. Coatings will crack, promoting pit and fissure corrosion, and expose what may not be biocompatible metal that was treated to receive the coating.

The implant is now seated and a progress periapical radiograph is done to verify all positioning.

Implanting New (or Healing) Extraction Sites

An implant may be placed immediately after an extraction provided there has been no purulence, curettage of all granulation tissue has been thorough, and there is adequate available bone on either side of the extraction site. This is also true in the case of a partially healed recent extraction site. The base of the implant abutment head is ideally seated against healed cortical bone on the ridge crest, not unsup-

ported over the extraction site (Fig 9–23). It is preferable, however, to wait for final healing prior to implantation.

Gingival Plastic Surgery

Often, the gingival flaps at the anterior portion of the mandible and in most areas of the maxilla are excessive and mobile. This indicates a need for plastic surgery. The amount of tissue is reduced along the incision line as required for a snug, firm apposition of both sides of the flap, retaining adequate attached gingiva. In the maxilla, the tissue may be too thick and cover too much head height. With a scalpel a wedge of tissue is removed from between the periosteum and the gingival crest. This will reduce tissue thickness but maintain both the tough gingival epithelium at the crest, and the valuable periosteum against the bone. Excess tissue is trimmed from the closure line, and the tissue punched (Fig 9–24).

Preparation of Gingival Tissue Around Abutment Head(s)

Single-Stage Systems.—Abutment heads occupy space. Removal of gingival tissue on the buccal and lingual side of the abutment heads prevents the tissue from bunching around them and encourages good gingival contour and healing. Essentially, the gingiva is wrapped around the abutment heads to create the optimal peri-implant cuff in the attached gingiva.

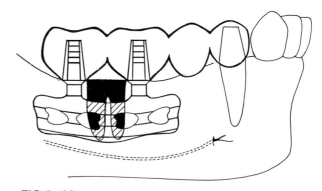

FIG 9–23.
The implant post is placed against the healed ridge crest in the area of recent extraction.

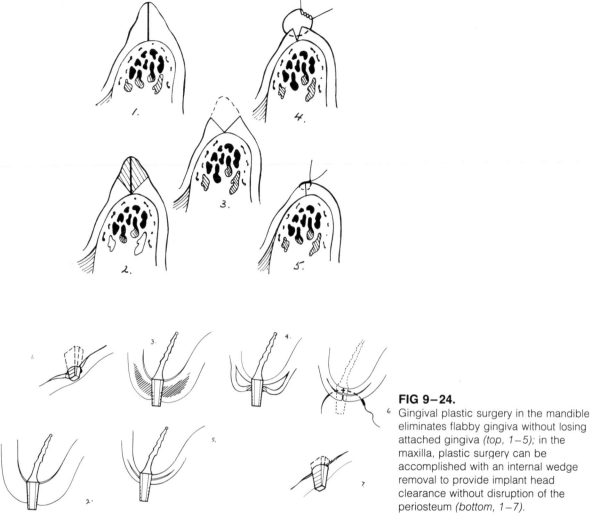

FIG 9–24.
Gingival plastic surgery in the mandible eliminates flabby gingiva without losing attached gingiva *(top, 1–5);* in the maxilla, plastic surgery can be accomplished with an internal wedge removal to provide implant head clearance without disruption of the periosteum *(bottom, 1–7).*

To properly excise this tissue, a semilunar tissue punch is used. First, the flaps are positioned against the abutment heads, and the tissue opposite the midline is marked with a felt pen to indicate precisely where the tissue should be removed. The tissue punch is placed and the tissue cleanly excised. The edges of the flaps are repositioned around the abutment head(s) (Fig 9–25). Accuracy is checked and correction made if necessary.

Two-Stage Systems.—If the option of total submerging is chosen, no tissue punching is done. When the semisubmerged option is chosen, tissue punching is done.

Final Closure

Single-Stage Systems.—The portion of the receptor site between the ridge crest and the implant shoulder is now filled with the same anorganic bone graft mixed with harvested bone (if any) as was used to fill the vents during the early stages of final seating. The flaps are coapted for suturing.

Suturing is an extremely important part of the procedure. An atraumatic needle is used, triple zero or its equivalent. The first suture is placed directly anterior to the anterior head of the implant, and the second distal to the abutment head, or distal to the distal abutment head in a two-headed implant. The

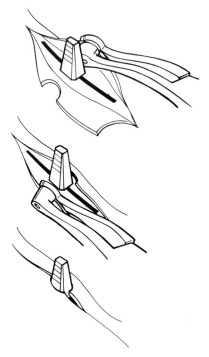

FIG 9–25.
A semilunar tissue incision ensures an optimal gingival cuff.

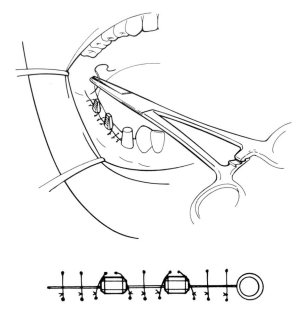

FIG 9–26.
Suggested suturing pattern for blade implants.

next sutures go between the abutment heads. Then, a suture is carefully placed adjacent to the natural abutment tooth, followed by interrupted sutures to close the incision securely at all points. When in doubt, extra sutures are placed (Fig 9–26).

Wet gauze is pressed against the sutured areas to hold the tissue down evenly. Direct pressure is applied for about 30 seconds. This completes the insertion procedure, and the case is now ready for temporization, if required. In selected single implant cases, when natural abutments have been prepared, final master impressions and interocclusal registrations may now be taken. During the administration of local anesthesia, no fluid was injected into the area where the pontics of the final bridge will be located in order to prevent edema. After the tissue is pressed down against the bone, it assumes the final position it will have after healing. There is not yet any natural edema. Hence, master impressions can now be taken. If one is placing an implant abutment for a restorative dentist, the patient appears for final impressions within 2 hours, before natural edema occurs. If

not, impressions may be taken approximately 2 weeks after final healing, subsequent to suture removal.

Two-Stage Systems.—If the option of total submerging is chosen, the final abutment head(s) is removed, and the healing collar is placed into position. Flaps are now coapted and suturing is completed.

When the option of semisubmerging is chosen, suturing is accomplished with the final abutment head(s) in position. After suturing is completed, the final abutment head(s) is removed and a healing collar or cap is inserted. The gingival tissue is carefully placed and pressed around the healing collar so that its upper surface is flush with or at most 1 mm above the tissue. Semisubmerging facilitates early attached gingiva formation around the abutment head during healing.

Temporization and Function During Healing

Single-Stage Systems.—Provisional prostheses for small fixed bridges utilizing both implant and natural abutments are fabricated in the same way as prostheses over natural abutments. Accurate margins, wide embrasures, careful occlusal adjustment, and high polish are all desirable. Provisional cement is placed only under natural abutments. No cement should be used in association with implant abutments. Frictional fit will be adequate. This protects the implant during healing, and when the provisional bridge is removed to facilitate suture removal or trial of final seating of the new prosthesis.

In the case of posterior bridges, where the implant abutment is not in an esthetically important area, the implant is allowed to heal freestanding. In the opinion of many, this is the method of choice. The most carefully made provisional prostheses can be weak, may break, or may have delicate margins. Any one of these may interfere with healing. In esthetically important areas, the implant abutments are always included under the provisional prosthesis.

Postoperative Home Care.—In extensive cases, an ice pack may be administered in the office immediately postoperatively, followed by a recommended ice pack regimen for home use, usually for 1 day. For all types of cases, gentle rinsing with warm saline solution is suggested, starting on the second day, to be performed three to four times daily for 1 week.

Prophylaxis of the provisional prosthesis at home is done with a soft brush. Sutures must not be disturbed.

A soft diet is recommended, that is, anything liquid or that turns to liquid. Soup, yogurt, ice cream, cooked cereals, milk and the like are taken until 1 or 2 weeks after insertion of the final prosthesis. Prepared nutritional supplements or full-value liquid protein regimens may be helpful. Patients with digestive problems should receive advice from their physician.

Provisional prostheses for complete-arch cases totally supported by implants always include all implant abutments. No provisional cement is placed. The fit is entirely frictional.

In general, the implant does not require splinting or extra protection during healing. If the residual alveolar ridge is narrow or the basic occlusion is not optimal, including the implant in a strong well-made provisional prosthesis is desirable. In marginal cases requiring protected healing due to extremely thin ridges, two-stage implants and submerged healing are preferred. A conservative approach is best. Marginal cases, except in very experienced hands, are probably best treated with conventional dentistry.

Two-Stage Systems.—There is a wide variety of removable, and rarely fixed, provisional appliances utilized to provide function for patients during the extended healing period. In general, all appliances are relieved as they pass over the submerged or semisubmerged abutment head area, to ensure adequate protection for the implant during healing. Soft relining is often recommended.

Suture Removal.—The first postoperative visit is to remove sutures. Earlier visits are not required unless there is reason. Patients are encouraged to call with questions, for advice, or for an appointment if they wish one for any reason.

Sutures are usually removed 7 to 12 days after the operation. In cases of single plate or blade form insertions, 7 days is adequate. In more extensive cases a longer wait is recommended. In extensive cases, and for patients with a friable gingiva, it is advisable to remove every other suture after 10 to 12 days, and the remainder 4 to 5 days later to prevent dehiscence.

When necessary, the provisional prosthesis is removed to facilitate suture removal. Movement or excessive trauma will disturb the healing implant. In posterior single-implant abutment cases, the sutures are removed without removing the provisional prosthesis from the natural abutments.

A valuable instrument in suture removal is the suture scissors. The hooked end slips atraumatically under the suture to sever it. College pliers are used for gentle withdrawal. An antiseptic is applied. This procedure causes little or no discomfort.

HEALING TIME AND SEQUENCING ONE-STAGE AND TWO-STAGE SYSTEMS

Following suture removal, healing is evaluated. If the provisional prosthesis was removed, it should be replaced now. In one-stage systems, if master impressions were not taken at the time of the implant insertion, an additional week is allowed for healing. In two-stage systems, 3 to 6 months' healing in the mandible and 6 to 9 months' healing in the maxilla are recommended. The length of healing time is affected in part by the length, width, and depth of the implant inserted. In general, a longer healing time is required in cases with smaller implants, greater angle bends between abutment heads and implant bodies, for implants that will function opposite a natural dentition or fixed prosthesis, and for the elderly.

EXPOSURE OF TWO-STAGE IMPLANT AFTER HEALING

Semisubmerged Option

In cases where the semisubmerged option was chosen, the healing collar is simply removed. In ideal configurations, the gingival cuff will be healed and exhibit a circumference that is compatible with that of the final abutment head.

The final abutment head is fastened according to the manufacturer's recommendations. Interocclusal clearance and parallelism have already been provided and checked. In the team approach, this procedure is best done by the restorative partner.

It is recommended that final attachment be accomplished at this time, followed by fabrication of a new prosthesis or adjustment of the previous provisional prosthesis, as circumstances require. This will avoid the use of analog systems and more certainly ensure the correct and passive fit of new prostheses. An effort should be made to avoid the use of analog systems. Continued removal and reinsertion of abutment heads and healing collars causes unnecessary trauma to the tissue. The fastened final abutment heads are treated as one would treat natural abutments. Elastic impressions, as customarily performed, can be utilized.

Submerged Option

Where the submerged option was chosen, anesthesia is administered, and the healing collar or cap is surgically exposed according to the manufacturer's recommendations. Some systems require a secondary healing collar or cap to clear the gingival crest and allow for formation of a healed cuff. Others advise placement of the final abutment head, which also promotes formation of the gingival cuff. This is the preferred technique.

Chapter 10

Periodontal Considerations for Implantology

Roland M. Meffert, D.D.S.

This chapter is concerned with the periodontal aspects of dental implantology and how to prevent "peri-implantitis" both before and after the restorative phase of endosseous implantology. The endosseous dental implant is divided into two phases: the first phase is within bone and the implant-bone interface must be maintained to remain healthy and functional; the second phase of the system exists through the gingiva, is perimucosal, and is totally dependent on a biological seal and optimum home care for achievement of a healthy bordering tissue.

The contradictory theories of fibro-osseous integration and osseointegration in terms of endosseous implant retention are discussed with the rationale and philosophy of each. Step-by-step bone healing after injury (placement of an implant system) is presented and correlated with the theories of implant retention.

Finally, case selection and treatment planning from the periodontist's viewpoint, to achieve optimum success, and maintenance techniques and therapy related to dental implants are covered in detail.

PERIODONTAL CONSIDERATIONS FOR IMPLANTOLOGY

A prerequisite to a successful endosseous dental implant should be to obtain a perimucosal seal of the soft tissue to the implant surface. Failure to achieve or maintain this seal results in the apical migration of the epithelium into the implant-bone interface and the possible complete encapsulation of the endosseous or root portion of the implant system.

Perimucosal or Transgingival Area

In the natural dentition, the junctional epithelium provides a seal at the base of the sulcus against the penetration of chemical and bacterial substances. If the seal is disrupted or the fibers apical to the epithelium are lysed or destroyed, the epithelium migrates apically, forming a periodontal pocket after cleavage of the soft tissue from the radicular surface. Since there is no cementum or fiber insertion on the surface of an endosseous implant, the perimucosal seal is all-important. If it is lost, the periodontal pocket extends to the osseous structures.

Is a perimucosal seal possible in the case of the endosseous dental implant? Gould et al.[1] reported that epithelial cells attach to the surface of titanium in much the same manner in which the epithelial cells attach to the surface of a natural tooth, i.e., via a basal lamina and the formation of hemidesmosomes. Schroeder et al.[2] observed that if the post of the implant were situated in a region of immobile, keratinized mucosa, a sign of adhesion of the epithelial cells to the titanium-sprayed surface would be apparent. Stallard et al.[3] and Skerman et al.[4] also reported that tissue culture and animal and human experiments confirmed a dynamic epithelial attachment between gingival epithelial cells and the smooth surface of vitreous carbon.

McKinney et al.[5] confirmed an ultrastructural level attachment complex (basal lamina, hemidesmosomes) between the gingiva and the aluminum oxide (single-crystal sapphire) implant—an attachment analogous to that seen around natural teeth.

Jansen[6] disputed the findings of Gould et al. and reported a hemidesmosomal attachment only on polystyrene or apatite specimens and never on carbon or metallic substrates. He attempted to explain the difference in findings by theorizing a difference in substrates or cell population between his study and that of Gould et al. Wennstrom[7, 8] also disagrees with Schroeder in the respect that attached gingiva around natural teeth is not necessarily a prerequisite for gingival health. He speculates that movable mucosa around the transepithelial extension of an endosseous implant is not necessarily a vulnerable situation. Clinical experience demonstrates that keratinized tissue at the transgingival area of a dental implant renders the area more accessible to optimum home care procedures and therefore more maintainable. Furthermore, the patient with dental implant(s) is not only hesitant to accomplish an effective oral hygiene regimen because of the fear of "causing it to fail" but is left with prosthetic devices and superstructures quite different from the normal gingival-tooth contours and relationships, a situation requiring special attention and instruction in terms of home care procedures.

If it is true that junctional epithelial attachment to the implant substrate is not predictable in a metallic system, can anything be done to retard epithelial invagination? Von Recum et al.[9] used collagen and fibronectin to promote fibroblast proliferation and mitotic activity in a series of laboratory animal experiments. Kleinman et al.[10] demonstrated that collagen bound fibronectin provided an excellent substratum for cell attachment in vitro. Von Recum et al. reported that the fibronectin, so closely associated with fibroblast attachment, actually retarded healing rather than promoted adhesion. Their studies showed that epithelium migrated apically at the rate of up to 2 mm/wk in an animal model and predictably ended at the crest of the bone when using a metallic substrate. Lowenberg et al.[11] reported on use of bovine

collagen on titanium alloy (Ti-6Al-4V) to enhance fibroblast attachment and mitotic activity in a 14-day study; a comparison of the uncoated substrate to coating with collagen and using a demineralized root slice as a control demonstrated a close comparison between the coated metal and the root slice control. The uncoated alloy did not compare favorably and no attachment was evident. Another study by the same group[12] compared the attachment of fibroblasts to Ti-6Al-4V and a zirconium alloy; there was no difference between the materials in terms of fibroblast growth. The study also showed a better attachment to a smooth surface but a better orientation of the cells to a porous or rough surface.

Laminin has recently been associated with epithelial cell adhesion. Seitz et al.[13] described predictable adhesion to Bioglass (a silica-based glass) when the surface was treated with laminin.

Most implant materials are biocompatible, but microporosity in the neck area will often result in failure. Klawitter et al.[14] placed porous alumina implants in mongrel dogs and stabilized them with acrylic splints for 8 weeks; after 6 months only 2 of the 44 implants were still in place and all the failures were associated with severe inflammation and pocket depths. DePorter et al.[15] placed implants in dogs, porous not only in the radicular portion but also in the transgingival area. Severe bone loss was noted after 7 months in more than half of the implants placed due to plaque retention and marked inflammation. Both Klawitter et al. and DePorter et al. proposed that a rough surface at the gingival-implant interface is extremely detrimental to tissue health.

As stated earlier, loss of the biological seal begins the inevitable failure of the dental implant. The junctional epithelium migrates apically into the bone-implant interface (Figs 10–1 and 10–2), eventually progressing to complete encapsulation of the osseous portion of the implant (Fig 10–3). An inflammatory response will ensue and typical periodontal-type bone loss with loss of the attachment apparatus through osteoclastic activity will result (Fig 10–4). It is recognized that there is no direct connective tissue attachment to the surface of an implant to keep gingival tissues adapted to the surface, but recent work by de Lange et al.[16] with hydroxylapatite-coated titanium implants revealed the devel-

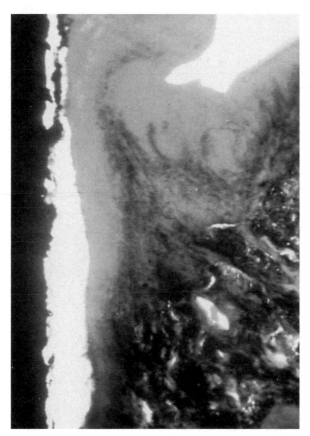

FIG 10–1.
Separation of soft tissue from the titanium surface.

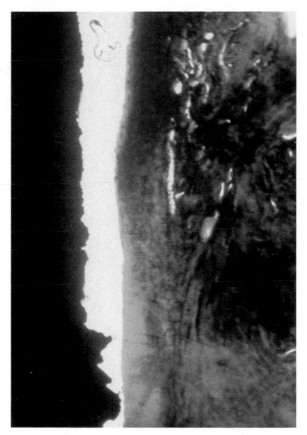

FIG 10–2.
Deep separation from the titanium surface (epithelial invagination).

opment of a supra-alveolar connective tissue attachment apparatus, with bundles of gingival fibers perpendicularly ending on the hydroxylapatite implant surface and embedded in a calcified layer covering the implant. This osteophilic or osteoconductive nature of hydroxylapatite has been confirmed in subsequent unloaded studies (Fig 10–5).

Endosteal Area

In a healthy endosteal implant, the only supporting structure is bone. Any fibrous encapsulation around an endosseous dental implant does not mimic the periodontal ligament. Whereas the periodontal ligament is constantly adapting to changes and collagen remodeling, the encapsulation around an implant is just that: it does not remodel, and when movement

ensues the encapsulation continues to expand. Linkow and Wertman[17] believe that the deeper structures initiate situations leading to implant failure; failure does not occur initially at the surface or perimucosal area.

The two basic means of retention of an endosteal dental implant in function are fibro-osseous retention and osseointegration. According to the American Association of Implant Dentistry (AAID) glossary[18] the term *fibro-osseous retention* is defined as tissue-to-implant contact: interposition of healthy dense collagenous tissue between implant and bone.

Weiss[19] defends the presence of collagen fibers at the interface between the implant and bone and interprets it as a peri-implant membrane with an osteogenic effect. He speculates that the fibers invest the implant, originating at a trabecula of cancellous bone

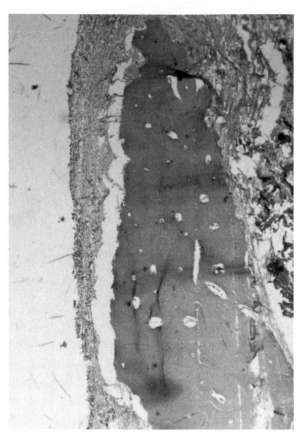

FIG 10–3.
Fibrous tissue encapsulation around the implant (implant removed).

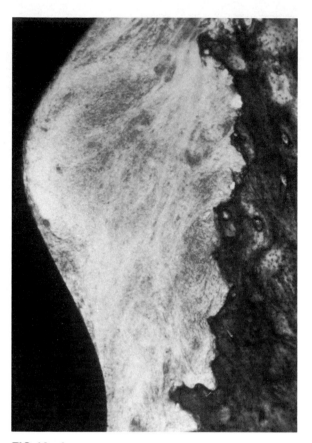

FIG 10–4.
Progressing bone loss (osteoclastic activity around the implant).

on one side, weaving their way around the implant, and reinserting into a trabecula on the other side. When function is applied to the implant, tension is applied to the fiber(s); forces closest to the implant interface cause a compression of the fibers, with a corresponding tension on the fibers placed or inserting into the trabeculae. The difference between the inner aspect (compression) and the outer aspect (tension) of the connective tissue components results in a bioelectric current and this bioelectric current (piezoelectric effect) induces differentiation into connective tissue components associated with bone maintenance. Hence the premise of the fibers being osteogenic.

Weiss[19] further speculates that the cylindrical or root form of implant now in common use would be invested with a fiber that is too long, in which the occlusal forces transmitted would be dissipated and the beneficial bioelectric effect would not be produced; however, fibers around a spiral, blade, or pin-type implant would be short enough for the piezoelectric effect. It is the prime theory of fibro-osseous integration that connective tissue at the interface is functional and desirable; that it is directly related to implant design along with the intentional preparation of bone with controlled, slightly elevated temperatures and placement of the implant in function early after insertion.[20]

On the other hand, *osseointegration,* as defined, is a contact established between normal remodeled bone and an implant surface *without* the interposition of nonbone or connective tissue.[18] The word was

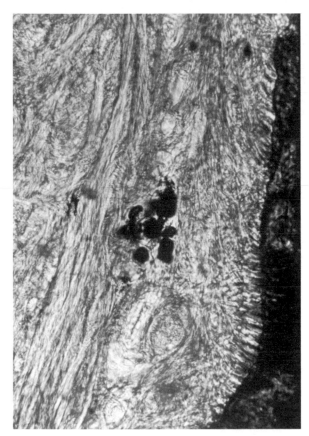

FIG 10–5.
New gingival fiber insertion into osteoid on the hydroxylapatite surface.

coined by Per-Ingvar Brånemark and is explained in detail in the text, *Tissue-Integrated Prostheses: Osseointegration in Clinical Dentistry*.[21]

The term *osseointegration* was used in conjunction with surgical titanium and Brånemark reported that the bone was not separated from the titanium surface by any fibrous tissue membrane but rather that normal bone components grow to within 100 to 200 A of the metallic surface with the interface between the metal and the bone consisting of a titanium dioxide layer and a protein glycosaminoglycan.[21] The development of a surface oxide—TiO_2 in the case of titanium or titanium alloy—is supposedly one of the reasons for the excellent biocompatibility of the metal. The tightly adherent oxide layer, called passivation, covers the implant and prevents a direct contact be-

tween the potentially harmful metallic ions and the tissue.[33] Brånemark et al.[21] believe that contact of the base metal with bone may result in corrosion. Albrektsson et al.[22] observed that the thickness of the proteoglycan layer was inversely related to the biocompatibility of the implant material; stainless steel, which has to be chemically passivated or subjected to a series of chemical baths, has a layer that is thousands of angstroms thick whereas titanium, passivated during the machining process, is surrounded by a layer less than 100 A thick. Much attention is given at the present time to sterilization of the implant surface. Baier[23] has advocated RFGDT (*r*adio*f*requency *g*low *d*ischarge *t*reatment) for the titanium material. This ion bombardment of the surface not only cleanses the implant material from organic debris but imparts increased surface energy and wettability, factors which supposedly induce cell growth, cell adhesion, and implant fixation.

FIBRO-OSSEOUS INTEGRATION VS. OSSEOINTEGRATION

The proponents of the two theories of implant retention and stabilization (fibro-osseous integration vs. osseointegration) are entirely at odds in their philosophies of tissue maintenance as related to function. According to Weiss[24] it is the difference between afunction and hypofunction or between submerging the endosseous portion of the implant or protecting it. Weiss[24] agrees that an afunctional, submerged system will allow for direct bone apposition (osseointegration). But he believes that submerging the system will result in retarded healing while the protected or hypofunctional implant (one-stage) is subjected to forces of low duration and magnitude. He speculates that the submerged implant, out of function for 3 to 6 months, will soon fail when placed in full function. According to the clinical application of the fibro-osseous theory, implants are placed in full function 1 to 2 months after insertion after being in a protected or hypofunctional mode since the day of insertion. This is in stark contrast to the Brånemark philosophy of avoiding loading before 3 to 6 months postinsertion.

Exactly what does happen when an implant is placed into bone? Roberts et al.[25] report that a bridging callus originates within a few millimeters of the implant site and a lattice of woven bone reaches the implant surface in approximately 6 weeks. They believe that this bridging callus requires complete stability of the two segments and has very little load-carrying capability.

The degree of bridging is dependent not only on stability but also on the distance between the bone and the implant surface. Harrell[26] observed in studies on Bioglass that bone will not bridge predictably more than 0.5 mm so it is absolutely essential that the implant fit the site.

The lattice structure of woven bone is filled with well-organized lamellae and maximum load-carrying capability in the human is not achieved before 18 weeks. A maximum compact or composite bone interface is achieved in the human in approximately 1 year.

So the work of Roberts et al.[25] seems to correlate very closely with the rationale of Branemark. Maximum load-carrying capability is achieved in 4 to 5 months and Branemark advocates protecting the system for 3 to 6 months before placing it in function. Weiss[24] advocates placing the implant in full function in 1 to 2 months, long before the lamellar latticework is in place and the load-carrying capability is reached.

What may cause the formation of a connective tissue interface? The following may account for a lack of osseointegration (definition: lack of connective tissue at the bone-implant interface at the light microscopic level) and development of the fibrous interface:

1. Premature loading of the system (earlier than 3 months, mandible, and 6 months, maxilla)
2. Invagination of epithelium (common in the one-stage system)
3. Overheating the bone during site preparation (above 47° C is detrimental)
4. Placing the implant with too much pressure (causes bone necrosis)
5. Implant not fitting the site exactly (needs 0.5 mm or less space)

What will happen if we have a connective tissue interface? If the implant is mobile, the connective tissue encapsulation continues to expand in width and mobility increases. If the implant is nonmobile and the width of the interface is minimal, the implant will continue to function.

Fibro-osseous integration may be present as a functioning entity *only* in the subperiosteal implant; in the endosseous systems, the connective tissue is present in varying widths only as a parallel fiber arrangement (Fig 10–6) or as a complete encapsulation (Fig 10–7). There is no functional arrangement of the fibers in any case (Fig 10–8) and it is difficult to discern the difference between a proposed peri-implant ligament with theoretical osteogenic potential and a so-called pseudarthrosis which is identified with a failing implant.[24]

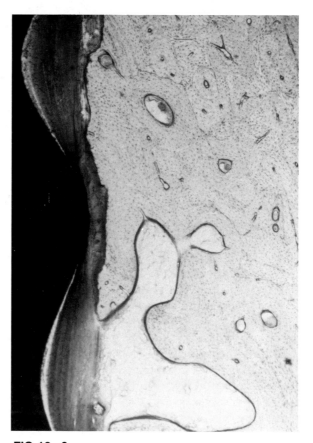

FIG 10–6.
Parallel fiber arrangement between implant *(left)* and bone *(right).*

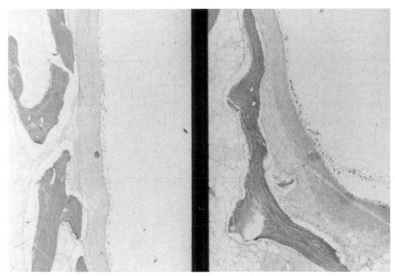

FIG 10–7.
Complete fiber encapsulation around the implant (implant removed).

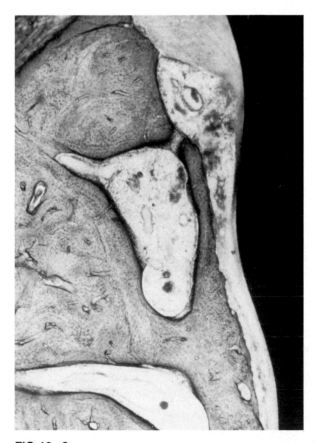

FIG 10–8.
Lack of fiber orientation between bone *(left)* and implant *(right)*.

OSSEOINTEGRATION VS. BIOINTEGRATION

Recent research has redefined the retention means of dental implants in the terminology of osseointegration vs. biointegration. De Putter et al.[27] observed that there were two ways of implant anchorage or retention: mechanical and bioactive.

Mechanical retention basically refers to the metallic substrate systems such as titanium or titanium alloy. The retention is based on undercut forms such as screws, blades, vents, slots, etc. and involves direct contact between bone and implant, either directly after implantation or before loading.

Bioactive retention can be achieved with bioactive materials such as hydroxylapatite or Bioglass which bond directly to bone, similar to ankylosis of natural teeth. Bone matrix is deposited on the hydroxylapatite layer as a result of physicochemical interaction between bone collagen and the hydroxylapatite crystals of the implant.[28]

Animal research has shown that not only do we have the possibility of the development of a supraalveolar connective tissue apparatus with new gingival fibers inserting into new osteoid, but also the coronal growth of new bone on the surface of a material such as hydroxylapatite (Fig 10–9) and lamellar bone forming in close apposition to a bioactive surface (Fig 10–10). The latter finding would seem

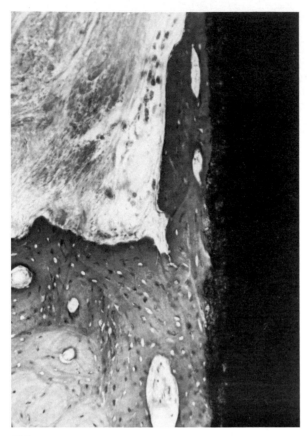

FIG 10–9.
Coronal osteoid activity on the hydroxylapatite surface (moving from the original crest).

FIG 10–10.
Lamellar bone formation on the facial surface and vent area of a hydroxylapatite-coated implant.

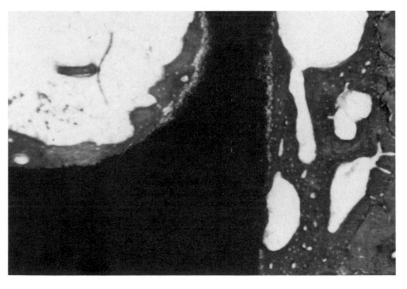

to support the hypothesis that the formation of a lamellar layer on the surface of the implant affords better retention in an area of spongy (cancellous) bone where retention is only gained through direct mechanical contact of bone with an undercut form. Research is being directed at this time to the response of a bonded material when load is applied over a period of time.

HYGIENE INSTRUMENTATION

How to maintain the dental implant? Hygienic techniques and armamentaria such as motorized interdental brushes and antimicrobial agents are often indicated because of the importance of the perimucosal seal, but how do we treat the periodontal pocket associated with the transgingival area of a dental implant and how do we treat the osseous defect attendant to an implant endosseous portion?

Studies[29] are demonstrating that ultrasonic instruments should not be used subgingivally because of scarring, grooving of the implant surface, and in the case of the titanium implant coated with hydroxylapatite, actually removing the hydroxylapatite itself. Any instrument used subgingivally on the implant surface should be Teflon-coated or plastic to prevent contamination or altering of the implant surface. The stainless-steel curet and even the titanium curet should be used sparingly and only on the soft tissue wall, never on the implant itself.

In the case of the actual osseous defect surrounding the dental implant, grafting materials such as synthetic alloplastic grafts and allografts are used. In my experience, none are totally effective in salvaging the failing implant but only in effecting some repair and delaying the inevitable. Once the implant is mobile as a result of loss of osseous support, no amount of grafting or stabilization, or both will restore the supportive apparatus.

DISCUSSION

The periodontal aspect of dental implantology in terms of avoiding or preventing "peri-implantitis" can be addressed from the prerestorative and post-restorative phases.

Initially, injury to the soft tissue must be minimized. This not only involves the preservation of keratinized tissue (or soft tissue grafting preimplant insertion to gain keratinized tissue) but also careful surgical incision and mucoperiosteal flap reflection. Smiler[30] observes that the osteogenic capacity of the periosteum must be preserved through the careful avoidance of excessive overstripping of periosteum from bone and by using lateral, instead of crestal, incisions if at all possible.

Branemark et al.[21] theorize that the prime reason for implant failure before the restorative phase is the frictional heat generated during surgery. Eriksson et al.[31] measured the temperature at 0.5 mm away from the drill edge when preparing for skull plates in humans. In spite of copious cooling with saline, the temperature was 89° C. The heat was so severe that a few seconds at that temperature was sufficient to prevent bone healing around the screws stabilizing the plate. Eriksson and Albrektsson[32] heated threaded titanium implants for a minute at 44°, 47°, and 50° C, and placed them in rabbit tibias. When examined after 4 weeks, implants heated for 1 minute at 50° C showed no bone formation, those heated at 47° C showed partial bone formation, and those heated at 44° C showed complete investment with bone. In order to minimize frictional heat during surgery, it is recommended that the drill be run at speeds no greater than 2,000 rpm, cooled with saline (internally if possible), and use a graded series of drill sizes instead of a one-step procedure. Much more heat is generated with a one-step drill even with internal irrigation.[21]

The implant must fit the site exactly. Harrell[26] reported that bone will not bridge predictably more than 0.5 mm. There is a difference of opinion in terms of implant "fit." Linkow and Wertman[17] propose that the implant fit passively without pressure. Weiss[19] advocates making the implant site slightly smaller than the implant so it can assume a tight frictional fit. There is no doubt, however, that if the implant is mobile on the day of insertion or if the space between implant and bone is marked, connective tissue will soon encapsulate the system and it will fail.

Assuming the endosseous portion of the dental implant has been submerged and protected with a mucoperiosteal flap for a time, what could cause failure of the implant *after* the restorative phase? Branemark et al.[21] believe that the second reason for implant failure is not allowing for an adequate healing time of 3 to 6 months before subjecting it to loading. Bone differentiation cannot take place in the face of mobility over a period of weeks. Weiss[19] advocates placing the system in full function in 1 to 2 months depending upon the theory of fibro-osseous integration and the presence of an osteogenic peri-implant ligament, instead of stability of the segments (bone and implant). The work of Roberts et al.,[25] suggesting that the initial callus reaching the implant surface in 6 weeks has very little load-carrying capability and that maximum load-carrying capability is reached in approximately 18 weeks in the human, would seem to support the premise of Branemark and colleagues.

The presence and maintenance of a perimucosal seal is all-important in endosseous implant predictability. The finding by Gould et al.,[1] that epithelial cells attach to titanium, is disputed by Jansen[6] and it is probable that there is no biological attachment of a predictable nature between the soft tissue and the implant surface and that the adaptation of the soft tissue at the transgingival area is due more to the circular fibers providing a tonus and close tissue approximation rather than to any epithelial cell attachment.

Various agents such as fibronectin and collagen[9, 11, 12] and laminin[13] have been used to coat the implant transgingival area to facilitate epithelial cell adhesion and fibroblast growth, but results have been contradictory to this point.

It is also apparent that the transgingival or perimucosal area of the implant should be smooth and not porous, as demonstrated by clinical studies in dogs.[14, 15] This negates not only the prospect of plaque retention but also the formation of a fibrous tissue capsule around the implant.

Hygiene is all-important in maintaining the dental implant. It is essential that the transgingival unit have a straight-emergence profile, eliminating any areas of plaque retention. Antimicrobials such as chlorhexidine digluconate are extremely effective in reducing plaque, and interdental brushes, motorized cleaning devices, are often indicated for optimal home care. It is essential that a period of home care instruction be instituted immediately after insertion of the superstructure or prosthesis and the patient seen every 3 months to check gingival health, plaque indices, and probing depths. If possible, the superstructure should be retrievable or removable so that it can be removed yearly to check mobility, pocket depths, and gingival health around the implant post. It is important to remember that the dental implant is a weak unit without connective tissue and epithelial cell attachment so that any gingival changes due to inefficient home care would soon be translated into disaster and failure of the system.

The theories of fibro-osseous integration and osseointegration have been discussed in detail. In the author's opinion, the formation of a connective tissue interface is dictated by surgical trauma, poor fit of the implant in the surgical site, and premature loading, and really has no function in terms of support.

SUMMARY

An endosseous dental implant must first of all penetrate the mucogingival tissues. Although most implant materials are biocompatible, they do not afford the soft and hard tissue attachment mechanisms that are present in the natural dentition. Thus a perimucosal seal, probably mediated more through the tonus of the circular gingival fibers surrounding the

transgingival unit than through any type of epithelial cell attachment, is all-important to maintain. This seal is understandably weak and optimal home care, often with the use of specialized devices and antimicrobial agents, is a necessity.

Second, the bone-implant interface is quite different from the bone-tooth interface. The latter is a functionally arranged collagen fiber arrangement attached to tooth and bone and able to adapt very well to any afunctional forces. The former consists of either a very close adaptation (osseointegration), a sling-type connective tissue interface (fibro-osseous integration), or actual chemical bonding (biointegration). The nature of the interface and connection needs more study in determining adaptability.

Finally, maintenance of the tissue interface is dependent on restorative considerations and a realization that if the device is overloaded in magnitude or direction of force, it cannot adapt and is doomed to failure.

REFERENCES

1. Gould TR, Brunette DM, Westbury L: The attachment mechanism of epithelial cells to titanium in vitro. *J Periodont Res* 1981; 16:611–616.
2. Schroeder A, van der Zypen E, Stich H: The reactions of bone, connective tissue, and epithelium to endosteal implants with titanium-sprayed surfaces. *J Oral Maxillofac Surg* 1981; 9:15–25.
3. Stallard RE, El Geneidy AK, Skerman HJ: Current research findings on the vitreous carbon tooth root replacement system. *Dtsch Zahnartzl Z* 1974; 29:746–748.
4. Skerman HJ, El Geneidy AK, Stallard RE: Periodontal implications of the surface characteristics of dental implants in the area of the gingival junction. *J Periodontal* 1974; 45:731–738.
5. McKinney RV, Steflik DE, Koth DL: Evidence for a junctional epithelial attachment to ceramic dental implants—a transmission electron microscopic study. *J Periodontal* 1985; 56:579–591.
6. Jansen JA: Ultrastructural study of epithelial cell attachment to implant materials. *J Dent Res* 1985; 65:891–896.
7. Wennstrom J: *Keratinized and Attached Gingiva: Regenerative Potential and Significance for Periodontal Health* (thesis). University of Göteborg, Sweden, 1982.
8. Wennstrom J, Lindhe J: Plaque-induced gingival in-

flammation in the absence of attached gingiva in dogs. *J Clin Periodontol* 1983; 10:266.

9. Von Recum AF, Schreuders PD, Powers DL: Basic healing phenomena around permanent percutaneous implants, in Proceedings of International Congress on Tissue Integration in Oral and Maxillofacial Reconstruction, May 1985, Brussels. Current Practice Series no. 29. Amsterdam, Excerpta Medica, 1985, pp 159–169.

10. Kleinman HK, Klebe RJ, Martin GR: Role of collagenous matrices in adhesion and growth of cells. *J Cell Biol* 1981; 88:473–485.

11. Lowenberg BF, Aubin JE, DePorter DA, et al: Attachment, migration and orientation of human gingival fibroblasts to collagen-coated, surface-demineralized and non-demineralized dentin in vitro. *J Periodont Res* 1985; 65:1106–1110.

12. Lowenberg BF, Pilliar RM, Aubin JE, et al: Migration, attachment, and orientation of human gingival fibroblasts to root slices, naked and porous-surfaced titanium alloy discs, and zircalloy 2 discs in vitro. *J Dent Res* 1987; 66:1000–1005.

13. Seitz TL, Noonan KD, Hench LL, et al: Effect of fibronectin on the adhesion of an established cell line to a surface reactive material. *J Biomed Mater Res* 1982; 16:195–202.

14. Klawitter JJ, Weinstein AM, Cooke FW: An evaluation of porous alumina ceramic implants. *J Dent Res* 1977; 56:768–775.

15. DePorter DA, Friedland B, Watson PA, et al: A clinical and radiographic assessment of a porous-surfaced, titanium alloy dental implant system in dogs. *J Dent Res* 1986; 65:1071–1077.

16. de Lange GL, de Putter C, de Groot K: Permucosal dental implants: The relationship between sealing and fixation, in Proceedings of International Congress on Tissue Integration in Oral and Maxillofacial Reconstruction. May, 1985, Brussels. *Current Practice Series* no. 29. Amsterdam, Excerpta Medica, 1985, pp 278–287.

17. Linkow LI, Wertman E: Re-entry implants and their procedures. *J Oral Implantol* 1986; 12:590–626.

18. Glossary of terms. *J Oral Implantol* 1986; 12:284–295.

19. Weiss CM: A comparative analysis of fibro-osteal and osteal integration and other variables that affect long term bone maintenance around dental implants. *J Oral Implantol,* 1987; 13:467–487.

20. Weiss CM: Tissue integration of dental endosseous implants: Descriptive and comparative analysis of fibro-osseous and osseointegration systems. *J Oral Implantol* 1986; 12:169–187.

21. Branemark PI, Zarb G, Albrektsson T: *Tissue-Integrated Prostheses: Osseointegration in Clinical Dentistry,* Chicago, Quintessence Publishing Co, 1985.

22. Albrektsson T, Branemark PI, Hansson Ha, et al: Osseointegrated titanium implants. *Acta Orthop Scand* 1981, 52:155–172.

23. Baier RE: Conditioning surfaces to suit the biomedical environment: Recent progress. *J Biomed Eng* 1982; 104:257–271.

24. Weiss CM: Tissue integration of dental endosseous implants. Description and comparative analysis of fibro-osseous and osseo-integration systems. *J Oral Implantol* 1986; 12:169–214.

25. Roberts WE, Turley PK, Brezniak N, et al: Bone physiology and metabolism. *J Calif Dent Assoc* 1987; 54(Oct): 54–63.

26. Harrell H: Thickness of bioglass bonding layers, in *Transactions of the Fourth Annual Meeting of the Society of Biomaterials,* San Antonio, 1978, p 70.

27. de Putter C, de Lange GL, de Groot K: Permucosal dental implants of dense hydroxylapatite: Fixation in alveolar bone, in Proceedings of International Congress on Tissue Integration in Oral and Maxillofacial Reconstruction, May 1985, Brussels. *Current Practice Series* no 29. Amsterdam, Excerpta Medica, 1985, pp 389–394.

28. Denissen HW, Veldhuis AAH, van den Hooff A: Hydroxylapatite titanium implants, in Proceedings of International Congress on Tissue Integration in Oral and Maxillofacial Reconstruction, May 1985, Brussels. *Current Practice Series no. 29.* Amsterdam, Excerpta Medica, 1985, pp 389–394.

29. Thomson-Neal D, Evans GH, Meffert RM: Effects of various prophylactic treatments on titanium, sapphire, and hydroxylapatite-coated implants. *Int J Periodont Rest Dent* 1989; 9:301–315.

30. Smiler DG: Evaluation and treatment planning. *J Calif Dent Assoc* 1987; 54(Oct):35–43.

31. Eriksson RA, Albrektsson T, Albrektsson B: Temperature measurements at drilling in cortical bone in vitro. *Acta Orthop Scand,* in press.

32. Eriksson RA, Albrektsson T: The effect of heat on bone regeneration. *J Oral Maxillofac Surg* 1984; 42:701–711.

33. Van Orden AC: Corrosive response of the interface tissue to 316 L stainless steel, titanium-based alloys and cobalt-based alloys, in McKinney RV Jr, Lemons JE (eds): *The Dental Implant.* Littleton, Mass, PSG Publishing Co Inc, 1985, pp 1–24.

PART II

Endosteal Implant Systems

Chapter 11

The Plate/Blade Oratronics Implant System

Charles M. Weiss, D.D.S.

THE IMPLANTS

The Oratronics Standard Blade Implant System

The Oratronics Standard Blade Implant System (Table 11–1), is the only plate/blade form implant system with provisional acceptance from the American Dental Association. Acceptance was granted, in part, as a result of independent prospective randomized controlled clinical trials conducted by the Veterans Administration (VA), and replicated at five VA hospitals, with a 95.8% 5-year implant survival rate.[1–3] No natural tooth co-abutments were lost during the 5-year study. This survival rate is remarkable when one considers that the implants were placed in generally narrow and shallow posterior bone, and withstood *four times* the magnitude of chewing forces that are applied to cylinder/root forms. The implants of this system, available in both one- and two-stage models, are illustrated in Figure 11–1. The labial- and buccal-lingual width of each implant is 1.2 mm, making them the implant of choice for marginally narrow ridges.

Oratronics Generation Ten Blade Implant System

The Generation Ten Blade Implant System was introduced some years after the Standard, when early computer studies and years of clinical experience suggested certain dimensional configuration changes to promote increased bone maintenance and ease of use.[4] The implants of this system, available in both one- and two-stage models, are illustrated in Figure 11–2. The labial- and buccal-lingual width of each implant is 1.35 mm, making them the implant of choice for narrow and medium narrow ridges.

Oratronics Osteo-Loc Plate Form Implant System

Combining form and function became the goal of a 6-year development cycle utilizing university-based research data that resulted in the Osteo-Loc Plate Form implant. Each Osteo-Loc Plate Form was designed to achieve a more homogeneous and equalized stress distribution as chewing forces are absorbed throughout the integrating body tissues (Figs 11–3 and 11–4,A). Data related to the limits of physiologic health between hypo- and hyperfunction were generated.[5] It became apparent that reduction of peak stresses, as well as homogenization of force transfer, neutralization, and transfer to investing tissues was a prime requisite to achieve more predictable long-term bone maintenance around the implant (Fig 11–4,B), as well as to achieve a significant increase in the margin of safety (Fig 11–5). The Tissue-Tac configuration, built into the surface of the titanium, increases interface area by 300%.[6]

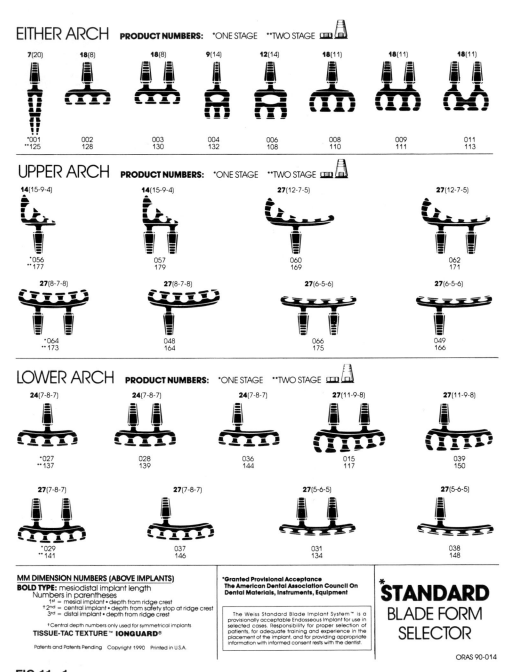

FIG 11–1.
American Dental Association provisionally accepted Oratronics Standard Blade Implant system.

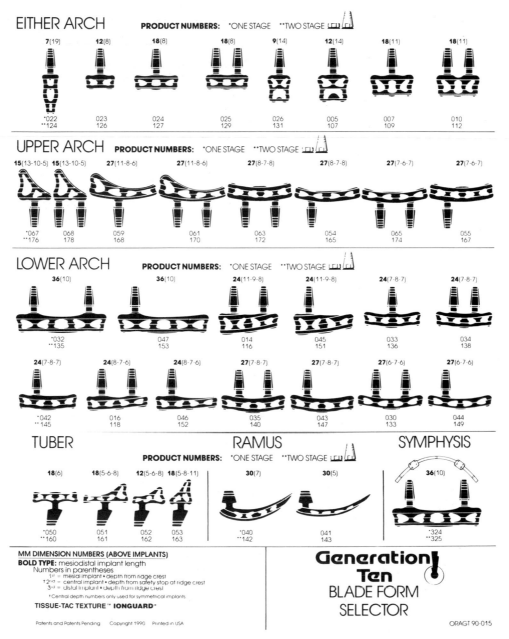

FIG 11–2.
Oratronics Generation Ten Blade Implant system.

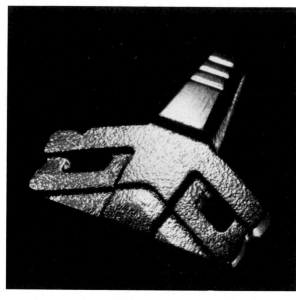

FIG 11–3.
Physiologically developed Oratronics Osteo-Loc Plate Form Implant.

Measurements compared with previous models indicate that the new Tru-Fit Profile of Osteo-Loc Plate Form implant affords a 400% increase in direct bone contact with the receptor site at the time of insertion. In comparison with implants of the same length and depth, utilizing the same volume of available bone, three-dimensional finite element computer analysis of Osteo-Loc Plate Form implants indicates average reductions in peak stress of 85% to 91% in tension, compression, and shear; a 203% increase in implant volume; a 50% increase in macroscopic interface area; and a 59% increase in the axial load-bearing area (Fig 11–6).[7]

The Osteo-Loc Plate Form implant is available

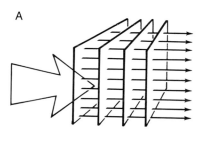

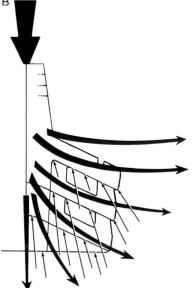

FIG 11–4.
A, conceptual representation of force homogenization. **B,** conceptual representation of stress neutralization and transfer to investing tissues

TABLE 11–1.

Plate/Blade Oratronics Implant Systems and Instruments*

	Average Cost	Material
Oratronics Standard Blade Form Implant		
One-stage	$100	CP titanium
Two-stage†	$150–$170	CP titanium
Oratronics Generation Ten Blade Form Implant		
One-stage	$125	CP titanium
Two-stage†	$175–$195	CP titanium
Oratronics Osteo-Loc Plate Form Implant		
One-stage	$150	CP titanium
Two-stage†	$200–$220	CP titanium
Plate/Blade Form Instrument Starter Kit	$900–$1,200	Solid titanium or titanium-tipped

*Manufactured and distributed by Oratronics, Inc., 405 Lexington Avenue, New York, NY 10174.
†Two-Stage Implants are supplied complete with Healing Collars and Final Abutment Perio-Heads
 CP = chemically pure.

with both one-stage and two-stage (submerged and semisubmerged) options (Fig 11–7). Angled heads to ease parallelism, and offset heads to promote optimum anterior-posterior prosthodontic abutment positioning are provided.

The Oratronics Systems

Blade implants can function as predictable prosthodontic abutments in over 90% of the areas of available bone in partially or totally edentulous alveolar ridges when compared with root-cylinder form systems (Fig 11–8). The ultimate mode of tissue integration must be determined by the clinician, and should be optimal, long-term, and predictable with

reasonable technical sensitivity and case sequencing. Prosthodontic restorative procedures should complement the practitioner's current practices and techniques. An esthetically pleasing appearance, a varied choice of materials, and simplicity are essential.

Controlling resorption of bone closest to the implant interface promotes and ensures predictability and long-term survival. Hypo- and hyperfunction can cause bone resorption. Stress levels between hypo- and hyperfunction are considered to be within the physiologic limits of health (Fig 11–5).

Sophisticated computer modeling of implants, bone, peri-implant ligaments, and other tissues permits controlled combinations of these to provide data on tension, compression, and shear stress distribu-

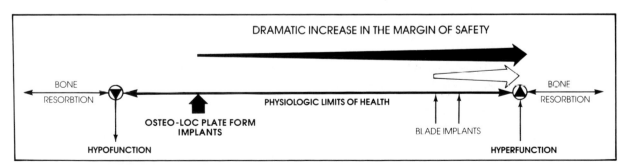

FIG 11–5.
Osteo-Loc Plate Form implants can now effectively distribute greater functional force within physiologic limits of health.

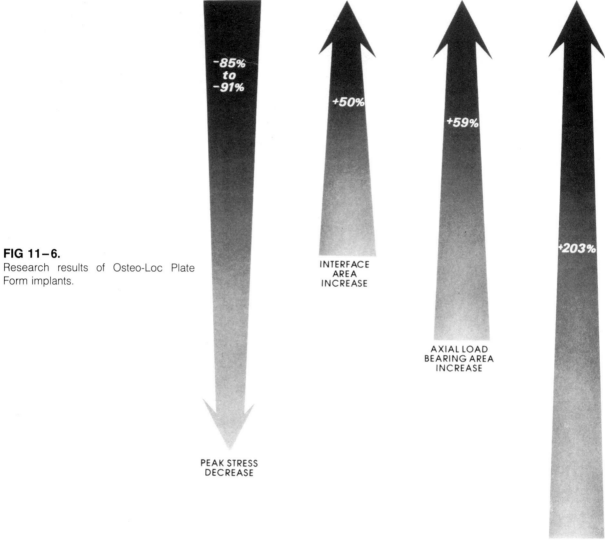

**UTILIZING THE SAME LENGTH AND DEPTH OF AVAILABLE BONE
WEISS OSTEO-LOC PLATE FORM IMPLANTS OFFER DRAMATIC BENEFITS**

−85% to −91%

PEAK STRESS DECREASE

+50%

INTERFACE AREA INCREASE

+59%

AXIAL LOAD BEARING AREA INCREASE

+203%

IMPLANT VOLUME INCREASE

FIG 11–6.
Research results of Osteo-Loc Plate Form implants.

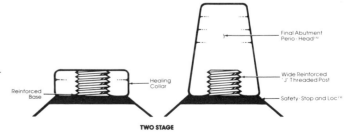

Final Abutment Perio-Head™

Healing Collar

Reinforced Base

Wide Reinforced "J" Threaded Post

Safety-Stop and Loc™

TWO STAGE

FIG 11–7.
Two-Stage (submerged and semisubmerged) options.

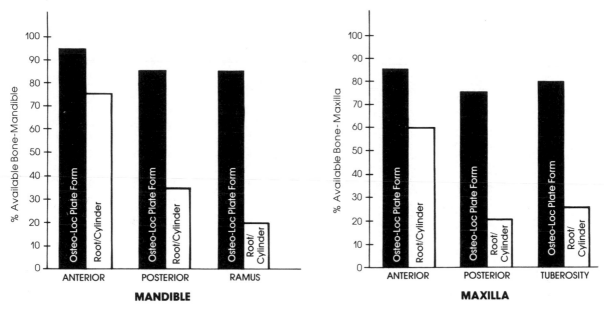

FIG 11–8.
Percentages of usable available bone compared between plate/blade-form and cylinder/root-form endosteal implants.

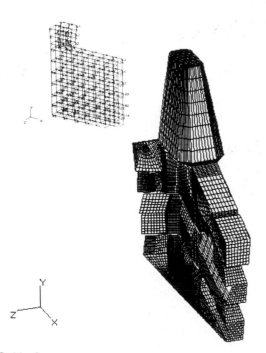

FIG 11–9.
Finite element models afford a vast array of data points.

tion in and around dental implants. Information on stress levels and patterns was developed to calculate the relationships governed by implant length, depth, and width (Fig 11–9).[8]

Metallurgy and Interface Texture

Grains, or crystals, are of varied geometric shapes and lie in their matrix with crystalographic pathways that are a result of their formation, geometric shape, and orientation (Fig 11–10). Metals can be coined or squeezed into desired shapes when sufficient pathways exist along which relative grain movement can occur without disrupting integrity.

Due to a paucity of crystalographic pathways, it is extremely difficult to coin titanium. The Oratronics coining process permits geometrically planned modifications of grain size and orientation. The procedure also positions the grains of titanium more nearly parallel to the lines of maximum force, thus increasing strength. This reduces long-term metal fatigue, and promotes ease and increased safety during the insertion bending adjustments to the implant.

Stress is equal to force divided by unit area. As the implant interface area increases, stress decreases.

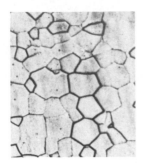

FIG 11–10.
Titanium grain structure.

One-Stage Sequencing

The Oratronics Osteo-Loc Plate Form implant design provides an increase in receptor site direct implant-bone contact area at the time of insertion, which results in an increase in implant-to-receptor site contact at insertion (Fig 11–13). When utilizing the one-stage configuration, the routine 4- to 6-week total treatment time is still advocated. One-stage cases requiring extended treatment time may be extended to 10 to 12 weeks prior to cementation.

The Tissue-Tac interface texture, utilizing the coining process, is built into the surface of the implant, not applied to it and increases surface area over 300% (Fig 11–11). Implants with this interface can be bent, handled safely with minimal threat of contamination, and easily sterilized. It has reasonable technique sensitivity.[6]

Retrieval studies indicate that the Tissue-Tac texture is an effective implant interface.[9] It is conservatively estimated that 800,000 Tissue-Tac implants have been placed worldwide, and well over 200,000 in the United States during the last 18 years. (Fig 11–12).[10]

Two-Stage Option

The two-stage configurations of Osteo-Loc Plate Form implants offer *submerged and semisubmerged options*. Each two-stage implant is supplied with universal abutment head(s) and collar(s).

Prior to final seating, with the universal abutment head in position, bending for parallelism is achieved with the aid of Titanium-Tipped head and body adjusting pliers. After final seating, the abutment head is removed, the healing collar is installed, and the gingival flaps are sutured over it (submerged healing) or the tissue is punched and sutured around it (semisubmerged healing).

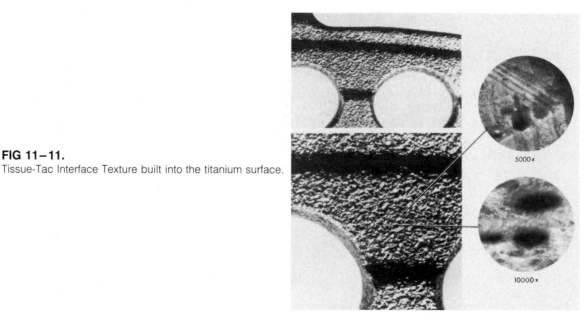

FIG 11–11.
Tissue-Tac Interface Texture built into the titanium surface.

United States Comparative Usage Oratronics Blades—Nobelpharma Fixtures

APPROXIMATE NUMBER OF BLADE IMPLANTS AND NOBELPHARMA FIXTURES PLACED IN THE UNITED STATES OVER YEARS*

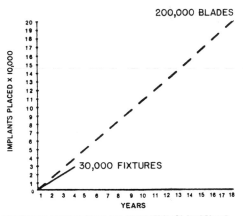
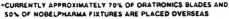

200,000 BLADES

30,000 FIXTURES

IMPLANTS PLACED x 10,000

YEARS

*CURRENTLY APPROXIMATELY 70% OF ORATRONICS BLADES AND 50% OF NOBELPHARMA FIXTURES ARE PLACED OVERSEAS

APPROXIMATE NUMBER OF PATIENTS WITH ORATRONICS BLADES AND NOBELPHARMA FIXTURES TREATED IN THE UNITED STATES OVER YEARS*

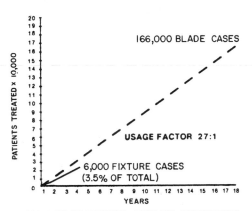

166,000 BLADE CASES

USAGE FACTOR 27:1

6,000 FIXTURE CASES (3.5% OF TOTAL)

PATIENTS TREATED x 10,000

YEARS

*COMPUTERIZED STATISTICS - ROOT LABS - SHOW THAT THE AVERAGE CASE UTILIZES 1.2 BLADES AND 5.0 FIXTURES

Comparisons of Replicated Studies

CONTROLLED REPLICATED STUDIES COMPARABLE SAFETY AND EFFICACY

VETERANS ADMINISTRATION	FIBRO-OSTEAL INTEGRATION			OSTEAL INTEGRATION			
	ORATRONICS STANDARD BLADE			NOBELPHARMA FIXTURE			
VETERANS ADMINISTRATION	VETERANS ADMINISTRATION		NIH - HARVARD	GOTEBORG		TORONTO	
SURVIVAL RATE	60 MONTH SUCCESS RATES		36 MONTH SURVIVAL RATES	5-9 YEAR SURVIVAL RATES		36 MONTH SURVIVAL RATES	
95.8% 60 MONTH	IMPLANT FPD	RPD	IMPLANT FPD	CANTILEVER FPD	CANTILEVER FTD	NO CONTROL	CANTILEVER FTD	NO CONTROL
INCLUDING ALL FAILURES	84.2%	74.0%	82.3%	–	70% MAXILLA* 76% MANDIBLE	–	83.2% W/SLEEPERS 87.5% W/O SLEEPERS	–
EXCLUDING EARLY FAILURES	91.5%	74.0%	91.0%	91.0%	81% MAXILLA 91% MANDIBLE	–	–	–
CLEARLY SUPERIOR PATIENT PREFERENCE	YES	NO	YES	NO				

RPD = REMOVABLE PARTIAL DENTURE
FPD = TOOTH/IMPLANT SUPPORTED FIXED PARTIAL DENTURE; ONE BLADE
FTD = IMPLANT SUPPORTED FIXED TOTAL DENTURE; FOUR TO SIX FIXTURES
* = JAMES ET AL...CRITICAL REVIEW, NYS DENT J 1986; 52(10):31-4

FIG 11–12.
Comparative usage and success rates of Oratronics and Nobelpharma implant systems placed in the United States.

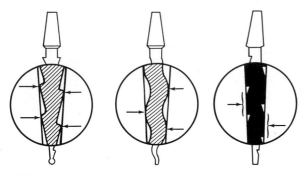

FIG 11–13.
Osteo-Loc Tru-Fit profile *(far right)* affords a 400% increase in implant-to-receptor site contact at insertion.

After complete healing and exposure, the healing collar is removed, and the restorative dentist replaces the original universal abutment head.

Prosthodontic Fulfillment

Parallelism.—As an adjunct to tapering and faceting of abutment heads on one-stage implants, abutment heads are angled (Fig 11–14). Parallelism is assessed by trial-seating, and transposition will determine which orientation of the abutment head is more nearly parallel.

Mesial and Distal Abutment Head Location.—Single and double abutment heads on models with asymmetric implant bodies are offset from center (Fig 11–15). Trial seating and envisioning the final

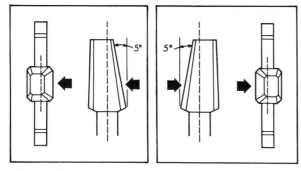

FIG 11–14.
Osteo-Loc Plate Form implants with symmetrical bodies have angled heads for greater ease of parallelism.

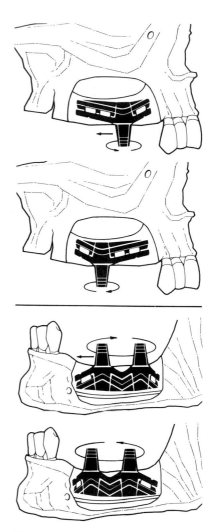

FIG 11–15.
Abutment heads of Osteo-Loc Plate Form implants with asymmetrical bodies are offset to promote ideal anterior-posterior prosthodontic positioning.

prosthesis will determine whether abutment head(s) are properly positioned under projected crown(s).

Osteo-Loc Plate Form Implants

Osteo-Loc Plate Form selectors are available in printed black on white or transparencies to overlay long-cone periapical films for implant selection compatible with available bone (Fig 11–16). The implants are separated into those suitable for both the mandible and the maxilla, those suitable for the

EITHER ARCH   PRODUCT NUMBERS: *ONE STAGE   **TWO STAGE

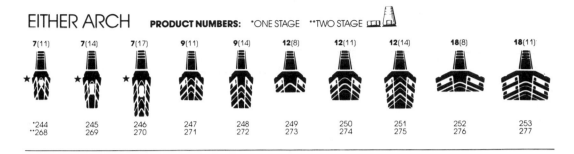

LOWER ARCH   PRODUCT NUMBERS: *ONE STAGE   **TWO STAGE

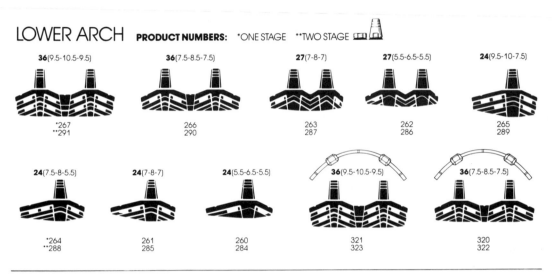

UPPER ARCH   PRODUCT NUMBERS: *ONE STAGE   **TWO STAGE

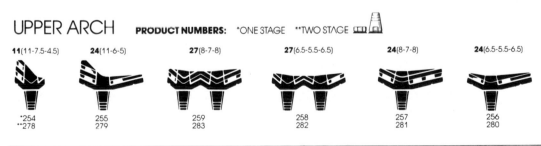

MM DIMENSION NUMBERS (ABOVE IMPLANTS)
BOLD TYPE: mesiodistal implant length
    Numbers in parentheses
        1st = mesial implant • depth from ridge crest
        †2nd = central implant • depth from safety stop at ridge crest
        3rd = distal implant • depth from ridge crest

        † Central depth numbers only used for symmetrical implants

    TISSUE-TAC TEXTURE™ IONGUARD®
   ★ Single Tooth and Cylinder/Screw Form Backup

    Patents and Patents Pending   Copyright 1990   Printed in USA

       IONINTEGRATION™

Osteo-Loc
Plate Form™
Selector

ORAOL 90-016

FIG 11–16.
Osteo-Loc Plate Form selector and implant dimension numbering key.

TABLE 11–2.

The Oratronics Osteo-Loc Plate Form Implant

1. Universal abutment Perio-Head (one-stage and two-stage)
   7 mm high from ridge crest
   Millimeter adjusting lines to aid interocclusal clearance
   Tapered to aid parallellism
   Faceted for cement retention (one-stage)
   Round to facilitate seating if utilizing analogs (two-stage)
2. Healing collar
   Compatible diameter with abutment head
   Suitable for full or semisubmerging
   Horizontal scribe line denotes top
3. Threaded post
   Stronger, larger diameter
   "J"-thread promotes enhanced retention
   Platform at beveled base for added protection
4. Safety-Stop and Loc
   Prevents overseating
   Protects landmarks
   Placed against the crest of the ridge
5. Neck
   Increased surface area reduces destructive peak stresses and saucerization
   Bordered by the Safety-Stop and Loc and shoulder set-slots
6. Plate Form
   Areas of parallel-sided metal reduce and redistribute stress
   Promotes homogeneity of stress transfer
7. Taper Form
   Areas of tapered-sided metal redistribute stress
   Promotes homogeneity of stress transfer
8. Tru-Fit profile
   400% increase in direct bone contact at insertion
   Provides increased one-stage working time
9. Stress Neutralization Contour
   Redistributes and neutralizes stress
   Oriented counter to stress contours
   Optimizes osteogenic effect
   Promotes homogeneity of stress transfer
10. Stress Elevation Groove
    Transfers stress to areas of insufficient distribution
    Oriented to synergize action of Stress Neutralization contours
    Promotes homogeneity of stress transfer
11. Vertical (Axial) Stress Absorption Ridge
    80% of applied stress is axial
    59% increased surface area for absorption
12. Vents
    Sized to optimize bone strength and vascularization
    Contoured to maximize resistance to axial loading
13. Shoulder Set-Slot
    Positioned 2 mm apical to Safety-Stop and Loc
    New contour eliminates pit and fissure corrosion

mandible only, and those suitable for the maxilla only (Table 11–2 and Fig 11–16).

An implant size numbering key indicates for each implant its mesiodistal length, and depths at the mesial, center, and distal of the implant (see Fig 11–16). For symmetrical implants, the length and depth at the center only are indicated.

Serial Placement of Osteo-Loc Plate Form Implants

Transverse and transverse-oblique anterior serial placement of Oratronics Osteo-Loc Plate Form implants with their 1.8-mm width places a far greater percentage of implant interface in direct contact with cortical bone at the insertion site as measured against the direct mesiodistal traditional placement of a single implant.[11] Chosen as a primary system, the concept is also often utilized as an important secondary back-up for root/cylinder form implants. The 7- and 9-mm-mesiodistal-length implants vary in depth from 11 to 17 mm (see Fig 11–16). The anterior implants can be used in combination with posterior implant placement (Fig 11–17). Distal cantilevering of no more than two pontics on a side is advocated only when insufficient available bone exists above the mandibular canals or under the sinuses to permit additional implantation for total support. When root/cylinder forms are contemplated, but ridge exposure at the time of insertion reveals areas with insufficient width of available bone, Osteo-Loc Plate Forms are often the second implant of choice (Fig 11–17,D). These implants should always be sterile and available for immediate back-up use as required.

ARMAMENTARIUM

All instruments without moving parts, and the Implant Remover Reverse Mallet with Tip are available in solid titanium. These include the Single-Head, Double-Head, and Shoulder Set-Slot Seating Instruments, as well as the Implant Carrier, and Channel Curette, Depth Gauge, and Bone Harvester. The Tissue Marker, Periosteal Elevator, Scalpel Handle, and Tissue Retractor are also available in solid titanium.

New additions in solid titanium are two sizes of the Bone Augmentation Carrier and Seater, and three Curettes for implant abutment head prophylaxis. A new set of two Titanium-Tipped Vise-Loc Adjusting Pliers, to hold the implant during bending for paral-

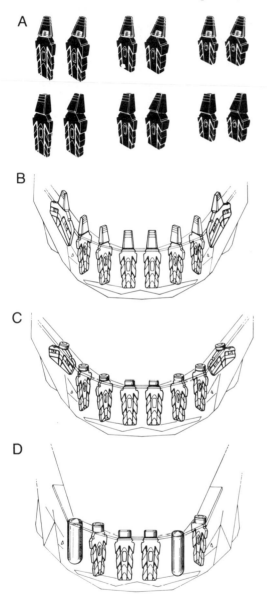

FIG 11–17.
A, Osteo-Loc Plate Form implants suitable for anterior serial placement. **B** and **C,** anterior serial placement of Osteo-Loc Plate Forms. **D,** use of Osteo-Loc Plate Forms as back-up when there is insufficient bone available for cylinder/root forms.

lelism, has been developed. The Vise-Loc Head Pliers grasp each implant under the Safety-Stop and Loc, thus protecting the threaded posts of two-stage implants. The Vise-Loc Body Pliers are positioned at the level of and parallel to the Shoulder Set-Slots.

Needle holders, scissors, tissue holders, suture assist forceps, and the like are also indispensable.

Listed in the general order of use, the instruments are depicted in Figure 11–18 and described in Table 11–3.

Coordinated burs in both parallel and tapered configurations are available to prepare receptor sites for the Osteo-Loc Plate Form implant system. Each bur is available in both XL and XXL lengths, high-speed friction grip, or low-speed latch-type, for use with external coolant and low-speed latch-type only with internal coolant (Fig 11–19).

TABLE 11–3.
Titanium Instruments

Fine-Line Tissue Marker
Marks the path of initial incision for receptor site; marks the exposed bone for length and buccal- or labial-lingual position of receptor site; marks tissue to be removed by tissue punch

Tru-Control Scalpel
A scalpel handle molded to nest fingers for optimal control during incising; weight-balanced

Multi-Access Tissue Scissors
Trims edges of reflected flap to ensure even coaptation for suturing; serrated to prevent slip during use

Noyes Scissors
Superior for general tissue trimming; aids during suturing

Shaping and Trimming Rongeur
Bayonet design allows for clearance of natural teeth; removes tissue tags to prevent bur clogging; removes spiny ridges from bone crest; conservatively widens narrow ridge if necessary

Regular Periosteal Elevator
Reflects tissue of average thickness; thin to protect friable tissue, semiblunt to prevent laceration, curved to follow osseous contours, narrow to limit force

Heavy-Duty Periosteal Elevator
Reflects tissue of greater thickness (maxilla); wider to increase force as required

Manual Tissue Retractor
Securely retracts flap during receptor site preparation; flat portion firmly controls and protects tongue

Automatic Tissue Retractor
Retracts both flaps securely; frees hands of surgical team

Tissue Holder
Blunt-ended interlocking teeth totally and atraumatically secure tissue for trimming, punching, etc.

Channel Curette, Depth Gauge, Bone Harvester
Atraumatically curettes the receptor site; harvests bone for use with bone augmentation procedures; checks depth of receptor site to assure complete seating

Implant Carrier
Carries implant to and from receptor site for required adjustments during receptor site preparation, and for final seating

Abutment Head Height Adjuster
Reduces head height for required interocclusal clearance; use followed by polishing

Single-Head Seating Instrument
Horizontally seats single-head implant; eccentrically seats double-head implant

Double-Head Seating Instrument
Horizontally seats double-head implant

*Shoulder Set-Slot Seating Instrument
Eccentrically seats mesial or distal of an implant to correct positioning toward horizontal; main seating instrument for all implants when a bend of 15 degrees or more is required for parallelism; ensures that all seating forces are in long axis of implant body
Insertion Tapping Mallet
Weighted and balanced for atraumatic seating; nylon inserts muffle sound
*Reverse Mallet Implant Remover with Tip
Protects lateral walls of receptor site during implant removal for further adjustment
*Vise-Loc Adjusting Pliers (Head Pliers and Body Pliers) (set of two)
Head pliers engages safety-stop at base of implant head or threaded post; body pliers engages at level of shoulder set-slots; bends for parallelism with implant locked in position; also used to bend implant body to adjust to receptor site curvature of bone
X-ray Grid (in mm)
Prints out millimeter control grid on radiographs
Semilunar Tissue Punch
Contours gingival cuff around implant abutment head or healing collar
Master Semilunar Tissue Punch
Double-action heavy-duty tissue punch for extrathick tissue.
*Bone augmentation carrier and seater (set of two sizes)
Used to pick up and set bone augmentation material in and over vents and shoulders
Grip-Loc Needle Holder
Affords positive needle control during all suturing procedures
Suture Assist Tissue Forceps
Holds and positions tissue for optimal needle penetration during suturing; after penetration, grasps and pulls needle through tissue
Grip 'N Snip Suture Scissors
Cuts and trims sutures during suturing
*Perio-Implant curettes (set of three)
Titanium curettes for curettage and other gingival health procedures associated with the perigingival sites around healed implant abutment heads*

*Indicates that entire instrument is of solid titanium.

PROSTHETIC PROCEDURES

In the case of three- to six-unit fixed bridges utilizing one single-stage implant in conjunction with one or more natural abutments, master impressions may be taken either at the insertion visit after suturing, or 2 to 3 weeks post-operation after gingival healing has occurred. Either of these choices will lead to optimal results. In the case of two-stage implants, the final abutment universal Perio-Head is affixed to the implant following healing of 3 to 6 months in the mandible and 6 to 9 months in the maxilla.

All endosseous plate/blade-form implant abutment heads are included in master impressions in the same manner as prepared natural abutment teeth. In size they are comparable to prepared mandibular central and lateral, and maxillary lateral incisors.

Use of analogs and transfer copings is possible but not required. Any accepted elastic impression material may be used. When required, gingival retraction around an implant abutment head is achieved in the same manner as with natural abutments. After removal of the impression, the sulcus is examined and any residual impression material is removed. Occlusal (bite) registrations are executed as for conventional prostheses. In short, implant abutments are treated as though they were natural abutments.

If the master impression has been taken at the implant insertion visit, the final prosthesis can be fabricated during the period of soft tissue healing. Then, when sutures are removed 7 to 10 days post-operation, individual castings or an assembled prosthesis can be ready for its initial try-in. Facings may also be waxed or porcelain biscuit–baked so that fit, occlusion, and esthetics are all checked and cor-

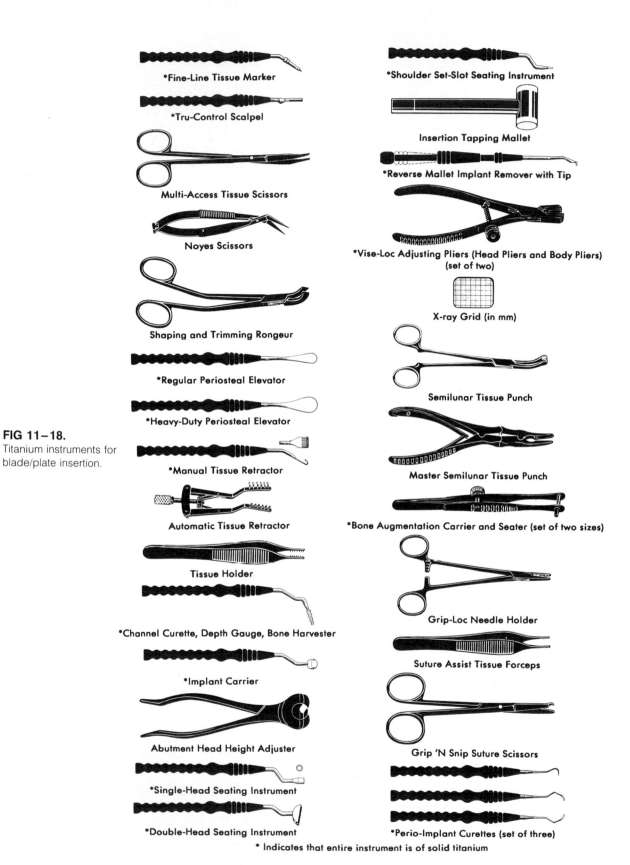

FIG 11–18.
Titanium instruments for blade/plate insertion.

*Fine-Line Tissue Marker

*Tru-Control Scalpel

Multi-Access Tissue Scissors

Noyes Scissors

Shaping and Trimming Rongeur

*Regular Periosteal Elevator

*Heavy-Duty Periosteal Elevator

*Manual Tissue Retractor

Automatic Tissue Retractor

Tissue Holder

*Channel Curette, Depth Gauge, Bone Harvester

*Implant Carrier

Abutment Head Height Adjuster

*Single-Head Seating Instrument

*Double-Head Seating Instrument

*Shoulder Set-Slot Seating Instrument

Insertion Tapping Mallet

*Reverse Mallet Implant Remover with Tip

*Vise-Loc Adjusting Pliers (Head Pliers and Body Pliers)
(set of two)

X-ray Grid (in mm)

Semilunar Tissue Punch

Master Semilunar Tissue Punch

*Bone Augmentation Carrier and Seater (set of two sizes)

Grip-Loc Needle Holder

Suture Assist Tissue Forceps

Grip 'N Snip Suture Scissors

*Perio-Implant Curettes (set of three)

* Indicates that entire instrument is of solid titanium

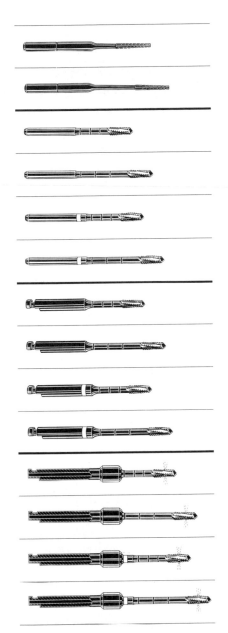

FIG 11–19.
Low- and high-speed, internally and externally cooled receptor site burs. Choice of latch type or friction grip.

rected. Thus, 3 to 5 weeks post-operation, the final restoration may be seated, checked, and often sealed with hard cement. If further corrections are required, or provisional seating is desired, cementation can be delayed. In the case of two-stage submerged or semisubmerged healing, the sequence is

extended for the 3 to 9 months required for healing.

Provisional cement is not used under implant abutments in order to protect the healing implant when tapping to remove a provisional or final prosthesis for try-in or final cementation. Frictional retention is adequate. Final cementing should be done utilizing any accepted crown and bridge cement for both implant and natural abutments.

In the case of one-stage implants, optimal tissue integration is best achieved with early firm cementing of the final prosthesis. Gradual, slowly increasing function promotes healing. Such sequencing affords a clear advantage to both dentist and patient.

Prosthodontic Considerations

Central Fossa–Ridge Crest Relationships

When natural teeth are removed, resorption occurs at the expense of the labial and buccal plates of bone. Edentulous alveolar ridges resorb medially as they lose height. After healing, the clinical crest of the ridge is somewhat lingual to its original position when the teeth were present (Fig 11–20). When a

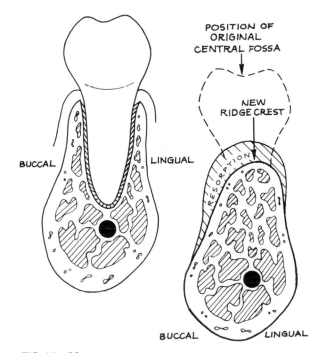

FIG 11–20.
Healed ridge crest is lingual to position of central fossa when tooth was present.

plate/blade implant is inserted, the receptor site is started through this healed ridge crest, bisecting the cortical plates of bone. The implant abutment head therefore protrudes through the gingiva directly over the healed clinical ridge crest, somewhat lingual to the original position of the natural teeth.

In positioning replacement teeth, the central fossae generally should be placed where they originally were, to ensure ideal occlusion and esthetics. Therefore, replacement teeth will be partially labial or buccal to the healed ridge crest. As a result, implant abutment heads will project under the lingual portion of the crown (Fig 11–21). In severely resorbed maxillary cases, it may be necessary, especially posteriorly, to establish an edge-to-edge or crossbite occlusion. In severely resorbed mandibular cases, occlusion may be established primarily between the tip and the buccal incline of the maxillary lingual cusp and the central fossa and lingual incline of an extremely narrowed mandibular buccal cusp.

Ridge-Lapping Implant Abutments

Because of the resorption pattern, it may be necessary for esthetics, and often for function, to *ridge-lap* the labial or buccal border of the implant abutment crown, especially in esthetically prominent areas. Patients are instructed in proper home care, and good health is thereby maintained.

One cannot successfully ridge-lap crowns or porcelain jackets placed over natural abutment teeth. The gingival sulcus becomes periodontally involved, no matter how well hygiene is performed. This is *not true* of implant abutments. For over 20 years, plate/blade-form prostheses have functioned with ridge-lapped implant abutments with routinely successful

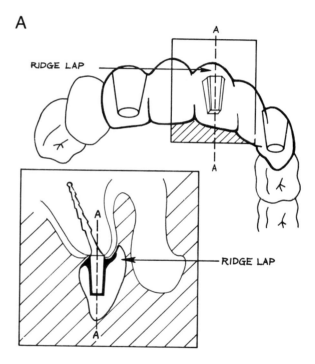

A

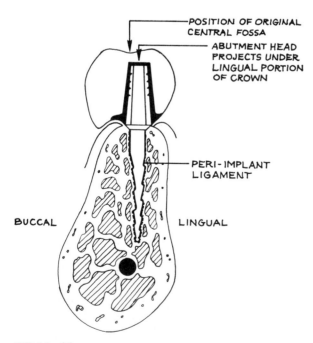

FIG 11–21.
Lingual position of implant abutment head under abutment crown.

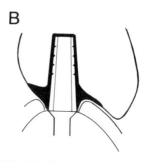

B

FIG 11–22.
A, maxillary anterior ridge-lapping. **B,** mandibular posterior ridge-lapping.

clinical results. Good hygiene is essential, and easily accomplished. In esthetic areas, ridge-lapping is always performed.

In forming a ridge lap, all proximal and lingual implant abutment casting margins are created as they would be against natural teeth (Fig 11–22). Only the labial and buccal areas are extended. This is best accomplished in the laboratory by setting replacement teeth as though they were pontics, with the abutment heads taking their place under the teeth as esthetic contouring dictates. In the area of the ridge lap, the metal casting margin is placed at or slightly above the gingiva and the metal extended 2 mm shy of the projected contour of the final acrylic or porcelain ridge lap to allow ample room for adjustment for esthetics without exposing metal during try-in.

In nonesthetic areas ridge-lapping is optional. Bullet-shaped crowns with wide embrasures are often used, depending on the practitioner's preference and patient acceptance (Fig 11–23).

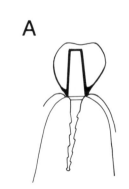

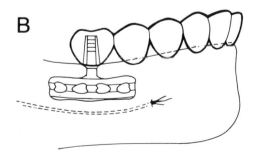

FIG 11–23.
A, profile of bullet-shaped abutment crown over implant. **B,** implant bridge: bullet-shaped abutment crown and pontics.

Finishing Lines

In the area of the ridge lap, the finishing line of the crown is placed at or 1 mm above the gingival margin, to allow for proper flossing and flow of water during rinsing. All other margins are placed above, at, or below the free gingival crest, in accordance with the same policy utilized for natural crowned abutments.

Embrasures are also created in accordance with the practitioner's fixed-bridgework experience. Excellent prosthetics is essential, as always, to success.

Occlusion

Occlusion is established in accordance with the techniques and principles currently providing success with one's conventional fixed prostheses. There is no single best technique. Narrow buccolingual dimensions, anatomic or semianatomic cuspal relations, group function, cuspid protection, long-centric, and gnathologic principles have all been successfully utilized with dental implants.

Materials

Vast numbers of porcelain-to-metal prostheses have been utilized successfully, as have gold with acrylic veneers and gold frames with entire teeth of baked acrylic. Softer gold or plastic occlusal surfaces transmit less trauma through the implant into bone. In ideal cases, porcelain may be routinely used. In marginal cases, gold or acrylic may be more suitable. (*Caution:* In porcelain fused to metal cases, use gold-based alloys. Nickel-chromium-beryllium nonprecious alloys, when cemented over titanium, may cause an adverse gingival reaction.)

DISCUSSION

In the VA Cooperative Dental Implant Study,[1] the Oratronics Standard Blade Implant System was utilized exclusively to provide distal implants as co-abutments with natural teeth in support of unilateral fixed partial dentures. The controls in this prospective randomized study were removable partial dentures, utilizing splinted natural teeth as abutments. Eliminating the few failures that occurred *before* the insertion of final prostheses, the 5-year survival rate of the implants was 95.8%. The success rate went up from the third to the fifth year, in part because implant mobility *decreased* with time. No natural tooth co-abutments were lost during the study. In contrast, in younger adults, the 5-year failure rate of the removable partial dentures was approximately 20% higher than for the implants supported by fixed prostheses. Some natural abutments supporting the removable partial denture were lost. One must conclude that unilateral fixed bridges, in part supported by blade implants, are true *preventive dentistry*. They interrupt the cycle of tooth loss well known to occur in association with the use of removable partial dentures.

The Plate/Blade Oratronics Implant System has been developed for use by general practitioners as an integral part of everyday practice.[4] One envisions the insertion of single-implant co-abutments as routine as the performance of periodontal and endodontic therapy.

The Plate/Blade Oratronics Implant System also features prosthodontic simplicity. While analogs and transfer copings may be utilized, they are by no means required. The implant abutment head, once placed into position, is treated as though it were a natural abutment. Provisional teeth can be fabricated over them, especially in esthetic areas. They are impressioned as natural teeth are for fixed bridge fabrication. The usual and customary techniques are all that are required.

Thousands of complete arch cases totally or partially supported by Plate/Blade Oratronics implants have been functioning for more than 20 years.[10] Severely troubled patients can and are being helped.

REFERENCES

1. Kapur KK: VA Cooperative Dental Implant Study—Comparisons between fixed partial dentures supported by blade-vent implants and removable partial dentures. Part II: Comparisons of success rates and periodontal health between two treatment modalities. *J Prosthet Dent* 1989; 62:685–703.
2. Weiss CM: Overview of new studies of fibro-osseous integrated implants and osseointegrated screw implants (German). *Quintessenz* 1988; 39:1475–1480.
3. Weiss CM: Dental implants: Physiological and clinical comparisons of fibro-osteal and osteal integration. *J Acad Gen Dent* 1988; 36:243–248.
4. Weiss CM: The physiologic, anatomic and physical basis of oral endosseous implant design. *J Oral Implantol* 1982; 10:459–486.
5. Bidez MW: *Oratronics Industrial Research Reports,* vols 1–5. Unpublished data, 1977–1988.
6. Weiss CM, Judy KWM, Chiarenza AR: Precompacted, coined titanium endosteal blade implants. *J Oral Implantol* 1973; 3:237–260.
7. Bidez MW: Personal communication, August 1989.
8. Bidez MW, Stevens BJ, Lemons JE: An update on finite element analysis in implant dentistry: The effect of modeling slip at the implant-tissue interface. Presented at the Third International Congress of Implantology and Biomaterials in Stomatology, Osaka, Japan, April 1988.
9. Lemons JE: Personal communication, October 1989.
10. Weiss CM: Fibro-osteal and osteal integration: A comparative analysis of blade and fixture type dental implants supported by clinical trials. *J Dent Educ* 1988; 52:706–711.
11. Chiarenza A: Personal communications, July 1987, December 1989.

Chapter 12

The Ultimatics Blade-Vent Implant System

Leonard I. Linkow, D.D.S.

This chapter discusses the Ultimatics Blade-Vent endosseous implants and their architectural designs with respect to the biomechanical and physiologic relationships at the implant bone interfaces and the rationale for their use.[1, 2]

BACKGROUND

With the removal of multiple teeth the underlying bone resorbs vertically and horizontally. In many situations this leaves insufficient bone, especially posteriorly, to place root form implants. After seeing numerous implant cases become mobile with soreness upon chewing, it was suspected that there were penetrations of screws and pins through the labial or buccal plates of bone which were camouflaged by the extremely thick mucoperiosteal tissues that prevail in the maxilla.

Thus I began to incise the tissues in both jaws, especially in the maxilla, to visualize the suspected perforations. Seeing the shallow knife-edge ridges of bone flaring obliquely from the horizontal plane, it became apparent that something had to be created to fit into the knife edge and shallow ridges. Screw-type implants or tripodial pins could no longer be used in those situations. The time had come to move completely from trying to duplicate or simulate the natural roots of our own teeth. We are prone to the loss of bone at the expense of the labial and buccal

plates; very seldom is there loss of the lingual or palatal bone. Thus, nature made a mistake—it gave us a maximum amount of bone on the lingual and palatal cortices, where it is needed less, and a minimum amount of bone flanking the teeth labially and buccally, where it is needed to resist lateral and anterior thrusts of the tongue and premature contact of teeth during lateral and eccentric movements. When the teeth are lost, the bone has no more periodontal stimulation, so it resorbs due to hypofunction. This continuous resorption reduces the height of the residual ridge and the width at the expense of labial and buccal cortices of bone.

THE IMPLANT

Thus, the Linkow Blade-Vent implant was created (Fig 12–1 and Table 12–1).[3] It was designed with openings, or vents, in its body to allow for osteogenesis to take place. Further, it was designed in such a way that a wedge-shaped body could be angled obliquely off the horizontal plane, to bisect the severely angled bone that usually exists in the maxillae; and with a bendable neck so that the posts of the implants could be paralleled to one another, or to remaining teeth.[4, 5]

Tuber blades were introduced by the author in 1980 to be used as posterior supports in the maxil-

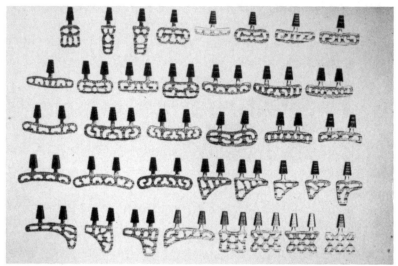

FIG 12–1.
A variety of Ultimatics Blade-Vent plate form implants.

lary tuberosities (Fig 12–2).[6] The multipurpose Blade-Vent implant, introduced in 1981, can be fashioned into 34 different designs (Fig 12–3).[7] A two-stage Blade-Vent implant was introduced in 1988 (Fig 12–4,A–C). This implant allows submersion of the device with subsequent attachment of the superstructure (see Fig 12–4,C).

The Blade-Vent implant is currently constructed of pure titanium (see Table 12–1). The post has retention circumflex grooves and is only 8 mm in height to help minimize preparation for insertion (Fig 12–5). The post neck is 2.5 mm in diameter for post support. The blade is devoid of any sharp line

angles, has a textured surface to provide more interface area, and large closed vents for bone ingrowth. The vents are closed for maximum stress distribution apically (Fig 12–5).

Principles

For success in blade vent implantology, four basic principles must be followed:

1. The architectural design of an implant must be correct. It must be able to withstand both lateral and occlusal forces and must be able to be placed in

TABLE 12–1.
The Ultimatics Blade-Vent System

Product name	Ultimatics Endosseous Blade-Vent Implants	
Manufacturer/supplier	Ultimatics, Inc.	
	P.O. Box 400	
	Springdale, AR 72765	
	1-800-872-7070	
	(501) 756-9200	
Implant composition	Pure titanium	
Approximate costs	Standard blade-vent implant	$100
	Submergible blade-vent implant	$150–$185
Armamentarium kits	Economy starter kit includes three standard implants	$810
	Deluxe starter kit includes three submergible implants and depth gauge	$975
	Economy submergible starter kit includes three submergible implants	$1,050
	Deluxe submergible starter kit includes five submergible implants and depth gauge	$1,375

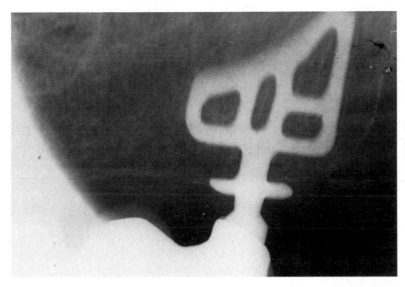

FIG 12–2.
A periapical radiograph of a tuber blade implant in the posterior maxilla.

resorbed knife-edge ridges as easily as in ideal ridges. Its mesiodistal dimensions (not depth in bone) must be depended upon for retention (Fig 12–6). It must have large openings or vents within its framework to allow bone to grow through. It must also be relatively simple to insert and must al-

ways be inserted into a groove which should be made on the palatal side of the crest in the maxilla and on the lingual crest in the mandible. By doing this, any possible impingement on the antral floor or inferior alveolar canal can be avoided. Lingual placement also allows a maximum amount of bone

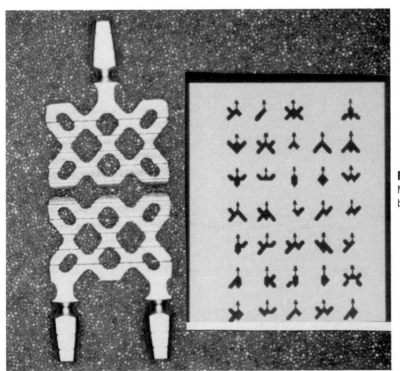

FIG 12–3.
Multipurpose Blade-Vent implants can be fashioned into 34 individual designs.

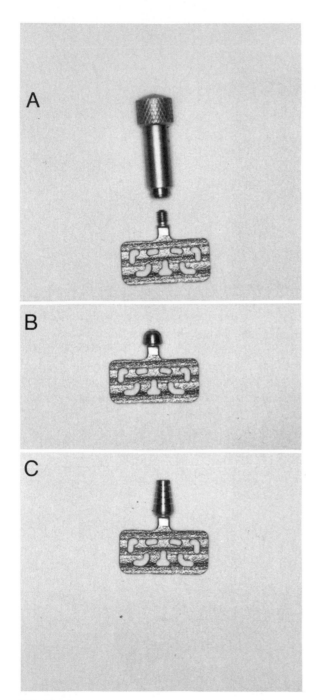

FIG 12–4.
A, a semisubmergible Blade-Vent implant with the corresponding instrument to screw on the healing cap. **B,** the semisubmerged Blade-Vent implant with its healing cap in position. **C,** the prosthetic post screwed into place on a semisubmergible Blade-Vent implant.

to flank the blade-vent implant labially and buccally where it is needed to resist the anterior and lateral thrusts of the tongue, as well as eccentric movements of the mandible. The blade must be thin, have flexibility in its body so it can be bent to fit passively into a curved groove, and the neck should allow bending in order to parallel the posts.

2. There must be enough available bone to be able to correctly insert the implant. An improperly placed blade implant will fail. A good implantologist is one who knows what types of implant(s) are contraindicated, as well as what types are indicated in a specific case.

3. There should always be a minimum amount of abuse to the hard and soft tissues, as well as the implant itself, from the moment of its insertion to the moment the final prosthesis is cemented into position. Even if the surgical phase went perfectly well, reckless abuse can cause adverse effects to the bone implant interface. The operator should not allow impression materials to be left beneath the mucoperiosteal tissues or in the unhealed groove. Another potential problem may be the forcing of a tight-fitting metal framework over the implant, thus causing the blade to be dislodged. If rapid loosening of the implant or implants occur, they must be removed from the groove and the operative site reestablished by making the groove longer mesiodistally and, when possible, a little deeper. A new implant of greater dimension should then be immediately inserted.

4. The completed prosthesis must fit properly and passively, and the occlusion must be precisely balanced and articulated with complete accuracy. Oral implantology, as we know it today, is both a science and an art. When techniques for implant intervention are carefully followed with every recommended detail, success ultimately follows. When the art is abused, failure is inevitable (Fig 12–7).

The Blade-Vent implant requires experience and clinical skills to accomplish the appropriate insertion techniques. In addition to the artistic aspects of the procedure, the scientific knowledge of why it must be done in a certain manner is of prime importance and must be carefully understood by the dentist.

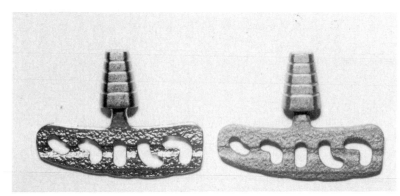

FIG 12–5.
The Blade-Vent implant. It can function successfully in a shallow, knife-edge ridge and the large internal body vents allow for ingrowth of bone.

Principles of Design and Rationale for Blade-Vent Implants

Because of the multiple perforations or vents in the blade implant, it offers the possibility of a rapid natural vascularization of the bone traumatized during drilling and regeneration of the bone through the vents and around the entire implant blade. With the very thin Blade-Vent implant, a minimum of bone substance is lost buccally and lingually, so minimal debilitation of bone occurs (Fig 12–8). The horizontal design of the implant gives optimal security against torsional effects on the implant from the strong muscular pressures existing in the mouth and the antagonist contacts between the teeth. The design of the Blade-Vent implant is such that when it is correctly inserted into the bone, it develops very strong mechanical retention.

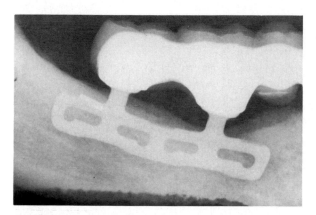

FIG 12–6.
A Blade-Vent implant of narrow height functioning in a severely atrophied mandible.

PATIENT CONSIDERATIONS

Choosing the Implant Site

The ideal site for each implant is determined by prosthodontic considerations; however, bone morphology may force its location elsewhere. This should not be a drawback since it is the post of the implant, not its body, that must complement the dental arch. The implant's body can be placed into the best bone and if the post does not protrude into a desirable plane, it can be bent into the desired plane.

Blade-Vent implants should be placed as far lingually and palatally as possible. Bone resorption usually does not affect the palatal and lingual surfaces of the bone in edentulous jaws but resorbs buccally and facially, especially in the anterior portion of the jaws.

Modification of the Blade-Vent Implant

If there is adequate bone available and the properly designed blade has been chosen, there should be no need to change any portion of the blade design by grinding. The shapes of the blades have been carefully designed from observation of hundreds of patients and then reduced in overall dimensions to allow room for error by the operators. Blade design specifically allows the maximum amount of metal to the maximum amount of bone available. Blade symmetry is also a very important factor as it helps to distribute the occlusal forces brought to bear upon it equally in all directions, spreading and dissipating these forces over as wide an area as possible. When the symmetry of one of these implants is compro-

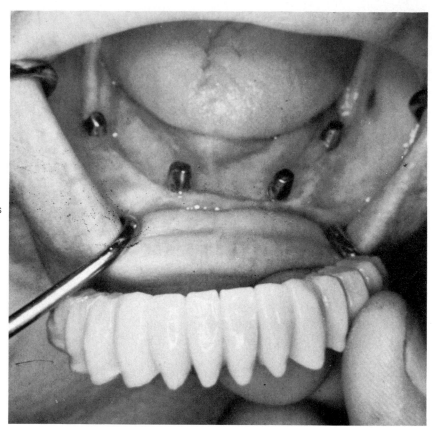

FIG 12–7.
Four Blade-Vent mandibular
implants 3 weeks after the implants
were inserted and just prior to
cementation of a full-arch fixed
prosthesis.

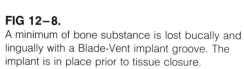

FIG 12–8.
A minimum of bone substance is lost bucally and
lingually with a Blade-Vent implant groove. The
implant is in place prior to tissue closure.

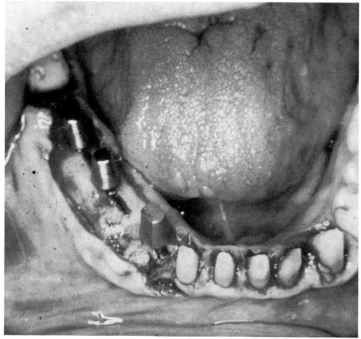

mised by reshaping, the equal force distribution is reduced and the blade might not be able to withstand the lateral and occlusal forces. Therefore, rather than changing the symmetry of a blade in order to fit it into a severely atypical situation, it is advisable to select a more appropriate design for that particular case. Once blades have been cut with titanium-tipped cutters, the rough surfaces and edges must be carefully smoothed down and the sharp line angles and point angles must be rounded off with pure aluminum oxide stones. The blade-vent implant should then be placed in an ultrasonic cleaner for cleaning and sterilization.

Whenever possible the bending of a blade should be done with titanium-beaked pliers. In this manner there is less chance of transference of dissimilar metal ions from the pliers to the implant. Never overbend a blade so that it has to be unbent in order to fit a curved groove. This can weaken any metal. When the body of the blade is bent, it is done by holding each end of the blade with two wide-nosed pliers. When a neck is to be bent, then one pliers holds the blade while the other grips the post.

Sterilization

The latest procedures regarding sterilization of implants seem to be shying away from the autoclave. The reason for this is that if the implant is touched by the human hand and then immediately placed into an autoclave unit, the bacteria that were transferred to the implant become baked onto the implant's surface. When the implant is then placed in the body it becomes almost impossible for phagocytic cells to clean off this material. This may contribute to possible failure of an implant because it prevents close adaptation of bone and fibrous tissue to the implant. The sterilization and cleaning of the implant surface should be accomplished by a radiofrequency glow discharge unit or plasma cleaner.

Treatment of the Blades During Insertion

At no time should the malleting forces be directed to an implant post in situations where the neck was severely bent. In these situations a specially designed titanium inserting instrument that engages the tiny horizontal grooves located along the superior surface of the blade's shoulders should be used. The inserting instrument should never touch the alveolar bone flanking the shoulders of the groove as this may cause chipping or fracturing of bone. However, the blade implant must be tapped down enough that the bottom of the post is resting on or very close to bone. By doing it in this manner, the shoulders are buried to their proper depth of 2 to 3 mm below the crest. With this technique, bone will fill in over the shoulders and through the deeper vents within 3 months. Blade reentry procedures have proved this.

BLADE-VENT IMPLANT INSERTION

The Blade-Vent implant's uniform design simplifies insertion. However, insertion procedures must be rigidly followed for correctly seating the implant. The Blade-Vent implant must be immediately stable upon insertion and the bottom of the post must meet or come close to the alveolar crest.

Clean rapid, atraumatic surgery is used to incise straight down to the bone in a single stroke. A broad-faced periosteal elevator will reveal enough bone to visualize the morphology of the site.

Making the Osteotomy Groove

The dimensions are as follows:

Length (Mesiodistal).—The groove must be as long or slightly longer than the mesiodistal length of the Blade-Vent implant.

Depth.—The groove must be deep enough to bury the implant in bone to the bottom of the post. This often requires a groove 5 mm or more deeper than the blade depth to allow for gentle spreading of bone. When the bone is porous, the osteotomy is made slightly shallower. Tapping the implant will break the few skimpy trabeculae under its base until it reaches its proper depth. No. 700XL and 700XXL stainless steel burs are preferred. Carbide burs are too brittle.

Width (Buccolabial, Linguopalatal).—The groove width should be as narrow as possible, preferably no wider than the bur's diameter. This is essential to take advantage of the blade's wedging action. The only bur to use is the 700XL. When the osteotomy requires a deeper groove, the 700XXL is substituted. The bur must always be sharp and used with a water coolant to prevent burning of bone. A slow-running contra-angle utilizing sterile saline or sterile water is always preferable.

Location.—The groove should always be made on the palatal side of the crest in the maxilla and on the lingual side of the crest in the mandible in order to avoid the maxillary sinus and inferior alveolar and mental nerves respectively.

Seating the Blade-Vent Implant

If the groove was made correctly, the Blade-Vent implant will not seat more than 0.5 mm. However, gently tapping on the blade post and shoulder with the appropriate instruments will easily seat it to the proper position. The bottom of the blade post must rest on or be close to the alveolar crest.

If the groove is curved, then the implant must be bent to fit passively into the groove. This is accomplished with two titanium-tipped pliers. If the groove has not been precisionally cut, the blade when placed in the groove will lodge about one third to one half of the way into the socket, which is not acceptable.

At this point parallelism of the post with other abutments is checked. Adjustments are made by withdrawing the blade along the axis of the channel and bending or twisting the neck of the post outside the mouth. Parallelism may also be created by using the 700XL carbide bur around the posts after the implants are seated.

The Blade-Vent implant is gently tapped, never hammered, to its correct depth. If the post has been bent, tap only the shoulders. If the implant resists being correctly seated, remove it and use the bur to deepen the channel or remove the interfering bone.

The wound is cleaned and closed with simple, interrupted 000 surgical silk sutures. These may be removed in 5 to 8 days.

Healing

When the mucoperiosteal tissues are neatly incised and carefully reflected without tearing the periosteum, and when the blades are gently tapped into the bone without forcing the bone beyond its physiologic capacity, healing becomes uneventful. Vertical incisions delay healing and must be avoided. Healing of soft tissues can also be delayed from underlying bone sequestration. Until these loose fragments are removed, the soft tissue will not completely heal.

Necrosis of the bone is due mainly to excessive trauma to the hard tissues during insertion of Blade-Vent implants. Trauma to the bone is caused by:

1. Excessively heavy tapping of the implant into the bone.
2. Lack of passive fit into a curved groove.
3. Occlusal trauma.
4. Severe overheating of bone.
5. Poor dissection and reflection of the mucoperiosteal tissues.
6. Placing a temporary provisional splint over nonparallel blade-vent implant posts and tapping it out during the early stages of bone healing.

Postoperative Considerations

A temporary prosthesis is rarely necessary unless desired for functional or esthetic reasons. Impressions should be taken over healed tissues. Ideally, 5 to 6 weeks after the implant surgery the final prosthesis should be in place.

Implant Selection and Bone

The amount and nature of bone in a prospective site determines whether or not a prospective implant can be used, and if so, which type (Fig 12–9). Alveolar bone is highly responsive to mechanical stimulation or the lack of it. Tolerable internal tension is osteogenic while concentrated external pressure causes resorption. When a Blade-Vent implant is inserted into alveolar bone, it operates with the natural forces in the area. Residual alveolar bone tends to be more porous and fragile in the maxilla than in the

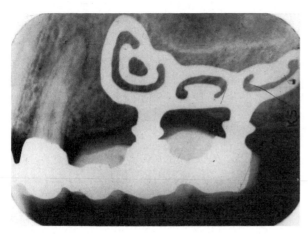

FIG 12–9.
Radiograph of a Blade-Vent implant selected to fit in the maxilla below the prominent maxillary sinus.

mandible, necessitating additional caution while drilling and tapping. Further, in the maxilla the occlusal surface of the alveolar crest often lacks a covering of cortical bone, making the clean retraction of the overlying soft tissues a bit more difficult.

Resorption following extractions may leave a sharp or uneven ridge in either arch. A sharp ridge can be reduced until it is broad enough to accept a blade implant, but leveling an uneven ridge is rarely necessary because a desirable occlusal plane may be achieved by adjusting the heights of the posts.

In the maxilla there is usually ample bone for blade implants from the lateral incisor to the first premolar region. The midline should be avoided. Most problems occur posteriorly because of bone loss and sinus expansion. Posterior maxillary areas are also the most difficult operative sites. Great care must be taken incising and retracting palatal tissues because of the greater palatine foramen and local tendinous attachments. Sinus penetration should be avoided, although some safety margin is provided by the tendency of the sinus membrane to be easily pushed up intact from the bone. Tomographic radiograms can illustrate the exact mesiodistal length and the depth to which a blade is buried. Anteriorly, a single- or double-posted Blade-Vent implant can be placed, preferably in the canine area or either side of the midline; posteriorly, two more Blade-Vent im-

plants are inserted, one on either side of the arch (Fig 12–10).

Ideally, a long specially designed double-posted maxillary Blade-Vent implant can be set in the bone below the sinus, the posts protruding into the premolar and molar regions. When sinus expansion or bone fragility prohibits seating the posterior implants in the normal dental arch, the tuberosity may be wide enough to accept a specially designed Blade-Vent implant seated buccopalatally or a thicker asymmetric blade such as the Tuber Blade-Vent Implant (see Fig 12–2).

In the mandible the anterior regions provide relatively simple implant sites. There are no major blood or nerve vessels anteriorly. The bone at the symphysis is solid and is reinforced by the mental protuberance. Because of the bone's density, care must be taken not to burn it with rotary instruments. Posteriorly, the location of the mandibular canal is

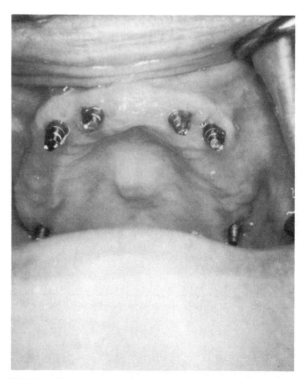

FIG 12–10.
The healed tissues around two double-posted anterior Blade-Vent implants and two single-posted posterior Blade-Vent implants in the maxilla.

important because implant procedures should not impinge upon its neurovascular bundles. The vessels are also threatened when the soft tissues are incised and reflected in the region of the mental foramen. A bony shelf overhanging a concavity is not an appropriate site for a Blade-Vent implant because of the ease in fracturing such a prominence. It is almost always possible to use Blade-Vent implants anteriorly for abutments (Fig 12–11); these may extend from two single implants set on either side of the midline, or from one double-posted design curved across it.

When Blade-Vent implants are used anteriorly, the posterior abutment posts on either side of the arch may be supplied by a long double-posted Blade-Vent implant set into the bone over the mandibular canal. It provides two abutments in a single surgical site (see Fig 12–11). The body of the Blade-Vent implant should be as long and deep as insertion requirements allow. Very often Blade-Vent implants are inserted directly into fresh extraction sites by preparing a groove through the intervening bone. This type of mandibular posterior blade-vent placement can also be used for posterior free-end prosthetic support when only anterior teeth remain.

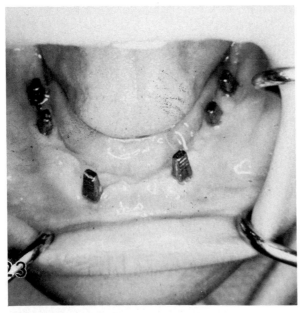

FIG 12–11.
Two mandibular single-posted anterior Blade-Vent implants and two double posted-posterior Blade-Vent implants.

FORCE DISTRIBUTION AND PROSTHETIC CONSIDERATIONS

The possibility of breakdown of the bone buccally or labially due to lateral thrusts of the tongue upon the bridge as a whole must not be discounted. A number of factors, some of them dependent on the restorative work that has been done, determine the presence or absence of bone destruction, and, when it is present, the course it will take. There will be, for example, less destruction of alveolar bone if the opposing jaw houses a full or partial denture.

The length, shape, and design of the implant, as well as the general periodontal condition of the mouth as a whole, are factors. The longer the implant, the better the prognosis for the retention of the implant. The amount of alveolar bone around the blade portion of the implant is also a significant factor; the more bone present, the better the chance that the blade will remain securely anchored. The number of anterior teeth that are splinted to a Blade-Vent implant and their ability to withstand lateral thrusts must be considered in determining the prognosis. Whether the splint is on a curved or straight arch is of significance. A mandibular curved-arch splint is far more advantageous for an implant than a straight-arch splint. In the curved-arch splint, occlusal forces on the buccal slopes of the posterior crowns covering the implant produce a lingual force. This force may pass through or near the center of rotation, which is usually lingual to the implant, causing little or no torque.

In a straight splint, the vertical forces on the buccal slopes of the crowns covering the implant result in forces being created perpendicular to these inclines. These forces produce lingual rotation of the splint about the center of rotation that passes through the apical third of the blade portion of the implant. Therefore, even though the splinting of a Blade-Vent implant to other teeth in the arch is a great aid in resisting occlusal forces in a straight-arch splint, lateral movements may not be as well accepted in knife-edge and shallow ridges since the center of rotation will also pass through the apical third of all the splinted teeth. Occlusal pressures result in the creation of forces perpendicular to the incline of the impact area.

The direction of the occlusal force on the maxillary splint is usually buccal, while on the mandibular splint it is usually lingual. In the maxillary curved-arch splint the same occlusal force that created little or no torque in the mandibular curved-arch splint produces more torque. The resultant force is buccal in direction, while the center of rotation is palatal and usually passes near the apical third of the terminal abutments. In the maxillary curved-arch splint, the resultant line of force may be at a greater distance from the center of rotation than in the mandibular straight-arch splint. With all types of implants, however, the full-arch rather than partial-arch splints are still the prosthesis of choice.[4]

PHYSIOLOGY OF ALVEOLAR BONE BREAKDOWN AROUND IMPLANT FAILURES

It is my opinion that the failure of an implant starts from within and not from without. Failure of an endosseous implant can occur for a number of reasons.

From a surgical point of view, failure can result from traumatizing the bone tissue beyond its physiologic limits. Causes of this trauma are overheating the bone tissue with rotary instruments causing tissue necrosis; spreading the bone beyond its viscosity limit by trying to insert blade implants into a groove which is not deep or wide enough to accept the implant; not burying the shoulder of the blade implant below the crest of the ridge; not bending a blade to fit passively into a curved groove; and perforating the labiolingual or buccopalatal cortices of bone.

In the prosthetic phase, failure can result from (1) forcing impression material into the implant crypt; (2) forcing a provisional or permanent restoration over nonparallel implant posts, causing dislodgment of the implant or improper transmission of occlusal forces to the bone; (3) traumatic occlusion on the temporary or permanent prosthesis, or loading the implant beyond its physiologic limit; (4) poor patient oral hygiene and maintenance, or (5) poor self-cleansing prosthesis design, leading to gingival tissue breakdown and periodontal disease around the implant.

Capillary stasis occurs, resulting in swelling and edema. Once this occurs the bone undergoes necrosis or resorption due to lack of functional stimulation between the implant and bone. Mobility of the implant becomes apparent with tenderness upon vertical pressures. When the implant is in function, a pumping action occurs, drawing oral fluids and debris into the implant alveolus. Outside bacterial invasion occurs, resulting in infection.

Because of some of these problems, the author developed various reentry implant systems in order to continue to treat patients with implant procedures.

REENTRY IMPLANTS

With all types of surgical procedures there are risks involved. Dental implant procedures also have their shortcomings and at times an implant must be removed. Therefore, reentry implants have been designed so patients can be maintained with continuous fixed appliances, eliminating both physically and psychologically the disadvantages these patients may have to experience.[8]

Reentry implants can be used to replace a group of teeth, failing screw-type or basket-type implants, or failing Blade-Vent implants. The procedures are the same.

1. A full-thickness incision is made along the anteroposterior extent of the soft tissue and should extend 10 mm mesially and distally from the failing implant.
2. The failing teeth or implants are removed.
3. The granulation tissue is judiciously curetted out from the inflamed sockets, or from the groove if a blade implant was involved.
4. Round burs of various diameters are used to freshen up the bone groove and shape it as a relatively wider groove than the original. First the bony floor of the groove is adjusted, then the crypt buccolingual and labiopalatal walls are gently adjusted until a new groove is attained.
5. A 700XXL bur is used to straighten the

buccolingual and labiopalatal walls. At this time, the operator can choose the type of reentry implant.

Different Types of Reentry Blade Implants

Biblades.—These are made of titanium and can be loaded immediately. If an unloaded phase of healing is desired; then the submergible Biblade is used. Because the titanium metal of the Biblade is extremely soft, it is relatively simple to mold the two horizontal support systems directly to the surrounding alveolar walls without spreading the bone beyond its physiologic capacity. The inside walls of the new osteotomy need not be parallel. A Biblade

of a slightly wider width is used and squeezed slightly in order to fit it into the wider portion of the osteotomy. Then, by gently tapping from the central structure, the implant seats to the base of the new crypt while the twin blades gently spring back to snugly fit flush with the surrounding walls. Their shoulders should be buried 3 mm or more below the crestal bone (Fig 12–12,A–C).

Corrugated or Snakelike Reentry Devices.—These implants are fabricated as titanium strips. They come in 3- and 5-mm superoinferior heights and 3- or 5-mm buccolingual widths (Fig 12–13).

Figure-of-8 Reentry Implants.—This implant is fabricated in long strips with protruding necks and

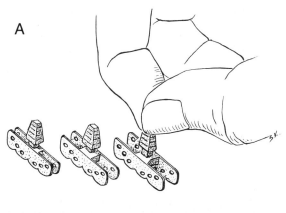

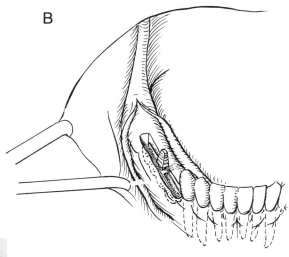

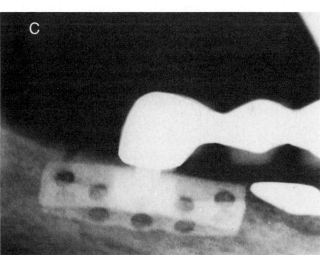

FIG 12–12.
A, Biblade implants are manufactured in three different widths. **B,** a diagram illustrating the narrowest Biblade in its new osteotomy site. **C,** radiograph of the Biblade implant after insertion and restoration.

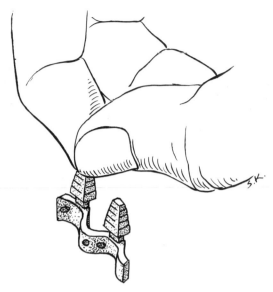

FIG 12–13.
The corrugated reentry blade implant device.

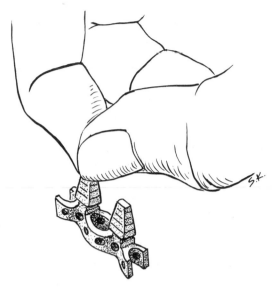

FIG 12–14.
A figure-of-8 reentry implant that measures 5 mm high and five mm wide. Both the corrugated and figure-of-8 reentry systems are manufactured in long strips that can be cut to the desired lengths that are required to fit into a particular site.

posts, and the interface body of the implant strips can be cut at any length to accommodate the antero-posterior length of the osteotomy. The superior surface must be buried 3 mm below the buccal and lingual plates of bone. The implant is 5 mm at the widest portion buccolingually and is available in 3-, 4-, or 5-mm blade heights (Fig 12–14).

Horizontal Basket Reentry Implants.—These reentry implants can be fully submerged or placed into immediate function. Synthetic or autogenous bone can be placed inside the body of the implant prior to insertion. An exact fit of the implant into the bony crypt is essential (Fig 12–15).

External Oblique Blade-Vent Implants.—This implant is designed specifically for use in the resorbed mandibular posterior ridge where the superior position of the mandibular nerve will inhibit insertion of the standard Blade-Vent implant into the body of the mandible proper, or in a situation where there is an extremely concave submandibular lingual fossa preventing implant insertion near the mandibular canal.

The uniqueness of this implant lies in the offset of the post of the implant toward the lingual (Fig

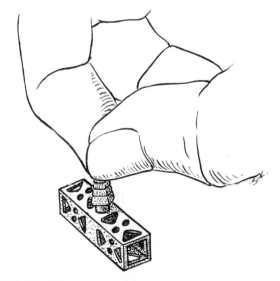

FIG 12–15.
The horizontal basket reentry implant can be fully submerged or placed into immediate function.

12–16,A). By positioning the post to the lingual of the body of the implant, the operator inserts the implant buccal to the external oblique ridge, avoiding the mandibular nerve, while still being able to construct the final mandibular prosthesis in proper occlusal relationship. This implant is designed with two types of lingual extensions. One has a single horizontal lingual extension, to be used in the mandible where sufficient bone is available for burying the extension above the canal with a T groove (Fig 12–16,B). The other design has a shallow V-shaped extension which can be used as a subperiosteal portion where the anatomy does not permit an endosseous insertion.

Unlike the osseointegration system, which calls for a 9-month bone healing period of failing implant sites before reentry can be attempted, the blade-vent implant reentry system provides immediate reentry, and has proved to be 98% successful. Sometimes these implants can be fitted directly into the existing bridge and placed into immediate function.[8]

SINUS-LIFT IMPLANTS

The inferior position of the maxillary sinus floor in the extensively resorbed maxillary arch has traditionally presented a restorative problem for the implantologist. Preoperative radiographs will reveal the maxillary sinus location and if adequate bone is available both mesial and distal to the antrum, the insertion of a sinus-lift Blade-Vent implant might be indicated. The sinus-lift implant was designed to take advantage of maxillary anatomy and the osteogenic potential of the schneiderian membrane. It is designed with a mesial and distal endosseous Blade-Vent portion, which is connected by a perforated basket-shaped sinus-lift portion (Fig 12–17). This sinus-lift design is either fixed in position or can be elevated away from the body of the implant to lift the membrane.

Upon insertion, the hollow basket is filled with hydroxylapatite nonresorbable material, or the artificial bone can be mixed with bone taken from the symphysis with hollow mill trephines (Fig 12–18). Often, the floor of the membrane is inverted upward into the sinus cavity. In these situations, the bone in

A

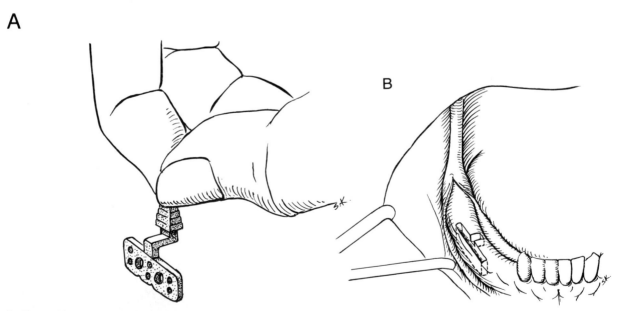

B

FIG 12–16.
A, a specially designed external oblique blade-type implant with a fairly broad buccolingual strut. **B,** the buccolingual bisecting groove made for the external oblique blade-type implant.

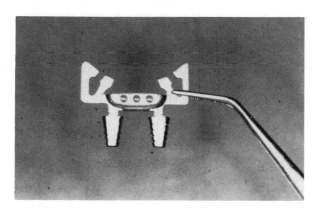

FIG 12–17.
A blade or plate form sinus-lift implant with a basket for autogenous bone or hydroxylapatite material.

the basket and inversion of the schneiderian membrane protect the membrane while at the same time a posterior abutment is created.

DISCUSSION

Although current designs are manufactured and distributed by Ultimatics, the name *Blade-Vent* has become a generic term for all blade- or wedge-shaped implants, which are now manufactured by

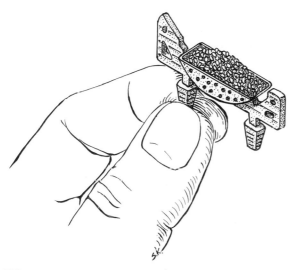

FIG 12–18.
The sinus-lift implant filled with nonresorbable hydroxylapatite prior to insertion.

various companies around the world.[9] Some original Blade-Vents that were inserted in the beginning of 1968 are still in function today, even though the prosthesis may have been changed (Fig 12–19).[10] The Blade-Vent implant can be used in most areas of either jaw, can be immediately inserted into multiple socket areas, and placed into functional loading from the day of insertion with excellent long-term success.[11] For the past 20 years, the Blade-Vent has been the most widely used implant in the world. Dentists who were against implants and happened to remove unsuccessful implants did not see the hundreds of thousands of implants that were successfully functioning without the need of their services.[11, 12]

In 1979, an evaluation of 564 implant patients, representing 1,540 implants, only 77 of which were mandibular subperiosteal implants, was carried out.[13] Women outnumbered men by two to one; 302 of the patients were partially edentulous and 51 patients were totally edentulous, while 206 patients were totally edentulous in one arch.[13]

Results of the evaluation showed that of the 487 patients, 269 had Blade-Vents in one arch, 188 had them in both arches, and 30 were totally edentulous and restored with four blades in each arch. There were 860 blade insertions in the maxilla and 603 blade insertions in the mandible. Of 115 seven-year cases, 11 were removed due to mobility, radiologic bone loss, and slight discomfort. In the 6-year follow-ups of 309 implants, 4 were removed and 14 showed radiographic resorption beneath the shoulders of the implants. The 3- to 4-year groups began to reflect the utilization of more sophisticated treatment planning. The implant channel preparation was changed by going to the palatal side in the maxilla and more to the lingual side in the mandible. This gave the Blade-Vents a maximum amount of bone flanking them bucally and labially where the bone was needed to resist the thrusts of the tongue and the eccentric movements of the mandible. Only 32 implants out of the total of 1,463 were removed.[13] A review of my patient records on a total of 91 cases representing 171 endosteal blade implants (implant duration 1–5 years) reported a success rate of 91.2%.

Within the past few years, two-piece submergible Blade-Vents have been used with much success

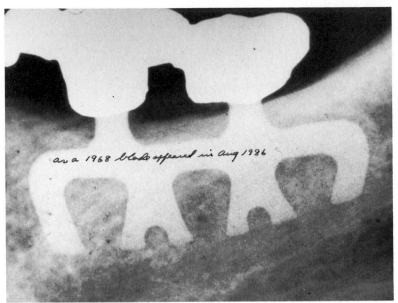

FIG 12–19.
A periapical film showing the radiologic appearance of a Blade-Vent implant that was inserted in 1968. This x-ray film was taken in August 1986.

in implant dentistry.[14] The process involves submerging the blade in the mandible for 3 months or in the maxilla for 6 months or more before reentering the implant site to screw on the abutment posts. Some believe that proceeding in this manner allows the bone to adapt itself closer to the implant's interface. Regarding Blade-Vent implants, however, only time will tell whether placing the implant into immediate function is any less beneficial than the prescribed submerged healing period.

Endosseous blades have existed in standard stock forms for more than 21 years.[3] Many types of custom designs have been utilized clinically since about 1968 and most types of biomaterials have been used. The blade design concept evolved in part because of the anatomy of edentulous bone.

Blade-Vent implants can be placed into immediate function, can be semisubmerged, or totally submerged, depending on the particular situation. Blade-Vent implants can be used in shallow or narrow ridges and in wide edentulous ridges. Their long-term success is technique-sensitive and highly dependent upon the skills of the clinician, not the least of which is the ability to cut an atraumatic free-hand groove in bone and get maximum contact of the implant with bone, thus maximizing the amount

of direct bone contact formed at the implant-to-bone interface. This good initial macroretention in an atraumatically prepared bone site, coupled with aseptic surgical conditions, a clean passivated implant surface, appropriate healing protocol, and prosthetic reconstructive procedures, is ultimately responsible for the long-term success and integration of an implant.

In all likelihood, a successful endosseous implant is both "osseous" and "fibroosseous-integrated" or osseovariegated (patches of fibrous tissue in bone osteoid, hematopoietic marrow, blood vessels, osteoclasts in various percentages and configurations) at different points along its surface. A Blade-Vent implant can function well with a fibrous tissue interface but moderate amounts of fibrous tissue can doom a cylindrical implant.

Our profession can now present to the public highly predictable prognoses in much the same manner in which the medical profession has given their patients a high rate of success in open heart bypass surgery. More than enough time has passed for us to realize that we have the means at our grasp to help millions of edentulous and partially edentulous sufferers obtain a normal, happy life.

REFERENCES

1. Linkow LI, Chercheve R: *Theories and Techniques of Oral Implantology,* vols 1 and 2. St Louis, CV Mosby Co, 1970.
2. Linkow LI: Implants for edentulous arches, in Winkler S (ed): *Essentials of Complete Denture Prosthodontics.* Philadelphia, WB Saunders Co, 1979, pp 633–694.
3. Linkow LI: The Blade Vent: A new dimension in endosseous implants. *Dent Concepts* 1968; 11:3–18.
4. Linkow LI: *Maxillary Implants.* North Haven, Conn, Glarus Publishing Co, 1978.
5. Linkow LI: *Mandibular Implants.* North Haven, Conn, Glarus Publishing Co, 1978.
6. Linkow LI: Tuber blades. *J Oral Implantol* 1980; 9:190–216.
7. Linkow LI: The multipurpose blade: A three year progress report. *J Oral Implantol* 1981; 9:509–529.
8. Linkow LI, Wertman E: Re-entry implants and their procedures. *J Oral Implantol* 1986; 12:590–626.
9. Linkow LI, Rinaldi AW: Evolution of the vent-plant osseointegrated compatible implant system. *Int J Oral Maxillofac Implants* 1988; 3:109–122.
10. Acevedo IA: Success and survivability of endosteal blade implants managed in the practice of Dr. Linkow. *J Oral Implantol* 1987; 13:488–491.
11. Schnitman PA, Shulman LB (eds): *Dental Implants: Benefit and Risks. An NIH Harvard Consensus Development Conference.* Bethesda, Md, US Department of Health and Human Services, DHHS Publication No (NIH) 81-1531, 1980, pp 326–339.
12. Smithloff M, Fritz ME: The use of blade implants in a selected population of partially edentulous adults. A five-year report. *J Periodontol* 1976; 47:19–24.
13. Linkow LI: Evaluation of 564 implant patients (1540 implants). *Implantologist* 1980; 9:33–37.
14. Viscido AJ: Submerged functional predictive endosteal blade implants. *J Oral Implantol* 1974; 5:195–209.

Chapter 13

The Startanius Implant System

Ralph V. McKinney, Jr., D.D.S., Ph.D.
Jack Wimmer

The Startanius implants are a series of blade or plate form and threaded cylinder form endosseous implants provided in two-stage application devices.

The Startanius implants have been developed and are manufactured and distributed by Park Dental Research Corporation of New York, N.Y. (see Table 13–1).

THE IMPLANTS

The Startanius Blade Implant

The Startanius blade implants are biologically innovative submerged blade or plate implants that are designed for the anatomic configuration of the maxilla and mandible. Thus an adequate assortment of the devices are available in order to match the various jaw configurations (Fig 13–1). The implants are made from commercially pure (cp) titanium in the form of a fully enclosed perforated blade. The blade post has a smooth cylindrical shape and contains internal threads for eventual attachment of one of the various threaded second-stage posts. The posts (heads) are available in prebent angled shapes, straight post, and a bendable post that allows numerous bends for alignment in difficult prosthetic draw situations. Healing closure plugs are used to close the internal threaded collar during healing of the first stage.

The Startanius blade was developed using a finite element analysis of 298 finite elements with computer-simulated loading in excess of 430 psia. The final design showed no simulated occlusal distortion of the implant.

The Star Vent Implant

The Star Vent multipurpose implants are cylindrical with exterior threads on the radicular portion of the implant (Fig 13–2). The threads are of a self-tapping type since the prepared bone socket is not tapped. A vent exists in the lower one third of the implant to allow bone ingrowth. The cervical or collar area is composed of a smooth metal surface and an approximately 1-mm-wide collar that is countersunk into bone. The implant can be used in a fully submerged application or the head may be inserted for immediate loading of the implant. The heads screw into internal threads in the radicular portion of the implant. Screws and heads are available to fit most prosthetic retention systems such as removable appliances retained by screws, magnet retention, or dolder bar retention.

INSTRUMENTATION

For the Startanius blade implants, the instrumentation is that generally used for the insertion of all

TABLE 13–1.

The Startanius Implant System

Product name	Startanius Submerged Blade Implants; Star Vent Multi-Purpose Implant Screws
Manufacturer/supplier	Park Dental Research Corporation
	19 West 34th Street
	Suite 301
	New York, NY 10001
	(212) 736-3765
Material	Commercially pure titanium
Implant cost	Startanius blade implants, $145–$165
	Post (head) for blades, $35–$65
	Star Vent screw implants, $100
	Post (head) for screws, $35–$65
Armamentarium	Startanius blade implants: No special kit is available, individual specialized instruments for insertion average approximately $700–$900 depending on needs of the dentist
	Star Vent screw implants: Kit A for fixed bridgework is available for $1,094, which includes four screw implants and posts of the operator's choice
	Kit B is for star vent fixed/removable or overlay denture techniques and costs $1,383, including four screw implants and posts

blade implants. No. 700XL and 700XXL burs are used to create the blade channel, and seating instruments are used for tapping the implant into place. A unique instrument offered by Park Dental Research Corporation is a special bending instrument for precise paralleling of the removable implant heads (item Star 17 in the Park catalog). Special wrenches are also available to seat the various abutment heads.

Special instrumentation kits for Star Vent screw implants have been prepared (Figs 13–3 and 13–4). These instruments include burs and reamers to prepare the socket. No tapping instruments are used; the implant screws are self-tapping.

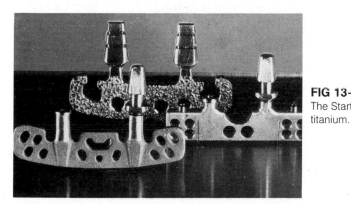

FIG 13–1.
The Startanius blade or plate form implants composed of cp titanium.

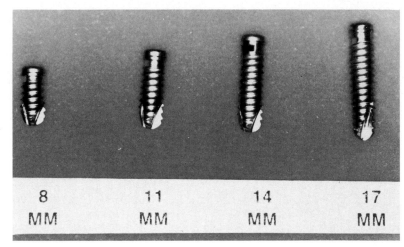

FIG 13–2.
The Startanius Star Vent Multi-Purpose Implant Screw composed of commercially pure titanium.

SURGICAL PROCEDURES

Startanius Blade Implants

The following is a step-by-step insertion protocol for the blade implant. These procedures are presented in Figure 13–5,A–C.

An incision is made along the crest of the alveolar ridge and full-thickness flaps are reflected buccal and lingual. The implant is held against the bur for purposes of drilling orientation. The short 700XL high-speed carbide bur is used for the initial preparation and a 700XXL is used to complete the socket to

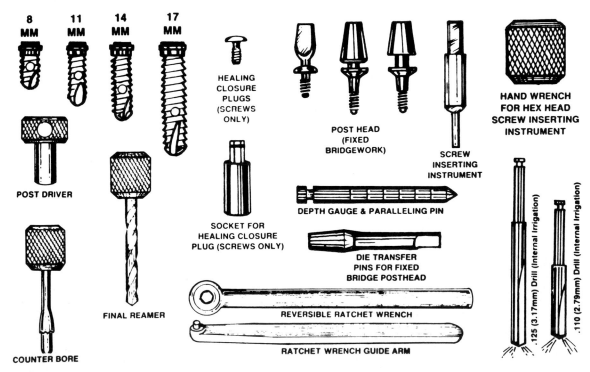

FIG 13–3.
The Star Vent kit A armamentarium set.

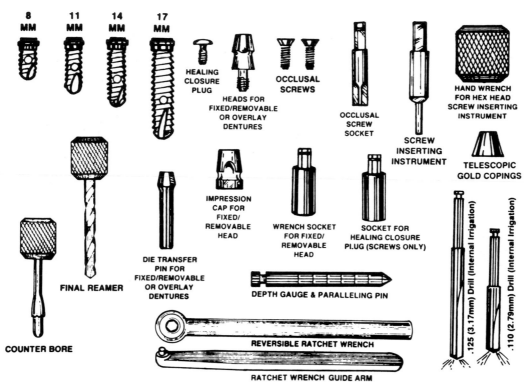

FIG 13–4.
The Star Vent kit B armamentarium set.

an appropriate depth. The drilling should be carried out with a sterile water-irrigated handpiece. The bur or handpiece should be used with a gentle sweeping motion, as with a paintbrush. The central area of the groove should be enlarged slightly to accommodate the oversize implant neck and post.

The mesiodistal length of the osseous preparation should be longer than the size of the implant. The groove depth can be verified with the depth gauge and then the implant is checked alongside the depth gauge.

The implant should be checked in the osseous groove, making certain the implant seats passively into the prepared site. If there is any resistance, the implant blade may have to be contoured to fit into the site. If the body of the implant requires bending, titanium-faced contouring pliers must be used, or the special Park Dental Research bending instrument can be used.

The implant can usually be seated with finger pressure to within 0.125 mm of the shoulder. The single-headed inserting instrument is used for final seating. The permanent implant post must be completely seated to the neck of the blade implant *before using the implant seating instrument*. The counterseating instrument is used for final positioning and appropriate alignment of the implant.

Final seating is achieved when the implant shoulder is 1 to 2 mm below the alveolar crest. The healing closure plug is inserted at this time. Suturing of the soft tissue flaps is achieved with 3-0 black silk sutures.

Once healing is complete, the covering mucosa is excised and the healing closure plug is removed with the square driver and the implant internal threaded neck is irrigated. If the Startanius blade is not perpendicular to the occlusal plane, the abutment head can be bent at this time from 5 to 10 to 15 degrees in any direction to achieve parallelism. Bending the abutment head is done by using a pair of titanium-faced bending or contouring pliers. The abutment head is inserted into a spare

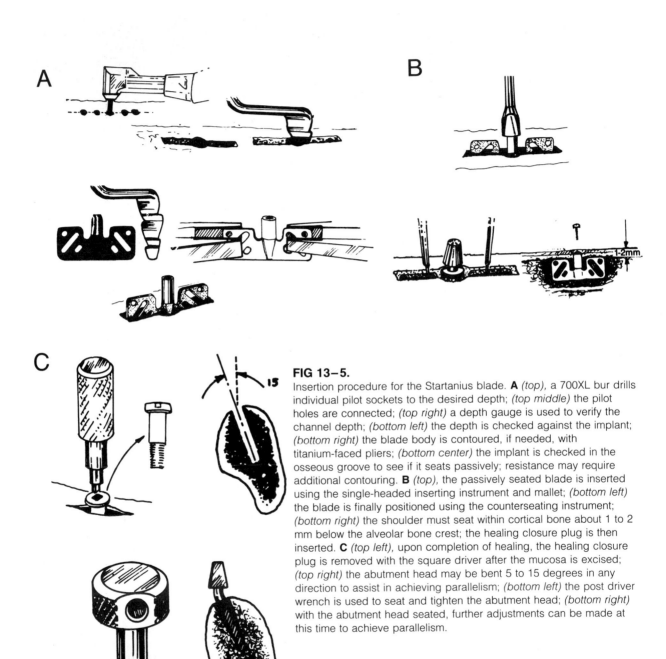

FIG 13–5.
Insertion procedure for the Startanius blade. **A** *(top),* a 700XL bur drills individual pilot sockets to the desired depth; *(top middle)* the pilot holes are connected; *(top right)* a depth gauge is used to verify the channel depth; *(bottom left)* the depth is checked against the implant; *(bottom right)* the blade body is contoured, if needed, with titanium-faced pliers; *(bottom center)* the implant is checked in the osseous groove to see if it seats passively; resistance may require additional contouring. **B** *(top),* the passively seated blade is inserted using the single-headed inserting instrument and mallet; *(bottom left)* the blade is finally positioned using the counterseating instrument; *(bottom right)* the shoulder must seat within cortical bone about 1 to 2 mm below the alveolar bone crest; the healing closure plug is then inserted. **C** *(top left),* upon completion of healing, the healing closure plug is removed with the square driver after the mucosa is excised; *(top right)* the abutment head may be bent 5 to 15 degrees in any direction to assist in achieving parallelism; *(bottom left)* the post driver wrench is used to seat and tighten the abutment head; *(bottom right)* with the abutment head seated, further adjustments can be made at this time to achieve parallelism.

Startanius blade to carry out the bending procedures.

The post driver wrench is used to tighten the abutment head into position. When the abutment head is seated into the final implant site, further adjustments can be done at this time to achieve parallelism. The Startanius endosteal blade implant with abutment head is now in position and ready for final restoration.

Startanius Star Vent Implants

The following step-by-step protocol for the cylindrical form implant can be followed using Figure 13–6 as a guide.

A guide hole is drilled with the .110-diameter (2.79 mm) or smaller drill. The first hole is enlarged with the .125-diameter drill (3.17 mm). The finger final sizing reamer is used to ream the .125 socket to a final finish size of .130 (3.3 mm). The hand counterbore reamer is used to form the countersink on the crest of the ridge with gentle finger pressure. The calibrated depth gauge and paralleling pin are used to determine the exact depth of the Star Vent screw site.

The one-piece Star Vent screw insertion instrument fits into the screw post headhole and engages in the groove placed there for this purpose. The hex post on the top of the screw insertion instrument fits the reversible ratchet wrench and the Star Vent screw hand wrench. To seat the Star Vent screw implant, the hand wrench is used to start the Star Vent screw into the prepared implant site. Then the reversible ratchet wrench with guide arm threads the screw into final position. As an alternative, the hand wrench can be used to entirely seat the Star Vent screw instead of the reversible ratchet wrench.

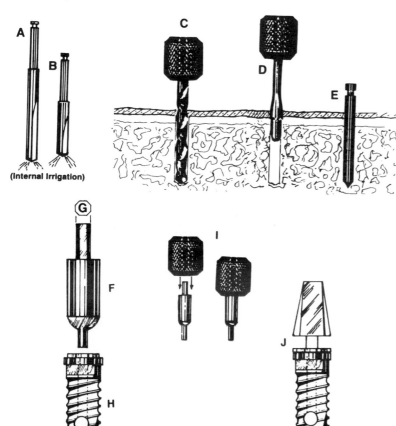

FIG 13–6.
Insertion procedure for the Startanius Star Vent implant. *(A)* The guide hole is drilled with the 2.79-mm internal irrigated drill and enlarged with the 3.17-mm drill *(B)*. *(C)* The finger reamer is used to size the socket site to a final 3.3 mm. *(D)* The counterbone reamer is used to form the collar countersink. *(E)* The calibrated depth gauge is used to determine the exact depth of the implant socket. *(F)* The insertion instrument is set into the screw post hole and the implant *(H)* carried to the socket and inserted. The ratchet wrench (not shown) or the hand wrench *(I)* can be placed over the hex end *(G)* of the inserting instrument and used to thread the screw implant into place and tighten it. Following seating, the healing closure plug can be used for a two-stage implant, or *(J)* an abutment head can be inserted for immediate loading.

When the Star Vent screw is seated to the required depth, the healing closure plug is inserted using the healing closure plug socket and hex head hand wrench. If immediate loading is desired, the proper head is inserted for restoration.

DISCUSSION

The Star Vent multipurpose screw implants are made of pure titanium. The implants and heads can be used in fully submerged applications or for immediate loadings for either fixed or removable bridgework restorations. The Star Vent screws are also adaptable to most denture retention systems, such as dolder bar, magnets, and other universal systems. Prosthetic procedures employed are those normally used for indirect impression techniques. Transfer copings and die transfer pins are available from Park Dental. The selection of impression material is left up to the practitioner.

The Startanius blade implants are also made of pure titanium and are designed to be used either in a one-stage or two-stage insertion mode, depending on the choice of the operator. The blade or plate form provides for better anchorage in the jaw bone because of the increased implant bone contact area. A positive feature of the Startanius blade is the numerous options of removable heads, many of which are already bent to various angles, thus facilitating establishment of parallel prosthetic draw for the practitioner. Both the blade proper and the head can be custom-bent to fit the jaw contours and prosthetic problems of the individual case. Again, transfer copings and transfer pins are available to match the Startanius blade implants. Routine indirect prosthetic procedures are employed.

Chapter 14

The Omnii Implant System

O. Hilt Tatum, Jr., D.D.S.

THE IMPLANT AND ITS BACKGROUND

The Omnii system of dental implants is uniquely different from those offered by any other source. This system offers a variety of designs necessary to fit into the anatomic, bone quality, functional, and restorative differences presented in clinical practice. The horizontal fin design of the root and sinus implants maximizes the amount of surface area that is available to load the bone vertically and allow ingrowth of bone around the implant. This allows the implants to be placed in thinner ridges than other systems and distributes the occlusal stresses over a large surface area of bone. The implants are designed to conform to the shape of the bone found in edentulous areas or to the sockets which are made possible by bone manipulation[1] (Fig 14–1,A and B) or grafting (Fig 14–2,A–D). Another feature of this system is the removable posts and filler screws that allow the implant radicular portion to be placed into a closed or submerged environment during the healing period to lessen or eliminate the potential for trauma during the healing phase. The posts can then be placed and shaped with burs when the restorative phase of treatment is begun to give multiple restorative options for the crown and bridgework. Root form and sinus implants are made of a titanium alloy for added strength. The blade and frame implants are made of pure titanium which has more malleability so the implants can be bent to conform with the contour of the bone.

This system is the product of over 30 years of restorative and surgical experience and over 20 years of implant experience. The system had its origin in 1968 when implants were individually hand-machined from titanium to fit the needs of each patient. From this experience, a large number of different designs were made, used, and the results observed. Bone grafting was added in 1971 to enhance deficient areas. This was followed by ridge expansion techniques for root forms and, in 1975, the sinus elevation or lift procedure was developed to further enhance receptor sites.

The Omnii system was introduced to the dental profession in 1981 by Omnii Products International.[2] This included the first submergible titanium root form implants available to American dentistry. Omnii reports that by mid-1990 over 35,000 of their implants have been placed (see Table 14–1). Four different types of endosteal implant designs make up this system: root forms, sinus, blade, and frame.[2]

ROOT FORM IMPLANTS

The R (root) series has seven sizes and has been recently redesigned. Beginning in September 1989, the R series has available three diameters: 3.2, 4.0, and 5.0 mm (Fig 14–3). They are numbered R1, R2, and R3, and are round and tapered (Fig 14–4). These implants come in lengths of 14, 16, 18, and 20 mm. Numbers D1, D2, D3, and D4 have a D shape and are tapered (Fig 14–5). These are all 3.5

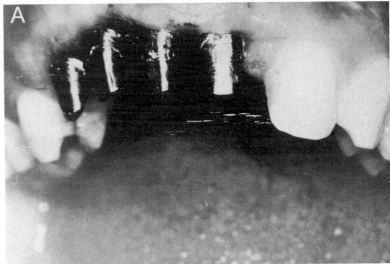

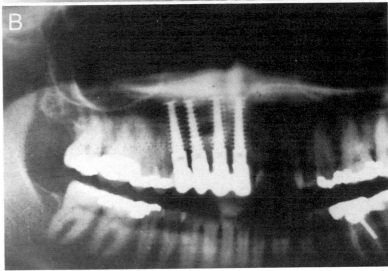

FIG 14–1.
A, photograph showing four implants with posts in place at time of restorative preparation. Implant placement was done 6 months previously by spreading the thin anterior maxillary bone to create adequate sockets to receive the implants. **B,** a radiograph of the implants in **A,** 7 years after placement.

mm in buccolingual width but vary in mesiodistal width. The widths are 4.0, 5.5, 7.5, and 10 mm. A set of graduated tapered internally irrigated burs are available to prepare the sockets for the three round implants. These sizes also have a set of hand augers (Fig 14–6) for use in spongy maxillary bone. A set of three channel formers (Fig 14–7) are available for starting the maxillary sockets for the D-shaped implants. All sizes of implants have a set of three socket formers (Fig 14–8) which are graduated to the full size of each implant. The round implants are indicated for ridges that are wide enough to allow for a minimum 3.2-mm socket preparation. The taper is designed to fit the normal narrowing of the jaw.

The D sizes offer unique opportunities to place implants with exceptional surface areas and physiologic stress transfer capacities into thin ridges.[1] This is extremely important because most edentulous alveolar ridges are 4 mm or less in buccolingual width. In this type of thin maxillary ridge, the sockets are formed with bone expansion techniques (Fig 14–9,A) for implant placement (Fig 14–9,B and C). The maxillary socket is usually formed without the removal of any bone.

The expansion technique used for thin mandibles requires the use of burs to prepare the mesiodis-

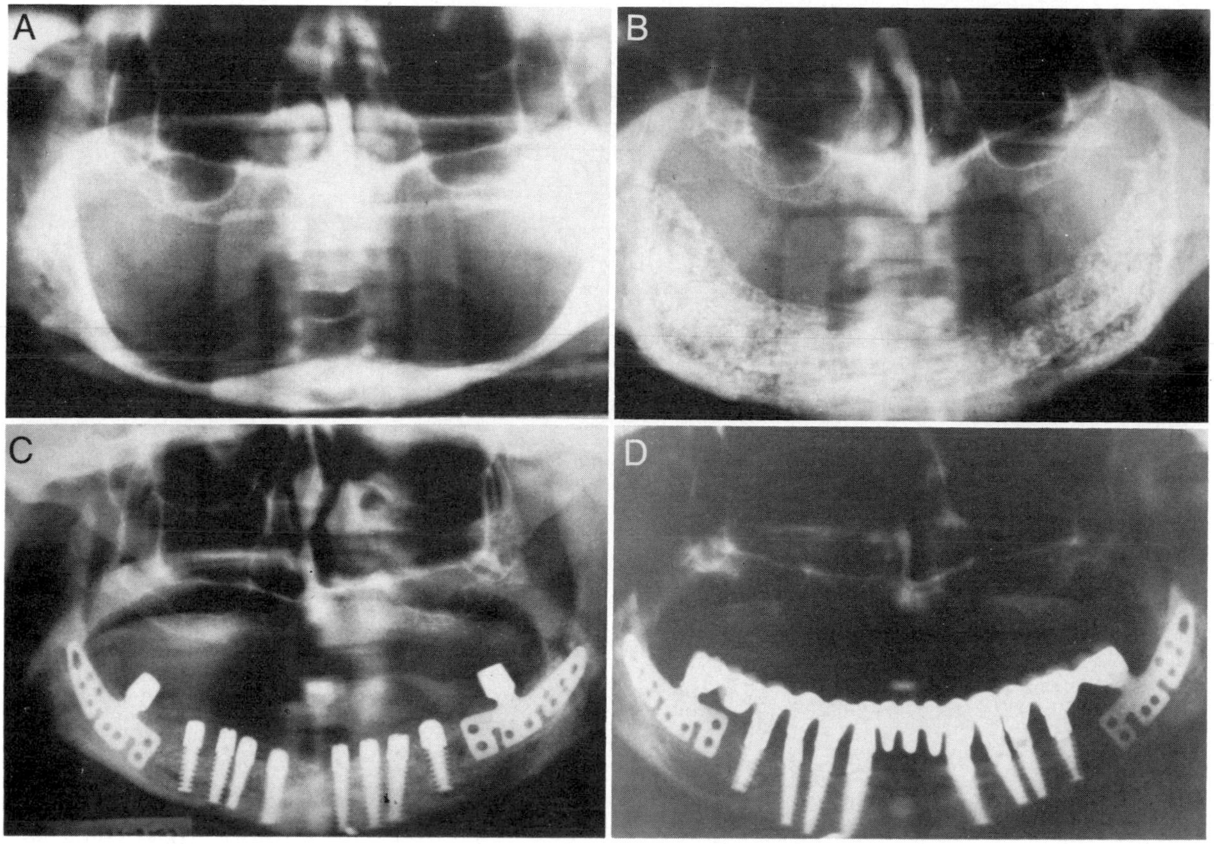

FIG 14–2.
A, a severely atrophic mandible. **B,** the same mandible immediately after a bone graft done with 50% autogenous bone and 50% beta tricalcium phosphate ceramic. **C,** the mandible 6 months after the bone graft and at the time of implant placement. **D,** same patient seen in **C** 9 years after the original bone graft was done.

tal width and depth of each socket (Fig 14–10,A). The careful use of the socket formers can then finish the socket form if the buccal wall is not too inflexible (Fig 14–10,B and C). The R series implants can be used in any location where a proper socket can be created. Healing time is 6 months for the maxilla and 4 months for the mandible (Fig 14–10,D). They are supplied with either a straight or angled post and oversize posts are available (Fig 14–11).

The posts have left-hand threads to prevent the bur rotation from unscrewing the posts during crown preparation. The body of the implant usually extends 2 to 3 mm superiorly from the bone crest (see Fig 14–10,C). This allows the margin of the crown preparation to cover the connection of the post to the implant, and still permit a proper biological zone to be maintained. When the root implants are used for overdenture support, Zest attachments, magnets, or O ring posts are available to screw into the implants. Also available is a bar technique for use in an overdenture situation.

SINUS IMPLANTS

The sinus series (S) is supplied in eight sizes and is made of titanium alloy[1] (Fig 14–12). There are also eight socket formers (Fig 14–13) matching the exact size of each implant. This series is specific for use in the posterior maxilla, and the selection of sizes is in harmony with the normal range of alveolar bone formation found in this area. The widths are

TABLE 14–1.

The Omnii Implant System

Manufacturer/supplier	Omnii International 442 94th Avenue North St. Petersburg, FL 33702 1-800-284-4123 (813) 576-9100
Material composition	Omnii R series and mucosal inserts are composed of titanium alloy (Ti-6Al-4V) Omnii custom blades and ramus frames are composed of cp titanium
Individual implant costs	R series $125 each S series $175 each Mucosal inserts $4.50 each Custom blades $120–$140 each Ramus frames $250 each
Kits/armamentarium	A complete armamentarium kit with basic supply of implants is available as follows: R series kit $1,000 S series kit $1,200 Mucosal insert kit $250 Ramus frame kit $795

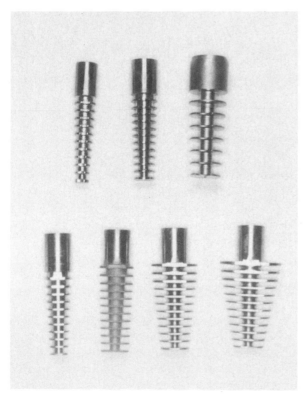

FIG 14–3.
The seven sizes of root form implants in 20-mm lengths.

3.2 and 4.2 mm and there are four lengths of 15, 20, 25, and 30 mm. The sinus implants are numbered as follows: S31, S32, S33, S34, S41, S42, S43, and S44. When the maxillary sinus limits the vertical bone height (Fig 14–14,A), these implants can be placed simultaneously with the elevation of the sinus floor (Fig 14–14,B–D). Sinus implants may also be placed after new bone has been formed following a sinus augmentation procedure. The sockets are then normally prepared with hand curets. The bone that is

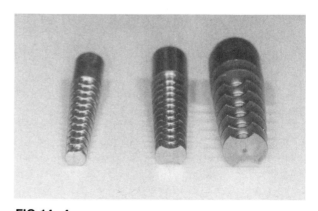

FIG 14–4.
An apical view of the three round root form 20-mm-long implants with key locks to prevent rotation.

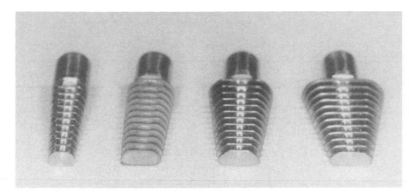

FIG 14–5.
Apical view of four D-shaped implants in 20-mm lengths.

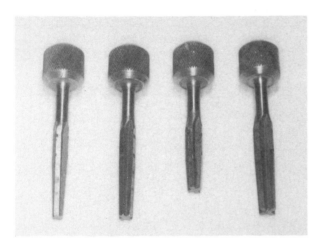

FIG 14–6.
Lateral view of the hand augers used for round implants. Lengths are 19 and 20 mm.

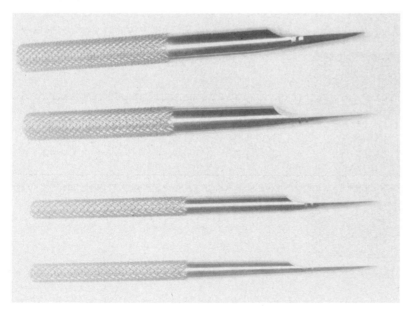

FIG 14–7.
Lateral view of the four channel formers showing the thinness of each instrument.

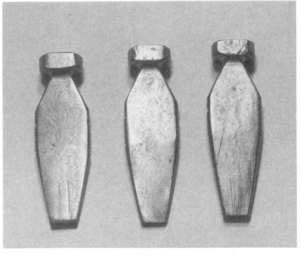

FIG 14−8.
Lateral view of the thread socket formers for the D4 implant.

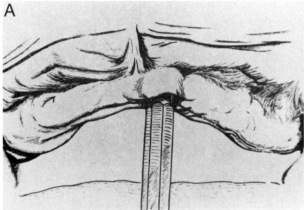

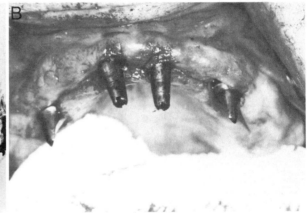

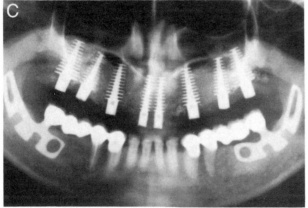

FIG 14−9.
A, view of a channel former fully inserted into a thin edentulous anterior maxilla with the bone expanded to the form of the instrument. **B,** view showing freshly placed implants following bone expansion with the posts in place to verify alignment and position. **C,** radiograph showing full arch of root form implants placed with bone manipulation of the thin crestal ridge. Bilateral sinus augmentation with tricalcium phosphate ceramic was done 9 months prior to implant placement. The mandibular blades were placed and restored 9 years previously.

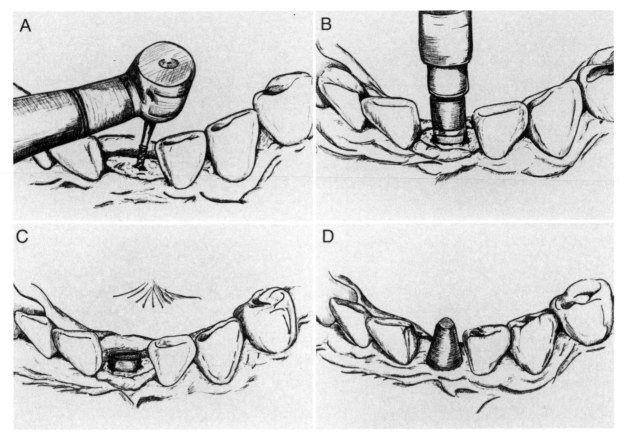

FIG 14–10.
A, mesiodistal width of bone showing the initial preparation utilizing a no. 699 carbide bur with copious irrigation, high speed, and light pressure. **B,** socket formed and the implant being seated following the bone preparation and manipulation with burs and socket formers. **C,** implant fully seated with the body of the implant extending 2 to 3 mm above the crestal bone. **D,** post in place following a 4-month healing period and prior to post preparation for a single crown.

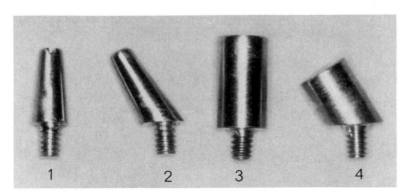

FIG 14–11.
Four of the posts that are available: *1* is a standard straight post, *2* is an angled standard post, *3* is a blank straight post, *4* is a blank angled post. Each of the implants is furnished with either a straight or angled post such as *1* or *2*.

FIG 14–12.
Lateral views of the eight types of sinus implants.

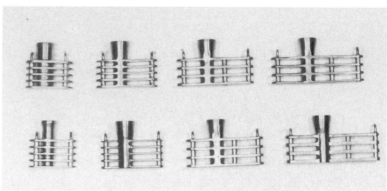

removed is packed into the implant fins (see Fig 14–14,B). Bone or an appropriate resorbable graft material is placed adjacent to the sinus membrane where the sinus floor has been elevated. This graft material is also placed over the implant to the ridge crest. A layer of hydroxylapatite (Osteograf, by CeraMed) or HTR (hard tissue replacement) is then placed over the entire ridge crest and the full-thickness palatal flap is placed over the ridge. Sutures and

a periodontal dressing are placed and removed after 2 weeks. A 6-month healing time is normal. When the posts are placed, it is frequently desirable to reduce the thickness of tissue found in the tuberosity area. Straight, angle, or oversize posts can be used and prepared to the final crown preparation form. If the implant post will exit in mucosa rather than attached gingiva, a split-thickness laterally positioned flap can be used at the time that the implant is ex-

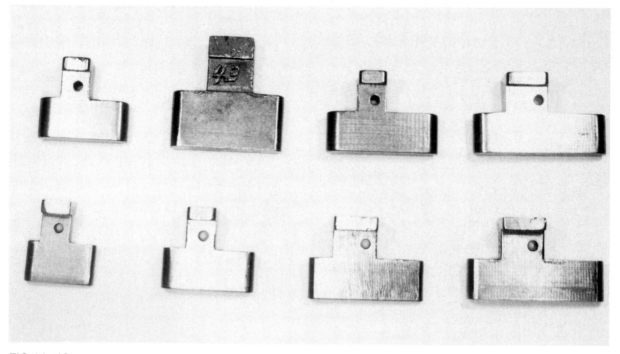

FIG 14–13.
Lateral views of the eight sizes of socket formers available for forming the sockets of the sinus implants.

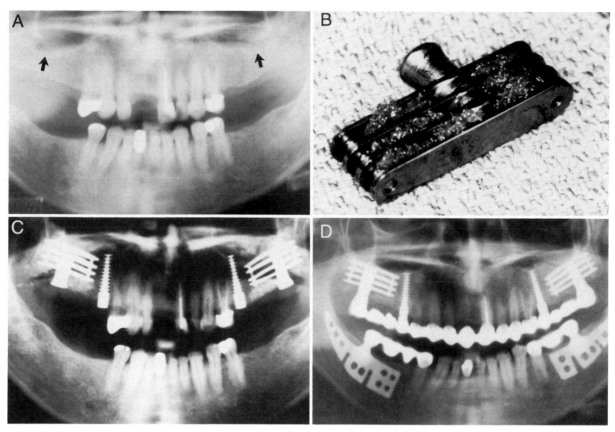

FIG 14–14.
A, *arrows* indicate the preoperative level of bone present in the floor of the sinus. **B,** a sinus implant packed with bone that has been harvested during the socket preparation placed into the fins of the implant. **C,** immediate postoperative radiograph showing the sinus floor elevated and grafting apical to the root form and sinus implants bilaterally. **D,** radiograph showing the same patient **(C)** 7 years after the implant placements.

posed and the post is placed. The sinus implants are used to support fixed restorative treatment.

BLADE IMPLANTS

The blade implant is made of titanium and is primarily indicated for use in the mandible distal to the mental foramen (Fig 14–15). This edentulous area is usually quite thin, with the bone loss occurring from the buccal. This blade is three-dimensional, fits into the mandible lateral to the mylohyoid space, and curves outward in the ascending ramus. The implant to be used is predetermined by the use of mounted study models and a good-quality pan-

oramic radiograph which clearly shows the mandibular canal. The degree of magnification present in the radiograph can be determined by measuring the vertical height of the same point on the patient and the radiograph. (It should be noted that Omnii allows the clinician to send in transparencies for fabrication of custom-designed metal blades). The burs used should be measured against the implant and marked to denote how deep the bone incision should be in each area. The incision should bisect the keratinized tissue and go lateral to the retromolar pad as it extends into the ascending ramus area. The bone incision is made with a 1557 or 1558 surgical bur and copious amounts of sodium chloride solution or water. The surgeon should palpate the lingual wall of

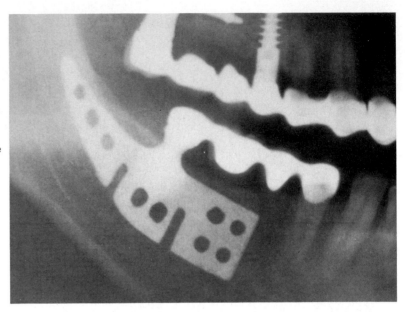

FIG 14–15.
A blade implant designed to fit into the available bone and placed 6 years previously.

the edentulous space to determine the angle of the bur penetration when preparing the site. The bur should be in harmony with the thickness of the implant. Light pressure on the bur with continuous movement will maintain adequate coolant in the cutting area. With the osteotomy completed, the implant is inserted into the bone in the ramus and rotated downward into position. The angles of the implant are modified if necessary and the implant is tapped to a seated position. Tricalcium phosphate ceramic (Augmen, by Miter) is placed to the ridge crest and hydroxylapatite or HTR is placed on the crest of the ridge and around the implant. Each implant should be nonstressed during its 4-month healing period and the posts are prepared at the time that the restorative treatment is started. Each implant can be one piece or have a removable post.

FRAME IMPLANTS

This is a one-piece titanium implant indicated for placement in edentulous mandibles (Fig 14–16). Implants are prefitted using mounted study models and a panoramic radiograph which has the retromolar pads identified on the film. The surgical steps are directed by correctly using anatomic landmarks. Retromolar pads, external oblique ridges, the mental foramen, the anterior ridge crest, and midlines are all used to place the bone and soft tissue incisions. Tricalcium phosphate ceramic and hydroxylapatite granules are placed above the bone to form a pad between the tissue and bone. A provisional denture is fitted following the closure of each incision and left in place for 2 weeks. At that time, sutures are removed and the denture is usually kept out during the night, but worn for limited function during a 3- to 4-month healing period. A new lower denture is made, and if an upper denture is being worn, a new denture is also fabricated at the same time. This implant provides an implant-supported prosthesis and has proved to be an exceptional device for the edentulous atrophic mandible.

SUMMARY

The Omnii system is comprised of different designs of implants which are used in different edentulous areas of the mandible and maxilla to allow restorative results that are in harmony with the bone and esthetic desires of the patient. Each implant is

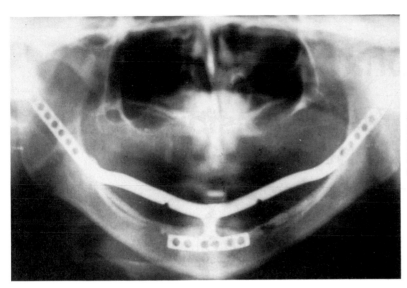

FIG 14–16.
Radiographic of a custom-fitted frame implant in place with the posterior arms lateral and superior to the nerve entry of each ramus area.

designed to maximize the use of available bone to allow the maximum bone implant interface for stress transfer capabilities. The system has very versatile prosthetic reconstructions and has proved to be extremely successful in implant practice.

REFERENCES

1. Tatum OH: Maxillary and sinus implant reconstructions. *Dent Clin North Am* 1986; 30:207–229.
2. Tatum OH: The Omnii Implant System, in Hardin JF (ed): *Clark's Clinical Dentistry,* vol 5. Philadelphia, JB Lippincott Co, 1984, chap 68.
3. Tatum OH: Endosteal Implants. *Calif Dent Assoc J* 1988; 2:71–76.

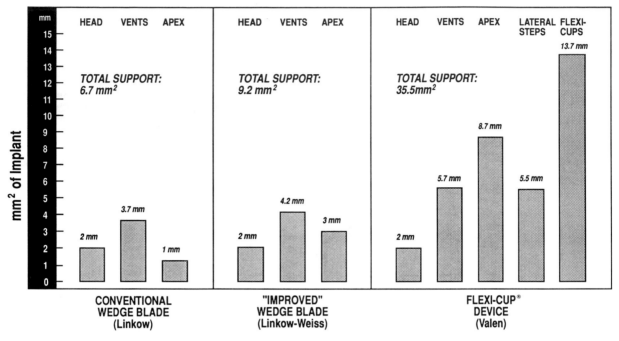

FIG 15–2.
Early (Linkow) blade or plate designs had limited horizontal areas to resist compressive or occludal loading as evaluated by computer analysis of their surface area. The Flexi-Cup device increases (300%–500%) the surface area. The ability of an endosteal implant device to resist occlusal loading is directly related to the implant's horizontal surface area as support values in square millimeters. The additional surface areas come from the activated flexible cups and the lateral subspinal step.

an endosteal implant[2], especially if it is immediately and rigidly secured within the alveolar bone by three-dimensional mechanical means.[1] Ironically, the use of standard one-stage blades or submerged healing implants does not result in controlled bone stimulation before loading, owing to their inability to resist bone deformation at the surrounding interface. One-stage blades have minimal horizontal surface areas to resist compressive loading and submerged blades simply are not loaded at all during healing. The characteristic bone at the implant interface following initial healing is classified as woven bone. Woven bone has relatively low mineral content, its fibers are more randomly oriented, and it provides minimal support or strength.[3]

IMPLANT SELECTION

In order to overcome the abovementioned limitations, we propose consideration of new criteria for implant selection.

Consider the case where an implant device becomes the distal abutment for a bridge (Fig 15–3). The mechanical principles by which splinted abutments or splinted natural teeth function in bone can be called physiologic biodynamics. It should be noted that these principles do not apply to the complete natural dentition since the teeth are not splinted. In nature, healthy bone is the result of the static equilibrium of the gnathodynamic muscular system and the harmonious state of occlusal interdigitation. All moments and forces equal zero and the muscles and the occlusal dentition are "equilibrated," or in equilibrium.

The masseter, temporalis, and medial pterygoids are the main closure muscles which generate the applied force. When abutments are splinted, the mechanics of mastication influenced by these muscles should be viewed as dynamic. This is because from the incisor region to the first molar, the mandible functions as a Class III lever with a mechanical advantage of less than one. From the first molar back to the condyle, the mandible functions as a Class II

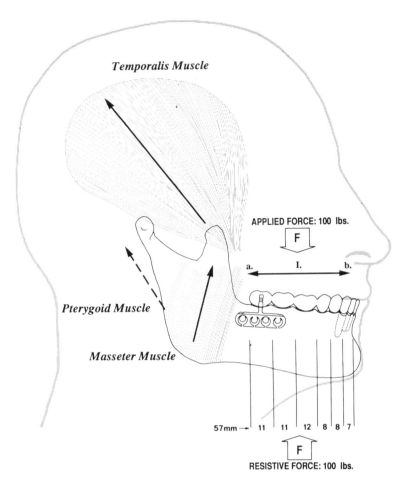

Temporalis Muscle

APPLIED FORCE: 100 lbs.

F

a.   I.   b.

Pterygoid Muscle

Masseter Muscle

57mm →   11   11   12   8   8   7

F

RESISTIVE FORCE: 100 lbs.

FIG 15–3.
If the hypothetical implant prosthesis pictured above is analyzed from a physiologic and biodynamic view, the distance from point *a* to point *b,* or the classic "cantilever," is termed the *moment arm* and is measured in inches. It is represented by the letter *l.* The total muscular applied force (100 lb) to the prosthesis, directly over the implant, is represented by the letter *F.* When multiplied, the resultant is termed the *moment torque,* in this case 200 lb (2 in. × 100 lb). The abbreviation for moment torque is Γ. We are utilizing this concept when there is a loss of equilibrium (unacceptable movement of an implant prosthesis). However, this loss of equilibrium, (i.e., a failing bridge) should be anticipated years in advance. Implant selection should be realistically based on an evaluation of the potential moment torques(s) in each individual case.

lever with a mechanical advantage greater than one.[4] This differential in mechanical advantages must be compensated for by implant selection, altered occlusal schema, and splinting ratio, severally or individually. If teeth and multiple implants are to be joined together, moment torques should be clinically estimated, and there should be a plan to equilibrate all abutments in the bone, before beginning. Equilibration in this application does not mean selective occlusal treatments, but rather balancing applied forces with known surface support areas of given implants or specific teeth.

Forces must be considered in pairs. The *resistive force* (that of the periodontium-gingiva, periodontal ligament, cementum, alveolar bone–tooth structures, temporomandibular joint, etc.) dissipates the *applied force.* In a given case the harmonious state of physiologic equilibrium is disturbed if the implant abutment has minute apical movement due to fibrous

encapsulation or even to cement breakdown at the natural abutment. When the apical movement of an implant is greater than the physiologic movement of a natural abutment to which it is splinted because of a thick fibrous capsule around the implant,[5] the relationship between the two abutments results in a loss of equilibrium and clinical failure. This frequently occurs with one-dimensional blades which have inadequate resistance to occlusal forces (see Fig 15–2).

The moment arm, or cantilever distance between natural and implant abutments, becomes the moment torque when placed in function (see Fig 15–3). This biodynamic physiologic state can be expressed mathematically as follows:

$$\Gamma = FI \text{ (lb in.)}$$

where Γ is the moment, its unit in engineering is the pound inch (lb in.), F is the applied force in pounds,

TABLE 15–4.

Approximate Comparative Support Areas (mm²) in the Bone for Various Endosteal Implants in a Compressive Mode (Valen)*

Mesiodistal Length (mm)		Head (mm)	Vents (mm)	Apex (mm)	Grooves (mm)	Flexi-Cup (mm)	Total Support (mm)
25	Wedge blades (Linkow)	2	3.7	1.0	—	—	6.7
25	Improved blades (Linkow-Weiss)	2	4.2	3.0	—	—	9.2
30	Large plate implants	3	15.0	3.7	—	—	21.7
25	Flexi-Cup (Valen)	2	5.7	8.7	5.5	13.6	35.5
	Conventional ramus implant	4	30.0	—	—	—	34.0
	Improved ramus implant	6	37.0	—	—	—	42.0

Diameters	Length	Names	Head	Vents	Apex	Threads	Total
5.5	16	Biotes	0.3	2	1.0	10	13.3
5.5	16	Core-Vent	0.5	21	2.5	1	25.0
4.0	12	Steri-Oss	0.5	—	1.5	9	11.0
4.0	14	TPS Screw	—	—	3.0	15	18.0
4.0	14	DB 1000	—	23	2.0	—	22.0
4.0	14	Star-Vent	—	—	1.2	12	13.5
4.0	13	LaminOss	(Valen)	—	10	40	50.0
4.0	14	Flexi-Root	—	—	10	10	20.0
4.0	14	Vent-Plant	0.5	3	3.0	12	18.5

*This table gives approximate surface support areas of implants in square millimeters as determined in a compressive mode. Bone implant interface can be calculated as the total support value for any given device. Data are determined from occlusal force registration obtained from the patient using transducer instrumentation.

ARMAMENTARIUM

There are only two unique items necessary to insert Flexi-Cup implant devices: a Surgical Profile Bur (Fig 15–4) and Flexi-Cup pliers (Fig 15–5). If a practitioner is experienced with one-dimensional blade or plate form implant placement, few additional skills are needed to use these instruments.

SURGICAL PROCEDURE

Two-Step Technique

Three-dimensional implant placement is a two-step procedure. The first step is identical to the simple insertion technique for one-dimensional plate or blade form implants.

Step 1 begins with the evaluation of available bone, through oral examination, appropriate radiographs, and finally, by direct vision of the surgically exposed edentulous ridge or implant site. For ideal three-dimensional placement of Flexi-Cup devices, ridges of approximately 3 to 4 mm in width are required.[17] Careful evaluation of the degree of bone density should be noted.

A simple crestal incision is made and full-thickness flaps are raised buccally and lingually. Care should be taken not to separate the periosteum from the overlying tissues. The anatomy of the ridge over its entire length should be carefully noted, realizing that an increased buccal flare is likely as one proceeds posteriorly.

A Surgical Profile Bur is utilized to prepare a bone channel 2 mm deeper than the intended implant body. The channel should also be the exact mesiodistal length or slightly longer than the intended implant. It should follow the general curvature of the ridge. With thinner ridges, it is helpful to make the channel slightly to the buccal to allow for lingual opening of the flexible cups. The precision fit of the implant spine with the prepared ridge crest and bone immediately subjacent to it will provide for substan-

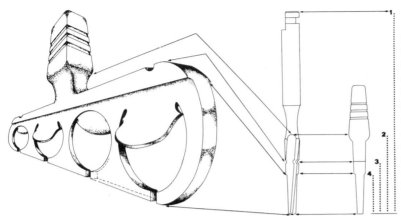

FIG 15–4.
Once a standard channel has been made with a high-speed rotary (700XXL or the equivalent) bur, a latch-type Surgical Profile Bur *(1)* is used to definitively refine the channel. Accuracy of implant-bone fit is critical and is achieved by carefully utilizing the implant channel depth marker *(2)*, the spinal step cutting area *(3)*, and the conformed body cutting and/or step *(4)* of the Surgical Profile Bur.

tial resistance to occlusal and lateral forces. Titanium bending pliers are used to conform the Flexi-Cup implant body to any ridge curvature. At this point the implant should be able to be almost completely seated with gloved finger pressure or gentle tapping with appropriate shoulder and abutment head seating instruments (Fig 15–6,A). Emphasis must be placed upon the gentle atraumatic nature of this initial seating and tapping.

Interocclusal clearance and abutment head parallelism should be noted and checked now, since adjustment can be made extraorally. Titanium-tipped instruments, usually pliers or a reverse mallet, are used to remove the implant from the channel. Step 1 is now completed. Any primary adjustments in height and angulation of the abutment head(s) are made at this time.

Step 2 of the three-dimensional implant insertion now begins. Again, the initial step is one of evalua-

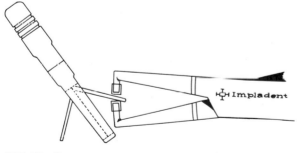

FIG 15–5.
Special pliers are necessary to activate the lateral "winglike" platforms of Flexi-Cup devices. The implant spine should be grasped firmly with standard titanium-tipped pliers.

tion of available bone, but this time the clinician should carefully note ridge width as well as depth and anatomy. Reformatted axial tomographs are particularly helpful in this regard.

Special pliers are used to activate individual flexible cups to their respective sides (Fig 15–6,B). The exact number and location of cups to be activated is based on direct visualization of available ridge width and tomographic analysis. Each cup should be opened laterally 0.5 to 1.0 mm. The "opened" implant is then placed directly into the bone channel, so that the flexible cups rest on the ridge crest (see Fig 15–6,B). Each cup site must be accurately marked on the adjacent bone by slight notching with a bur taking the implant in and out of the channel until all sites can be easily and correctly identified. The Surgical Profile Bur is used to finalize the half-moon notches in the alveolar crest. This final bone preparation for the outspread cups is only for the removal of cortical bone at the ridge crest, not down into the alveolus (see Fig 15–6,B).

The selected Flexi-Cup implant is then placed into the channel with finger pressure. Great care should be taken to see that the outspread cups clear the notched ridge, when viewed occlusally. The implant is then tapped into place firmly with a mallet, recalling the initial evaluation of bone density. The abutment head should only be used for seating if it has not been bent out of parallelism with the body. Several firm mallet taps will be necessary to properly seat the implant, relevant to the quality of available bone (see Fig 15–6,B). Initial cup spreading of 0.5 to 1 mm (20 degrees) from the vertical axis of the

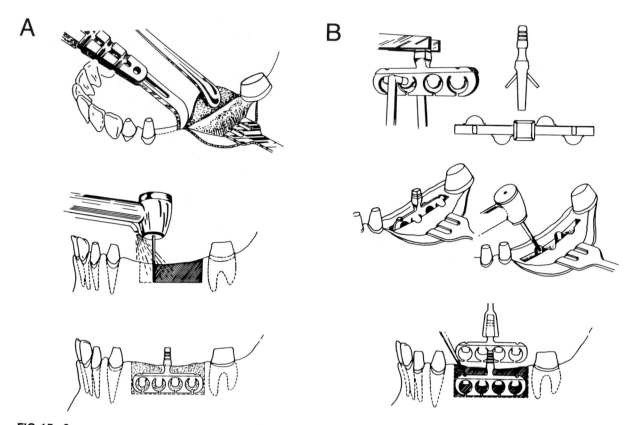

FIG 15−6.

A, Flexi-Cup implant insertion. *Step 1:* A standard crestal incision and full-thickness buccal and lingual flaps expose the alveolar ridge *(top)* so the operator can visualize its thickness and trajectory. A bone channel is made with a low-speed bur *(middle)* with proper cooling, or simply with the Surgical Profile Bur (recommended method). The channel should be 2 mm deeper than the body of the Flexi-Cup device, or simply, the total cutting surface of the Surgical Profile Bur. Using standard seating instruments the implant is gently tapped into place *(bottom)*. Step 1 is now complete. **B,** *step 2:* The implant is removed and Flexi-Cup pliers are used to activate individually chosen flexible cups outward, in conformity to the evaluation of ridge width *(top)*. The implant is reinserted into the top of the channel *(middle)* and a bur is used to mark the exact sites where the flexible cups engage the ridge crest. The implant is again removed and the marked crestal sites are fully notched. The implant is then tapped firmly into place with standard abutment head and shoulder seating instruments *(bottom)*. Step 2 is now complete.

implant body will be transformed into partially or fully spread cups, greater than 45 degrees, by insertion into bone.

When seating Flexi-Cup devices, bone is actually moved and compacted under the cups and within the vents of the implant. Therefore, more force is required in seating the implant in the mandible than in the maxilla owing to more internal support at the junction of the cancellous and cortical bone (see Table 15−3). Flexi-Cup implants will guide themselves into place and lock into bone in a three-dimensional manner dependent upon internal variations in bone

density. Step 2 (see Fig 15−6,B) is now complete.

The superior aspect of the bone channel is routinely filled with a resorbable hydroxylapatite such as OsteoGen. Often, especially in the maxilla, additional resorbable hydroxylapatite is placed in the implant channel prior to final seating to compensate for lack of trabeculation and to provide physical support under the implant.

The incision line is closed routinely with sutures according to the preference of the clinician. Excess tissue at the percutaneous sites is removed.

The most crucial individual step for correct

placement of Flexi-Cup devices is the channel refinement to accept and guide the opened flexible cups. This notching process should be carried down through any dense bone on the crest of the ridge, but *not* down into the trabecular bone or for the full depth of the body of the implant. The final insertion of a Flexi-Cup device must be viewed as a dynamic placement, rather than as a passive or neutral process.

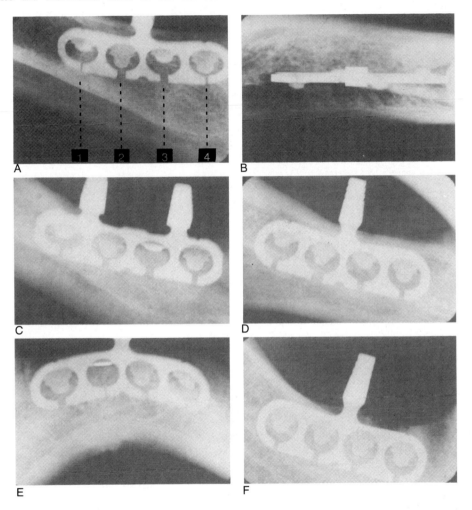

FIG 15–7.
Immediate postinsertion radiographs. Certain anatomic characteristics of inserted Flexi-Cup devices should be noted. **A** represents a three-dimensional blade device inserted in 1980. Cups *1* and *3* (all cups numbered left to right) open to the buccal. Cups *2* and *4* open to the lingual. Note compression of both the anterior and posterior legs, in contrast to the "opening" of the legs immediately under the abutment head. **B,** an occlusal view clearly shows the initial lateral spreading of all four flexible cups prior to the final seating. **C,** cups *1* and *3* open to the buccal greater than 45 degrees. Cups *2* and *4* on the lingual aspect do not appear opened to the same extent. Note slight compression of the distal legs which protects against encroachment or overseating into the mandibular canal. **D,** cup *3* is opened greater than 45 degrees. Cup *3* was placed into an extraction site. **E,** a Flexi-Cup blade is placed in the mandibular symphysis. Note that the shape of the implant body conforms to the arch curvature. Also, cup *2* is opened greater than 60 degrees and cup *4* greater than 45 degrees, thus providing tremendous resistance to anterior vertical loading. Cup *1* was placed into an immediate extraction site. **F,** use of a Flexi-Cup blade in an extremely narrow ridge. Note that the implant has been placed one-dimensionally (no cups are spread), although there is slight compression of the distal legs.

PROSTHETIC CONSIDERATIONS

Flexi-Cup implants should not be left freestanding prior to construction of definitive prostheses. The authors recommend routine provisional prosthetic construction techniques.

Care should be taken, however, not to engage abutment head and neck undercuts or cement grooves when bulk or reline temporary acrylics harden. One of the advantages of Flexi-Cup implant abutment heads are their square corners, which provide for superior primary prosthetic retention. However, additional care is necessary to guarantee that provisional prostheses fit well and can be inserted and withdrawn

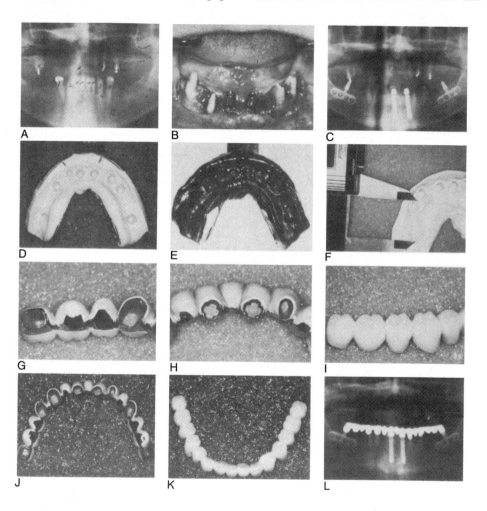

FIG 15–8.
A full-arch fixed prosthodontic case supported posteriorly by single-head Flexi-Cup blades. **A,** only two maxillary teeth can be retained for an overdenture prosthesis. The panoramic radiograph has been utilized to explain available bone concepts and benefit-risk factors to the patient. **B,** two TPS screws replace the incisors. Extractions, periodontal therapy, root canals, and implant placement are done at the same visit. **C,** note activation of all the flexible cups. **D,** the relieved heavy silicone impression should be used as a tray to carry light-body silicone and obtain a final impression 6 weeks after implant placement. **E,** this healing time should be adequate to prevent compression of the impression material subgingivally. **F,** moment arms are measured prior to instructing the laboratory about the desired occlusal schema. **G,** the "squared" head of Flexi-Cup abutments provide superior retention, as do the slotted heads of the TPS screws. **(H).** The final prosthesis **(I–K)** has a pinpoint cusp-fossa relationship and narrow occlusal tables in order to compensate for the patient's strong musculature. **L,** final panoramic x-ray film.

passively, especially with multiple abutment cases (Fig 15–7). Prior to suture removal, temporary cement is not usually recommended. Ideally, 6 to 8 weeks should elapse before final impressions.

Plastic transfer copings are supplied by the manufacturer and can be used as an abutment head; the transfer coping should be used with laboratory analogs (replica dies) of the Flexi-Cup heads. When significant preparation of an abutment head(s) has been made for parallelism or interocclusal clearance, the transfer coping(s) is best used to carry a light body impression material at the time of final impressioning. If additional reduction of an implant head(s) is advisable, the laboratory can furnish "cutdown" coping(s) for intraoral adjustment. The rigidity in bone of healed Flexi-Cup devices makes this a riskless procedure, which should result in a passive final casting insertion path.

The authors recommend a two-stage impression technique. A full-arch, heavy silicone impression is taken after placement of the transfer coping(s). It is allowed to harden, withdrawn, and then hollowed out with acrylic trimming burs. Cyanoacrylate cement is used to secure the transfer coping(s), which also may be slightly hollowed out, to the air-dried heavy-body silicone "custom tray." A light-body silicone is injected into the relieved coping(s) and into the relieved heavy-body impression, which has been coated with an appropriate adhesive. Additional light-body silicone is injected around the implant(s) and the natural abutment teeth after removal of retraction materials. The heavy-body custom tray impression is then inserted and placed under slight compression and stabilized until hardening of the light-body silicone. An exquisite impression usually is the result (Fig 15–8).

Castings should be returned ideally on an unbroken model. If solder connections are necessary, it is advisable to maintain the original master model. A general tissue pickup impression can also be taken. While this takes additional time and effort, the result should be an elegant final prosthesis.

DISCUSSION

Flexi-Cup endosteal blade implant devices have been utilized by many practitioners for over 10 years with a high clinical success rate. Without question, the greatest single variable that alters the time of good clinical service is the quality of initial selection. The use of the Flexi-Cup implant is a predictable procedure owing to the standardized uniformity of the implant height and a universal system of implant-to-bur interface for the preparation of the osteotomy.

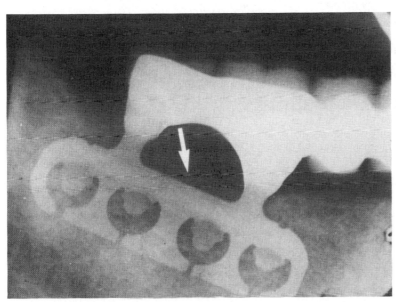

FIG 15–9.
A recent clinical case showing use of a double-headed Flexi-Cup blade as a posterior abutment. Current designs have a thickened or strengthened horizontal spine when compared to earlier implants *(arrow)*. The first anterior abutment is the canine. This results in a long moment arm or cantilever.

Flexi-Cup implants have been shown to provide maximum resistance to occlusal forces and are clearly indicated when there is sufficient width of available alveolar bone (Fig 15–9). Because of the three-dimensional nature of engagement of the cancellous bone, the implants can also be used to "bridge" recent extraction sites or older alveolar defects. These areas can be filled with autogenous bone or various synthetic resorbable hydroxylapatite materials. Correct utilization of the Surgical Profile Bur significantly helps to ensure initial intimate bone-to-implant fit which is critical for short-term as well as long-term implant success. Flexi-Cup devices can be utilized for immediate replacement of many forms of failing or already failed one-dimensional implants.

While Flexi-Cup devices have been designed to be inserted three-dimensionally, they can also be utilized one-dimensionally. In fact, the completion of step 1 of three-dimensional insertion represents one-dimensional placement.

Clinicians can utilize a Flexi-Cup device, which will be later inserted three-dimensionally, to evaluate the bone density or trabeculation of a given ridge, by the process of completing step 1.

Utilization of Flexi-Cup devices in their three-dimensional mode requires knowledge of the principles of bone preparation, movement, compaction, healing, and intended functional support. More time must be allocated to properly insert three-dimensional devices. The intimate fit and maximum resistance to occlusal loading that result justify the additional effort, and extend the life of the functioning prosthesis.

When adequate alveolar width exists, implant devices that are truly three-dimensional is clearly warranted. This selection is scientifically based on knowledge of the occlusal loading capacity of three-dimensional implants.

REFERENCES

1. Valen M: The relationship between endosteal implant design and function: Maximum stress distribution with computer-formed, three dimensional Flexi-Cup blades. *J Oral Implantol* 1983; 11:49–71.

2. Linkow LI, Chercheve R: *Theories and Techniques of Oral Implantology,* St Louis, CV Mosby Co, 1970.

3. Roberts WE, Turley PK, Brezniak N, et al.: Bone physiology and metabolism. *Calif Dent Assoc J* 1987; 15:54–61.

4. Mansour RM: *Forces and Moments Generated During Maximum Bite in Centric Occlusion* (master's thesis). Drexel University, Philadelphia, 1972.

5. Brunski JB, Hipp JA: *In vivo* forces on endosteal implants: Measurement system and biomechanical considerations. *J Prosthet Dent* 1984;51:82–90.

6. Ismail YH, Pahountis LN, Fleming JF: Comparison of two dimensional and three dimensional finite element analysis of a blade implant. *Implantologist* 1987;4:25–31.

7. Atmaram G, Mohammed A, Schoin FJ: Stress analysis of single-tooth implant using finite element method. *J Dent Res* 1977;56(special issue A):abstract 296.

8. Kakudo A, Ishida A, Yoshimoto S: Strains in dog jaw bones following implant insertion, a photoelastic study. *Implantologist* 1976; 1:67–77.

9. Mohammed H: Photoelastic stress analysis of single tooth implant with different root configurations, in *Transactions of the Third Annual Meeting of the Society for Biomaterials and Ninth Annual International Symposium,* 1977, pp 1–17.

10. Weinstein AM, Klawitter JJ, Anand SC, et al: Stress analysis of porous rooted dental implants. *J Dent Res* 1976;55:772–777.

11. Weinstein A: Implant-bone interface characteristics of Bioglass dental implants. *J Biomed Mater Res* 1980; 14:23–29.

12. Farah JW, Craig RG, Yapp RA: Stress distribution caused by blade type dental implants. *Implantologist* 1979;1:82–85.

13. Yanagisawa S: Clinical effects of the endosseous implant to the supporting bone and to the opposing teeth and jaw bone. *J Oral Implantol* 1979;8:643–653.

14. Vajda T, Fung J: Comparative photoelastic stress analysis of four blade-type endosteal implants. *J Oral Implantol* 1979;8:257.

15. Mohammed H, Atmaram GH, Schoen FJ: Dental implant design: A critical review. *J Oral Implantol* 1979;8:393–410.

16. Martin J, Valen M: *In Vitro Comparison Between*

Wedge-Blade and Flexi-Cup Implants Using Human Mandibles. Newark, University of Medicine and Dentistry of New Jersey, 1982.

17. Misch C, Judy K: Classification of partially edentulous arches for implant dentistry. *Implantologist* 1987; 4:7–13.

18. Knoblauch KR: *In Vivo Occlusal Force Determination* (master's thesis). Drexel University, Philadelphia, 1971.

19. Hastings GW, Ducheyne C: *Natural and Living Biomaterials*. Boca Raton, Fla, CRC Press, Inc, 1984.

Chapter 16

The Stryker Precision Dental Implant System (Root Form Series)

Thomas D. Driskell, B.S.

The Stryker precision implant system (Table 16–1) is the culmination of 22 years of design, development, and research experience with osteointegrated dental implants.[1-7] The Stryker root form implant configuration offers a number of exclusive design features which facilitate maximized function, periodontal health, prosthetic versatility, optimal esthetics, and ease of surgical placement.[8] All implantable components are provided in double-packaged sterile condition. Two root form surface preparations are available: (1) the original uncoated version with carefully cleaned and passivated surfaces, and (2) with a high-bond-strength hydroxylapatite coating (Osteobond) (Fig 16–1). Three diameters, 3.5, 4.0, and 5.0 mm, as well as three lengths, 8, 11, and 14 mm, in both the plain and hydroxylapatite-coated versions are offered.

Of particular significance are the improvements seen in the periodontal response to the implant. This is due to the unconventional head, neck, and shoulder contours used in the design. These features appear to markedly enhance preservation and maintenance of the crestal bone surrounding the implant.[8]

Stryker implants are the first specifically intended to be used in conjunction with a crestal autogenous graft (harvested during socket preparation).[1] The autogenous material is used to cover the sloping shoulders of the implant up to the alveolar crest. This technique virtually assures complete bone coverage over the implant early on, appears to inhibit epithelial downgrowth, and helps prevent bone cratering from occurring. The sharply downward sloping shoulders of the root components are also designed to favorably stress and therefore help maintain and stimulate the regenerated crestal bone. Clinicians confirm that if the recommended surgical protocol is followed, cratering or saucerization around the implant can be substantially eliminated.[9-13]

Stryker's ultraprecision locking taper attachment of implant head to root components permits angled heads to be locked in any rotational position required to obtain parallelism. It also provides a hermetically sealed, high-strength attachment. The locking taper attachment eliminates the rotational alignment and fluid percolation problems inherent with screw thread attachments as well as the mess, biodegradation, and potential periodontal problems associated with cemented attachments.

"Protected healing" is an important aspect of the Stryker design philosophy. The root component is surgically placed 1 to 2 mm below the crest of the alveolar ridge. This is much deeper and therefore more protected compared with other submergible implant systems. A small black plastic healing plug obturates the ultraprecision locking taper socket in the root component during the 3-month passive healing period. The plug can be easily shortened with scissors to prevent its protrusion too far above the alveolar crest and possibly irritating the gingiva.

This technique assures complete submergibility

TABLE 16–1.

The Stryker Precision Implant System

Product name:	Stryker Precision Implants
Manufacturer/supplier	Stryker Corporation
	Surgical Division
	420 Alcott Street
	Kalamazoo, MI 49001
	1-800-253-3210
Material	All implantable components are fabricated from surgical-grade titanium alloy (Ti-6Al-4V ELI) except for temporary healing plugs which are injection-molded, surgical-grade, ultra-high-molecular-weight polyethylene; all are supplied in sterile packaging, ready for implantation
Cost of typical implant	Root component (uncoated) $110
	Straight head component $ 50
Cost of instrumentation	Surgical instrumentation kit for anterior and posterior placement $800

and minimizes the possibility for dehiscence during the critical protected healing phase. Furthermore, the black healing plug can usually be seen through the overlying, somewhat translucent, healed gingiva. Thus, it facilitates ease of locating the submerged implant prior to head placement (Fig 16–2).

The Stryker system offers 26 interchangeable implant head options. All Stryker implant head styles and sizes will mate with any Stryker root component regardless of length or diameter. The subgin-gival contours of the head components are designed for improved periodontal maintenance and are provided in straight and angled versions in a variety of diameters and lengths for esthetic considerations.

Stryker root form implants are used as freestand-

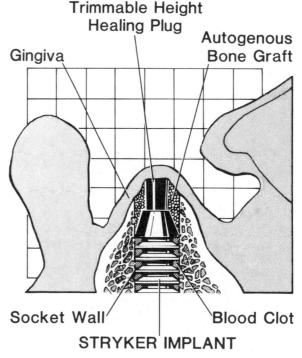

Trimmable Height Healing Plug

Gingiva

Autogenous Bone Graft

Socket Wall

Blood Clot

STRYKER IMPLANT

FIG 16–1.
Uncoated *(left)* and hydroxylapatite-coated *(right)* Stryker root components.

FIG 16–2.
Submerged Stryker root component.

ing single tooth replacements, as abutments for bridgework, and for overdentures. Outstanding occlusal load-bearing capacity results from the use of serrated (multifinned) root surfaces. Figure 16–3 shows two photomicrographs of an undecalcified section of an osteointegrated serrated root form implant in function for 5½ years recovered from a human. This highly efficient serrated "Christmas tree" (finned) configuration with horizontal undersurfaces (not a screw) results in a high degree of predictability toward osteointegration of the implant.

The Stryker system was the first to offer a complete surgical instrumentation system made from the same material as the implants. This innovation anticipated the growing concern among biomaterials researchers over the use of unlike metal instruments in the preparation of implant placement sites. Recent studies at the University of Alabama in Birmingham have identified traces of metallic residue from stainless steel socket-forming instrumentation on cut bony surfaces.[14] This dissimilar metal contamination could be expected to result in electrolysis occurring at the cut bony surfaces and elicit an inflammatory response at the bone-implant interface. Because Stryker's instrumentation components are now fabricated from titanium alloy, as are Stryker's implantable components, the possibility for an adverse tissue reaction from dissimilar metal contamination at the implant site has been eliminated.

Two instrumentation options are offered for creating implant sockets. One incorporates Stryker's atraumatic single-fluted hand reamers, which, in addition to their accuracy in socket sizing, provide a "feel" of the bony structure being instrumented. For example, in the maxilla, the thin cortical plate apposing the sinuses can be felt when using the hand reamer before inadvertently cutting too far and perforating into the sinus. Hand reamers are also useful when instrumenting a fresh extraction site for placement of an implant.

The second option is a set of specially designed ultra-low-speed latch-end drills intended to be operated at no more than 50 rpm. At this speed, and because of their special design, overheating when cut-

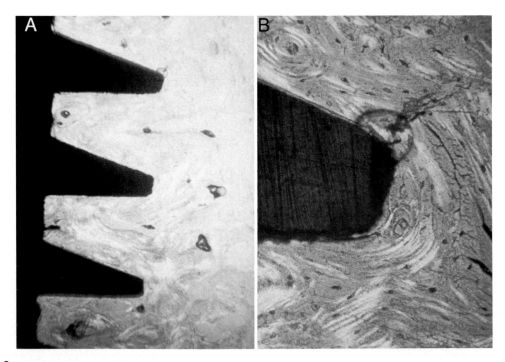

FIG 16–3.
A and **B,** photomicrographs of an undecalcified section of an osteointegrated serrated root form implant in function for 5½ years, recovered from a human.

ting the bone is not a problem. Remarkably, the speed of drilling is not compromised. Irrigation during socket formation is not needed or recommended when using either the hand reamers or latch-end drills. Both options are designed to collect the particulate autogenous cutting debris which is used as a graft to cover the shoulders of the implant root component.

A simple second-stage procedure for exposing the healed root component for head placement is used. It incorporates guided tissue punches for excision of the overlying gingival tissue, and guided sulcus reamers for removal of any interfering underlying crestal bone. This approach to buried root components ensures a perfectly fitting gingival sulcus. The method is fast and does not require a second flapping procedure or suturing.

PATIENT CONSIDERATIONS AND SELECTION

Stryker root form components are available in three lengths so that length adjustment by cutting is not necessary (Fig 16–4,A). This avoids the potential for contamination of the passivated surface as

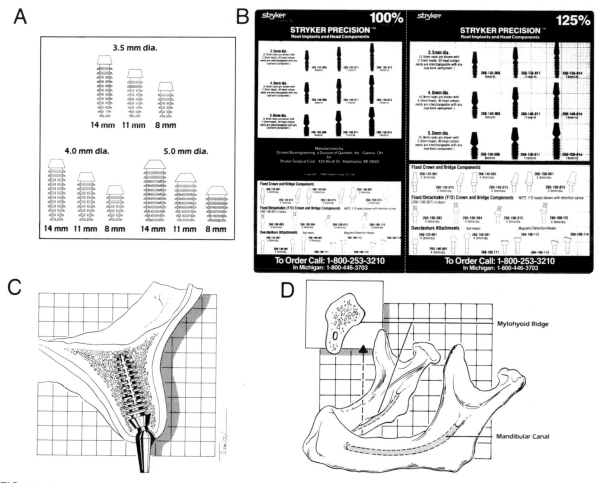

FIG 16–4.
A, available root component sizes. **B,** a transparent overlay showing implant outlines full size and one showing them 25% oversize to allow for radiographic distortion. **C,** it is often necessary to angle a root component to accommodate to the available bone. An angled head component may then be needed to permit proper alignment of the finished case. **D,** illustration of mandible showing mental foramina, mandibular canals, and mylohyoid concavities.

well as loss of sterility. The longest length possible, commensurate with the depth of bone available, should be chosen for maximum crown-root ratio. The short (8 mm) root components should not be used for single tooth replacements, distal abutments, or as freestanding abutments for overdentures. They should be used only as pier abutments in combination with other implants or natural teeth. The crown-root ratio is inadequate for other applications.

Panoramic and bite-wing radiographs are used to determine if enough mesiodistal space and vertical bone height free of anatomic problem areas exists to place the implant safely in the proposed receptor site.

A transparent overlay showing implant outlines full size and one showing them 25% oversize to allow for radiographic distortion are used to select an appropriately sized implant (Fig 16–4,B). Size distortion is corrected with radiographs and an appropriately sized implant is selected with this in mind. As a rule, the greater the diameter and the greater the length, the better. However, there must be adequate lateral bone width so that the root component chosen does not impinge on cortical bone labially or lingually. If there is any doubt, the use of a Stryker submergible osteointegrating blade form implant should be considered, as well as the possibility that an endosteal implant is not indicated in this site at all.

In the upper anterior, it is often necessary to angle the root component toward the palate to avoid the thin labial cortex. In such cases, an angled head component will usually be required to permit proper alignment of the finished case (Fig 16–4,C).

Figure 16–4,D illustrates a mandible showing the mental foramina, mandibular canals, and mylohyoid concavities. When placing implants, care must be taken to avoid the mental foramina in the premolar regions. Also, the mandibular canals are often inclined coronally in the mandible in these same areas.

It should also be recalled that the submandibular fossa is located below the mylohyoid line. This concavity of the lingual plate may be penetrated if the implant socket is not oriented toward the buccal appropriately.

Figure 16–5,A illustrates the maxillary sinus. The location of the sinuses must be positively identified to avoid penetration by the socket or the implant. In general, at least 2 mm of bone should separate the apex of implant sockets from the sinuses or the mandibular canal. A frenectomy may be advisable if frenum pull around the implant is likely.

Recently, computed tomography (CT) has been found to be of great value in determining the best placement sites when there is concern as to the exact location of these anatomic danger zones and whether there is adequate bone for safe placement of endosteal implants.

Clinical experience has shown that it is preferable to have implants precisely fitted into their sockets to ensure osteointegration. We recommend a condition best described as a "passive, intimate fit."

PREOPERATIVE PROCEDURES

All surgical instruments should be sterilized, preferably by dry heat or steam autoclave. Stryker implantable component surfaces have been specially treated to remove organic contaminants and are supplied in a passivated and sterile condition in a plastic bag within a tear-open blister package. The components require no further preparation prior to placement.

A radiograph of the proposed placement site should be checked to verify depth of bone and all anatomic features (Fig 16–5,B). The transparent implant radiograph overlays, one showing implant outlines at their actual size, another showing them 25% oversize to allow for radiographic distortion, will prove helpful in selecting the properly sized implant components. This will aid substantially in averting trauma to adjacent roots, sinuses, mental foramina, cortical plates, mandibular canals, etc.

The width of the alveolar ridge is checked with a periodontal probe to be sure that enough bone exists to permit the safe placement and long-term maintenance of the root component selected. It is important to retain as much labial bone as possible in order to retain a good blood supply to this easily traumatized bone. The patient should close his mouth so that the proposed implant-bone alignment in regard to the opposing occlusion may be determined.

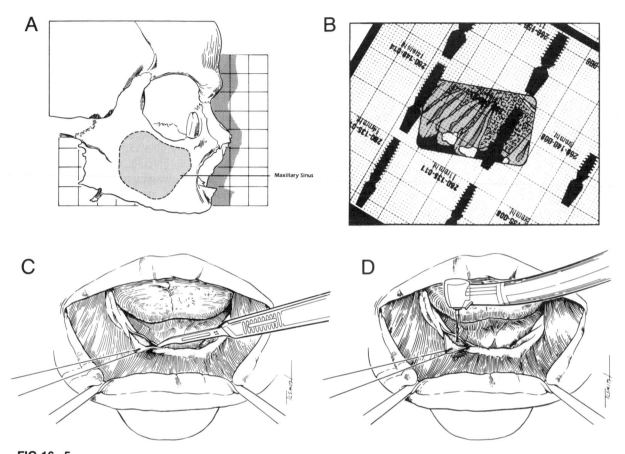

FIG 16–5.
A, the location of the sinuses must be positively identified to avoid penetration by the socket or the implant. **B,** transparent implant radiograph overlays, one showing implant outlines in actual size, another showing them 25% oversize to allow for radiographic distortion, will prove helpful in selecting the properly sized implant components. **C,** an incision is made along the crest of the alveolar ridge to the bone. **D,** the center of the implant site is determined and the crestal cortical plate pierced with a small fissure bur such as a 700XL or a no. 2 round bur.

FIRST STAGE: ROOT COMPONENT SURGICAL PROCEDURE

The patient is draped and anesthetized and the surgical site prepared using standard aseptic techniques. The importance of good sterile surgical procedures cannot be overemphasized. The incision should be made along the crest of the alveolar ridge to the bone (Fig 16–5,C). The incision must be long enough to permit adequate reflection of the tissue without tearing it. Some dentists prefer to create an envelope flap so that the closure is not directly over the implant. We have not been able to determine clinically whether one technique is preferable to the other.

The dissection is continued using a periosteal elevator to reflect the mucoperiosteal tissue on both the buccal and lingual aspects. The dissection should be sufficiently extensive to completely expose the alveolar ridge faciolingually. Any tissue tags are excised to promote healing. The mucoperiosteal tissue should be retracted away from the surgical site using sutures or other appropriate means of retraction. The center of the implant site is determined and the crestal cortical plate pierced with a small fissure bur such as a 700XL or a no. 2 round bur (Fig 16–5,D).

The penetration is continued using a pilot drill in a low-speed handpiece rotating at 500 to 1,000 rpm. A small piece of rubber tubing or an endodontic-type stop is slipped onto the pilot drill and is used to gauge the proper depth of penetration, taking care to obtain the desired socket location and angulation. The pilot hole should be deep enough to permit the root component to be placed 1 to 2 mm below the crest of the ridge (Fig 16–6,A).

A radiograph should be taken with the pilot drill in situ to verify proper alignment and depth. If the radiograph indicates improper alignment, the correction should be made by realigning the pilot drill and redrilling at the proper angulation. Another radiograph should then be taken with the pilot drill in its new position to be sure that the proper orientation has now been achieved.

If multiple implants are being placed, paralleling pins should be inserted consecutively into the completed pilot holes to help guide the angulation of the

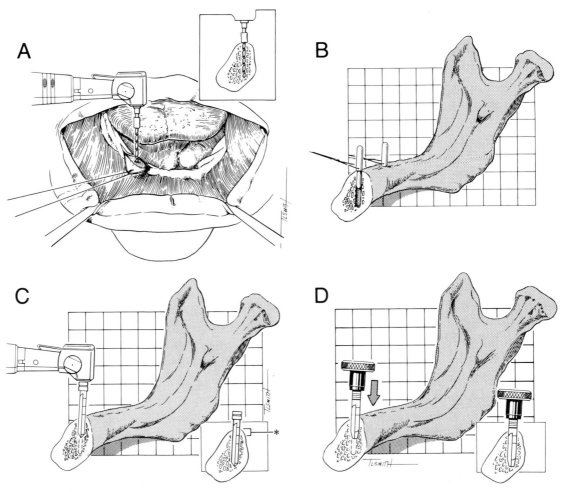

FIG 16–6.
A, the pilot hole should be deep enough to permit the selected root component to be placed 1 to 2 mm below the crest of the ridge. **B,** paralleling pins should be inserted into completed pilot holes to help guide the angulation of the pilot drill in additional sites. **C,** a hand-driven or ultra-low-speed intermediate drill is used to enlarge the socket. **D,** to place the implant to the desired 1 to 2 mm below the crest of the ridge, it is necessary to insert the reamer or drill to that distance beyond the indicator mark for the implant length chosen.

pilot drill in additional placement sites as they are drilled (Fig 16–6,B). This will help ensure that the degree of parallelism needed will be attained.

A hand-driven or ultra-low-speed intermediate drill is used to enlarge the socket (Fig 16–6,C). The depth is easily determined as there are three depth indicator marks on the shank of the intermediate drills corresponding to the three available root lengths. Prior to insertion, when using the hand system, it may facilitate initial penetration if a small round bur or 700XL fissure bur is used to enlarge the opening made by the pilot drill. Care should be exercised to follow the previously determined alignment and depth.

The paralleling pins can be used inverted, if desired, in sites drilled with the intermediate drill to confirm that parallelism has been achieved. Because of their unusual design, these drills, as well as the hand reamers, tend to "track" accurately and create a truly precision-cut socket. The depth indicator marks represent the exact length of the root component. Thus, the intermediate drill and, subsequently, the hand reamers and ULS drills must be inserted 1 to 2 mm beyond the desired depth mark to obtain the proper implant depth.

A straight driver handle, a short knob, and a ratchet wrench are available for "hand-instrumenting" the hand intermediate drill and the successive hand reamers. No irrigation is needed while cutting with these hand instruments as no heat is generated. In addition, larger-diameter short knobs for greater torquing ability and a deluxe long "spinner knob" handle are available for easier instrumentation of the sockets using the hand-reaming system. The ULS latch-end drills are used with the Stryker low-speed handpiece or equivalent and can be used instead of the hand reamers to prepare the implant socket using the same sequence described for the hand-reaming system. (*Caution:* These drills should not be operated at speeds exceeding 50 rpm.)

The three hand reamers and ULS drills correspond to the three diameters of root components. The reamers or drills are used sequentially. For example, a 3.5-mm-diameter reamer or drill (blue color code), then a 4.0-mm (red), and then a 5.0-mm (yellow) would be used for a 5.0-mm-diameter root component. Only the first two reamers or drills

would be used for a 4.0-mm-diameter root component, while only the 3.5-mm reamer is needed for the 3.5-mm root component. A special wrench is provided to facilitate easy release of the hand reamers from the drivers.

The reamers and ULS drills have a cutting edge on the bottom. If it is determined that the socket is not deep enough, it is possible to increase the depth with the reamer. The three depth indicator marks on the reamers correspond to the exact lengths of the implants. Thus, to place the implant to the desired 1 to 2 mm below the crest of the ridge, it is necessary to insert the reamer or drill to that distance beyond the depth indicator mark for the implant length chosen (Fig 16–6,D).

Some dentists prefer to combine the hand and power methods using the ULS drills, except for the final sizing which is accomplished with the appropriately sized hand reamer. Reamers or drills must be removed frequently during socket preparation and the cutting debris removed from the flutes (saving it for grafting later). Failure to do so will cause difficulty in cutting the bone, possibly resulting in high resistance to rotation, burnishing of hard mandibular bone, and oversize sockets in the maxilla.

The implant depth gauge corresponding to the diameter of the implant chosen is used to ascertain that the implant will insert into the prepared socket correctly and deeply enough. The three 1-mm-wide depth indicator grooves indicate the normal placement depth for the three lengths of implants (Fig 16–7,A). For example, the middle groove is used for gauging the normal depth for an 11-mm implant. All cutting debris is removed from the socket to ensure that the depth gauge will insert to the desired depth.

A radiograph should be taken with the depth gauge in situ to ascertain that correct positioning has been attained. If all seems proper, the depth gauge is removed but the socket is not flushed out to remove the blood.

The sterile blister package containing the selected root component is removed from its folder by the circulating assistant. The assistant then tears open the backing on the blister package and carefully drops the sterile inner plastic bag containing the root component and the plastic healing plug onto the ster-

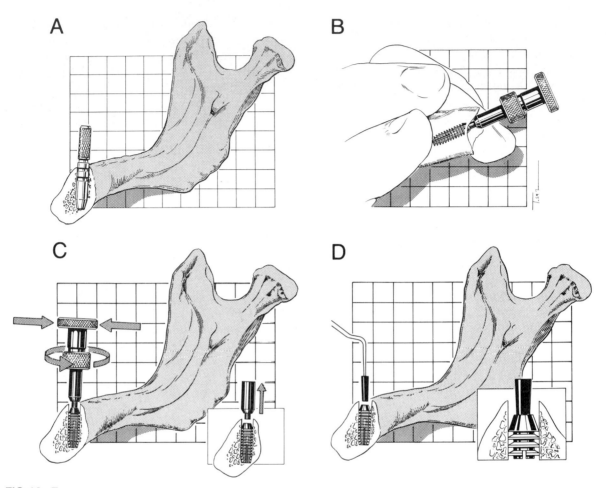

FIG 16–7.
A, the implant depth gauge corresponding to the diameter of the implant chosen is used to ascertain that the implant will insert into the prepared socket correctly and deeply enough. **B,** the implant insertion instrument is inserted into the opened bag, and into the locking taper socket. **C,** the inserter is released by rotating the lower knob counterclockwise while preventing root rotation with the top screw-on knob. **D,** the plastic healing plug is inserted.

ile instrument tray. The scrubbed assistant or surgeon grasps the implant through the plastic bag and opens the package with a pair of scissors.

The implant inserter with the rotary knob (or any of the other screw-on drivers) attached is inserted into the opened bag (Fig 16–7,B), and then into the locking taper socket of the root component, pressing them together lightly so that the root component is firmly affixed to the implant inserter. The assembly is then removed from the bag. Care must be taken during this maneuver not to lose the sepa-

rately bagged plastic healing plug included with the implant component.

The implant, attached to the inserter assembly, is carefully inserted into the prepared socket and seated. The implant should not contact anything prior to being placed into the bleeding prepared socket. The socket is not irrigated during preparation or flushed out because it is essential for uneventful rapid healing that a good undiluted blood clot form within the implant placement site. During seating, rotating the assembly while pressing apically will help to bottom the root component. The inserter is released by rotating the lower knob counterclockwise while preventing root rotation with the top screw-on knob (Fig 16–7,C). After separation of the inserter, some dentists prefer to additionally seat the implant by using the straight driver or the offset driver with the implant seating tip attached, and gently impact the root component into the socket. This step is optional and is usually not needed nor is it recommended.

The locking taper socket in the root component should be flushed with sterile saline, using a syringe with needle attached and then thoroughly dried. The plastic healing plug should now be inserted (Fig 16–7,D).

A periodontal probe may be inserted into the small drilled hole in the plug to place and seat it into the socket, or a pair of forceps may be used. Little pressure is required to obtain adequate seating. The residual space over the shoulders of the implant should now be filled with the autogenous bone particles recovered from the flutes of the reamers (Fig 16–8,A).

The plastic healing plug is trimmed with a pair

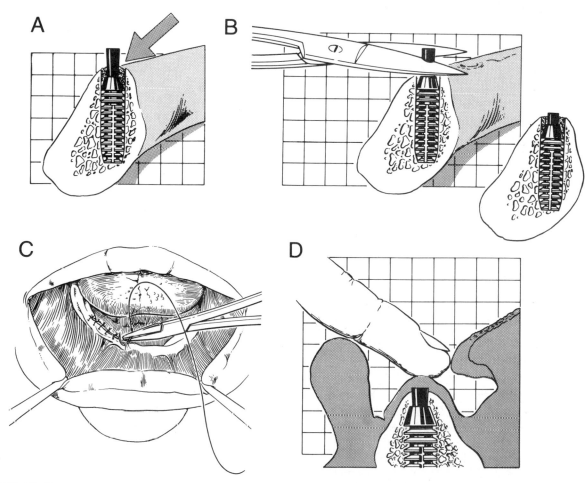

FIG 16–8.
A, the residual space over the shoulders of the implant is filled with autogenous bone particles. **B,** the plastic healing plug is trimmed with a pair of scissors to extend just above the crest of the ridge. **C,** the mucoperiosteal flaps are closed and approximated with interrupted sutures. **D,** the buried healing plug extending through the crest of the alveolar ridge should be located.

of scissors to extend just above the crest of the ridge (Fig 16–8,B). The plug is made too long so that it may be adjusted to the proper height. As bony healing occurs, the plug will be long enough to remain slightly protruded above the bone but short enough to avoid dehiscence of the overlying gingiva. The plastic plug must not be submerged at this point, as it will be very difficult to locate later when attempting to place the head component.

The mucoperiosteal flaps are closed and approximated with interrupted sutures (Fig 16–8,C). Care should be taken to ensure that tight closure is achieved to prevent seepage of oral fluids into the implant site or the loss of the overlying autogenous graft particles.

Healing should take place for at least 3 months before restoration is attempted. Healing may be slower in postmenopausal women or others whose healing ability may be compromised for any reason. In most cases patients may wear their old bridges or dentures during the healing period. Extreme care should be taken to make sure that these are relieved or otherwise adjusted so that no traumatic forces are transmitted to the healing implant.

SECOND STAGE: PLACEMENT OF HEAD COMPONENT

The buried healing plug extending through the crest of the alveolar ridge should be located. As it is black, it can often be seen through the somewhat translucent gingiva. If it is not visible, a radiograph can be useful or, often, the plug can be felt through the gingival tissue (Fig 16–8,D). A plastic stent prepared prior to the initial surgery with pilot holes for initially positioning the implant(s) can also be useful for this purpose. The location of the plug can then be marked with an indelible pencil on the gingival tissue. A no. 6 round bur in a high-speed handpiece or a scalpel with a no. 12 blade can be used to remove a plug of tissue over the healing plug, eliminating the necessity for creating a flap (Fig 16–9,A).

The plastic plug can be removed by pressing a 700XL or a no. 2 round bur into the center hole in the plug and retracting while turning the bur clockwise slightly (Fig 16–9,B). The intent is to jam the bur into the soft plastic plug so that it can be extracted by retracting the bur. Some dentists may prefer to use forceps. In any case, care should be taken to avoid scratching the shoulders of the root component should they, by chance, be slightly exposed.

The guide pin is inserted, split tapered end first, into the root component's locking taper socket. The Stryker guided tissue punch (color-coded), corresponding to the diameter of head component to be used, is mounted onto the guide pin (Fig 16–9,C). The tissue punch is then rotated between the thumb and forefinger while being pressed toward the alveolar crest. The rotating and pressing should continue until the reamer is solidly pressing the crestal bone. The guided tissue punch and the guide pin are removed. The tissue plug, being attached gingiva, may require the use of a small bone curet to remove it.

The guide pin is reinserted into the locking taper socket of the root component. The guided sulcus reamer (color-coded), corresponding to the diameter of head component to be used, is mounted onto the seated guide pin (Fig 16–9,D). The sulcus reamer is rotated clockwise between the thumb and forefinger while pressing it toward the alveolar crest (all Stryker cutting instruments must be pressed into the bone in order to cut). The rotating and pressing should continue until no more bone is removed. There is an automatic stop on the guide pin to prevent too much bone from being removed. The guided sulcus reamer is then removed and the guide pin decoupled from the root component socket.

The sterile blister package containing the selected head component is removed from its folder by the circulating assistant. The assistant tears open the backing of the outer package and carefully drops the sterile inner plastic bag containing the head component onto the instrument tray.

The inner package is opened by the scrubbed assistant or surgeon with a pair of scissors. The surgeon then removes the head component from the plastic bag with a pair of forceps, grasping it from the head end (Fig 16–10,A). The surgeon, after making sure that the root component socket is thoroughly flushed with sterile saline, free of blood, and dried, inserts the mating end of the head component into the root component socket.

The head component is turned to the desired ro-

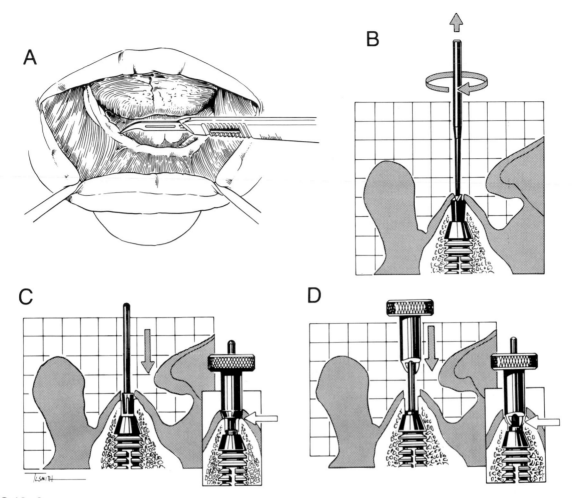

FIG 16–9.
A, a no. 6 round bur in a high-speed handpiece or a scalpel with a no. 12 blade can be used to remove a plug of tissue over the healing plug. **B,** the plastic plug is removed by pressing a 700XL or a no. 2 round bur into the center hole in the plug and retracting it while turning the bur slightly clockwise. **C,** excising a plug of tissue with the guided tissue punch. **D,** removing crestal bone to accommodate the abutment head with the guided sulcus reamer.

tational orientation and checked for proper alignment and angulation in relation to the patient's other implants or natural teeth (Fig 16–10,B). The straight driver handle or offset driver handle with a head seating tip attached is used for seating the head component. The seating tip and driver assembly is positioned on the implant head and in alignment with the root component; a light tap with a surgical mallet will lock the head into place (Fig 16–10,C). If the guided tissue punch and sulcus reamer have been used, no further closure is needed once the implant head has been seated (Fig 16–10,D).

Instructions for taking impressions and proper prosthetic techniques are covered in detail in the Stryker prosthetics manual.

IMPLANT HEAD OPTIONS

The Stryker implant system offers an extensive array of implant head options. They provide prosthetic versatility, esthetics, high strength, and stability coupled with surgical simplicity. Machined-in angled heads are available in all varieties of Stryker

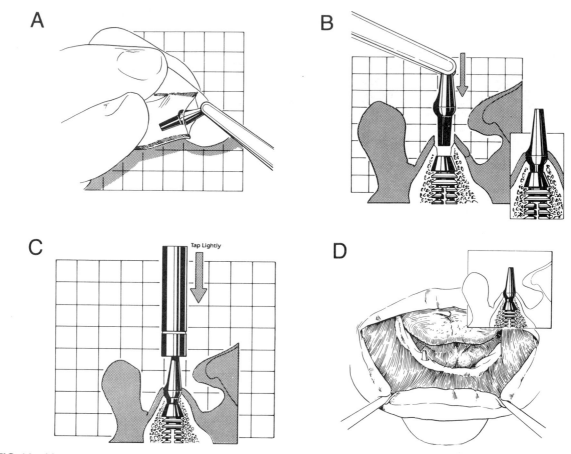

FIG 16–10.
A, removing the head component from the plastic bag with a pair of forceps. **B,** the head component is turned to the desired rotational orientation and checked for proper alignment and angulation in relation to the patient's other implants or natural teeth. **C,** the head-seating tip and driver assembly is positioned on the implant head; a light tap with a surgical mallet locks the head into place. **D,** if the guided tissue punch and sulcus reamer have been used, no further closure is needed once the implant head has been seated.

heads where needed. They feature the same subgingival contours as straight Stryker heads.

It is, unfortunately, often necessary to place implants in a less-than-ideal position from the standpoint of parallelism, simply because that is where the bone is. In these cases, achieving parallelism so that a path of insertion for the prosthesis is possible can sometimes be difficult and may often be an almost insurmountable problem with some implant systems. However, when using a Stryker angled fixed crown and bridge head, it is possible to surgically place the root form component up to 15 degrees off axis, while, with minor preparation of the

head, up to 25 degrees of correction can be obtained. If a fixed or detachable prosthesis is desired, a Stryker straight fixed or detachable head can correct up to 18 degrees while the available 15-degree angled head can correct up to 33 degrees.

Stryker straight and angled fixed crown and bridge heads are used in a similar way to the mounting and cementing of crowns and bridges on natural abutments in that the crown margins are feathered and can stop at the gingival margin or insert slightly subgingivally. A choice of three head diameters, 3.5, 4.0, and 5.0 mm, are available. These are all interchangeable and will fit any Stryker root form

TABLE 16–2.

Stryker Precision Abutment Head Choices and Prosthetic Options

Fixed crown and bridge abutment heads, straight and 15-degree-angled, in three diameters, and *extra-long fixed crown and bridge abutment heads,* straight and angled, for cemented attachment of:
a. Crowns for single tooth replacement
b. Partial bridges including those in conjunction with natural abutments
c. Full arch restorations
d. Custom-cast bars for partially tissue-supported overdentures
e. Custom-cast bars for implant-supported overdentures
Fixed or detachable abutment heads, straight and angled, in two lengths, for facultatively removable:
a. Bridges
b. Full arch restorations
c. Custom-cast bars for tissue-supported overdentures
d. Custom-cast bars for implant-supported overdentures
O ring retained overdenture heads, straight and angled, in three lengths for retention of:
a. Tissue-supported overdentures
b. Implant-supported overdentures
Ball overdenture heads, in three lengths, for retention of tissue-supported overdentures
Magnetically retained overdenture heads, straight and angled, in two lengths for retention of tissue-supported overdentures
Zest Anchor overdenture abutment heads, designed to accept Mini Zest anchor components

component. Thus, one can easily tailor gingival contours and dimensions based on the most appropriate head diameter to achieve optimal crown esthetics with minimal overhanging margins. Longer straight and angled versions are available for situations where the root component is placed deeper than normal or the overlying gingiva is inordinately thick.

Like their fixed crown and bridge heads, mounting of prosthetic crowns on Stryker fixed or detachable heads is similar to placing them on natural abutments in that the crown margins are feathered and can stop at the gingival margin or insert slightly subgingivally. Their tapered shoulders permit stable, self-centering mounting of the prosthesis and also permit adjusting the contour of gingival margins for optimal esthetics where required.

Where esthetics are not a prime consideration, the margins can be supragingival if desired. In these areas and also where the gingival tissue may be inordinately thick, extra-long straight and angled fixed and detachable heads are offered, featuring a longer locking taper pin to raise the head above the implant root an additional 2 mm. Because of the typically low or slightly subgingival margins required where

optimal esthetics are desired, it is recommended that a provisional cement be used when seating the prosthesis on the implant heads. This will help seal the margins and prevent percolation of oral fluids into the interspace between the implant heads and crowns.

There are no appreciable lateral loads on the retention screws so that fracture or elongation of these screws is not a problem. Even if the retention screws are loose, the prosthesis tends to remain rigid and stable. Fixed or detachable heads are also used as abutments for custom-cast bars for overdenture retention. Stryker abutment head options are listed in Table 16–2.

REFERENCES

1. Driskell TD: *The DB Precision Implant System, 1000 Series: Evolution and Rationale.* Galena, Ohio, Quintron, Inc. Driskell Bioengineering, 1985.
2. Driskell TD, O'Hara MJ, Greene GW: Surgical tooth implants, combat and field, Report no. 1. Contract no. DADA17-69-C-9118, 1971. Supported by US

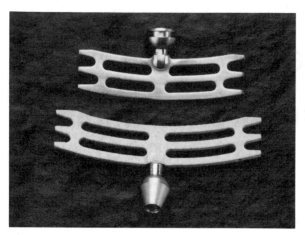

FIG 17–1.
Two blade form surface preparations are available: *(top)* the original uncoated version or with a high-bond-strength hydroxylapatite coating *(bottom)*.

in effecting removal. This instrument is available from Stryker Surgical. As is true with Stryker's root form abutment heads, it is always possible to safely remove a Stryker blade form head at any time owing to its noncemented locking taper attachment to the blade component.

Stryker blade form implants are currently provided in eight anatomic shapes, two of which have double heads. These suffice for most blade form implant indications. More shapes will be made available as demand is indicated (Table 17–1).

PATIENT CONSIDERATIONS AND SELECTION

Stryker blade form implants are available in various shapes and sizes so that reshaping by cutting is minimized (Fig 17–2). The largest size possible, commensurate with the depth, anatomy, and mesiodistal length of bone available, should generally be chosen for maximal crown-root ratio and load distribution. Blade form implants should only be used as distal or pier abutments in combination with other implants or natural teeth.

Panoramic and bite-wing radiographs are used to determine if enough mesiodistal space and vertical bone height free of anatomic problem areas exist in the proposed receptor site.

Transparent overlays, one showing implant outlines full size and one showing them 25% oversize to allow for radiographic distortion, are used to select an appropriately sized implant (Fig 17–3,A). The Stryker blade form component most appropriate in size and shape for the available anatomy at the proposed implant site is chosen, mindful of the size distortion in the radiographs when selecting the implant. There must be adequate lateral bone width so that the blade does not impinge on cortical bone buccally or lingually. If there is sufficient lateral bone width and vertical height, a root form implant may, in fact, be a better choice, particularly if mesiodistal space is limited. Finally, if there is any doubt as to

TABLE 17–1.
The Stryker Precision Blade Form Implant System

Product name	Stryker Precision Implants	
Manufacturer/ supplier	Stryker Corporation Surgical Division 420 Alcott Street Kalamazoo, MI 49001 1-800-253-3210	
Material	All implantable components are fabricated from surgical-grade titanium alloy (Ti-6Al-4V ELI) supplied in sterile packaging, ready for implantation	
Cost of typical implant	Blade component	$150
	Straight head component	$ 50
Cost of instrumentation	Blade form instrumentation kit for anterior and posterior placement	$420

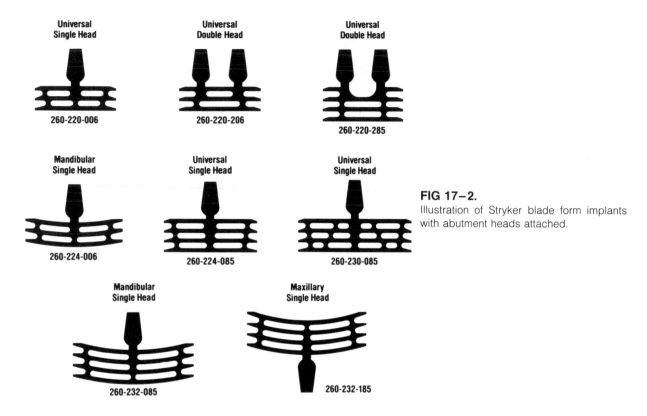

FIG 17-2.
Illustration of Stryker blade form implants with abutment heads attached.

the adequacy of the available bone, the possibility that an endosteal implant is not indicated in this site should be considered.

In the upper anterior, it is often necessary to angle blade components toward the palate to avoid the thin labial cortex. In such cases, angled head components will usually be required to permit proper alignment (Fig 17–3,B). As mentioned earlier, root form implants are generally a better choice in this region if sufficient bone exists. A frenectomy may be advisable if frenum pull around the implant is likely.

Extreme care must be taken to avoid the mental foramina in the premolar regions. The mandibular canals are often inclined coronally in these same areas. It should also be recalled that the submandibular fossa is located below the mylohyoid line (Fig 17–3,C). This concavity of the lingual plate may be penetrated if the implant trough is not inclined toward the buccal appropriately. An angled head will often be needed in these cases.

The location of the maxillary sinus must be pos-

itively identified to avoid penetration by the socket or the implant. In general, at least 2 mm of bone should separate the implant socket from the sinuses or the mandibular canal (Fig 17–3,D).

Recently, computed tomography (CT) has been found to be of great value in determining the best placement sites when there is concern as to the exact location of these anatomic danger zones and whether there is adequate bone for safe placement of endosteal implants.

Clinical experience has shown that it is preferable to have implants precisely fitted into their sockets to ensure osteointegration. We recommend a condition best described as a "passive, intimate fit."

PREOPERATIVE PROCEDURES

All surgical instruments should be sterilized, preferably by dry heat or steam autoclave. Stryker implantable component surfaces have been treated to tissue should be retracted away from the surgical site using sutures or other appropriate means of retraction (Fig 17–4,B, inset).

The length and location of the proposed blade placement channel is marked on the alveolar ridge with a scalpel, small bur, or other marking device (Fig 17–4,C).

After determining the placement location, the cortical plate is penetrated along the channel location line with a series of pilot holes 3 to 4 mm apart with a 700XL fissure bur. The holes are then carefully connected using the same bur (Fig 17–4,D). *(Caution: Irrigate with copious amounts of sterile saline or sterile water during all blade implant bone-cutting procedures.)* It is sometimes necessary to curve the proposed implant trough to accommodate to the curvature of the jaw at the placement site. If this is required, the blade must be bent mesiodistally with a set of titanium-tipped bending pliers to conform the implant to the curvature of the trough.

The channel is deepened with a fresh 700XL or a 700XXL bur. The same method of gently drilling a number of holes using a series of light thrusts and withdrawings may be used, ensuring the while that sufficient cooling water is flushing the area being cut. An endodontic stop to gauge depth in relation to the blade form chosen may be used. The depth of the holes should be approximately 2 mm deeper than the depth of the implant. Care should be exercised to follow the previously determined alignment and depth of the implant channel and that it is in proper angulation with respect to anatomic problem areas such as the submandibular fossa. The individually deepened holes are connected with the same bur to obtain the desired channel dimensions to accommodate the blade form component (Fig 17–5,A).

The channel may have to be enlarged slightly at the point where the butt of the locking taper post penetrates the crest of the ridge. (Many dentists replace cutting burs several times during this channeling procedure to avoid any possibility of burning the bone. This is an excellent idea.)

The sterile blister package containing the selected blade form component is removed from its folder by the circulating assistant. The assistant opens the backing on the blister package and carefully drops the sterile inner plastic bag containing the blade component and the healing head(s) onto the sterile instrument tray.

The scrubbed assistant or surgeon grasps the implant through the plastic bag and opens the package with a pair of scissors. The blade implant inserter is inserted into the opened bag and then onto the tapered post of the blade component, pressing it lightly so that the blade component is firmly affixed to the blade implant inserter (Fig 17–5,B). The assembly is then removed from the bag. The intent is that the implant should not contact anything prior to being placed into the prepared socket.

The implant, attached to the blade implant inserter and held by the knob, is conveyed to the surgical site. The blade component is then carefully inserted into the prepared socket (Fig 17–5,C). The blade should fit tightly into the prepared trough. It should also be at least 2 mm below the crest of the ridge. If the implant is too loose, it may be possible to bend it slightly to bind it in the trough better. The use of tricalcium phosphate ceramic particles, freeze-dried bone, or autogenous bone particles to fill in any large voids is recommended. The use of hydroxylapatite particles in and around the load-transmitting areas of implants is not recommended as this may inhibit normal bone remodeling in these areas.

The base of the blade implant inserter is identical dimensionally to the spherical base of the implant head component and healing head component. The blade implant inserter is also located in the same position on the blade-locking taper post. Often, to seat the blade component to the depth desired, it will be necessary to carefully remove with a round bur a little bone at the crest of the ridge at the point of insertion of the post. This will permit complete seating of the healing head component. Thus, the blade component with the attached inserter can be used as a trial for proper crestal preparation for assuring that the healing head will seat. The blade implant inserter is then removed by rotating the upper knob clockwise while preventing outer sleeve rotation with the lower knob (Fig 17–5,D).

If necessary, after separation of the blade inserter instrument (or sometimes before), the implant is additionally seated by using a surgical mallet and the straight driver or offset driver with the blade

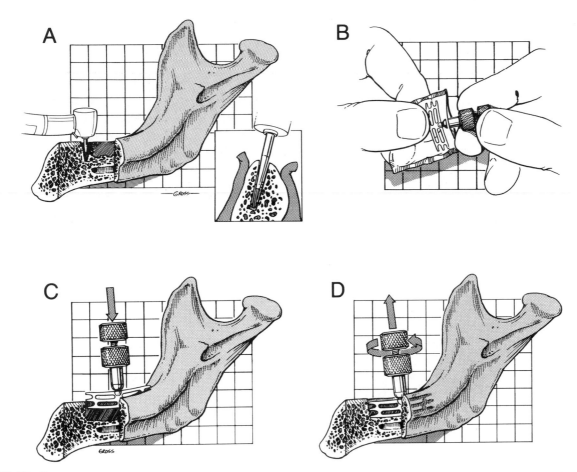

FIG 17–5.
A, the channel is deepened with a fresh 700XL or 700XXL bur. **B,** the blade implant inserter is inserted into the bag and then onto the tapered post of the blade component. **C,** the implant, attached to the blade implant inserter, is carefully inserted into the prepared socket. **D,** the blade implant inserter is removed by rotating the upper knob clockwise while preventing outer sleeve rotation with the lower knob.

seating tip attached. The blade component is then lightly tapped into final position in the socket. The shoulders of the blade component should be about 2 mm below the crest of the ridge (Fig 17–6,A).

The blade component is tapped only when the seating tip is centered within the countersunk dimples located on the shoulders of the blade or on the top of the locking taper post. Damage to the blade or trauma to the implant site can result if care is not taken to assure proper seating tip positioning before tapping.

The blade-locking taper post and the implant site may now be flushed with sterile saline, using a sy-

ringe with a needle attached. Next, the temporary healing head is removed from the sterile plastic bag using titanium-tipped pliers, being careful to orient it properly, flat side coronally, so that it will mount properly on the blade-locking taper post. It is then lightly pressed on with the pliers or *very lightly impacted* with a driver to ensure that it will remain in place (Fig 17–6,B).

The residual defect over the shoulders of the implant should be filled with one of the hydroxylapatite bone grafting materials, freeze-dried bone, or autogenous bone particles. This helps to ensure that the shoulders of the blade component will be covered

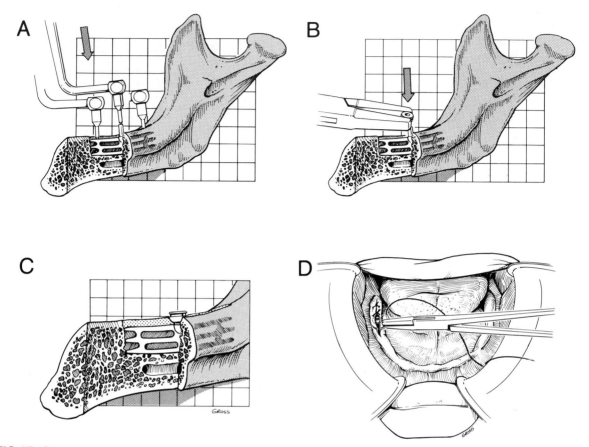

FIG 17–6.
A, the blade component is lightly tapped into final position in the socket. **B,** the temporary healing head is removed from the sterile plastic bag. It is then lightly pressed on the implant post. **C,** the residual defect over the shoulders of the implant should be filled with one of the hydroxylapatite bone grafting materials, freeze-dried bone, or autogenous bone particles. **D,** the mucoperiosteal flaps are closed and approximated with sutures.

with bone and help preserve the height of the alveolar ridge (Fig 17–6,C).

The mucoperiosteal flaps are closed and approximated with sutures (Fig 17–6,D). The temporary healing head should be submerged. However, in some cases, this may not be possible or, during the passive healing period, the overlying tissue may dehisce, thus slightly exposing the healing head. If this is the case, the patient must be cautioned to avoid "tongueing" the implant or otherwise traumatizing the site. Exposure of the healing head is not uncommon and does not appear to affect healing adversely.

Healing should take place for at least 3 months before restoration is attempted. Healing may be slower in postmenopausal women or others whose healing ability may be compromised for any reason. Patients may wear their old bridges or dentures in most cases during this healing period. Extreme care should be taken to make sure that any prosthesis is relieved or otherwise adjusted so that no traumatic forces can be transmitted to the healing implant.

STAGE II: PLACEMENT OF HEAD COMPONENT

The implant healing head can usually be visualized or palpated (Fig 17–7,A). If not, a radiograph should be taken to locate the blade component precisely and to determine the status of the alveolar

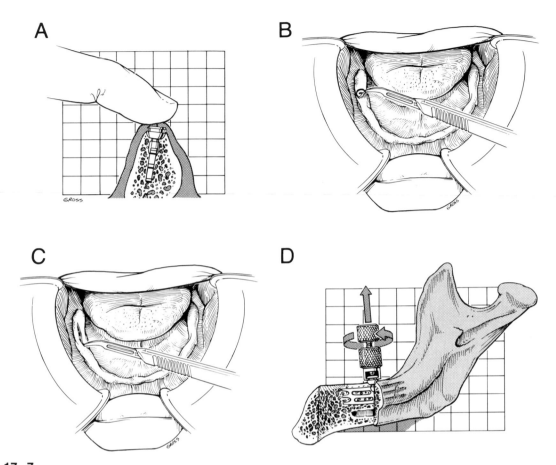

FIG 17–7.
A, the implant healing head can usually be visualized or palpated. **B,** it will often be possible to expose the healing head by carefully excising the gingival tissue from around the head. **C,** If the condition of the crestal bone is of concern, or the implant has been placed very deeply and the healing head cannot be easily accessed, a flap is laid to the bone and the mucoperiosteal tissue is reflected. **D,** the temporary healing head can then be removed by sliding the healing head remover onto the exposed groove in the head. Rotating the ejector screw knob clockwise will release the head from the locking taper post.

crest at the site. Crestal bone should cover the blade shoulders. Depending on the depth of the healing head beneath the gingiva, one of the two following procedures will be required to remove the healing head and expose the blade-locking taper post for placement of the head component.

The coronal surface of the healing head will usually be clearly identifiable beneath the gingiva, or it may have become slightly exposed during the healing period. In the latter case the gingival tissue will be found to have grown tightly into the removal groove, which is the secondary purpose of the groove. The groove assists in stabilizing vertical

movement of the interfacial soft tissue, thus helping to protect this critical area from trauma.

It will usually be possible in these circumstances to expose the healing head sufficiently for removal merely by carefully excising the gingival tissue closely from around the head with a no. 11 or 12 scalpel blade (Fig 17–7,B). Contacting the healing head surface with the scalpel blade is required to obtain a perfect circle. This contacting with an unlike metal should not be of concern, however, as the healing head will be discarded upon removal.

If the condition of the crestal bone is of concern, or the implant has been placed very deeply and the healing head cannot be easily accessed, an incision can be made along the crest of the ridge to the bone and the mucoperiosteal tissue reflected as before. However, this time the reflection need not be extensive and only the area precisely at the location of the healing head should be exposed (Fig 17–7,C). The coronal surface of the healing head should be visible.

The temporary healing head can then be removed by sliding the healing head remover onto the exposed groove in the head. When the healing head remover is fully slipped into place, the ejector screw

should be located directly over the dimple centered on the end of the locking taper post. Rotating the ejector screw knob clockwise will release the head from the locking taper post (Fig 17–7,D).

Some dentists may prefer to remove the healing head using forceps. In removing it, the healing head should be rotated slightly while simultaneously lifting with the forceps to loosen it. Extreme care should be taken to avoid scratching the locking taper post of the blade component.

The exposed tissue around the blade component locking taper post is flushed with sterile saline from

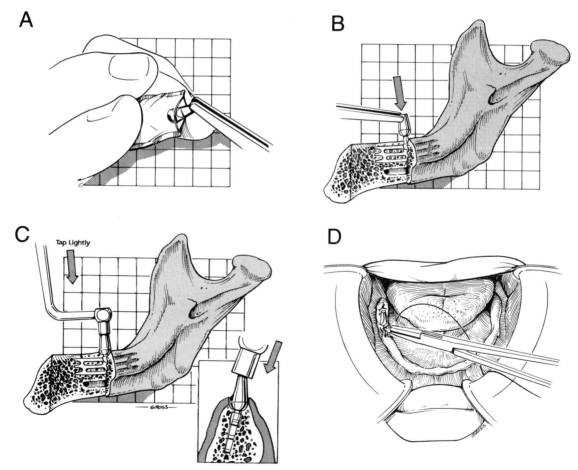

FIG 17–8.
A, the head component is removed from the plastic bag with forceps, grasping it from the head end. **B,** the head is mounted onto the blade component locking taper post and rotated to the desired orientation. **C,** the head is seated by impaction using the head seating tip, driver handle, and a light tap with a surgical mallet. **D,** the mucoperiosteal flaps are trimmed with scissors or a semilunar punch to accommodate the protruding implant head and then closed and carefully approximated with interrupted sutures.

a syringe with an 18- or 20-gauge needle attached. The sulcus formed by the presence of the temporary healing head is then inspected. Rarely, it may be necessary to chamfer or reduce the bony perimeter above the socket with a small round bur to permit the head component to seat properly.

The sterile blister package containing the selected head component is removed from its folder by the circulating assistant. The assistant then tears open the backing of the sterile outer package and carefully drops the sterile inner plastic bag containing the head component onto the sterile instrument tray.

The package is opened by the scrubbed assistant or surgeon with a pair of scissors. The surgeon then removes the head component from the plastic bag with a pair of forceps, grasping it from the head end (Fig 17–8,A). The surgeon, after making sure that the blade component locking taper post is thoroughly flushed with sterile saline and free of blood, inserts the mating end of the head component onto the blade component locking taper post.

The head, mounted onto the blade component locking taper post, is rotated to the desired orientation for proper parallelism and angulation in relation to the patient's other implants or natural teeth (Fig 17–8,B). An angled head may often be needed to accomplish this.

The head is then seated by impaction using the head seating tip, driver handle, and a light tap with a surgical mallet (Fig 17–8,C). When seating angled heads, the direction of impaction should be in align-ment with the buccolingual axis of the blade component (Fig 17–8,C, inset), not the axis of the head!

If a mucoperiosteal flap was laid, the edges are trimmed with scissors or a semilunar punch to accommodate the protruding implant head and then carefully approximated with interrupted sutures (Fig 17–8,D). A temporary bridge may be fabricated and used during the interim while the permanent bridge is being constructed.

STRYKER PRECISION BLADE FORM IMPLANT HEAD OPTIONS

The Stryker system offers an extensive array of blade form implant head options. They provide prosthetic versatility, esthetics, high strength, and stability coupled with surgical simplicity. Machined-in angled heads feature the same subgingival contours as do straight Stryker heads (Table 17–2).

It is often necessary to place implants in a less-than-ideal position from the standpoint of parallelism simply because that is where the bone is. In these cases, achieving sufficient parallelism so that a path of insertion is possible can sometimes be difficult and may often be an almost insurmountable problem with some implant systems. To avoid this problem, many blade form implants (and a few root forms) rely upon bendable necks to obtain parallelism, a practice which may severely compromise neck strength and fatigue resistance to fracture. Neck fracture is a more significant concern with blade form

TABLE 17–2.

Stryker Precision Blade Abutment Head Choices and Prosthetic Options

---

Fixed crown and bridge abutment heads, straight 15- and 25-degree head angles, for cemented attachment of:
    a. Partial bridges including those in conjunction with natural and root form implant abutments
    b. Full-arch restorations including those in conjunction with natural and root form implant abutments
    c. Custom-cast bars for implant-supported overdentures

Fixed or detachable abutment heads, straight and 15-degree angles, for facultatively removable:
    a. Partial bridges
    b. Full-arch restorations
    c. Custom-cast bars for implant-supported overdentures

---

implants that osteointegrate as compared to the older types which did not. The reason is that osteointegrated blade form implants, while able to more effectively transmit occlusal forces to the bone, do not flex or move appreciably within the bone. Thus the implant neck is forced to absorb substantially higher stresses and must be designed with this fact in mind. The older traditionally styled blade form implants, because of their design, induce a fibrous encapsulation between the implant and the surrounding bone; thus, they manifest a slight-to-moderate overall implant mobility within the bone. This mobility helps reduce the strain at the neck on this style of implant. However, neck fractures as a result of bending the implant neck are still a factor, even with these older designs. Therefore, it is our philosophy that bendable necks on implants are no longer an acceptable or safe method for obtaining implant head parallelism.

Stryker angled fixed crown and bridge blade form heads are available in 15- and 25-degree angles. Thus, it is possible to surgically place blade form components off axis in any required position by those amounts, owing to the locking taper attachment's 360-degree locking ability. If a fixed or detachable prosthesis is desired, a straight fixed or detachable head can correct up to 18 degrees while the available 15-degree angled head can correct up to 33 degrees.

Like the fixed crown and bridge heads, mounting of prosthetic crowns on fixed and detachable heads is similar to placing them on natural abutments in that the crown margins are feathered and can stop at the gingival margin or insert slightly subgingivally. The supragingival conical portion of the head permits stable, self-centering mounting of the prosthesis and also permits adjusting the contour of gingival margins for optimal esthetics where needed. Because of the typically low or slightly subgingival

margins required where optimal esthetics are desired, it is recommended that a provisional cement be used when seating the prosthesis on the implant heads. This will help seal the margins and prevent percolation of oral fluids into the interspace between the implant heads and crowns.

There are no appreciable lateral loads on the retention screws so that fracture or elongation of these screws is not a problem. Even if the retention screws are loose, the prosthesis tends to remain rigid and stable.

A RATIONALE FOR THE USE OF BLADE FORM IMPLANTS

Currently, about 85% of the dental implants placed in the United States are said to be root form implants. If this is true, then it is probable that many implant candidates are receiving root form implants where not enough bone exists vertically or buccolingually to ensure safe placement. It is likely that many patients are being turned away as potential endosteal implant recipients because the value of osteointegrating submergible blade form implants in severely resorbed edentulous ridges is not, as yet, widely comprehended or appreciated. This will undoubtedly change as our awareness of the merits of these implants continues to grow.

REFERENCES

1. Hahn J: The Titanalloy endosseous implant. *Implantologist* 1981; 2:17–21.
2. Driskell TD: *A Rationale for the Use of Submergible Blade Form Endosteal Implants. An Overview of the Development and Rationale Behind the DB1000 and DB2000 Series Implant Systems.* Galena, Ohio, Driskell Bioengineering, 1985.

Chapter 18

The Bioceram Implant Systems

Ralph V. McKinney, Jr., D.D.S., Ph.D.
David L. Koth, D.D.S., M.S.
David E. Steflik, M.A., Ed.D.

THE IMPLANT

Bioceram dental implants are composed of single-crystalline alpha aluminum oxide (Al_2O_3) or polycrystalline aluminum oxide, or a combination of both ceramic materials, and manufactured in a variety of endosseous shapes and sizes but predominately as a threaded cylindrical implant.

The manufacturer, Kyocera Corporation of Kyoto, Japan, makes four types of cylindrical screw implants. Two of these are composed entirely of single-crystalline aluminum oxide material and are designated as S type and E type.

The other two cylindrical types are the A type, which is a polycrystalline post on a single crystalline radicular portion, and a porous rooted implant consisting of an application of porous polycrystalline ceramic on the radicular portion of an otherwise single-crystalline implant (see Table 18–1).

The S-Type Design

The S-type implant (Fig 18–1) has a threaded radicular portion, threaded from the cervical area to the apex (Fig 18–2). The coronal portion is flattened on one surface to allow keying of copings and crowns. Previously the company made an S-collared type which had a 1 mm-wide collar at the cervical area that was 2 mm greater in diameter than the radicular portion. The purpose of the collar was to provide greater implant stability when the collar was countersunk in bone. Although now discontinued by Kyocera, there are many collared S types still in clinical service.

The S-type implants come in two lengths, short, 19.5 mm, and long, 23.0 mm, and two diameters, 3.0 and 4.0 mm. These are the most commonly used ceramic one-stage endosseous dental implants and are employed in well-healed areas of the edentulous jaw.[1]

The E-Type Design

The E-type implants were designed primarily for immediate insertion in extraction sockets at time of surgery. The lands and grooves of the E-type screw have the pitch and angle of a self-tapping screw. In practice the implant is screwed into the trabecular bone without any tapping of the bone prior to insertion, thus making insertion simple. The implant (Fig 18–3) has a collar in the midsection to assist in stabilization in the socket and two vertical grooves through the threaded portion to allow bone ingrowth during healing and thus prevent rotation. The implant comes in three lengths, 19, 22, and 25 mm, and two diameters, 3.3 and 4.2 mm.

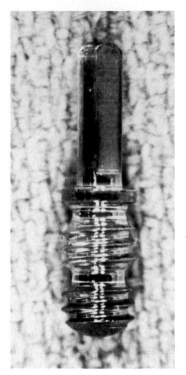

FIG 18-1.
The S-type Bioceram implant.

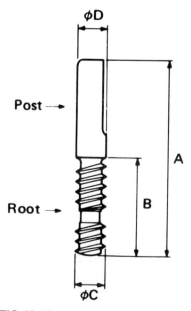

FIG 18-2.
Diagram of the S-type Bioceram implant.

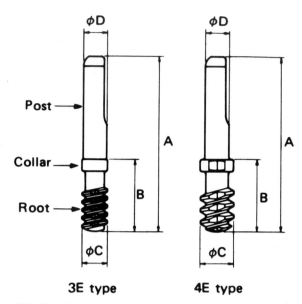

3E type **4E type**

FIG 18-3.
Diagram of the E-type Bioceram implant.

The A-Type Design (A9 and A1 Types)

This implant has a coronal portion made of polycrystalline ceramic in order to allow the implant coronal portion to be easily shaped for use in anterior regions of the jaws (Fig 18-4). The threaded roots are the same thread design as the S type for the A9 series and require tapping bone for placement in edentulous areas. An A1 type utilizing the self-tapping thread system of the E type is available for immediate use in extraction sockets. The implants come in one length of 25 mm and diameters of 3 and 4 mm for the A9 type and 3.3 and 4.2 mm for the A1 type.

The Porous Root Design

The porous root implant has a polycrystalline ceramic layer of aluminum oxide on the radicular portion surrounding a central core of single-crystal sapphire that is contiguous with the coronal portion (Fig 18-5). The polycrystalline material is constructed in a threaded root design and has an average pore size of 130 μm to allow ingrowth of bone to assist in stabilization of the implant. The implant comes in two lengths, 20.5 and 24 mm, and two diameters, 4.2 and 4.8 mm (Fig 18-6).[2]

TABLE 18–1.

The Bioceram Endosseous Dental Implant System

Product names	Bioceram Single Crystal Sapphire Dental Implant; Bioceram Porous Root Dental Implant; Bioceram Type II–Two-Stage Design Implant; Bioceram LaJolla Two-Stage Implant [prototype]	
Manufacturer	Kyocera Corporation, Kyoto, Japan	
Supplier	Kyocera America, Inc. Bioceram Division 8611 Balboa Avenue San Diego, CA 92123 1-800-421-5735	
Material composition	Alpha aluminum oxide ceramic in single-crystalline (sapphire) and polycrystalline forms.	
Costs	S type	$ 80
	E type	$ 80
	A type	$105
	Porous root type	$130
	Type II porous root	Approximately $165–$200
Armamentarium kits	Instrument set for S type	$225
	Instrument set for E type	$155
	Instrument set for A type	$165–$271
	Instrument set for porous root type	$438

Type II–Two-Stage Design

A new two-stage ceramic implant called the Bioceram Type II–Two-Stage Design has just been released by Kyocera. This implant utilizes the technology of the porous root implant with a polycrystalline radicular portion to be buried in bone with a single crystalline neck for cortical bone and soft tissue interface (Fig 18–7). The implant is not completely buried, but has a healing cap that extends through the tissue. The second stage is added after approximately 3 months' healing.

Other Implant Designs

The company makes blade implants in T, W, and U shapes from single-crystalline sapphire. These endosseous implants are widely used in Japan, but rarely used in the United States. Also made are single-crystal sapphire endodontic stabilizer implants and post and core implants for tooth restoration. The latter have single-crystalline posts and polycrystalline cores.

A new prototype two-stage implant is being developed by Kyocera that is called the Bioceram La-

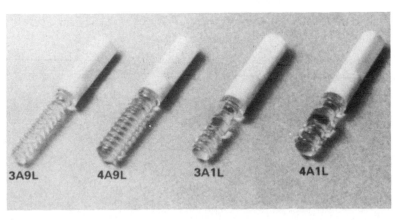

FIG 18–4.
The A9 and A1 A-type Bioceram implants.

3A9L   4A9L   3A1L   4A1L

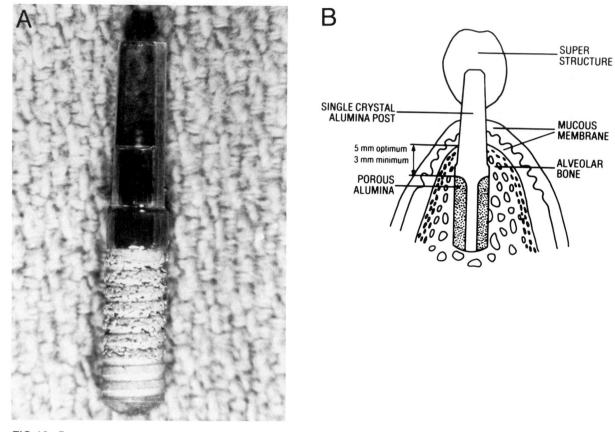

FIG 18–5.
A, the Bioceram porous root implant. **B,** diagram showing the construction of the Bioceram porous root implant and proper placement in the jaw so that the attached gingiva coapts against the single-crystalline cervical or post area of the implant.

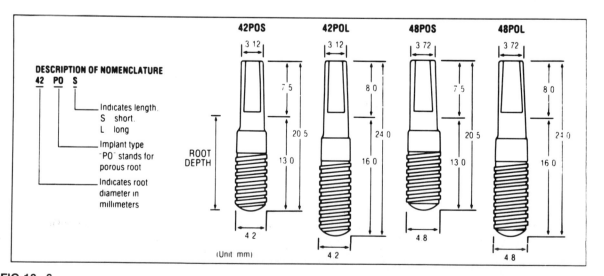

FIG 18–6.
Diagram of various configurations of the Bioceram porous root implant and indication of ideal depth placement in bone (root depth).

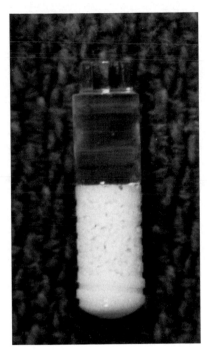

FIG 18–7.
The Bioceram Type II–Two-Stage Design radicular (stage 1) section implant. Note the cervical area is single-crystal ceramic.

Jolla type implant (submerged). The implant is a submerged two-stage implant that is completely covered by gingiva during the healing process. The first stage is composed of titanium alloy. The second-stage cervical collar area is composed of titanium alloy and single-crystal sapphire for soft tissue abutment. The coronal portion is angled for various directional draws and attaches to the second-stage collar. More on this implant will be forthcoming by late 1991.

THE CERAMIC MATERIAL

The implants are composed of single-crystalline alpha aluminum oxide. The material is obtained from aluminum oxide crystals artificially grown by a technique developed by Kyocera. The crystals were originally utilized as ceramic packaging in the semiconductor industry. Because of the extreme hardness and inertness of the material, consideration was

given to developing biomedical applications for the product. Initial experimental biomedical applications were developed in Japan and consisted of the fabricating of orthopedic pins and screws, as well as screw-type dental implants.[3–7] Because of the extreme hardness of the aluminum oxide single crystals, they exhibit excellent flexural and compressive strength throughout the lands and grooves of the screw configuration.

The artificially grown crystals are produced using the edge-defined film-fed growth method which facilitates crystal orientation and shape. This production methodology, which is carried out by Kyocera in Japan, makes possible the production of various ceramic shapes such as rod, ribbon, tube, filament, and disk or sheet shapes (Fig 18–8). Because of this flexibility in the mass production of artificially grown crystals, a great deal of cutting and polishing procedures are eliminated during manufacture.

The crystal is a rhombohedral single-crystal hexagonal system (Fig 18–9,A). The artificially grown crystals are identical in crystalline structure and hardness to natural gem sapphire; thus, the name that evolved for these products is single-crystal sapphire. The manufacturer has assigned the name Bioceram to these crystalline sapphire products.[3] The physical and thermal characteristics of the single-crystal sapphire implants are shown in Table 18–2 and Figure 18–9,B.

Although a *polycrystalline* aluminum oxide crystal can be grown and cut into desired shapes for dental implants, it does not have the flexural strength or modulus of rupture ($3.8 \text{ kg/cm}^2 \times 10^3$) that is found with the single crystal ($13 \text{ kg/cm}^2 \times 10^3$).[6] Thus polycrystalline sapphire implants may be more prone to rupture under biting stress. One advantage of the polycrystalline alumina material, however, is that it allows the dentist to more effectively adjust the length of the implant for occlusal clearance and thickness of crown coverage. When the single-crystal implant coronal portion must be reduced in height, the operator must do this by using a diamond disk. The roughened surface is difficult to polish and, as shown by Kawahara and Hirabayashi,[6] the grinding by diamonds leaves lattice imperfections on the surface which may cause fracture of the single crystal. In recognition of these problems, Kyocera is

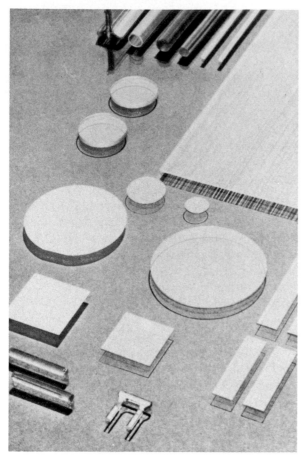

FIG 18−8.
The various configurations of artificially grown single-crystalline aluminum oxide (sapphire) material produced by the edge-defined film-fed growth method.

currently producing an implant with a single-crystal radicular portion and a polycrystalline coronal portion. This latter implant, called the A type, allows the operator to adjust and polish the implant at chairside for proper interocclusal height.

The sapphire single-crystalline and polycrystalline substrates have very desirable anticorrosion, antiabrasion, and antiheat properties. The single crystal has excellent light transmission which makes the material superior for use in the anterior jaw segments where the implant may be visible or show through tissues. The material has compressive, flexural, and tensile strengths generally far exceeding those of other currently used implant materials (see Fig

18−9,B). Because of the high anticorrosive property, there is minimal surface corrosive development on the implant surface and thus the constant concerns about passivation, pitting, fretting, and crevice corrosion are not major areas of precaution in the use of ceramic implants as is the case with various metal implants.

One of the material features of alpha aluminum oxide that contributes to its excellent biocompatibility and lack of tissue toxicity is the fact that the material has a high affinity for water molecules (hydrophilic).[5] Because of the tightly packed rhomboid crystal structure, the smaller aluminum ions are bound in voids between the oxygen ions (Fig 18−10). Since oxygen composes the outer surface of the crystal, it is an attractant for the water molecule (see Fig 18−10).

Sterilization.—The implants can be routinely steam-autoclaved. The porous root type is provided in a plastic sievelike container to facilitate sterilization and saline wetting prior to insertion. As an alternative, gas sterilization may be used.

Mechanical Damage.—Although the Bioceram sapphire implant has sufficient mechanical strength, its strength is adversely affected by superficial flaws or cracks. Therefore, *physical contact between implants, or impact against any hard material such as a metal object, must be avoided.* In storage, sterilization, or in cleaning, great care must be taken to avoid any mechanical damage to the implant. If vigorous cleaning such as an ultrasonic agitation method is used, *care should be taken to keep individual implants from ever coming into physical contact with one another.*

The surface of the single-crystal sapphire implants is highly polished and defect-free when received from the factory (Fig 18−11,A). Every attempt should be made to preserve this defect-free surface prior to insertion. The porous root implants need to be protected from dust or dirt contamination so adverse material will not get into the pores (Fig 18−11,B).

Cutting.—The single-crystal sapphire can be cut perpendicular to the axis to shorten the length.

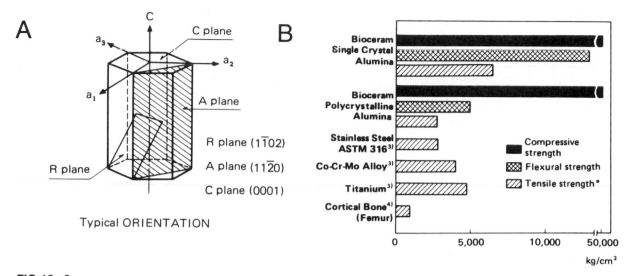

FIG 18–9.
A, crystalline structure of the hexagonal single-crystal (sapphire) alpha aluminum oxide ceramic material. **B,** mechanical strength comparisons of various implant biomaterials. The tensile strength is shown as 0.2% yield strength for the metals.

However, oblique cutting should be avoided, because it can lessen the mechanical strength. If the implant post must be cut obliquely, e.g., if it is to be used at the anterior portion of the upper jaw, a superstructure should be made (i.e., a crown) to cover the entire cut surface so that stress concentration will not occur on the surface. Special care should be taken not to damage any other portion during cutting. High-speed, rotating diamond-polishing instruments of fine grade should be used with abundant water coolant in cutting. After cutting, edges should be rounded off so that no sharp edges remain.

TABLE 18–2.

Physical and Thermal Characteristics of Single-Crystal Sapphire Ceramic (Al_2O_3)

Physical characteristics	
Crystallographic structure	Hexagonal system (rhombohedral single crystal)
	A plane = 4.763 Å
	C plane = 13.003 Å
Density	3.97 g/cm³
Hardness	Mohs 9 (diamond 10, quartz 7)
	Vicker hardness 2,300
Tensile strength	230 kg/mm² (diameter 0.25 mm, filament 25°C)
Compressive strength	300 kg/mm² (25°C)
Young's modulus	4.8×10^6 kg/cm²
Flexural strength	7,000 kg/cm²
Thermal characteristics	
Melting point	2,053°C
Coefficient of linear thermal expansion	5.3×10^{-6}/°C(25°C) (parallel to C axis)
	4.5×10^{-6}/°C (25°C) (perpendicular to C axis)
Thermal conductivity	0.1 cal/cm·sec·°C(25°C)
Specific heat	0.8 cal/g·°C(25°C)
Emittance	<0.02 (= 2.6–3.7μm at 880°C)

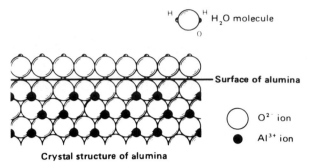

FIG 18–10.
Molecular model of the alpha aluminum oxide outer crystalline layer demonstrating the complexing with water molecules.

PATIENT CONSIDERATIONS—SITE SELECTION

The Bioceram implant systems can be used in combination with natural teeth as abutments for fixed prosthesis support. In fact, this is a superior way to utilize the Bioceram implants. Occlusal considerations are of great importance, and the patient with opposing natural dentition must have a mutually protected occlusion so that horizontal masticatory forces are well controlled. Adequate periodontal status and demonstrated satisfactory oral hygiene control must be present.

Site selection must include consideration of width of remaining alveolar bone, quality of the remaining bone, surgical access, proximity of the mandibular canal, inclination of the mandibular body, and potential angle of draw of the final prosthesis. Since it is not possible to bend the implant prior to insertion, as with metal blade implants, the inclination of the mandibular body and the path of draw become important in planning to keep the implant in trabecular bone and not undermine cortical bone.[1]

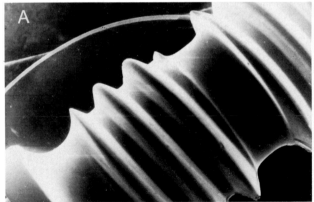

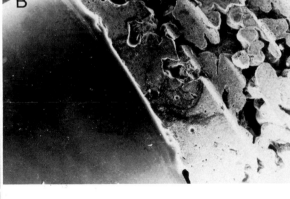

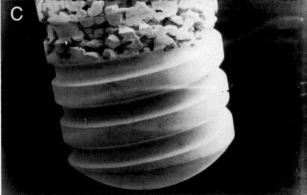

FIG 18–11.
A, scanning electron micrograph of the surface of a single-crystal sapphire Bioceram dental implant showing the extremely smooth crystalline surface of the radicular section. **B,** scanning electron micrograph of the polycrystalline porous structure of the Bioceram porous root dental implant, demonstrating the polycrystalline porous ceramic at the juncture with the single-crystalline ceramic. **C,** scanning electron micrograph showing the apex of the porous root implant composed of polycrystalline material without the presence of pores.

INSTRUMENTARIUM

Placement of sapphire endosseous implants requires a combination of routine dental and special instrumentation. The special instruments are available from the implant manufacturer.[8] These instruments are numbered and shown in Figure 18–12,A and B.

A *no. 5 round bur* is used to mark the implant location in bone, which then serves as a detent to position the guide drill.

The *guide drill* is used to prepare a guide hole in the desired path of insertion in the bone (Fig 18–13,A, instrument #16). The guide drill is available in straight and contra-angle models and is of one diameter, regardless of the implant root diameter.

The *bone drill* is used for the final creation of the implant socket. Bone drills are available in straight and contra-angle models and correspond to the diameter of implant selected for insertion, with allowance for vibration so the socket diameter will not be excessive. Bone drill #22 is used for 3-mm-diameter implants (Fig 18–13,A), bone drill #31 for 4-mm-diameter implants.

The *washer bur* is used to prepare the counterbore for the 3-mm-diameter S-type or A-type implants (Fig 18–13,B).

A *depth gauge* is used for measuring the socket depth while preparing the socket with the bone drill.

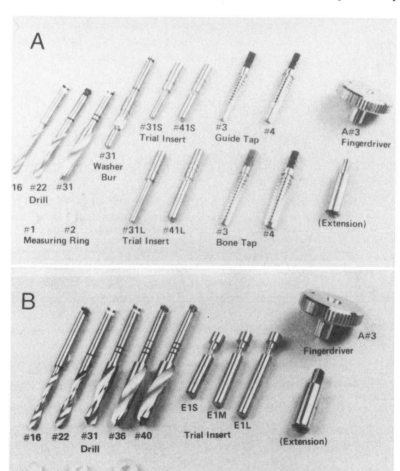

FIG 18–12.
A, display of the armamentarium used for surgical placement of the S-type implant. **B,** display of the armanentarium used for placement of the E-type implant.

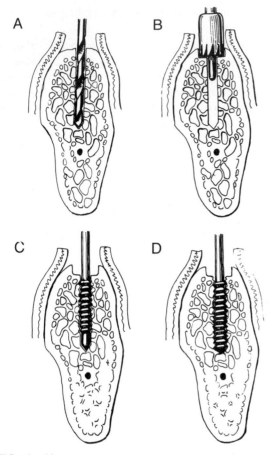

FIG 18–13.
Diagrams of the surgical placement of the Bioceram implant. **A,** use of the guide drill to prepare the initial channel for the implant and use of the bone drill corresponding to the implant size to establish the final trephined socket depth and width. **B,** use of the #31 washer bur to prepare the countersink channel for the 3S9 sapphire implant or the A-type implants. **C,** use of the guide tap to start the socket threads; note the tap-cutting threads do not go to the end of the tap. **D,** the bone tap is used for final preparation of the socket threads.

Trial inserts are used to check the final depth of the formed channel as well as occlusal clearance and path of draw for the prosthesis. These trial gauges are available in widths and lengths to match the selected implant. They may be used as a trial insert following drilling operations and as a final check after tapping prior to implant placement.

The *guide tap* is used to initiate the internal bone threads and is available in a diameter to match the implant (Fig 18–13,C).

The *bone tap* is used to prepare the final bone threads in the socket. These instruments also match the diameter of the implant (Fig 18–13,D).

The *fingerdriver,* with extension, is used to hand-turn the guide and bone taps and for the final implant insertion.

Also available are *plastic caps* for placement on the implant post prior to prosthetic impression taking. These allow the firm placement of dowel pins in the impression prior to pouring the final cast. The dowel pins have a slightly greater diameter than the implant posts to facilitate seating of the final prosthesis.

Also available are *ceramic inner caps* made of polycrystalline aluminum oxide. These caps are advised for use over sapphire implant coronal posts that have been reduced to provide occlusal clearance.[1]

SURGICAL PROCEDURE

The surgical procedure for implant insertion is relatively simple and can be carried out under local anesthesia.[8] Principles of sound surgical practice should be employed throughout the entire operative procedure.

Prior to surgery the implant site must be carefully selected, taking into account the quality of the remaining jaw bone, surgical access, interocclusal clearance, path of draw for prosthetic devices, and proximity of the mandibular canal for the lower jaw. The implant should be placed so it is surrounded by attached gingiva, even if a graft is necessary. Adequate study casts and radiographs are imperative for this preoperative planning. Size of implant, length and width, to be utilized is decided at this time.

An excellent aid for the surgeon is a clear vacuum-formed plastic template prepared on the study cast of the jaw to be implanted. Holes can be placed in this template with the no. 5 round bur to serve as a guide for accurate intraoral placement of the guide hole detents with the no. 5 bur.[1]

Under local anesthesia an incision is made on the crest of the edentulous alveolar ridge with a no. 15 Bard-Parker scalpel blade. The incision should be long enough to allow adequate retraction of the tissue without placing undue stress on it. This is followed by the insertion of the plastic template.

Mark dents are made in the cortical bone using the no. 5 bur. Following removal of the template, the guide drill is used to prepare the channel for the implant socket. The depth of the channel should be checked frequently with the depth gauge until the desired depth is reached.

The bone drill is then used to prepare the implant channel to its final diameter (see Fig 8–13,A). The trial insert can be used at this time to check the width, depth, interocclusal clearance, and angulation of the implant. The channel should be cleared of debris and bone chips by flushing with copious sterile saline.

The washer bur is next utilized to create a countersunk channel for the S-type 3-mm-diameter implants or A-type implants (see Fig 18–13,B). This step is eliminated for the 4-mm-diameter S-type implant (Fig 18–14).

The next step is the threading of the bony chan-nel. For this the guide tap is used first, being turned by the fingerdriver, and extension if necessary (Fig 18–13,C). Following removal of the guide tap, the channel is again irrigated with copious amounts of sterile saline. The bone tap is inserted next, *being careful to engage the starting threads made by the guide tap* (see Fig 18–13,D). The bone tap is advanced carefully until the tap reaches the bottom of the socket. If desired, a periapical radiograph can be made with the bone tap in place to check the socket depth. If undue resistance is encountered while turning the bone tap, the tap is reversed and completely removed, and the socket lavaged with sterile saline and suction to remove bone chips and debris. When reinserting the bone tap, care is taken *to engage the original threads*. After removal, the socket is again lavaged, and the trial insert used to check all aspects of the socket preparation, paying particular attention to interocclusal clearance. If interocclusal clearance is not sufficient, the selected implant should be shortened prior to placement.

The sterilized sapphire implant is then inserted to its proper length using the fingerdriver. The implant should be gently but firmly seated to its predetermined length. The operator can ascertain when the

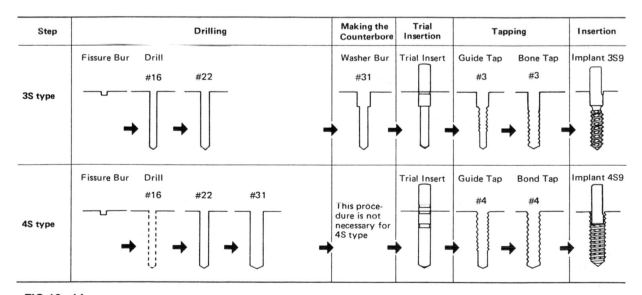

FIG 18–14.
Diagram showing the step-by-step operational procedure for the S-type Bioceram single-crystal sapphire dental implant. A similar procedure is used for the A type. For the E type, counterboring and tapping procedures are eliminated.

implant is completely inserted by tactile sense on the fingerdriver. Care should be used not to attempt to overtighten the implant as this may result in "stripping" of the bone threads and eventual loosening of the implant. Finally, the surgical area should be lavaged and the mucosa tightly sutured.

The implant *cannot be removed* once it has been placed because the bone has been spread by the implant threads and the same-size implant will not tighten again. If by chance, an implant socket is inadvertently overprepared, then an implant of larger diameter must be used and the socket appropriately reprepared. If the implant does not firmly seat or tighten upon placement but remains freely rotatable, the implant will not tighten upon healing. These cases must be removed and a larger-size implant used.

After placement, the implants are left freestanding and no postoperative splint or retaining devices are used. Previous studies indicate that splint devices contribute to severe plaque accumulation, gingivitis, and eventual breakdown of the periodontium.[9]

Following surgery the patient should be given the normal postoperative cautions concerning eating, drinking, and possible bleeding. In particular, the patient should be warned not to use the implant as a biting fulcrum. Also, patients should be warned about possible lip numbness or tingling following mandibular insertions. If the operator desires, or has reason to believe the operative procedure was not as aseptic as he or she would have liked, the patient may be placed on antibiotics for a period of 10 days. The patient should be recalled at 1 week, 2 weeks, and 5 weeks postoperatively. The sutures are removed at the 1-week appointment. If healing has progressed uneventfully, the final prosthesis preparation and placement should not be delayed beyond 6 weeks.[1] Oral hygiene instructions are of the utmost importance and the patient should begin gentle brushing of the surgery site with a soft brush as soon as the soreness has reduced.

Surgical Procedures for the Porous Root Implant.—The soft tissue at the implant site is reflected and the quality and quantity of bone examined. As an option, a tissue punch may be used to remove a circular section of soft tissue. The surgical site is kept small to prevent loss of blood supply to the bone and to minimize epithelial downgrowth. A round no. 5 bur is used to penetrate the cortical bone and create a detent for placement of the pilot drill. To prevent bone damage by frictional heat, a high-torque low-speed internal irrigation handpiece and engine are used. The recommended speed ranges are 500 to 1,000 rpm depending on the manufacturer's recommendation. Using the pilot drill, a channel is drilled to an initial depth of 5 to 7 mm. The parallel pin is inserted to check parallelism with adjacent natural teeth or other implants. Any paralleling adjustments are made with the pilot drill at the preliminary depth. Once parallelism is achieved, the pilot drill is used to complete the osteotomy to full depth. The *minimum* recommended depth of the osteotomy is 11 mm for the short implant and 14 mm for the long. If the specific anatomy of the surgical site permits, and to ensure that all the porous root is securely embedded within cancellous bone, the desired depth mark scribed on the pilot drill is carried below the alveolar crest. If indicated, the bone removed by the osteotomy is harvested for graft material. A final check for parallelism is made using the parallel pin.

The osteotomy is completed so that the porous portion of the implant is 5 mm below the alveolar crest. The *minimum* acceptable depth is 3 mm (see Figs 18–5,B and 18–6).

The osteotomy is enlarged with the internal irrigation cannon drill to the same depth drilled with the pilot drill. The desired depth marking scribed on the cannon drill is carried below the crest of the alveolar ridge. Any laterally directed force or other movement of the surgical drill is to be avoided. This can produce an irregularly shaped receptor site for the implant.

Before inserting the porous implant in dense bone, especially in the mandible, the osteotomy is enlarged and refined atraumatically with the expand reamer, which is placed in the receptor site with finger pressure. The fingerdriver marked EX(ANT) or EX(POS) is attached to the reamer (Fig 18–15). To complete the osteotomy, the fingerdriver is turned one full revolution and removed.

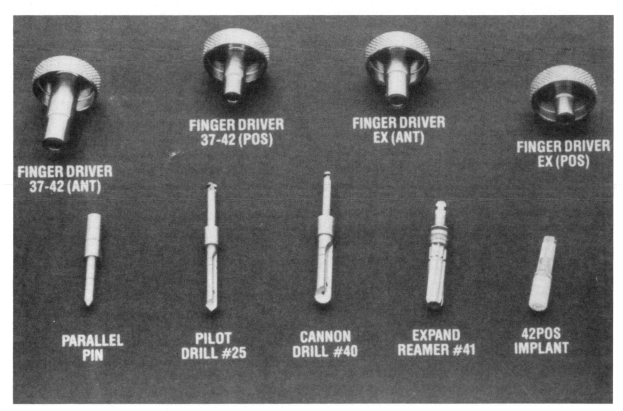

FIG 18–15.
Instrumentation set for the Bioceram porous root implant.

Parallelism is checked once again, this time using the broad end of the parallel pin. To make sure the osteomy is the correct minimum depth to receive the implant, depth markings are also scribed on the parallel pin.

The implant is flushed with sterile saline solution and the fingerdriver is attached to the implant. For the 42POS implant, the 37-42(ANT) or 37-42(POS) fingerdriver is used. The porous root portion of the implant is positioned so it is 5 mm below the crest of the alveolar bone. The porous root portion of the implant must not extend above the bone or contact soft tissue directly. Risk of infection and potential loss of the implant increases if this protocol is not followed.[8]

To create a dense receptor site, the harvested bone is packed and condensed into the osteotomy, using the fingerdriver to seat the implant firmly in the prepared surgical site. If the implant is mobile upon seating, a larger-diameter implant is used to obtain firm fixation.

Surgical Procedures for the Type II–Two-Stage Design Implant.—The new two-stage Bioceram Type II implant utilizes the technology of the porous root implant as the first stage of a two-stage technique. Figure 18–16 recaps the step-by-step procedure for placement of the implant. The radicular portion is placed using the same armamentarium as for the porous root implant. This portion needs to be set into the bone so that the porous outer surface is totally within the bone crypt and the single-crystal cervical area projects above the bone in order that the smooth sapphire surface interfaces the outside plate of cortical bone and the soft tissue periosteum and attached gingiva after it is sutured back in place.

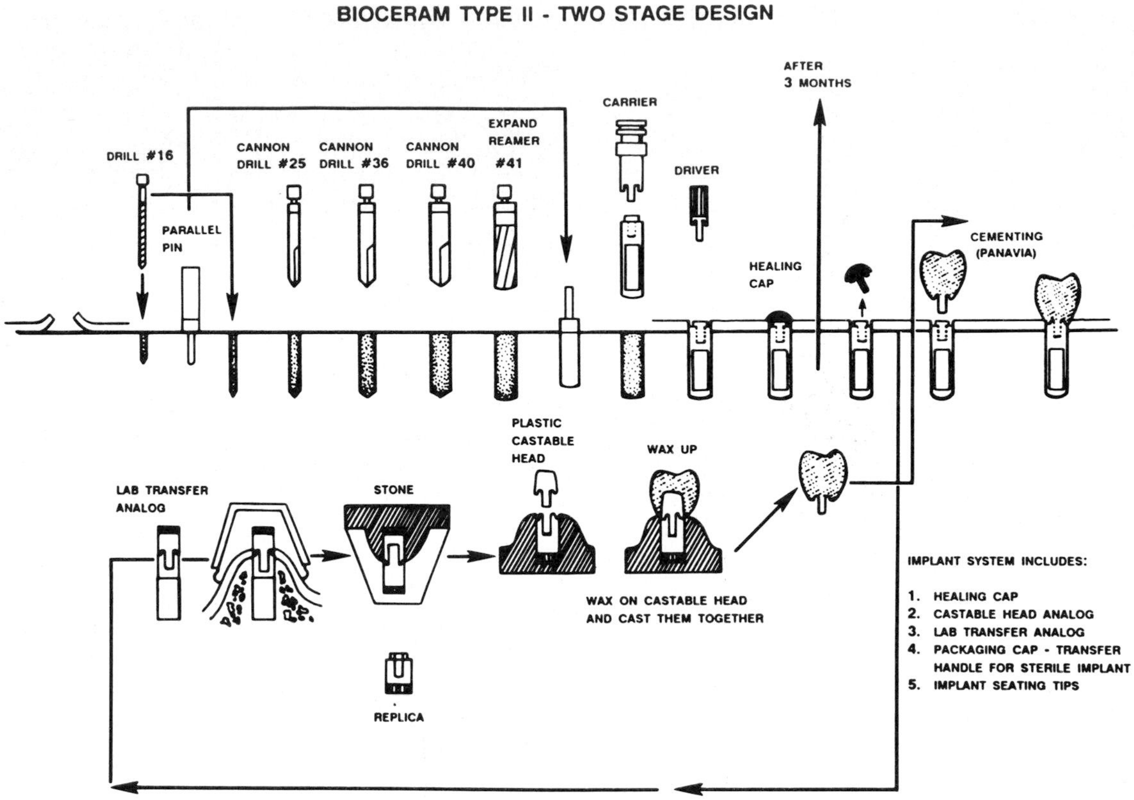

BIOCERAM TYPE II - TWO STAGE DESIGN

FIG 18—16.
Diagram showing the step-by-step surgical procedures, plus prosthodontic procedure, for the new Bioceram two-stage ceramic implant called the Type II—Two-Stage Design.

The implant first stage is not buried totally beneath the soft tissue as in other implant systems. The superior aspect of the first stage is allowed to protrude through the tissue and the tissue is coapted and sutured tightly around the implant. This takes advantage of the knowledge about the biological seal (see Chapters 1 and 5) and the fact that it has been scientifically shown that this biological seal develops against single-crystal sapphire material.[10] Prior to surgical coapting of the tissue around the implant post, a plastic healing cap is snapped into place on the hexagonal head of the implant (see Fig 18—16).

Following 3 months' postimplantation healing, the healing cap is removed and the second-stage superstructure is cemented into the first stage using Panavia luting cement (J. Morita USA, Inc., Tustin, Calif.) (see Fig 18—16).

PROSTHODONTIC CONSIDERATIONS

The conventional armamentarium is used for the prosthetic technique. Selected abutments are prepared for retainers using accepted modern principles of design. Prior to full-arch impressions, plastic caps, which are slightly larger in diameter than the coronal portion of the implant, are placed over the implant and subsequently become a part of the impression. Care is exercised so that no impression material remains in the cervical space surrounding the implants. Before casting the impression, a dowel pin is placed securely into the plastic cap and becomes the die for the implant. This dowel can be used for the wax-up and is 150 μm larger in diameter than the head of the implant. It is recommended that casts be mounted on adjustable arcon-type articulators using a face-bow transfer and interocclusal jaw registration records.

The most frequently encountered problem in the fabrication of the fixed prosthesis is the path of insertion. Because implant placement is dictated by jaw shape and size, some implants are not in alignment with the abutments, and, because of pulpal considerations it is not possible to always prepare abutment teeth so that a fixed prosthesis will draw with the implant(s). This problem can be overcome by the use of copings or semiprecision keyways, singly or in combination.[1]

Difficulty involving tight fit of the castings can be overcome by using a die spacer and by creating maximum expansion of the investment.

Fixed prostheses should be designed for optimal access for plaque removal. When the clinical crown length is sufficient, cervical margins of the abutments are prepared supragingivally. The buccal and lingual dimensions should not be overcontoured and, when possible, at least 1 mm of the implant is left exposed between the tissue and crown margin.

As mentioned previously, occlusion is a major consideration. In order to minimize horizontal forces, the concept of a mutually protected occlusion should be followed and an articulator adjustable for immediate side shift used whenever occlusal considerations require. Since a discussion of occlusal philosophies and articulators is not a primary purpose of this chapter, the reader should consult one of several special texts for this information.[15]

Initially, the fixed prosthesis can be temporarily placed using temporary cement (Optow Trial Cement, Teledyne Dental Products, Elk Grove, Ill.) for a period of 5 to 7 days so that occlusal and axial crown contours can be evaluated. After discrepancies are corrected, the prosthesis can be finally luted.

DISCUSSION

The Bioceram implant systems provide a simple, practical approach to implantology that is well within the skills of the general practitioner after in-

struction and preparation. The alpha aluminum oxide ceramic material, both single-crystal sapphire and polycrystalline, is one of the most biologically inert and kindest biomaterials that can be used in dental and oral implantology. The nontoxic nature of the material has been established.[3-5] The ability of gingiva to heal successfully around the material and create the important biological seal has been scientifically established (see Chapter 5).

Following completion of the prosthetic bridgework, the maintenance and oral hygiene is enhanced because oral plaque and debris does not readily adhere to the highly polished single-crystal sapphire surface. An oxide corrosion layer does not form. This facilitates maintenance and protects the delicate biological seal structure.

The clinical longevity of the Bioceram implant has been detailed in carefully controlled clinical studies with rigid evaluation criteria.[11-14] The implant is well tolerated, surgical placement causes minimal surgical trauma to the patient, and biological and clinical longevity has been well established scientifically.

REFERENCES

1. Koth DL, McKinney RV Jr: The single crystal sapphire endosteal dental implant, in Hardin JE (ed): *Clark's Clinical Dentistry*. Philadelphia, JB Lippincott Co, 1981, Chap 53.
2. Yamagami A, Kotera S, Ehara Y, et al: Porous alumina for free-standing implants. Part I: Implant design and in vivo animal studies. *J Prosthet Dent* 1988; 59:689–695.
3. Kawahara H, Yamagami A, Hirabayashi M: Bioceram—A new type of ceramic implant, in *The First Proceedings of the Japan Society of Implant Dentistry*. 1975, p 187.
4. Kawahara H: Today and tomorrow of bioceramics in artificial organ. *Jpn Artif Organ* 1977; 6:218.
5. Kawahara H: Today and tomorrow of bioceramics. *J Oral Implantol* 1979; 8:411–432.
6. Kawahara H, Hirabayashi M: Single crystal alumina for dental implants and bone screw. *J Biomed Mater Res* 1980; 14:597–605.
7. Yamane T, Yura Y, Matsuzawa K, et al: Fundamental and clinical studies on endosseous implant of new

sapphire (Al_2O_3) material. *J Oral Implantol* 1979; 8:232–256.

8. Kawahara H, Shebata K, Yamagami A, et al: *Surgical Technique of S-Type Bioceram Sapphire Dental Implants*. Kyoto, Japan, Kyocera Corporation, 1982.

9. Klawitter JJ, Weinstein AM, Cook FW, et al: An evaluation of porous alumina ceramic dental implants. *J Dent Res* 1977; 56:768–776.

10. McKinney RV Jr, Steflik DE, Koth DL: The biologic response to the single crystal sapphire endosteal dental implant: Scanning electron microscopic observations. *J Prosthet Dent* 1984; 51:372–379.

11. Koth DL, McKinney RV Jr, Steflik DE, et al: Clinical and statistical analyses of human clinical trials with the single crystal aluminum oxide endosteal

dental implant. Five year results. *J Prosthet Dent* 1988; 60:226–234.

12. Koth DL, McKinney RV Jr, Davis QB, et al: Single crystal Al_2O_3 endosteal implants: Nine year results. *J Dent Res* 1989; 68(special issue):911.

13. McKinney RV Jr, Koth DL, Steflik DE, et al: Statistical analysis of a nine year endosseous ceramic implant study. *J Dent Res* 1990; 69(special issue):267.

14. Long WG, Lightbody PM, McKinney RV Jr, et al: Nine year clinical study of alumina oxide endosseous dental implants. *J Dent Res* 1988; 67(special issue):142.

15. Malone WF, Koth DL (eds): *Tylman's Theory and Practice of Fixed Prosthodontics*, ed 8. St Louis, Ishiyaku EuroAmerica, 1989.

Chapter 19

The Titanodont Implant System

Alfred L. Heller, D.D.S., M.S.

The Miter Titanodont implant system (Table 19–1) was developed to take advantage of the submergibility feature, make use of titanium metal strength, and allow easy head placement on the implant after the recommended healing phase of the root portion of the implant. This chapter describes the step-by-step procedure of placing the Miter Titanodont as well as the head placement. Potential problems of the implant are discussed together with the reasons that led to the new Miter 2000 series being developed.

MITER TITANODONT IMPLANT DEVELOPMENT

In 1969, rhesus monkeys and baboons were used as experimental animals to place high-density aluminum oxide ceramic dental implants. These studies were conducted at the Battelle Memorial Institute in Columbus, Ohio, and the State University of New York (SUNY) at Buffalo. The studies were funded by the Dental Research Division of the US Army Medical Research and Development Command and were under the direction of Thomas D. Driskell.[1]

The first implants were similar to the shape of normal monkey teeth. The thought was to make the root form the same as the tooth form coming out of the socket. This did not work because the smooth-surface alumina did not allow for good bone-ceramic interface. Porous and particulate coatings were used with some success.

In 1971 a circumferential fin design with hori-zontal undersurfaces perpendicular to the occlusal force was developed.[2] Gross anatomic and histologic examination of block-sectioned implants recovered from the experimental animals revealed direct bone-to-ceramic interface with very little intervening soft tissue.[3] This phenomenon is now described as osseointegration, by Brånemark.[4]

Driskell and Heller[5] did several animal studies between 1971 and 1975 with the Miter Synthodont implant, which was designed for human use. Heller placed the first Synthodont in September 1975 in a 22-year-old man. This implant has functioned successfully for 15 years under normal occlusal chewing. The Synthodont became the first predictable freestanding single tooth replacement.

From 1975 to 1982 Heller placed over 500 of the Synthodont implants. Approximately 48 of the implants were lost due to fracture of the ceramic. The Synthodont limitations were the possibility of fracture as well as the need to be stabilized to the adjacent teeth for a period of 4 to 6 months. Keeping the implant solidly splinted was often difficult to accomplish.

By 1981, it became clear that endosseous implants would be more stable if the early healing phase were protected from occlusal forces. Driskell then designed the Miter Titanodont implant system with a submergible root.[6] The head would be attached to the submerged root after adequate healing took place over a period of 4 to 6 months. The basic root shape of the Titanodont implants was almost identical to the Synthodont implants. The major change was that the Titanodont was made out of tita-

TABLE 19–1.

The Titanodont Implant System

Product name	The Titanidont Implant System: a two-stage endosseous implant	
Supplier	Miter, Incorporated	
	P.O. Box 1133	
	Warsaw, IN 46580	
	1-800-325-8566	
	(219) 267-6662	
Material composition	Titanium alloy	
Implants and approximate costs	Titanodont system post	$90
	Titanodont subcortical blade	$125
	Miter System 2000 post	$90
	Implant head	$45–$79
	Basic instrument kit for root forms	$690
	Basic instrument kit for blade forms	$749

nium alloy and had a two-piece root-head system. It was felt by Driskell and Heller that the design of the Synthodont was very important to its success and should be incorporated into the Titanodont.

STERILE SURGICAL TECHNIQUE

It has long been the desire of dentists to be able to perform surgical procedures in the mouth under sterile conditions. The ability to work under surgically clean conditions could prevent autogenous infections. Rosen and co-workers,[7] in 1984, conducted a pilot study of ten patients utilizing povidone-iodine (Betadine) with a carefully planned regimen of scrubbing and wiping the teeth and soft tissues in the oral cavity. The study showed that intense aseptic treatment of the oral cavity with povidone-iodine before surgery causes a marked reduction in oral bacteria during the course of surgery. The data showed that this bacterial reduction occurred at every sampling with statistical significance being obtained at each time interval except the last procedure of suturing.

TECHNIQUE OF PLACING
A TITANODONT

Whether placing a single or multiple implants, the surgeon must design the incision preoperatively.

To keep the attached gingiva on the labiobuccal aspect of the implant, the incision is made lingual to the crest of the ridge. Figure 19–1 shows the incision line for a freestanding implant. The operator reflects the tissue buccally and lingually to reveal the underlying bone. If visibility of the bone is not sufficient to determine thickness or if a buccal bone defect is not visible, then the surgeon must make a vertical incision which usually includes a papilla or enough tissue that will help facilitate proper suturing after implant placement. Figure 19–2 shows placement of a vertical incision which will allow visualization of the underlying bone. The tissue must not

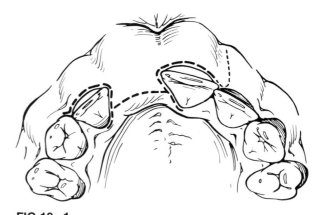

FIG 19–1.
Large dashed line indicates the incision pattern to be used for placement of a Titanodont freestanding dental implant. *Small dashed line* indicates position of a vertical incision if necessary for greater bone access or visualization.

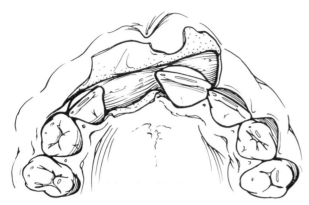

FIG 19—2.
Reflection of tissue using horizontal and vertical incisions shown in Figure 19—1.

be reflected more than is necessary to see the underlying bone. When the periosteum is reflected, the main blood supply to the cortical bone is compromised and excessive reflection results in needless bone loss (see Chapter 6).

After proper visualization of the bone the operator determines the angulation needed to place the implant. A 700XXL bur is used to drill a hole through the cortical crest of bone (Fig 19—3). Usually this opening bisects the buccolingual width of bone. If the bone is marginally thin buccolingually, it is suggested that the operator place the hole toward the lingual crest as it is more important to maintain

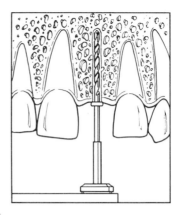

FIG 19—4.
Titanodont 1.5-mm pilot drill used for initial trephine. Note the endodontic rubber stop placed for correct depth at the alveolar crest.

a buccal thickness of bone after implant placement.

A 1.5-mm pilot drill is used to drill a hole at the proper angulation. An endodontic rubber stop is placed on the pilot drill at the desired depth. It is suggested that a radiograph be taken at this time to check the desired angulation and depth (Fig 19—4). A 2-mm intermediate drill is then used to enlarge the crypt, being careful to maintain the previously established alignment and depth (Fig 19—5).

A 3-mm bone reamer, placed on the driver handle, is forced to the desired depth of bone preparation, usually to the respective circumferential groove (Fig 19—6). As the bone reamer is removed, the bone caught in the vertical flutes is wiped onto a sterile amalgam squeeze cloth so as to save the bone

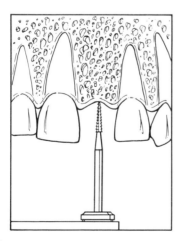

FIG 19—3.
Pilot hole drilled with a 700XXL bur through the cortical bone.

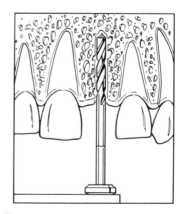

FIG 19—5.
Enlargement of the crypt with the 2-mm intermediate drill.

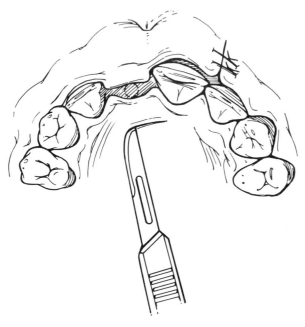

FIG 19–10.
The vertical incision is sutured first. A horizontal incision is made 10 mm off the ridge crest to free up alveolar mucosa to allow sliding of sufficient mucoperiosteum for primary closure of tissue over the ridge crest and implant.

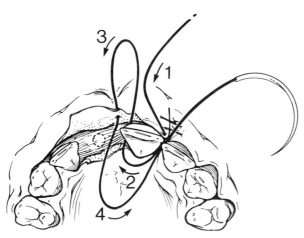

FIG 19–11.
A step-by-step diagram of the proper suture technique to close the mucoperiosteum. *(1)* Through interdental papilla, *(2)* around the tooth *not* engaging lingual tissues, *(3)* the suture is looped back *through* labial tissue, and around the lingual of the tooth, and *(4)* then under the tooth interproximal contact, but *not* through tissue. The suture is tightened up, the tissue positioned and tied off.

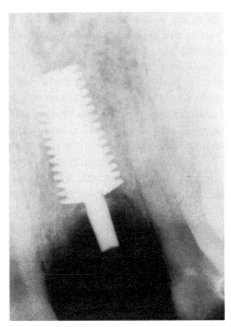

FIG 19–12.
Radiograph of first-stage implant in place. The Teflon healing collar does not show in the radiograph.

step suturing technique to reposition the papilla and labial tissue securely around the tooth adjacent to the surgical site.

It is recommended that a radiograph now be taken using a double packet to allow for proper documentation (Fig 19–12). One film can be placed in the patient's folder and one sent to the referring dentist for his or her records.

EXPOSURE OF HEALED, BURIED, TITANODONT IMPLANT

Healing of the Titanodont subcortical root implant is usually excellent because it is well protected during the passive 4- to 6-month healing period. It is suggested that a wait of 6 months is better than 4 months if excessive augmentation of buccolingual bony plates was necessary.

The Teflon healing collar may or may not be slightly exposed. If it is completely exposed, a periodontal probe or sharp explorer is inserted into the

Teflon and pulled coronally. This should easily remove the healing collar.

If the gingival tissue covers or partially covers the Silastic healing collar, the desired margins should be contoured by using a curved scalpel blade, making sure that enough tissue is removed to allow easy removal of the Teflon collar. It may be necessary to lay a buccal and lingual tissue flap to uncover the healing collar, but this is usually not the case.

Examination of the tissue site should reveal a well-shaped and healed space around the taperlock post, ready for final placement of the implant head structure. The implant site should be flushed with sterile saline solution because some bleeding will probably have occurred.

Care should be taken with the angled head of 20 degrees to be sure the head is rotationally aligned appropriately. The head should be placed by gently pushing with finger pressure. Care must be taken to not allow the patient to bite on the implant head as this might cause instant seating of the head in that position. If possible, adjustments of the head should be made outside of the mouth for the patient's comfort. Occlusal clearance in all movements must be checked closely.

Once the angled or straight head has been altered to accept the patient's occlusal schemes, the head is tapped in place using a driver handle and mallet (Fig 19–13). The tap should be sharp, but not necessarily heavy, and in line with the root portion. From this point forward a one-piece implant system is in place.

TREATMENT CROWN COVERAGE

It is suggested that the operator now place a treatment crown over the head of the implant. If necessary, the head can be altered in the mouth with a carbide bur or diamond stone to accommodate a treatment crown. Usually a tooth-colored shell crown is filled with quick-cure acrylic and placed over the head of the implant. After proper curing time the crown is fitted and adjusted for proper occlusion. It is suggested that the treatment crown be attached to the adjacent teeth by etching methods for a period of at least 1 month. Usually 1 month is sufficient time for tissue to adapt to the head of the implant, and recontour to a healthy acceptable level.

After 1 month's healing of the tissue around the implant head, the operator can use the normal restorative methods and techniques that have been shown to be effective when restoring implants. Electrosurgery is not acceptable for tissue retraction before the impression as the electrical current will damage the bone adjacent to the implant. A retraction cord, when placed with care, usually works nicely. It is also suggested that the final fixed crown have lingual wings that touch the adjacent teeth to help prevent labial occlusal forces. If tremendous protrusive forces are present, the operator may want to acid-etch the lingual surface of the adjacent teeth and lute the lingual tabs as if placing a Maryland bridge. It is better to be overprotected against occlusal forces than underprotected (Fig 19–14).

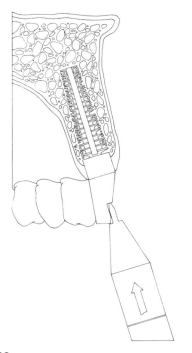

FIG 19–13.
Placement of the straight head on the implant using the driver handle which is struck with a mallet.

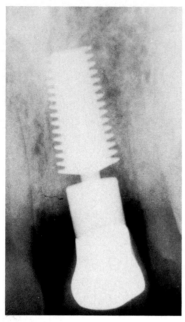

FIG 19–14.
Radiograph of the implant with the second-stage head and the crown restoration placed.

DISCUSSION

With over 300 Titanodont implants in service, it was noted that with some of the implants there was breakdown of bone over the top of the coronal fin. It would take 2 to 3 years to see evidence of bone breakdown in this area. Most of the bone breakdown would just involve the coronal fin.

If progressive breakdown occurs then the tissue is reflected sufficiently to see the area. A no. 4 round bur is used to remove the exposed fin or fins, the granulation tissue is curetted, hydroxylapatite is placed around the reduced fin, and the tissue is readapted to the implant. Most often this intervention procedure will stop or slow down the deterioration process to where the tissue and bone health is maintained.

MITER SYSTEM 2000 AND SUBCORTICAL BLADE IMPLANTS

Because of the potential problem of bone breakdown over the coronal fin, the Miter System 2000

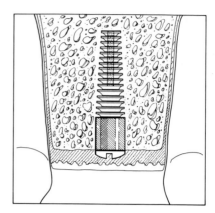

FIG 19–15.
The Miter System 2000 implant showing the enlarged coronal portion which has the same diameter as the most superior coronal portion of the first-stage implant.

implant was developed in 1985. The root form remained the same but the coronal portion was enlarged to the diameter of the implant (Fig 19–15). The neck of the implant then was large enough to allow cementing of a straight or angled head after healing of the root portion of the implant (Fig 19–16). Fifty prototype Miter System 2000 implants have been placed and the bone degradation around

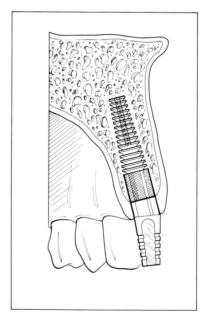

FIG 19–16.
An angled head placed on the Miter System 2000 implant.

the neck of the implant has been minimal.

The improved results are thought to be because bone now closely adapts around the neck of the implant and is not disturbed when placing the head to the implant. The other improvement is a healing screw that adapts closely to the implant during the healing phase. The surgical placement technique is exactly the same as for the Titanodont implant.

The Miter System 2000 implant appears to be a significant improvement over the Miter Titanodont implant system for the reasons stated above. Like any system that requires cementing the head in place, the problems of blood and moisture can be a disadvantage. If the tissue covering the implant is thick and fibrous, reflection of this tissue is usually difficult and results in bleeding from the tissue around the implant. Blood, of course, can cause a problem with the setting time and strength of cement used to attach the head to the implant. Care must be taken to reflect the tissue away from the implant sufficiently to diminish the bleeding problem.

A Titanodont subcortical blade implant system is also available. This is a two-stage blade form implant that uses standard blade or plate form surgical technique for insertion. The standard series of Miter second-stage heads fit all three Miter implants, the Titanodont root form, the Titanodont subcortical blade form, and the Miter System 2000 root form implant.

REFERENCES

1. Driskell TD, O'Hara MJ, Sheets HD, et al: Development for application of ceramics and ceramic composites for implant dentistry, in Hulbert SF, Levine SF, Young FA (eds): *Bioceramics—Engineering in Medicine*. New York, NY, Interscience Publishers, 1972, pp 345–361.
2. Driskell TD, O'Hara MJ, Greene GW: Surgical tooth implants, combat and field. Report No. 1. Contract #DADA 17-c-9181, 1971.
3. Driskell TD, O'Hara MJ, Greene GW: Surgical tooth implants, combat and field, report no. 2. Contract no. DADA17-69-C-9118, 1972. Supported by US Army Medical Research and Development Command.
4. Brånemark P, Breine U, Adell R, et al: Intraosseous anchorage of dental prosthesis—Experimental studies. *Scand J Plast Reconstr Surg* 1969; 3:81–100.
5. Driskell TD, Heller AL: Clinical use of aluminum oxide endosseous implants. *J Oral Implantol* 1977; 7:53–76.
6. Hahn J: Clinical experience with the Titanodont subcortical implant system. *J Oral Implantol* 1983; 11:72–88.
7. Rosen S, Ogg-Bell K, Heller A, et al: Use of an organic iodine compound to decrease oral microflora in the implant patient. *Ohio Dent J* 1988; 62:20–21.

Chapter 20

The ITI Implant Systems

Joel L. Rosenlicht, D.M.D.

The International Team of Implantologists (ITI) was established to develop endosseous implant systems to satisfy a variety of needs and applications for the totally and partially edentulous patient. The organization was established in 1974 and includes dental clinicians, bioengineers, metallurgists, histologists, and dental researchers from a variety of international academic backgrounds. Recognizing that the oral anatomy varies greatly in quality and quantity, one size or type of implant would not meet all situations. Basic guidelines were formulated to include not only size and shape but also material biocompatibility, implant surface coating, and surgical preparation. Utilizing the experience of the European Association of Osteosynthesis and the US Association for the Study of Internal Fixation, various designs and concepts evolved. Thorough testing of stress distribution analysis, photoelastic analysis, and corrosion were completed, followed by animal testing and histologic examination via electron and light microscopy. All ITI implants utilize the concept of initial primary stability upon insertion and the promotion of a bony-implant interface (ankylosis or osseous integration) without intervention of a fibrous connective tissue layer.

ITI has developed two distinctly different implant systems: the titanium plasma-sprayed screw (TPS Screw) and the titanium plasma-sprayed Hollow-Cylinder implants. For simplicity, each system is addressed separately.

THE IMPLANT

The Titanium Plasma-Sprayed Screw

The titanium plasma-sprayed screw (TPS Screw) implant was developed in conjunction with Dr Philip Lederman, ITI, and the Institut Straumann.[1] The titanium plasma-sprayed screw has been utilized since 1978. It is unique among contemporary implant systems in its application, surgical site preparation, and prosthetic loading. The initial protocol was that this implant system was to be used solely in the edentulous mandible in the symphyseal region between the mental foramina. However, its use has been expanded to include single tooth replacements, bridge abutments, and use in the maxilla.

The TPS Screw corresponds to the cortical traction screw used by the Association of Osteosynthesis (see Fig 20–1). It is manufactured from commercially pure titanium, ASTMB standard 265-58T, and is additionally plasma-sprayed with commercially pure titanium powder (see Table 20–1). The surface coating has been shown to be biocompatible, promoting significant direct bony healing, as well as increasing the surface contact area sixfold. This increase in surface area significantly increases the possible amount of bone-to-implant contact (see Fig 20–2). In in vivo experiments utilizing *Macaca* sp. monkeys, the bone applied itself without an intervening layer of connective tissue to the surface of the implant and, as revealed over periods of up to 21 months, remained directly interfaced to the loaded implant.[2, 3] The fibers of the connective tissue be-

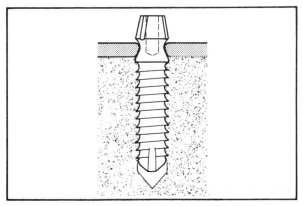

FIG 20–1.
The cylindrical TPS Screw developed by ITI and the Institut Straumann. The screw is cp titanium, ASTMB standard 265-58T, and is plasma-sprayed with pure titanium powder.

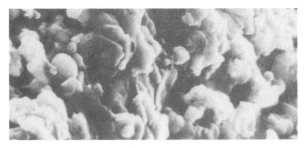

FIG 20–2.
Scanning electron micrograph of the TPS Screw plasma-sprayed titanium surface.

tween the bone and epithelium interface the titanium-sprayed surface and appear to be functionally oriented. If the post of the implant is situated in a region of immobile, keratinized mucosa, adhesion of the epithelial cells to the metal surface becomes apparent.[2]

The TPS Screw system is packaged in a fully autoclavable anodized container with all appropriate drills, wrenches, depth gauges, and prosthetic components (see Fig 20–3).

The TPS Screws are available in five lengths of 9, 11, 14, 17, and 20 mm and two widths of 3.5 and 4.2 mm diameter (see Fig 20–4). The implant has a 12-degree conical head with four slots to prevent rotation of the prosthesis and to aid in seating the implant. The slots aid in positioning the prefabricated transfer copings and stabilize them during impression taking. The head is also internally threaded with a 5-mm-deep socket, which will accept 4- or 8-mm-long, 2-mm-wide occlusal screws, which anchor the superstructure and allow it to be removed. Below the head is a highly polished neck, slightly concave to allow for good oral hygiene and gingival adaptation. The remaining portion is plasma-sprayed to increase the surface area and to allow ingrowth of bone cells to the implants. The screw threads have edges that are slightly rounded to cause compression of the cor-

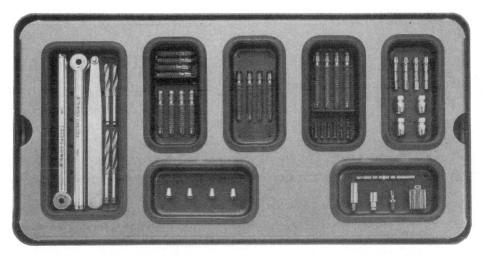

FIG 20–3.
A typical complete anodized TPS Screw tray setup that includes all screw components, wrenches, drills, implants, gold telescopic copings, master dies, transfer copings, depth gauge, occlusal screws, and hand screwdriver.

TABLE 20–1.

The ITI TPS Screw Implant and the TPS Hollow-Cylinder Implant

Name	Titanium plasma-sprayed screw implant (TPS Screw)	
	Titanium plasma-sprayed Hollow-Cylinder Implant	
Manufacturer	Institute Straumann, Waldenberg, Switzerland	
Supplier	Park Dental Research Corporation	
	19 West 34th Street, Suite 301	
	New York, New York 10001	
	(212) 736-3765	
Physical properties	Atomic weight	47.90
	Melting point	1660° ± 10° C
	Specific gravity	4.54
Mechanical properties	Annealing	Cold-worked, heat-tempered
	Modulus of elasticity	110,000 MPa
		1.59×10^7 psi
	Yield strength	485 MPa
	Ultimate tensile strength	550 MPa
	Shear modulus	46,000 MPa
	Elongation	15%
	Fatigue limit	170–300 MPa
	Brinell hardness	160 kg/mm^2
Corrosion properties	Insoluble titanium oxide layer	
Approximate costs, TPS Screw	Implant kit	$2,050
	Individual implants including accessories of copings, etc.	$110–165
Approximate costs, Hollow Cylinder	Implant kit costs	
	F	$2,995
	K	$2,380
	H	$2,510
	Individual implants	
	F	$125
	K	$235
	H	$250
	Gold copings	$70.75
	Transfer copings	$10.75
	Master dies	$21.00
	Occlusal screws	$ 6.50

tical and medullary bone, eliminating microfracture and compression necrosis. The apical tip is fluted and angled to 120 degrees to permit self-tapping of the threaded implant (see Fig 20–1 and 20–4).

PATIENT CONSIDERATIONS

Indications

The TPS Screw, when used as an overdenture with clip retention, is indicated when:

1. A conventional prosthesis is nonfunctional or difficult to retain.
2. The vertical symphyseal height is 9 mm or greater.
3. The genial tubercles are superior.
4. A severe gagging problem exists.
5. The patient is not suitable for long or complicated surgery.
6. Ease of hygiene is necessary for maintenance.
7. Restoration needs to be completed in a short period of time.

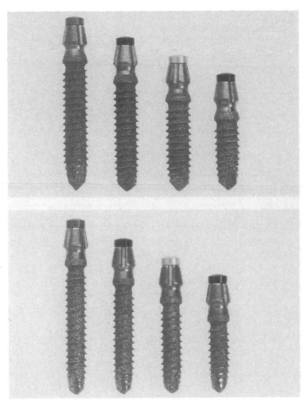

FIG 20–4.
The TPS Screw implants are available in lengths of 9, 11, 14, 17, and 20 mm and diameters of 3.5 and 4.0 mm.

Contraindications are:

1. Recent extraction site or any pathologic condition.
2. Vertical height less than 9 mm.
3. Crestal bone width not greater than 4 mm.
4. History of radiation treatment.
5. Medical or systemic contraindicating diseases.

The simplicity, both surgically and prosthetically, makes this a useful implant system for edentulous patients. The existing denture, if recently made, can be utilized. The cost is less than similar systems. Also, existing implants utilized with an overdenture can be converted to fixed and fixed-removable bridges. This convertibility is another advantage.

Surgical Procedures for the TPS Screw When Used as an Overdenture

Aseptic surgical technique and careful handling of both hard and soft tissue is imperative for all implant surgery. Preoperative medication of antibiotics and steroids is the operator's choice. An intraoral surgical preparation is advised.

The procedure is usually carried out in an office setting under local anesthesia and, if warranted, adjunctive inhalation or intravenous sedation. The procedure begins with careful palpation of the anterior mandible to assess the anatomic contours and the vertical dimensions and to assess the position of the neurovascular bundle. A crestal incision is made from the premolar region on one side to the premolar region on the other side at the crest of the ridge, trying to preserve, if possible, attached gingiva on both sides of the incision. The buccal and lingual tissues are then reflected to give good visibility to the crest of the ridge and dissection is carried out to identify the mental nerve. Any bony spicules or irregularities along the crest of the ridge, at this time, are reduced using appropriate rongeurs or a low-speed handpiece with copious irrigation. It is advisable to try to obtain a level ridge with a minimum of 5.5 mm of bone width and 9.0 mm of bone height. Once the alveoplasty is complete, a pilot hole is then drilled with a small bur placed at the crest of the ridge approximately 3 mm anterior to the mental foramen. This is then performed on the opposite side. Once the two distal holes are completed, the midline of the mandible is marked and the pilot hole for the two anterior implants is then drawn by bisecting the dimensions between the midline and the distal pilot hole (Fig 20–5). When this is done, the pilot holes are drilled and the two anterior implants can be appropriately placed. Next, the appropriate drill for the diameter of the implant to be used is selected, either the 3.0-drill for the 3.5-mm implant or the 3.2-drill for the 4.0-mm implant. It is imperative to use a high-torque, low-speed handpiece, which does not exceed 600 rpm, in the implant site preparations. Copious iced physiologic saline or other irrigant to maintain temperature within biological limits (below 43° C) is always used. Drilling should be done with a firm definitive deliberate motion, avoiding any ec-

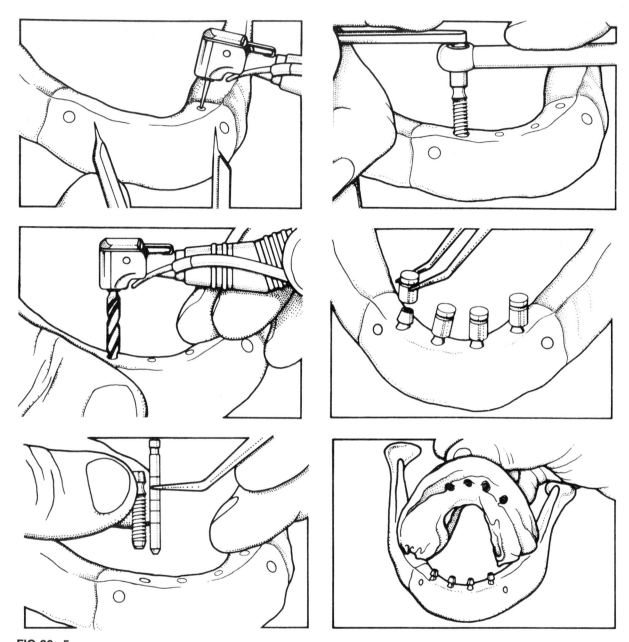

FIG 20–5.
Step-by-step surgical procedure for insertion of the TPS Screw implant. See text for details.

centric drilling. The drills can be marked for depth, or depth gauges can be used to ascertain proper depth and angle of inclination. All four sites are drilled, being careful not to perforate the inferior border or the buccal or lingual plates. The implants should be seated so that the shoulder is flush with the crest of the ridge. It is more important to have the shoulder seated than to use an excessive length of implants and risk perforation of the inferior border or buccolingual plates. The implants are handled within their sterile packaging and held in place with the titanium-tipped handling forceps. The ratchet wrench is used to gently position and insert all implants. After all implants are properly placed, any excess tissue that may be found as a result of the alveoplasty can be trimmed to minimize any bulging of tissue around the implant heads. Standard interupted suturing is used in order to get a well-adapted soft tissue closure around each implant head.

A transitional denture or the patient's previous prosthesis is then modified so that there is no loading on the implants when the prosthesis is placed in the mouth. Soft tissue conditioners can be used to maintain the soft tissue from becoming too edematous post-insertion. The patient can be discharged with this interim prosthesis. (see Fig 20–5).

PROSTHETIC TECHNIQUE

At the conclusion of surgery, transfer copings supplied in the kit are placed over the implant heads. Care is taken to make sure that they are well seated and that no tissue, suture material, or edema has misplaced them. At this point, an impression is taken using a stock tray and an elastic impression material strong enough to pull the transfer copings within the impressions. Securing the copings together with acrylic prior to the impression may assure the operator of an accurate transfer and removal in the impression. Once the impression is taken, master dies, which are also included in the kit, are inserted into the copings and secured with sticky wax. A master model is then poured. At that point, gold telescopic copings are placed over the die heads, which are exact replicas of the implant head. A variety of bars, either premade or cast, can be soldered to each gold coping rigidly fixing the entire system. This connector bar is then returned to the patient within 48 to 72 hours and placed onto the implants and secured with occlusal screws. The patient's existing denture can then be relined to fit over the connector bar to allow for function and esthetics during healing. It is possible, if desired, to have the patient's new denture processed from a master impression. Since the surgery is only confined to the anterior portion of the mouth, the posterior segments

remain unchanged. If this technique is done, the final denture with its retentive device can simply be fabricated and inserted. If the superstructure cannot be returned to the patient within 48 to 72 hours, a transitional acrylic splint will need to be fabricated. The placement of the superstructure over the implant heads usually takes only a few minutes and is secured with the occlusal screws. Anesthesia is usually not needed and the provisional denture can then be relined. Once all tissues are healed, a variety of prosthetic techniques can be applied to place a clip into the existing denture or fabricated into a new denture.

Important Considerations for the TPS Screw System

Securing the four implants within 48 to 72 hours is very important. If the laboratory cannot perform this service, then the dentist must anticipate and make an acrylic splint at the time of implant placement. Lack of splinting, premature loading, or perforation of the cortical plates certainly decreases the chances for successful integration. The longest span of the superstructure bar should be in the midline and the bar should be placed over the ridge. This eliminates a large bulk of acrylic to the lingual. The bar should also be positioned so that the denture can rotate symmetrically about it. Hygiene is a critical aspect with all implants and conventional prostheses. For this reason, the bar should be well above the gingiva so that hygiene can easily be maintained. Attempts should also be made to keep the bar level with the jaw. The denture should have some relief around the distal copings so that occlusal pressures are not placed on these implants, but the denture can rotate around the mesiobar.

The TPS System can be used as a single tooth replacement, as well as for fixed bridgework. This use has not been endorsed by the ITI to date. When the TPS Screw is used in this fashion, it is left out of function until integration occurs, which is 2 to 3 months in the mandible and 4 to 6 months in the maxilla. A temporary prosthesis can be relieved so that there is no function on the implant when placed in visible or esthetic areas. Since the implant is transmucosal, care in determining the implant placement with the line of draw or parallelism to the other teeth must be carefully planned. The final crown can be fabricated and cemented to the implant head or held in place with the occlusal screws available.

Discussion

The implant design, biocompatibility, and surface coating are well tolerated. Initial stability, immediate splinting, and prevention of premature overloading are critical to the integration of the implants. The fact that four splinted implants are used ensures distribution of forces over a large surface area and protection against lateral forces. It must also be remembered that the prosthesis is not entirely implant-borne. The saddle areas are tissue-borne and there is some tolerance for movement around the clip which is secured to the bar. The prosthesis is easily removed and the superstructure can be hygienically maintained with simple techniques. Although not a common problem, if an implant were to fail or not integrate, the superstructure can be easily removed, and the failed or problematic implant treated or removed without affecting the functional ability of the prosthesis. Some clinicians believe that since this is a one-stage procedure and the implant is not submerged, that there may be some potential reason for the implant to fail. There does not appear to be any correlation to the success or failure of any implant that is one-stage or submerged. The problems appear to arise as a result of improper surgical technique or premature loading.

Numerous international centers have participated in studies utilizing the TPS system for overdentures.[4, 5] It has been established that the success rate for each implant are 94.08% and 96.26%, respectively. It is interesting to note that in the longitudinal studies, the vast majority of implants which did not survive failed in the first 12 months. This leads one to suspect that poor surgical technique or inability to stabilize the implants caused the failure. Once integration occurs and the system functions, long-term success becomes highly predictable.

ITI HOLLOW-CYLINDER IMPLANTS

ITI, recognizing that different functions and stresses to which implants are exposed play an important part in implant design, sought to develop a series of endosteal implants capable of distributing the high dynamic forces that would have to be tolerated. At the same time, the implant system would be developed incorporating the principles of maximum available bone, biologically favorable materials, and surface finish. ITI was committed to single-stage implant systems with ease of prosthetic components to facilitate impression taking, as well as prosthetic construction. All ITI implants have incorporated the ability to be screw-retained for periodic examination of the implant and tissue health.

The quality, quantity, and shape of the maxilla and mandible are highly variable. Because of this, a series of implants evolved which could satisfy the objectives of the ITI system and the anatomic variations. Each design form was such that dynamic load extremes would be well distributed and shear forces minimized.[6] In order to achieve this goal, a geometric shape was chosen such that the physiologic forces are optimally transmitted in three dimensions (see

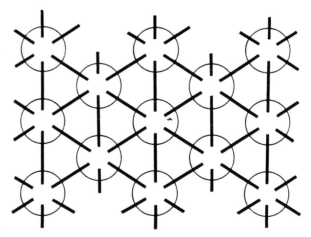

FIG 20–6.
The geometric layout of the perforations in the cylinder (planar projection) of the ITI Hollow-Cylinder Implant system. The perforations are important because they allow bone bridges to the inner core that reduce the shear forces between bone and implant.

Fig 20–6). Further important factors necessary for success were sufficient primary stability, precision fit of the implant in its prepared site, maximum contact area of implant to bone, minimal bone loss, and an implant surface that promotes bone interface.[7, 8]

From these factors a hollow geometric, titanium plasma-sprayed surface was developed. Three shapes have evolved, the F, K, and H. Each is designed to best serve the appropriate anatomic area (see Fig 20–7).

Surgical Indications and Placement Procedures

As discussed previously, aseptic surgical technique and careful handling of both hard and soft tissue are imperative for all implant surgery. Preoperative administration of antibiotics and steroids are the operator's choice. An intraoral surgical preparation is advised.

The procedure is done in the office under local anesthesia or, if warranted, with adjunctive inhalation or intravenous sedation. Careful x-ray analysis and palpation play an important part in the initial assessment as to the anatomy and morphology of the area. A midcrestal incision is made and tissue is reflected both buccally and lingually to assess the ridge. Depending on the amount of bone available buccally and lingually and the predetermined bone height, the appropriate implant is selected.

For all Hollow-Cylinder Implants, the basic soft tissue incision and preparation of the alveolar ridges are the same. What varies is the technique and instrumentation for each of the implant designs. The choice of implant is dictated by the anatomy of the area into which the endosseous implant will be placed. Tables 20–2 and 20–3 list the indications and contraindications, bone requirements, and prosthetic applications for the hollow-cylinder implants.

All drilling procedures should be done with copious irrigation with sterile saline and performed between 600 and 800 rpm.

F Implant Surgical Procedure

Flap Preparation.—After obtaining satisfactory local anesthesia, the patient is prepared and draped. A midcrestal incision, centered over the proposed implant site, is made with a no. 15 scalpel blade. The incision is carried down through the mucoperiosteum to the bone and the flap is gently elevated with a periosteal elevator to provide conservative but adequate exposure of the alveolar ridge. Releasing incisions are used as indicated when exposure is inadequate or there is a chance of tearing the flap. Lingual exposure should be limited only to provide adequate assessment of bone dimension and guidance for surgery. In the mandibular posterior region, cognizance of the lingual nerve is important.

Alveolar Ridge Assessment.—Frequently, when the flap is reflected, spinous processes or knife-edge ridge crests are revealed. Alveoplasty can be performed conservatively with a bone file or slow-speed side-cutting bur with copious irrigation.

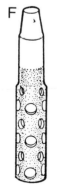 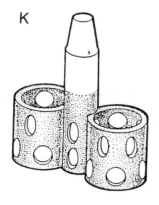 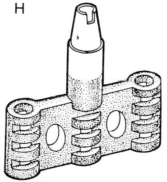

FIG 20–7.
Illustration of the F, K, and H design ITI Hollow-Cylinder Implant types.

TABLE 20–2.

ITI Hollow-Cylinder Dental Implant Series: Site, Indications, Contraindications, Complications

Implant	Site(s)	Indications	Contraindications	Complications
F	Maxilla or Mandible (anterior or posterior)	Single tooth replacement Fixed bridge prosthetics Lower denture support and retention	Inadequate bone dimension Inadequate oral hygiene/compliance Recent extraction (<4 mo) General poor health Oral pathology/history of radiation therapy to site	Oversized receptor site, poor primary stability Premature function; poor osseous integration (<8 wk mandible) <12 wk maxilla Bone necrosis secondary to drill >800 rpm, or poor irrigation technique
H	Maxilla or Mandible (posterior)	Narrow alveolar ridges Fixed-removable prosthetics	Inadequate bone dimensions Inadequate oral hygiene/compliance Recent extraction (<4 mo) General poor health Oral pathology/history of radiation therapy to site Patient unable to open mouth adequately for surgery	Oversized receptor site, primary stability Perforation of buccal/lingual cortex Premature function; poor osseous integration Bone necrosis secondary to drill >800 rpm, or poor irrigation technique Damage to neurovascular structures Perforation to maxillary sinus/nasal antrum
K	Maxilla or Mandible (posterior)	Single tooth replacement Abutment for fixed or removable prosthetics	Inadequate bony dimensions Inadequate oral hygiene/compliance Recent extraction (<4 mo) General poor health Oral pathology/history of radiation therapy to site	Oversized receptor site, poor primary stability Perforation of buccal/lingual cortex Premature function; poor osseous integration Bone necrosis secondary to drill >800 rpm, or inadequate irrigation Damage to neurovascular structures Perforation of maxillary sinus/nasal antrum

Creation of a plateau of adequate width is desired such that the most superior portion of the receptor site remains round and does not erode into the buccal or lingual plates on preparation. Vertical measurement for implant selection must be modified after alveoplasty has been completed.

Implant Site Preparation.—The first step is placement of purchase points on the crest of the ridge in the designated positions with a no. 4 or 6 round bur and the aid of a surgical template, if available. A twist drill is used to initiate a 4-mm-deep pilot hole with angulation guided by a prefabricated template or a visual estimate of angulation with respect to the available bone at prospective abutments. The drilling depth is correct when the shoulder of the drill is level with the alveolar crest. The operator's thumb or forefinger should cradle the ridge to aid in

TABLE 20–3.

ITI Hollow Cylinder Dental Implant Series: Minimal Skeletal Dimensions, Postoperative Function and Splinting Guidelines and Prosthetic Options

Implant Series	Implant Dimensions (mm)		Minimum Bone Requirements (mm) Buccal (Facial), Vertical* Lingual (Palatal)†	Postoperative Function and Splinting	Prosthetics
	Diameter	Length			
F	3.5, 4.8	7.0, 9.0 11.0, 15.0, 17.0	5.5, 6.0 length + 2 countersink + 2 anatomic clearance; 11.0 minimum	Nonfunction Maxilla >12 wk Mandible >8 wk	Fixed prosthetics: single tooth replacement or abutment for fixed bridgework Removable prosthetics:Dolder bar or similar technique for denture stabilization and retention
H	3.0 wide 15.0 long	3.0 head 4.0, 5.5 neck 5.5 body	5.0 + 5.5 implant body + 3.0 countersink + 2.0 anatomic clearance + 2.0 drill taper; 12.5 minimum	Nonfunction Maxilla >12 wk Mandible >8 wk	Fixed or removable prosthetics; posterior abutment
K	4.0 wide 10.0 long	3.0 head 4.0, 5.5 neck 5.5 body	6.0 + 5.5 implant body + 3.0 countersink + 2.0 anatomic clearance + 2.0 drill taper; 12.5 minimum	Nonfunction Maxilla >12 wk Mandible >8 wk	Fixed-removable prosthetics; posterior abutments

*Allow clearance of at least 2 to 3 mm from neurovascular structures, maxillary sinuses, nasal antrum, and inferior border of the mandible.
†Allow at least 1 mm buccal (labial) and 1 mm lingual cortex.

centering the drill and for detection of thinning of the cortex before perforation.

The site preparation is then completed with the end-cutting trephine mill of appropriate diameter using the standard guidelines for cutting speed and irrigation. The trephine has five rows of perforations that correspond to the implant length and can be utilized for simultaneous depth measurement as the site is being prepared. These levels also correspond to the color-coated depth gauge supplied. The trephine is sunk to the selected depth with the trephine depth holes showing their upper half when viewed at the level of the alveolar crest (see Fig 20–8).

Implant Placement.—The implant is passed sterilely to the operator, who only handles the implant by the head or neck region. Meticulous care is required to avoid contamination of the implant surface. The edges of the implant are rounded to ease insertion. The implant is press-fitted into place ini-tially with finger pressure and finally seated by a gentle tap with the implant insertion tool and mallet. This press-fit of the cylindrical section into the precisely prepared implant site provides primary stability.

Flap Closure.—The surgical site is irrigated with saline and the flap is repositioned and sutured with 3-0 silk under minimal tension. Excess tissue around the posts can be modified with a tissue punch or scalpel blade. A postoperative radiograph is recommended to confirm placement.

The implant should remain out of direct function for a period of 8 to 12 weeks and thus should be shielded by modifying an existing prosthesis or fabricating a temporary appliance. Suture removal, clinical examination, and oral hygiene are evaluated at 1 week. A follow-up schedule is outlined with the patient.

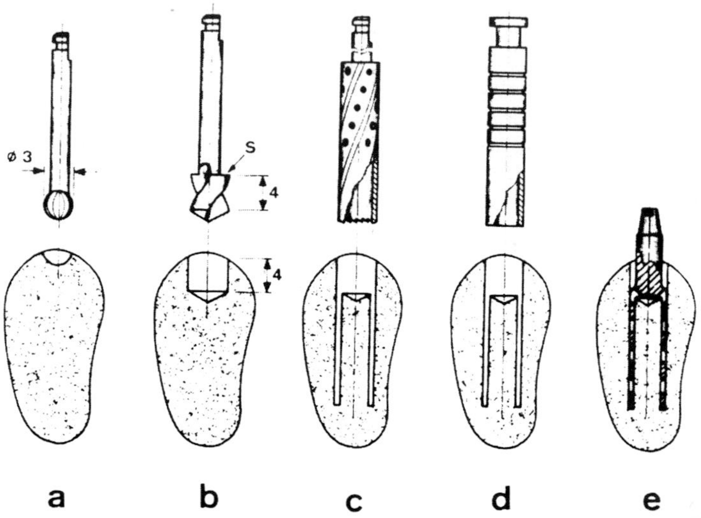

FIG 20–8.
Progressive steps of the surgery technique for the F design Hollow-Cylinder Implant. See text for details.

a   b   c   d   e

K Implant Surgical Procedure

Implant Site Preparation.—The first step is to drill the hole to receive the middle cylinder of the implant. The hole is made with the standard 3-mm-diameter drill. The depth is correct when the shoulder of the drill is level with the bone surface (Fig 20–9).

The peg on the drill guide for the outer holes fits into the 3-mm hole. The holes for the outer two cylinders of the K-type implant can then be prepared using the appropriate trephine mill. Once again, the depth is correct when the shoulder of the mill is level with the upper surface of the guide. As a further safety measure, the mill shaft acts as a stop, to prevent the shoulder from sinking more than 3.5 mm below the alveolar crest. Once the first outer cylinder site is prepared, the expandable temporary fixation device is fitted and clamped into place by tightening the central screw. This provides stability for the guide and allows parallel preparation of the second outer cylinder.

The depth gauge can be used to confirm that adequate depth throughout the profile has been obtained and that the shoulder of the implant will be countersunk 3 mm below the crest of the ridge. Bone fragments and debris should be thoroughly flushed from the receptor site with sterile saline irrigant.

H Implant Surgical Procedure

Implant Site Preparation.—The procedure begins with sinking of the first 3-mm-diameter hole; the no. 1 drill guide helps stabilize the first 3-mm twist drill. The correct depth has been attained when the shoulder of the drill (S) is level with the upper surface of the guide (Fig 20–10). As illustrated, the guide can now be stabilized by means of a peg (A) inserted into the first hole; the second outer hole can then be drilled. A second peg (B) is placed in this hole and the center 3-mm hole is completed.

The no. 1 drill guide is left in position. The drill guide has four smaller holes between the larger 3-mm-diameter drill guide holes. These guide holes are for preparation of the channel for the connecting arms. The four holes should be drilled with the 1.3-mm special flute twist drill (C). The holes should be sunk to the depth stop on the drill. They are then at approximately the same depth as the 3-mm holes.

The no. 1 drill guide is replaced by the no. 2 guide with its two rigid guide pins. A further six holes must then be sunk with the drill (C). The axis of these six holes are each one-half diameter displaced from the axis of the previous four 1.3-mm-diameter holes prepared. The result is a trench with wavy inner walls joining the three larger holes.

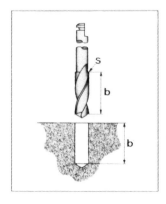
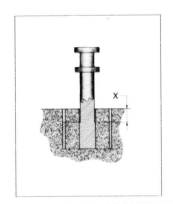
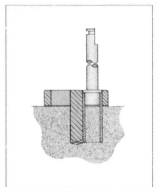
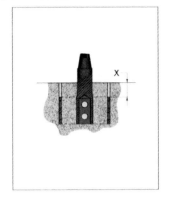

FIG 20–9.
The progressive steps of the surgery technique for the K design Hollow-Cylinder Implant. See text for details.

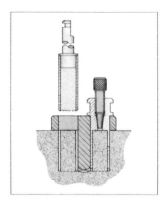
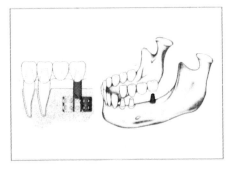

The depth gauge can be used to confirm that adequate depth throughout the profile has been obtained and that the shoulder of the implant will be countersunk 3 mm below the crest of the ridge. Bone fragments and debris should be thoroughly flushed from the receptor site with sterile saline irrigant.

Prosthetic Technique

All of the hollow-cylinder implant heads are identical. They have an internal threaded head with a small slot into which a prefabricated high-fusing gold coping can be placed. A small degree of tolerance between the implant head and the coping acts as a stress breaker. Each kit comes complete with

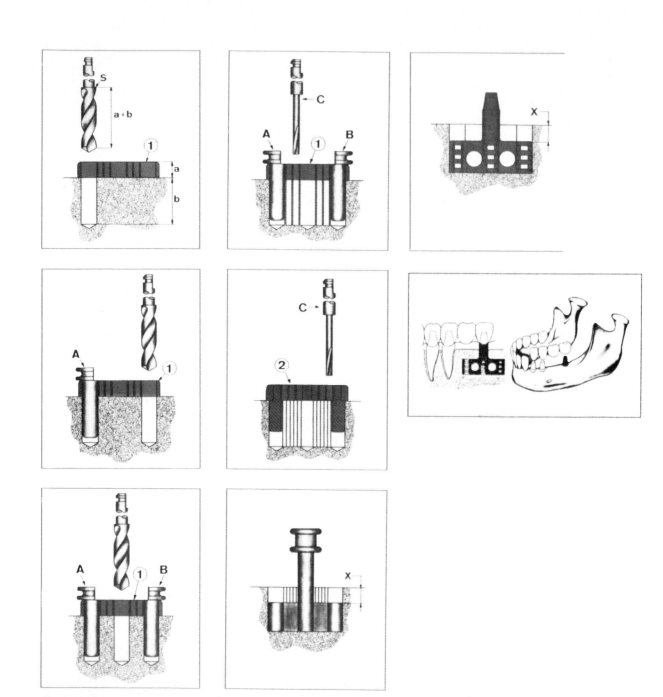

FIG 20–10.
The step-by-step surgical technique for the H design Hollow-Cylinder Implant. See text for details.

transfer copings, as well as master dies. After the implants have integrated, the transfer coping is placed over the implant head and an impression is taken. The laboratory can then fabricate a master model utilizing the master die. Wax-ups can be done over the gold coping maintaining internal accuracy, and standard crown and bridge techniques can be utilized. The internal threads permit the securing of the crown so that removal is possible. When natural teeth are involved in the restoration, precision or semiprecision attachments may be considered so as not to affect the removal of crowns permanently cemented.

Discussion

The Hollow-Cylinder Implant has been highly successful. A greater degree of clinical skill and diagnosis is necessary, however, to ensure long-term success. With both the F and K implants, the fragility of the core can lead either to an avascular necrosis or fracture within the trephine. A fractured core is best removed rather than used as a free graft. Another potential problem is that a perforation, either through the cortical plates or into the sinus, may induce a soft tissue ingrowth within the cylinder. For this reason, a careful assessment of the anatomic structures is necessary to position the implant totally within bone. The theory that the vents permit vascular communication to the core area and maintain a greater degree of vitality to the bone-implant interface is sound; however, many endosseous implants are plagued with a certain amount of crestal bone loss or disease. If this occurs to the depth of the vents, a difficult hygiene problem may arise.

It also must be noted that this is a one-stage implant with a fixed head that protrudes through the gingiva. Care must be taken that the implant is protected during healing. Endosseous implants need to be placed in areas of maximum bone and the direction of the implant placement is determined by the anatomy. The fixed head does not permit a significant degree of angulation to maintain parallelism when multiple implants or natural tooth abutments

	F–3	F–1	TPS	TPS	K	H
Outer diameter (mm)	3.5	4.0	3.5	4.0	–	–
Insert-length (mm)	18/16/14/ 12/10/8	18/16/14/ 12/10/8	20/17/14 11/8	20/17/14 11/8	8.5	8.5
Length over all (mm)	26/24/22 20/18/16	26/24/22 20/18/16	26/23/20 17/14	26/23/20 17/14	13.5/15	13.5/15
Width (mm)	–	–	–	–	4.0	3.0
Length (mm)	–	–	–	–	10.4	15.0

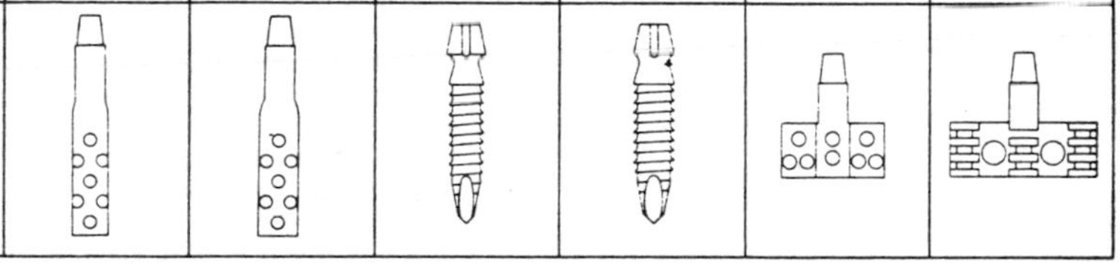

FIG 20–11.
Summary chart providing overall nomenclature and dimensions for the TPS Screw and ITI Hollow-Cylinder endosteal dental implants.

are utilized. In cases of severely angled implants, telescopic copings may need to be used which adds to the prosthetic component of the procedure.

These systems are best utilized when easy access to the patient's mouth is available to accommodate the instrumentation and when a sufficient amount of bone exists away from vital structures to ensure proper placement (see Fig 20–11).

Acknowledgments

Dr. Charles Babbush initiated and documented much of the information available today on the ITI systems. Dr David Altobelli provided much of the product information. Paul McMinn, C.D.T., Product Manager for Synthes, U.S.A., assisted with the prosthetic aspects.

REFERENCES

1. Ledermann PD: ITI-International Team für orale Implantologie, sechsjährige klinische Erfahrungen mit dem Titan-Plasma beschichteten ITI-Schraubenimplant in der Regio interforaminalis des Unterkiefers. *Schweiz Monatsschr Zahnheilk* 1983; 93(suppl):1070.

2. Schroder A, Stitch H, Straumann F, et al: Deposition of osteocementum at the surface of the load-bearing implant. *Schweiz Monatsschr Zahnheilk* 1978; 88:1051–1058.

3. Lederman PD: Titanium-coated screw implants as alloplastic endosteal retention element in the edentulous problematic mandible (1 + 11). *Quintessence Int* 1981; 12:484–491.

4. Babbush CA, Kent JN, Misiek DJ: Titanium plasma sprayed (TPS) screw implants for the reconstruction of the edentulous mandible. *J Oral Maxillofac Surg* 1986; 44:274–282.

5. Babbush CA, Kent JN: *United States Clinical Documentation.* Burlingame, Calif, Colmed, Ltd, 1984.

6. Sutter F, Schroeder A, Straumann F: *Engineering and Design Aspects of the ITI Hollow Basket Implants.* Heidelberg, Hiiting Verlag. 1981, pp 50–59.

7. Schroeder A, Pohler O, Sutter F: Tissue reaction to a titanium hollow cylinder implant with titanium sprayed layer surface. *Schweiz Monatsschr Zahnheilk* 1976; 86:713–727.

8. Hahn H, Palich W: Preliminary evaluation of porous metal surfaced titanium for orthopedic implants. *J Biomed Mater Res* 1970; 4:571.

Chapter 21

The Flexiroot Implant System

Andras G. Haris, D.M.D.

THE CONCEPT

The Flexiroot dental implant system was developed on the basis of the CODAR concept (*c*omplete *o*sseointegrated *d*ento*a*lveolar *r*eplacement) which is the replacement of the dental functional unit (lamina dura, periodontal ligament, dental root) with an osseointegrated implant. The Flexiroot dental implant system, because of its distinctive design, promotes the development and maintenance of osseointegration and mimics the natural dental functional unit in its entirety (Fig 21–1).

Components

The Flexiroot implant replaces the complete dentoalveolar unit, not just the dental root. A controlled mobility pattern is used to produce a range of motion similar to natural teeth. The concept uses physiologic principles to promote primary bone healing and biomechanical principles to ensure functional maintenance of the direct bone-implant interface. Histologic monitoring of the development of the osseous interface is carried out via the implant test kit (see Appendix) to prevent premature loading of the implant. Maximum esthetics can be achieved because no components of the implant are visible in the oral cavity. The conceptual changes incorporated in the Flexiroot implant system were developed jointly by Drs. Andras G. Haris and Peter G. Mozsary.[1, 2]

THE IMPLANT

The Flexiroot dental implant system simulates the natural dentition, and is applicable in every conceivable prosthetic situation where the replacement of the natural dental functional unit is required due to loss of teeth (see Fig 21–1).

The Flexiroot is a clinically proven two-stage implant system that provides not just direct bony interface but is equipped with an internally positioned artificial periodontal ligament (the flexible element), which is enclosed in a precisely fitting titanium component, and is able to provide limited mobility similar to the natural periodontal ligament. The design allows the changing of the mobility pattern of the implant and achievement of different degrees of movement. This mobility pattern allows the implant to be connected to other implant systems or to periodontally involved teeth (Fig 21–2). The flexible internal element allows motion up to the degree where metal-to-metal contact prevents further compression.

Titanium is used as the metal component because of its biocompatibility with bone and soft tissues. Titanium implants, in any shape or form, may develop direct interface with bone if they are protected from excessive mobility during the healing phase; however, for the cylindrical threaded implant, after loading, functional stress accumulation occurs at the edges of the threads. The Flexiroot system is designed with inside-outside radius threads to prevent this accumulation of stresses at the thread tips in bone.[1, 2]

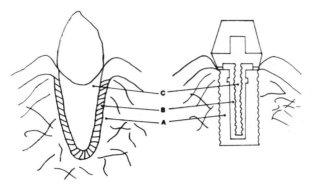

FIG 21–1.
The Flexiroot implant system replaces the entire dental functional unit. *(A)* lamina dura–osseointegrated part of the Flexiroot *(B)* Periodontal ligament–high-density polyethylene liner. *(C)* Root center screw.

The shock-absorbing unit installed within the Flexiroot system is composed of ultra-high-molecular-weight high-density polyethylene and represents the artificial periodontal ligament (see Fig 21–1) which transfers occlusal forces to the radicular portion of the implant unit. The shock-absorbing element does not have to be changed during the life of the implant. By introducing the concept of limited or controlled mobility, this system not only resolves the problems commonly associated with overly rigid implant-bone systems but also resolves the difficulties that occur in overly permissive mobility implant systems.

The design of the prosthetic implant heads promotes maintenance of gingival health, and allows placement of dental superstructures which cover all of the supragingival parts of the implant, achieving maximal esthetics.

A novel test implant, in vivo bone stain, and biopsy technique complement the Flexiroot system and provide histologic information about the maturing of the bone at the developing interface to prevent premature loading (see Appendix).

Additional features of the Flexiroot implant system include simplified surgical placement, simplified prosthodontics with two-piece angled heads that rotate 360 degrees, flexi-line attachments, a test implant kit, inserting instruments with specially calibrated internal irrigation burs that fit any low-speed, latch-type handpiece, and an internal irrigation system. Table 21–1 provides further information about the Flexiroot system. Over 5 years of clinical trials with the implant reveal satisfactory service.

The essential elements of the Flexiroot system are a threaded, hollow cylindrical endosseous screw, a high-density polyethylene (HDPE) inner sleeve, and a threaded internal post connected to a supragingival head (Fig 21–3).

The thread of the titanium hollow cylinder is provided with inside and outside radii. The inside of

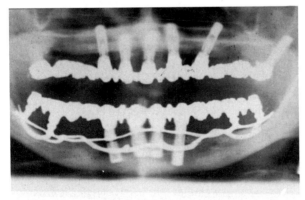

FIG 21–2.
The mobility of the Flexiroot implant provides for use with other types of implants. The compatibility is especially important in complex reconstruction when various methods must be used in combinations, e.g., sinus elevation, ridge augmentation, subperiosteal and Flexiroot implants.

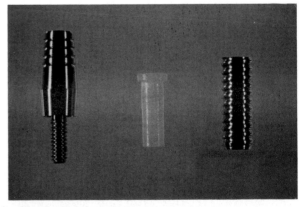

FIG 21–3.
The components of the Flexiroot implant. *Right to left,* threaded hollow-cylinder endosteal screw, polyethylene inner sleeve, and threaded superstructure gingival head.

TABLE 21–1.

The Flexiroot Dental Implant System

Product name	Flexiroot dental implant system (also known as complete osseointegrated dento-alveolar replacement, FAIR implant system)
Manufacturer/ supplier	Facial Alveo-dental Implant Rehabilitation, Inc. 101 Bala Avenue Bala Cynwyd, PA 19004
Material composition	Commercially pure, medical-grade titanium and ultra-high-molecular-weight, high-density polyethylene
Starter kit	Flexiroot implant system starter kit: 9 complete Flexiroot implants; all inserting instruments including special calibrated internal irrigation drills; an internal irrigation system; technique manual; test implant kit $1,975
Implant system	One complete Flexiroot implant system including titanium casing, sleeve insert, implant head with internal screw available in lengths of 9, 11, 14, or 17 mm $150

the hollow cylinder is designed to accept the HDPE sleeve through a tight friction grip; rotation is controlled by an internal hexagon. The diameter of the screw is 3.5 mm and the implant is available in lengths of 8, 11, 14, and 17 mm.

The polyethylene insert is threaded inside and has an outside retention rim (see Fig 21–3). The oc-clusal end of the sleeve that will partially overlap the occlusal surface of the endosteal screw (Fig 21–4). It fits tightly against the side of the hollow metallic cylinder screw and is open at the apical portion. The superstructure has a threaded extension on its apical end that screws into the internal HDPE sleeve. An undercut is machined on the apical end of the super-structure to partially cover the occlusal rim of the HDPE sleeve (Figs 21–1 and 21–5). The supragin-

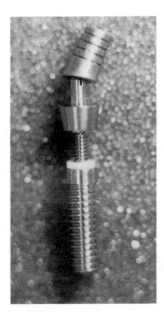

FIG 21–4.
The assembled components of the Flexiroot implant showing a two-piece rotating angulated head.

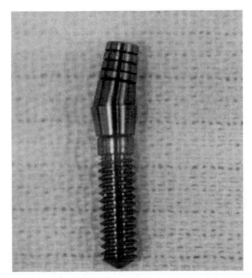

FIG 21–5.
Assembled Flexiroot implant with angulated head.

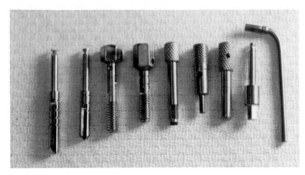

FIG 21–6.
Instrumentation. *Left to right,* internally irrigated channel drills (two lengths), bone taps (two lengths), implant positioner, sleeve inserter, sinus elevator, Allen wrenches.

gival part of the head (superstructure) is made in three different designs: a standard head (one piece); an angled head (two pieces); the upper portion, which rotates 360 degrees around a fixed post; and a fixed detachable head.

Instrumentation

The simplified instrument kit contains the following: an internally irrigated channel drill; tapping instrument; implant positioner; sinus floor elevator, depth guide and paralleling device; sleeve inserter; Allen wrench (motorized and hand-driven); and an adaptor for the handpiece (see Table 21-1). All instruments are made of stainless steel (Fig 21–6). The implant test kit for histologic assessment includes a test implant, bone tap, implant positioner, and trephine implant remover (Fig 21–7).

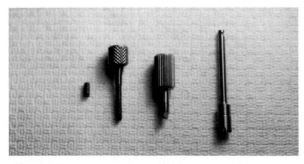

FIG 21–7.
Test implant kit. *Left to right,* test implant, bone tap, implant positioner, implant remover (trephine).

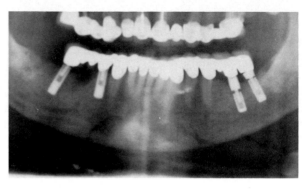

FIG 21–8.
Radiograph of a posterior partially edentulous mandible restored with Flexiroot implants and fixed prostheses in combination with natural teeth abutments.

INDICATIONS

The Flexiroot system can be used in any situation where a sufficient amount of bone is present, or can be created, to provide stable abutments for the fixation of any type of prosthodontic device (Fig 21–8). The ideal width of available bone is 5 mm or more and the depth 2 mm longer than the length of the selected implant. When there is not enough bone available to envelop the implant, special techniques may be used to correct the osseous deficiencies such as sinus elevation (Fig 21–9), retropositioning of the mental foramen, bone grafting, and bone augmentation.

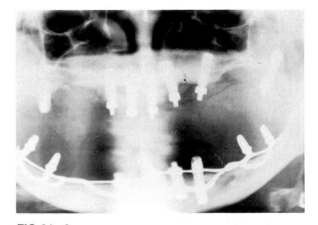

FIG 21–9.
The Flexiroot implant system used in a sinus elevation procedure showing the new bone growth which has occurred at the apex of the posterior maxillary implants.

The implant can be used as a freestanding replacement of a missing tooth or group of teeth; retention for an overdenture; as an abutment(s) for a fixed prosthesis in combination with natural teeth or other implants, and for the completely edentulous patient. The Flexiroot dental implant system should not be used in patients who cannot properly care for themselves and cannot follow postoperative instructions.

SURGICAL PROCEDURES

First-Stage Surgery

1. Sterile technique should be enforced.
2. The gingivoperiosteal flap should be a 1-cm crescent-shaped split flap with a large gingival and small periosteal base. The periosteal reflection should be slightly larger than the diameter of the implant to facilitate periosteal bone formation around the implant.
3. A no. 8 round bur in a contra-angle handpiece should be used to perforate the cortical bone and create a guide hole.
4. The final cavity is prepared with the 3.5-mm-diameter internal irrigation drill (Fig 21–10). The depth of the cavity should be equal to the length of

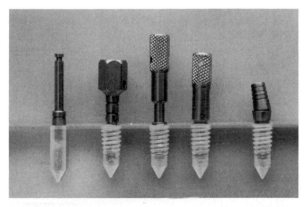

FIG 21–10.
The stages of surgical placement of the Flexiroot implant. *Left to right,* cavity preparation with the internal irrigation drill; hand tapping of the implant socket; implant positioning with the screwdriver; insertion of the high-density polyethylene sleeve with the sleeve inserter; the completely assembled implant.

the implant. During cavity preparation, copious irrigation is essential. The preparation should be completed slowly in ten to 12 or more increments using low-speed, high-torque or gear-reduction handpieces (1,500–1,700 rpm). Internal and external irrigation is recommended.

5. The cavity is tapped with a hand or motorized tap (see Fig 21–10). The tap should be turned backward several times during the threading. Hand tapping or extremely low speed (5–15 rpm) is used.

6. The screwdriver is inserted into the endosteal part of the implant while the implant is in the package. DO NOT TOUCH the implant with instruments or hands. The implant is driven into the cavity and the screwdriver removed. The top of the implant should be 1 mm under the bone. It is permissible to insert the implant with the polyethylene insert in place (see Fig 21–10). When that is done, the insert should be at the same height of the bone or 1 mm beneath.

7. One or two atraumatic sutures are used to close the flap.

Clinical Considerations

An edentulous area is seldom flat and since it is preferable that the implant be surrounded by bone, alveoplasty may be needed. Knife-edge ridges have to be trimmed to gain a flat area at least 4 mm in diameter. Alveolar bone grafting also may be used.

If the usable height of mandible is less than 8 mm the preparation should be stopped at the inferior border and the periosteum of the inferior border elevated with small curets through the cavity. After tapping, implant placement will keep the periosteum in an elevated position and bone formation will take place 4 to 6 months after surgery.

Narrow maxillary ridges present a special problem, especially in the maxillary anterior where the buccal plate of the alveolus has been resorbed or broken away by the surgical extraction. In these cases, we recommend the use of an 11-, 14-, or 17-mm implant leaving the occlusal half of the implant on the buccal area exposed and covering it with hydroxylapatite to achieve a healed barrier of dense connective tissue and hydroxylapatite. At least two thirds of the implant should be in bone.

The proximity of the mandibular canal may interfere with implant placement and nerve transpositioning may have to be performed as a separate procedure. Decortication of the lateral wall up to the molar area and retropositioning of the mental foramen is the procedure of choice. The first-stage implant surgery can be performed 2 or 3 weeks after the nerve transposition.

The amount of bone between the maxillary sinus floor and the maxillary ridge may be insufficient and require the use of a sinus lift procedure. The sinus floor bone is measured on a panoramic radiograph and socket preparation is stopped before penetrating the cortical plate of the floor of the sinus. The socket former instrument is inserted into the cavity and with hand pressure or careful malleting the sinus bone cortex is fractured. The mucoperiosteum of the sinus is elevated with a curet. Extreme care should be exercised not to perforate the sinus or detach the cortical fragment. The implant is inserted in the usual manner. Bone regeneration will occur from the osteogenic potential of the sinus wall and the bone, with bone formation being detected on the x-ray films (see Fig 21–9). Patients with compromised bone structure such as osteoporosis or with previous radiation therapy or osteomyelitis may have significant changes in bone metabolism, and in these medically compromised patients the test implant technique should be used (see Appendix).

Second-Stage Surgery

Four months after the placement of the implants, healing and maturation is usually completed and the implants exposed. The gingiva covering the implant is anesthetized, the implant is located with a probe or template and a circular incision or punch biopsy to the periosteum is made and the tissue removed exposing the occlusal surface of the implant. Tissue fragments or overlying bone have to be removed. As a practical manner, a midline horizontal incision provides sufficient uncovering of the implant.

The inserting instrument is driven into the plastic insert until it locks. The plastic is placed in the endosteal implant and pressed until it snaps into the retention groove of the implant (see Fig 21–1). All fluid must be removed from the internal implant cylinder which must be dry before inserting the sleeve.

Following removal of the inserting instrument, the superstructure is driven into the plastic with the screwdriver until a tight lock is achieved (Fig 21–11). Before completing tightening of the screw, the gingiva should be checked to ensure no gingival tissue is trapped between the plastic and the superstructure. The gingiva is closed with one or two sutures, if needed.

Clinical Considerations

In the Flexiroot system, we do not use a cover or healing cap as bone growth will not occur in the central implant cavity. On occasion, we have observed bone coverage on the edge of the implant; this bone is easily removed. The implant central cavity is usually filled with connective tissue which is easily removed.

Narrow attached gingiva should surround the intragingival part to assure the development of the epithelial seal. If the buccolingual dimension is insufficient, punch excision should be avoided and an incision parallel with the ridge is recommended.

In the molar area of the partially edentulous mandible, the thickness of the gingivoperiosteum is sometimes less than 2 mm, and therefore the titanium collar will only be partially covered. This condition is functionally satisfactory; gingivoplasty may be performed, however, if needed for esthetic reasons. Subgingival wedge resection or gingivectomy is recommended if the gingiva is excessively thick.

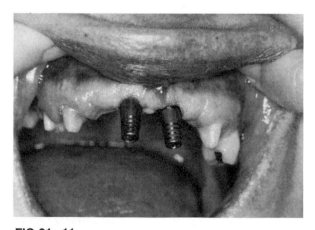

FIG 21–11.
Completed Flexiroot implants in situ following assembly after second-stage surgery.

Patient Evaluation—Case Selection

The placement of oral implants involves delicate and sometimes extensive surgery which at times necessitates hospitalization. Most oral implants, however, are placed in the dental office so the evaluation of the patient becomes the duty of the dentist who performs the surgery. After the surgical phase is completed, the patient generally receives a complex prosthetic structure supported by implants or implants and natural dentition; hence, the oral structures must be carefully judged from the standpoint of prosthetic reconstruction as well.

An implant planning package should include the following: trial setup—a preliminary wax try-in checks the esthetics of the restoration; clear stent—the stent or template acts as a guide for proper placement of the implants and angulation of the abutment heads; corrective panoramic tray—the tray is fabricated with six strategically placed 5-mm stainless wire segments or balls. It is used intraorally during the panoramic radiograph. The wire segments act as a reference to help correct the measurements taken on the processed film. Custom tray—a custom tray is used after the implant abutments are cemented into place. This impression facilitates placement of the brass analogs in the master model for construction of the restoration.

There is no typical implant case. The chronological age of the patient is not directly related to the success or failure of dental implants. However, in the process of establishing suitability, full consideration should be given to the patient's medical and dental status, and psychological, social, and habitual patterns.

PROSTHETIC REHABILITATION

There are many osseointegrated systems on the market today. Indeed, to achieve direct interface development between the bone and the titanium dental implant is a relatively easy task. The maintenance of the interface is considerably more difficult to achieve. In the process of interface maintenance, the surface geometry of the implant, as well as the attenuation of occlusal forces, plays an extremely impor-tant role. Because of the flexible, but controlled, mobility pattern of the Flexiroot implant system, practitioners can proceed with the prosthetic reconstruction in much the same fashion as they do with natural abutment teeth. The high-density polyethylene insert transfers the majority of the masticatory forces to their most natural location, namely, to the surface of the root structure.

The architectural design of the implant prosthesis, however, plays an extremely important role in assuring a lasting result. Special prosthodontic care during the healing phase is important. The buried implants and the developing interface must be protected from excessive stress and pressure by using generous amounts of soft liners inside the dentures of a fully or partially edentulous patient. If the implants are used as abutments in a partially edentulous patient and a fixed temporary bridge is constructed, it is preferable that the surfaces of the pontics not come in contact with the healing tissues. Sanitary pontics should be used in the posterior area.

When joining natural teeth to implant supports the practitioner faces the difficulty of placing prosthetics on abutments that have vastly differing amounts of rigidity. The problems this creates can be cracking at the cement margins and subsequent leakage. Clinicians approach this problem with the use of stress breakers and copings.

Another difficulty encountered is that second-stage superstructure alignment can be off anywhere from a few degrees to a severe angle. This presents an undesirable situation and renders the prosthetic tasks overly complicated. Different implant manufacturers have offered a number of solutions, ranging from bendable attachments to complex ball-and-socket designs. The Flexiroot implant rotating head allows up to 28 degrees correction of angulation in any direction. An angle larger than 28 degrees will usually lead to implant failure. The Flexiroot implant system can be used with conventional crown and bridge techniques with minimal effort.

Technique

1. Insert the plastic sleeve.
2. Insert the plastic prosthetic superstructure.

3. Place the angled coping (titanium cup) in the direction where the correction is needed.

4. Take a rubber impression and transfer the titanium cups into the impression. Insert the analog of the prosthetic superstructure (Fig 21–12).

5. Fabricate model and dies.

6. (a) Wax up or use Duralay to cast the second part of the head (abutment) for precise angulation (or to correct the path of insertion); or (b) the stock titanium cup may be reshaped by the laboratory (and can be used); or (c) wax up the entire head superstructure.

7. Trim, finish.

The superstructure with custom-cast abutment is now ready to be inserted into the implant. Before insertion an impression of this custom abutment will facilitate fabrication of the marginal die.

Implants can be used as distal abutments to replace removable partial dentures with bridges, or as additional abutments in long-span bridges.

Technique

1. The preparation of the natural abutments should be completed by the time of second-stage surgery.

2. An impression is taken using rubber base material with the titanium cups in place but not cemented. The titanium cups stay in the impression. As an alternative, the titanium cups are cemented and corrected for parallelism and gingival margin.

3. The occlusal table should not be larger than the largest diameter of the gingival part of the implant. Occlusal interference must be avoided.

4. It is mandatory that the prosthodontic effort achieve an absolutely passive fit of the prosthesis placed over the abutment fixtures.

5. After rechecking (3) and (4), the bridge is cemented.

If one-piece implant heads are used, a wait of at least 1 week after the second-stage surgery is recommended for adequate healing of the periosteal tissues. Then the dentist may prepare the head of the implant for parallelism. Optimal healing takes 6 weeks. During that time, the patient may wear the temporary prosthetic appliance, which obviously has to be modified to incorporate the new abutment heads. Because proper parallelism rarely can be achieved prior to modification of the posts, the part of the prosthesis which fits over the new head may be hollowed out and relined with a conventional self-curing acrylic. The head, during the relining process, should be generously lubricated and the relined bridge removed prior to the setting of the relining medium, reinserting the prosthesis several times while final polymerization occurs. If the patient wears a removable partial prosthesis during the healing period, the construction of an acrylic temporary bridge is recommended.

During cementation of the temporary bridge, special consideration must be given to the metallic implant heads. Only a very soft temporary cement, for example, Opotow, should be used over the implant heads because the metallic heads contain no natural moisture. Frequently the bridge crowns break loose from the natural abutments and the bridge remains fixed only to the implant head. This situation creates an undesirable load distribution and can culminate in implant failure. With use of the soft temporary cement, the bridge is easily removed and recemented. During construction of the final fixed prosthesis, the hexagonal hole inside the implant head may be filled with a loosely fitting cast post that is part of the overlay crown and will provide ex-

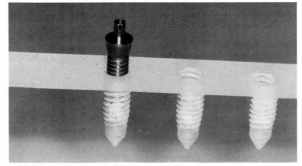

FIG 21–12.
The Flexiroot plaster analog head for prosthetic construction.

tra retention. It is also possible to fill the hole with cement during the final fixation rather than create an extra post. The utilization of detachable fixed bridgework that can be screwed on is also possible for the partially edentulous patient.

Follow-up Care

Meticulous plaque control is mandatory. Daily use of floss and proxy brush is recommended. Patients should be on a 3-month hygiene recall cycle and checked for calculus, gingivitis, and bone loss. Bone loss in the first 6 months is normal if it does not exceed 1 mm, but it rarely occurs because the radial surface of the screw threads creates extremely favorable stress distribution. If it is more than 1 mm, the gingiva has to be checked for infection and the occlusion for possible overload.

The Fully Edentulous Patient

In full upper or lower edentulous patients, six to ten fixtures are needed per arch for support of the fixed appliance. The second stage of surgery should proceed as previously described. Once the implant heads are positioned, one may proceed immediately with impression taking, but extreme care must be given to remove all the impression material from the gingival cuff area. If heads with removable titanium cones are used, the titanium cone must stay in the impression and be sent to the laboratory. If one-piece posts are used, the transfer die should be placed in the impression. In fully edentulous patients it may be desirable to use a detachable fixed prosthesis which can be fitted to the implant heads by an inner removable screw. These heads are available in the Flexiroot system. The fabrication of the prosthesis in this case would proceed first by the fabrication of a cast framework for the detachable fixed prosthesis. The distal portion of such a prosthesis may be cantilevered. During the impression process, the screws should remain in the posts. The final cast bar will have to have an uncovered occlusal portion so the screw may be placed properly into the head of the implants. The bar can be cast from any alloy certified for prosthetic reconstruction. The finished bar should not contact the tissues; enough space should

be left for thickness of acrylic underneath the bar as well as the abutment portions of the connecting structure. The metal framework should be kept light and, if extensive ridge resorption is present, used only to reinforce the prosthesis and firmly attach it to the implants.

The Overdenture Procedure

In fully edentulous patients, implants can be used to *stabilize* dentures. Used mostly in the mandible, the implants provide stability and the denture remains tissue-borne. A minimum of two implants have to be used in the canine-premolar area and the fabrication of the denture should be in the final try-in stage before the second-stage implant surgery is performed.

After the second-stage surgery is completed, a rubber-base impression is taken with the titanium cones in place, but not cemented. If removable cone posts are used, the titanium cones must stay in the impression and be sent to the laboratory. If a one-piece post is used, the transfer dies should be placed in the impression. The technician can make necessary adjustments in parallelism by modifying the sides of the titanium cups. The technician casts copings on the titanium or transfer dies and connects the copings with a Dolder-like bar. The denture is processed in the usual manner, except a 3-mm space has to be provided around the copings and the bar. Upon completion of processing, a permanent soft liner is polymerized in the space providing a tight, friction grip attachment between the cast and soft liner.

When the denture and casting are delivered, first the titanium cups are cemented on the central screw. When cementing the titanium cups, they should be placed in the casting. If the technician modified the titanium, there will be only one correct position, which must be maintained or the casting will not fit. As an alternative, the titanium cones may be cemented and handled as prepared teeth for the retention bar. The same procedure is followed as if one-piece posts were used.

Implants can be used to support an overdenture in combination with natural teeth. Splinted cast copings or crowns on the teeth and a variety of implant heads may be used. For denture-to-bar fixation a variety of clips, rings, and removable horizontal pins may be used depending on the clinical judgment of the prosthodontist.

It cannot be overemphasized that the complexities of the prosthodontic reconstruction be taken into consideration during the surgical phase by the implantologist or the performing dental team. An initial design of the prosthetic reconstruction should be established prior to surgery.

DISCUSSION

The Flexiroot system is designed on the basis of the CODAR concept which is a dynamic replacement of the missing functional unit of the lamina dura–periodontal ligament. One of the most important functions of the CODAR concept is occlusal load transmission to bone without causing breakdown in the supporting alveolar bone. It is achieved in the Flexiroot system with an HDPE plastic layer placed inside the hollow endosteal titanium screw.

Although shock absorption is needed to protect the bone, excessive elasticity may damage the natural teeth if the bridge is tooth-implant–borne. Elasticity becomes excessive if the mobility of the superstructure exceeds the mobility of the teeth. The Flexiroot system is designed to limit lateral mobility through the compression of the plastic and metal-to-metal contact between the implant and the superstructure. This limit on mobility makes the implant especially useful in prosthetic situations where implants and teeth will be connected. The specially designed undersurface of the superstructure partially encases the HDPE polymer resulting in limited mobility of the superstructure under physiologic load. This mobility is similar to the range of flexibility provided by the periodontal ligament of natural teeth.

The conical angled removable titanium cups and the central post provide versatility. The titanium cups can be cemented and modified if necessary; can be sent to the laboratory for precise marginal alignment; or can be eliminated and the central post used with a wide variety of attachments. The simplified technique and reduced number of instruments de-creases confusion during surgery and prosthetic reconstructions and provides a technique easy to learn.

Acknowledgment

I am grateful for the assistance provided by Drs. James Allen, John Brunski, Robert Craig, Walter Knouse, Peter Mozsary, and Ms. Joan Di Gironimo.

REFERENCES

1. Haris AG, Mozsary PG: A new concept: CODAR (Complete Osteointegrated Dentro-Alveolar Replacement) and a corresponding dental implant design (Flexiroot). *J Oral Implantol* 1986; 12:630–660.
2. Mozsary PG, Haris AG: Osteointegrated dento-alveolar replacement system (Flexiroot). *Implantologist* 1986; 3:15–30.
3. Roberts WE, Morey ER: Proliferation and differentiation sequence of osteoblast histogenesis under physiological conditions in rat periodontal ligament. *Am J Anat* 1985; 174:105–118.

APPENDIX

An in vivo fluorochrome stain-test implant-bone biopsy technique has been developed and utilized to gain detailed histologic information about the development of the bony interface around osseointegrated dental implants. The technique permits reliable timing of the second-stage surgery and loading of the implant. The principle is similar to *in vivo* staining techniques used by Roberts and Morey in their animal experiments.[3] Tetracyclines are widely used antibiotics suitable for bone labeling. They are taken up and stored by osteocytes active at the time the antibiotic was administered. If the bone is histologically evaluated under ultraviolet light, fluorescence is observed where the antibiotics are stored. Several kinds of tetracyclines given at different time intervals give multiple stains in different colors: oxytetracycline fluoresces orange, declomycin green, and chlortetracycline yellow.

The histologic evaluation provides information about the amount of bone formed during the period of investigation; maturity of the bone, i.e., whether

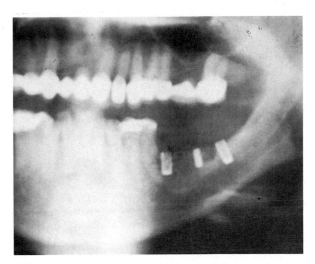

FIG 21–13.
Radiograph of a Flexiroot implant system test implant *in situ* between two first-stage Flexiroot implants.

repair, woven, or mature lamellar bone; completeness of the interface; and speed of bone formation.

The timing of the second surgery should be based on this information. This is especially indicated where compromised bone structure such as osteoporosis, previous radiation therapy, or osteomyelitis may cause a significant change in bone metabolism. In any case where delayed healing is suspected, a test implant and bone biopsy should be done.

The surgical procedure is carried out as for the implant surgery itself. A no. 8 round bur is used to prepare a 5-mm-deep cavity. After hand-tapping the cavity, the test implant is placed with a screwdriver and the flap is closed (Fig 21–13).

Immediately after surgery, declomycin is given for 2 days, 300 mg four times a day. The test implant is usually left in place for 3 months. Thirteen days before test implant removal, oxytetracycline is administered for 2 days, 300 mg four times a day. Four days prior to removal, a 2-day regimen of chlortetracycline is given, 500 mg four times a day. The test implant removal is performed under anesthesia using the 5-mm-diameter trephine with low speed, high torque, and copious irrigation. The specimen is fixed in formalin and sent to the oral pathology laboratory along with patient information. Histologic evaluation should be conducted by an oral pathologist or anatomist familiar with bone fluorescing techniques. Information is needed about the bone structure, the amount of bone formed between two labelings, and, most important, the implant-bone interface.

The timing of the second-stage surgery and loading of the implant should be determined from the histologic evaluation of the test implant and the surrounding bone. The test implant may be placed at the time of the first-stage surgery at a site near the actual implants (see Fig 21–13). In certain cases, when use of the implant is questionable, bone biopsy may be used as a separate, preliminary procedure.

Chapter 22

The Vent-Plant Osseointegrated Compatible Implant System

Leonard I. Linkow, D.D.S.
Anthony W. Rinaldi, D.M.D.

THE ORIGINAL IMPLANT

In 1963, Linkow[1-16] developed the Vent-Plant, an original vented screw-type implant, which was at first fabricated in cobalt chrome, stainless steel, or tantalum. Upon evaluating the performance of implants fabricated from various materials, it quickly became obvious that pure titanium or titanium-based alloys were the materials of choice.[17] By the end of 1964, all Vent-Plant implants were made from the titanium-based alloy Ti-6Al-4V.

The original Vent-Plant screw design implant was redesigned as a self-tapping implant (Fig 22–1). Unlike basket-type implants, which rely on a prepared core of existing bone with an avascular base, the Vent-Plant self-tapping device created medullary bone cuttings through the use of V-shaped sluiceways in the threads. These autogenous grafts were forced into the apical vents of the implant as it was self-tapped into the bone and mixed with blood inside the large, open, vented chambers and thus created a matrix for new bone growth.[17] The presence of autogenous graft material in the apical chamber was observed when self-tapping Vent-Plant implants were removed from residual ridges after it had been determined that a different implant design was better suited for the recipient site. Once initial healing occurred and the implant was loaded, new bone formed according to the functional demands.[17]

Early histopathologic studies[18] of tantalum Vent-Plant implants utilizing high-speed bone preparation with immediate loading protocols consistently showed bone deposition inside the open vented chambers, but fibrous tissues encapsulated the uppermost unthreaded portion of the implant shafts. The final diameter of the recipient site in bone was wider than the shaft, but narrower than the outside diameter of the threads. If the threaded portions of the shafts were buried deeply, the implants were generally successful; but it was then possible for a connective interface tissue to form along the shafts of the implants.

It will be recalled, that in the early 1960s, the technique of implant placement was to drill directly through the mucoperiosteal tissues and into the bone without incising and reflecting the tissues to expose the bone. This procedure had two distinct disadvantages: (a) the epithelial tissues were forced directly into bone, creating epithelial inclusions; and (b) the mucoperiosteal tissues, especially in the maxilla, with their extreme tissue thickness, camouflaged the often occurring knife-edge ridges of bone that existed beneath. In addition, early Vent-Plant implants were often too wide for the residual edentulous ridges or entered the ridges at inappropriate angles, causing many labial, buccal, and sometimes palatal bone perforations. Once some of the failures of the original Vent-Plant implants and tripodial tantalum

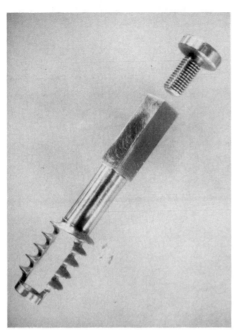

FIG 22–1.
The original Vent-Plant screw design implant.

pin implants (the latter used to circumvent the maxillary sinuses) were examined with the mucoperiosteal tissues fully reflected, it was realized that the implant designs and the true bone resorption patterns that generally took place in the edentulous maxilla and mandible were not always compatible.

Thus, by 1966, it became evident that for original Vent-Plant screw implants to become routinely successful:

1. Bone preparation needed to be done with slow speed, using latch-type round and helical burs with profuse external irrigation.

2. A prolonged healing time was important, thus necessitating two-stage protocols that utilized internally threaded shafts to allow for uninterrupted healing.

3. Self-tapping designs with sluiceways, coupled with an increased number of shaft threads to the uppermost unthreaded portion of the implant shafts, were necessary to create intimate bone contact, early stabilization, and the elimination of interfacial connective tissue, while seeding minute autogenous bone grafts into the vented chambers.

4. Adequate exposure of the recipient site was needed to determine the complete bony topography and adequacy of width and depth to accept screw-type implants.

5. Pure titanium or titanium-based alloy (Ti-6Al-4V) must be used because of its biocompatibility and superior physical properties.[17] (Machining techniques and the original designs of Vent-Plant screw-type implants limited their manufacture to the stronger titanium alloy and electron micrographs of the original Vent-Plant microstructure demonstrate micropits and tooled groovings running parallel to the surface of the screw threads.)

Vent-Plant screw design implants utilizing the above-mentioned techniques have been documented to be currently functioning without mobility or bone breakdown after more than 25 years.[17]

PATIENT CONSIDERATIONS

Nature made a mistake—it gave us a maximum amount of bone on the lingual and palatal cortices flanking our teeth, where it is needed less, and a minimum amount of bone flanking the teeth labially and buccally, where it is needed more to resist lateral and anterior thrusts of the tongue and premature contacts of teeth during lateral and eccentric movements of the mandible. When the teeth are finally lost, the bone has no more periodontal stimulation, so it resorbs due to hypofunction. This continuous resorption reduces the height and width of the residual ridge at the expense of the labial and buccal cortices of bone.

The knife-edge, obliquely flared, shallow ridges that existed in many edentulous maxillae covered with thick, mucoperiosteal tissues were not conducive to the placement of large vertically oriented, round, screw-type endosteal implants. Also, in the severely resorbed mandible, the existing medial knife-like mylohyoid ridge, with deep occlusal concavities, representing the resorbed alveolar ridge and laterally the depressed external oblique ridge, often joined together. These problems, coupled with the hazards associated with encroachment into anatomic landmarks, contributed to the lack of success and ac-

The Vent-Plant Osseointegrated Compatible Implant System

Implants	4.0/4.75mm	3.0/3.75mm	4.0/4.80mm	3.0/3.81mm	2.5/3.46mm	4.0mm	3.3mm	3.0mm
2mm Internally Threaded Attachment	X	X	X	X	X	X	X	X
Self-Tapping Screw	X	X	X	X	X			
External Hex Head	X	X	X			X		
Fixture Mount Required for Insertion	X	X	X					
Use Osseolock Healing Washer	X	X	X			X		
Internal Hex Drive for Insertion				X	X			
"Tap-in" Insertion						X	X	X
Built-in Osseolock Washer				X	X		X	X
Cortical Bone	X	X				X	X	X
Cancellous Bone			X	X	X	X	X	X
CP titanium Substrate	X	X	X	X	X	X	X	X
Bone Like Microstructure	X	X	X	X	X			
CP titanium/HA Coated						X	X	X
10,13,15mm Lengths	X	X	X	X	X	X	X	X
7mm Length	X	X	X	X		X	X	
Surgical Instrument Compatibility	Brånemark	Brånemark	Brånemark	Core-Vent/Denar	Core-Vent/Denar	IMZ/Integral	IMZ/Integral	IMZ/Integral
Unisize Abutments								
Standard Abutments,2.5,4.0,5.5mm hgts	X	X	X	X	X	X	X	X
25° Universal Robutment	X	X	X	X	X	X	X	X
20°or30°Robutments/Std Cap	X	X	X	X	X	X	X	X
20°or30°Robutments/Mini Cap	X	X	X	X	X	X	X	X
Direct Abut for Ext Hex Implants	X	X	X			X		
Direct Abut for Non Ext Hex Implants				X	X		X	X
Mini Abuts-3mm wide,1or2mm hgts	X	X	X	X	X	X	X	X
Short Abuts-4.5mm wide,1or2mm hgts	X	X	X			X		

Prosthetics	Standard Coping Standard Analog	†Use Standard Prosthetic Adaptors	Mini Cap Coping/Analog	Mini Cap Cyl or Mini Cap C&B	Mini Coping/Analog	Mini Cylinder	Ext Hex Impl Coping/Analog	Non Hex Impl Coping/Analog
Standard Abutments,2.5,4.0,5.5mm hgts	X	X						
25° Universal Robutment	X	X						
20°or30°Robutments/Std Cap	X	X						
20°or30°Robutments/Mini Cap			X	X				
Direct Abut for Ext Hex Implants							X	
Direct Abut for Non Ext Hex Implants								X
Mini Abuts-3mm wide,1or2mm hgts					X	X		
Short Abuts-4.5mm wide,1or2mm hgts			X	X				
Prosthetic Compatibility	Cyl/Screw	Cyl/Screw	Cyl/Screw	Cyl/Screw	Cyl/Screw	Cyl/Screw	Cyl/Screw	Cyl/Screw

Standard Prosthetic Adaptors†	Unisize Pan Head Screw	Resilient Abutment Screw	Magnetic Keeper Screw	Optional Chimney
4mm Fixed/Det Cylinder	X			X
3mm Fixed/Det Cylinder	X			X
C&B Extension	X			
"O" Ring Cylinder	X			
Resilient Abutment Adaptor		X		X
Magnetic Keeper			X	

Vent-Plant
Osseointegrated
Compatible Implant System

FIG 22–2.
The Vent-Plant Osseointegrated Implant System.

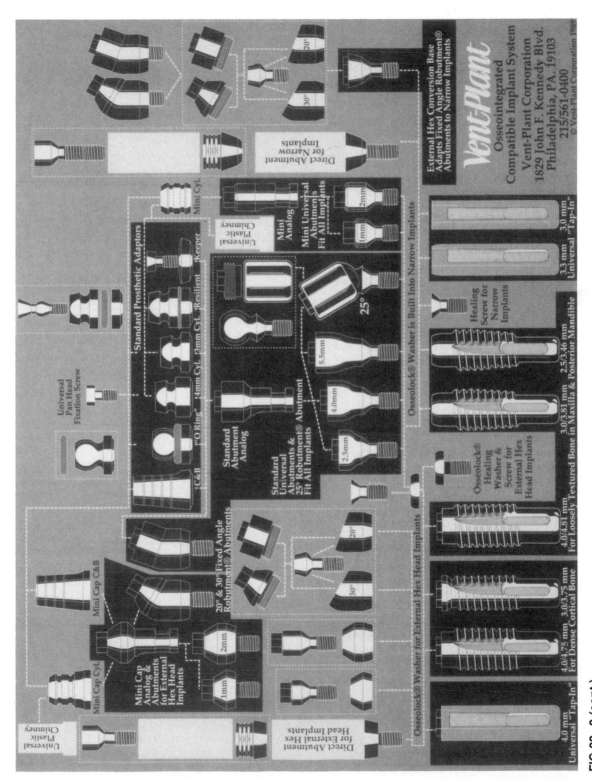

FIG 22–2 (cont.).

ceptance of screw-type implants at that time. Thus, in 1967, Linkow[19-30] introduced the horizontally designed Blade-Vent implants (see Chapter 12), which became commonly used in dental implantology.[31-33] By 1971, manufacturing techniques were developed that made it possible to fabricate Blade-Vent implants from pure titanium and since then, the majority of blade-type implants have been made from pure titanium. The Linkow Blade-Vent implant (Ultimatics Inc., Springdale, Ark) soon completely displaced the use of the original Vent-Plant screw-type implant.

CLINICAL VERIFICATION OF SCREW- AND CYLINDRICAL-TYPE IMPLANTS

In Sweden, Brånemark and his associates,[34, 35] in their research conducted during the past several decades, also found titanium to be an excellent implant material. Brånemark et al. combined the use of pure titanium threaded dental implants with slow-speed sequential bone drilling and tapping and prolonged submerged healing protocols similar to techniques developed by Cherchève.[14, 15] Long-term use and documentation of these techniques were published.[34-36] A fibrous tissue-free anchorage was reported with screw-type dental implants. The concept of osseointegration, or direct contact of bone to the oxide of titanium, was established.

In 1970, Hahn and Palich[37] developed flame plasma spray techniques for the application of molten titanium and other metals to implant substrates. This created a surface area that was six times greater for bony ingrowth in orthopedic implants. This coating technique was eventually adapted for use by many European dental implant manufacturers.[17]

A direct bone-to-hydroxyapatite interface has been discussed by Cook et al.[38] The adherence of the hydroxyapatite coating to bone has been shown to be stronger than to the underlying implant substrate. These results indicated that the hydroxyapatite-coated titanium material could be used in endosseous dental implant systems.

Current two-stage osseointegrated screw and cylindrical endosseous implants, coupled with controlled atraumatic surgical and drilling techniques

and prolonged submerged unloaded healing periods, have added greatly to the reliability and long-term success rates of these types of implants. The diameter of the prepared osseous recipient site is the same as the round inner shafts of the implants, so that the potential for epithelial downgrowth and the formation of connective tissue at the interface is minimized. These recent advances in implant protocols have helped to further demonstrate to the dental profession, and the general public, that dental implants can be predictable.

CURRENT VENT-PLANT IMPLANT DESIGNS AND SUGGESTED CLINICAL USES

In 1986, the original self-tapping screw-type Vent-Plant implant was redeveloped as a two-stage osseointegrated system (Fig 22–2). There are now eight patented commercially pure (cp) titanium implant designs, including three widths of cp titanium hydroxyapatite plasma-sprayed tap-in cylindrical im-

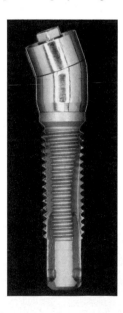

FIG 22–3.
A threaded 3.0/3.75-mm implant with tripodial struts, creating three large side vents which open into a larger vented chamber allowing for transimplant bone growth and additional support. A fixed-angle Robutment abutment is shown assembled to the external hex head of the implant.

TABLE 22–1.

Vent-Plant Osseointegrated Compatible Implant System

Product name	
	Vent-Plant Osseointegrated Compatible Implant System
	Trademarks Vent-Plant
	Osseolock
	Robutment
Manufacturer	
	Vent-Plant Corporation
	1829 John F. Kennedy Boulevard
	Philadelphia, PA 19103
	215/561-0400
	800/VPCORP 1
Material composition	
	Threaded implants cp Titanium
	Tap-in substrate cp Titanium with cp titanium plasma-sprayed mesh coat
	Tap-in final coating Hydroxyapatite plasma spray
	Abutment components Ti-6Al-4V ELI grade
	Prosthetic components Ti-6Al-4V ELI grade
Approximate cost	
	Threaded implant $145
	Tap-in implant $170
	Standard abutment $60
	Robutment abutment $153
	Prosthetic cylinder and screw $40
	Surgical kit (threaded implants) Compatible with all threaded implant instrumentation kits
	Surgical kit (tap-in implants) Compatible with all root form implant instrumentation kits
	Robutment tool kit $415

plants in various lengths, (7,10,13, and 15 mm)* (Table 22–1). These second-generation implants have multiple designs which provide good initial stability by gently creating the maximum contact at the implant-to-bone interface in loosely textured cancellous bone of the posterior mandible or thin residual alveolar ridges in the maxilla as well as in dense, symphyseal bone. Each implant has tripodial struts, creating three large side vents which open into a larger vented chamber allowing for transimplant bone growth and additional support (Fig 22–3). The narrowest (2.5 mm inner diameter, 3.46 mm outer diameter [2.5/3.46]) threaded Vent-Plant implants and the 3.0-mm tap-in cylindrical Vent-Plant implants are the only exceptions. These implants have two struts, creating two large side vents which open into their central vented chambers (Fig 22–4). All

*US patents 4,713,004, 4,842,518; 4,915,628; and 4,932,868. Other US and foreign patents pending.

Vent-Plant implants have open apical architecture to increase the blood supply to their vented chambers and lessen hydrostatic pressure created during insertion. Each implant has a correspondingly sized final drill which creates the exact bony crypt through sequential drilling preparation (Fig 22–5,A–C,E,F, I,M).

The threaded Vent-Plant implants have redesigned built-in inverted bone tap cutting sluiceways, allowing the implants to be gently cut and self-tapped securely into the residual ridges (Fig 22–5,D,G,H,O,P). End-cutting notches are present on these implants to assist in starting the self-tapping function while also serving to engage apical cortical bone where available. These features create immediate macroretention and intimate contact of the implant within bone, while depositing autogenous bone grafts through the vents and into the central vented chamber. The intimate contact of the threads and shaft of the implant with bone is thought to facilitate

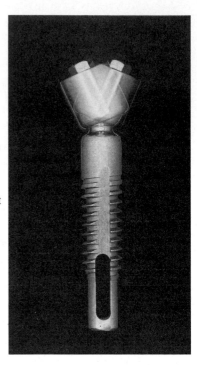

FIG 22–4.
A threaded 2.5/3.46-mm implant with two struts, creating two large side vents which open into a larger vented chamber allowing for transimplant bone growth and additional support. A universal Robutment abutment is shown assembled to the internal hex head of the implant and pivoting prior to locking into the most appropriate angle of emergence.

the healing of bone by primary intention at the implant-to-bone interface.[17]

Most implant systems crush bone as they are inserted creating "die-back" of the affected bone which may delay early healing.[17] Some implant systems require a separate bone-tapping procedure prior to placing screw-type implants into bone. The latter technique creates gaps at the implant-to-bone interface.[17] In some cases, this compromises the initial stability of the implant in bone, resulting in implant failure.

The large vented chamber of the threaded Vent-Plant implants initially acts as a reservoir for the deposition of cut bone. These harvested bone cuttings are thought to accelerate, or act as a scaffold for, new vascular bone growth into and through the vented chambers, thus creating additional areas of supporting bone, even in the sometimes thinner and loosely textured cancellous areas of the maxilla and mandible. Once healing occurs, the bone in the vented chamber increases the surface area of the implant-to-bone interface, while the bone in the sluice-ways acts as additional vertical support and antirotational pillars.

Vent-Plant cp titanium–hydroxyapatite plasma-sprayed cylindrical implants can be used by those who prefer a tap-in cylindrical implant. These tap-in cylindrical implants have outwardly extending antirotational, longitudinal pillars with end cutters, allowing the implants to be gently cut and securely tapped vertically into the residual ridges. A notch-cutting tool is used to start the grooves in dense cortical bone at the entrance to the initially prepared, round, bony crypt (Figs. 22–5,J,K,N). This feature creates immediate antirotational macroretention and intimate contact of the implant within bone, while depositing autogenous bone grafts through the vents and into the central vented chamber.

The large vented chamber of the Vent-Plant tap-in cylindrical implants initially acts as a reservoir for the deposition of cut bone. These harvested bone cuttings are thought to accelerate, or act as a scaffold for, new vascular bone growth into and through the vented chamber, thus creating additional areas of supporting bone, even in the sometimes thinner and loosely textured cancellous areas of the maxilla and mandible. Once healing occurs, this increases the surface area of the implant-to-bone interface, while

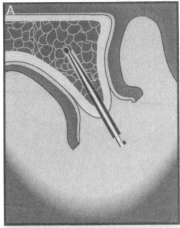
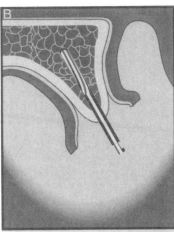
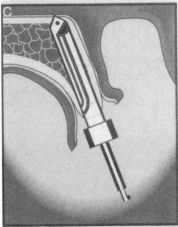
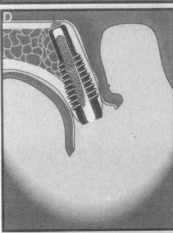
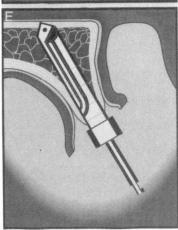
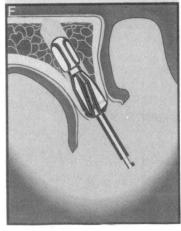

FIG 22–5.
A, initial pilot hole preparation. External irrigation is used. **B,** enlargement of pilot hole with 2-mm twist drill. External irrigation is used. **C,** sequential bone crypt preparation with 2.5-mm internally irrigated spade drill. Externally irrigated drills may be substituted to prepare this 2.5 mm width and any other subsequent crypt enlargement including 3.0, 3.3, and 4.0 mm. **D,** in narrow ridges, a 2.5/3.46-mm internal hex head threaded implant may now be inserted in this 2.5-mm-wide bone crypt. This implant is also indicated for average cancellous ridges to avoid apical perforation into extreme bony concavities or internal anatomic landmarks. **E,** sequential bone crypt preparation to 3.0 mm. In narrow ridges, a 3.0-mm tap-in cylindrical implant may now be inserted. This implant may require a notch-cutting tool to start the grooves for its two antirotational, longitudinal pillars. In average cancellous ridges, the 3.0/3.81-mm threaded implant can now be used. This implant requires a separate narrow countersinking operation (see **F**) or the final 3.0-mm countersunk bone crypt may be prepared with a one-step drill specifically designed for a 3.0/3.81-mm threaded implant in a length of 7, 10, 13, or 15 mm. **F,** narrow countersink preparation is only necessary in the two-step final crypt preparation for the 3.0/3.81-mm threaded implant. External irrigation is used. *(Continued.)*

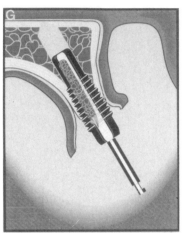

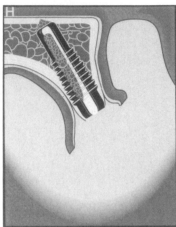

FIG 22–5 (cont.).

G, insertion of an internal hex head 3.0/3.81-mm threaded implant utilizing a slow speed (15 rpm), high-torque handpiece or hand ratchet. Note autogenous bone graft being deposited into the central vented chamber. **H,** a 3.0/3.81-mm threaded implant completely seated in the prepared bone crypt with the built-in Osseolock collar slightly below the crestal bone. In average dense ridges, the 3.0/3.75-mm threaded implant can be used. This implant requires the same 3.0-mm crypt but a different narrow countersink configuration. **I,** sequential bone crypt preparation to 3.3 mm. In narrow ridges, a 3.3-mm tap-in cylindrical implant may now be inserted. **J,** this implant may require a notch-cutting tool to start the grooves for its three antirotational, longitudinal pillars. **K,** insertion of a 3.3-mm tap-in cylindrical implant. Note the placement of a Robutment ballfitting to facilitate the tap-in procedure. **L,** insertion of a healing screw into a 3.3-mm tap-in cylindrical implant completely seated in the prepared bone crypt with the built-in Osseolock collar slightly below the crestal bone. *(Continued.)*

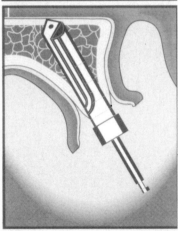

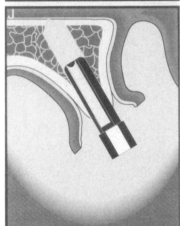

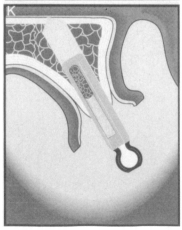

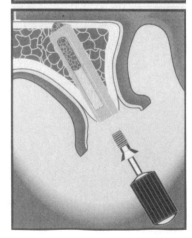

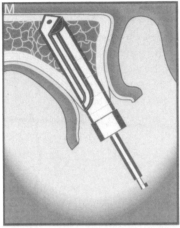

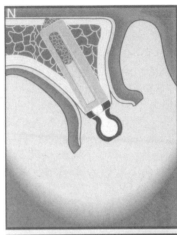

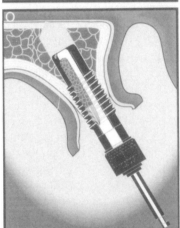

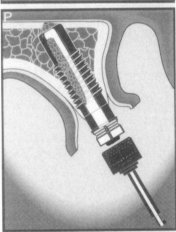

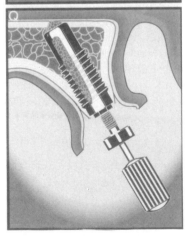

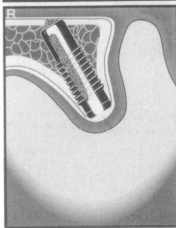

FIG 22–5 (cont.).
M, sequential bone crypt preparation to 4.0 mm. **N,** in wide ridges, a 4.0-mm tap-in cylindrical implant may now be inserted. In wide cancellous ridges, the 4.0/4.80-mm threaded implant can be used. **O,** insertion of an external hex head 4.0/4.80-mm threaded implant utilizing a slow speed (15 rpm), high-torque handpiece or hand ratchet. A handpiece connector is clipped to a fixture mount which is attached to the implant. Note autogenous bone graft being deposited into the central vented chamber. **P,** removal of the handpiece connector and fixture mount from a 4.0/4.80-mm threaded implant completely seated in the prepared bone crypt below the crestal bone. In wide dense ridges, the 4.0/4.75-mm threaded implant can be used. This implant requires the same 4.0-mm crypt. **Q,** insertion of an Osseolock healing washer and screw into a 4.0/4.80-mm threaded implant with an Osseolock insertion tool. **R,** initial healing after first-stage surgery.

the antirotational pillars resist the "spinner phenomena" associated with root form or cylindrical implants in general.

IMPLANT CLINICAL SELECTION

The 3.0/3.75-mm and 4.0/4.75-mm threaded Vent-Plant implants are used for average and wide dense cortical ridges, respectively, and the 4.0/4.80-mm threaded Vent-Plant implant for wide cancellous ridges. These implants have an external hex and fixture mount system to assist in self-tapping the implants firmly into bone and subsequently accommodate antirotational abutments (Fig 22–5,O,P). The 2.5/3.46-mm and 3.0/3.81-mm threaded Vent-Plant implants are designed with thin coronal heads and a built-in Osseolock collar with an internal hex to assist in self-tapping the implants into narrow and average cancellous ridges, respectively (Fig 22–5,D,G,H). All threaded Vent-Plant implants are inserted into bone with a high-torque, low-speed handpiece at 15 rpm or with a ratchet or with hand tools.

To standardize and simplify the surgical and prosthetic armamentarium, prosthetic components, and prosthodontic techniques for implants, minor additions of instrumentation can be made that the threaded Vent-Plant implants to be used interchangeably with the armamentaria of various other screw-type implant systems. Bone taps and widely flaring countersink burs are not necessary.

The 4.0-mm tap-in cylindrical implant has an external hex to accommodate antirotational abutments and can be used as a back-up, alternative implant when a thinner implant cannot be well secured. The 3.0- and 3.3-mm tap-in cylindrical implants are designed with thin heads and built-in Osseolock collars for narrow and average ridges, respectively. The cp titanium plasma-sprayed mesh coating on the implant surface cuts as it is tapped into the recipient site to establish good initial stability and implant-to-bone interface. The bone cuttings are embedded into the hydroxylapatite-impregnated mesh and act as autogenous bone grafts to assist in creating new peri-implant bone growth and support. Side vents and one apical vent open into a large central chamber allowing for transimplant bone growth and additional support. Minor additions of instrumentation will allow the Vent-Plant tap-in cylindrical implants to be used interchangeably with the armamentaria of other tap-in root form or cylinder implant systems.

Extended periods of healing, while currently well tolerated and equated with the term *osseointegration* and long-term success, in actuality are absolutely necessary with most other current osseointegrated-type dental implants, even in the mandibular symphysis, owing to limitations in their inherent designs and insertion techniques. Previously existing designs of other implant systems are either tap-in root form or cylinder implants that depend on microretention and long-term bony ingrowth into surface irregularities, or screw-type implants with threaded macroretention designed to be inserted into bone by methods that can create gaps at the bone-to-implant interface, or crush bone with poor self-tapping designs.[17]

Although the current threaded Vent-Plant osseointegrated compatible implant have been redesigned as part of a two-stage implant system, second-stage surgery may be eliminated in certain cases. The abutment can be connected at the same time the implant is placed (semisubmerged technique), where the implant is protected from premature loading by adjacent teeth, or where there is no opposing occlusion. Multiple sizes and designs allow for the immediate insertion of threaded Vent-Plant implants into selected noninfected extraction sockets, as long as the implants are wider and longer than the extraction site and are not loaded prematurely. The intimate and secure initial stabilization and macroretention established by the threaded, true self-tapping Vent-Plant implants make these expanded treatment modalities available for selected cases. The semisubmerged technique, however, is not recommended for Vent-Plant cp titanium–hydroxylapatite plasma-sprayed cylinders.

The Osseolock collar, a two-piece cp titanium cover screw system, is installed over submerged 3.0/3.75-mm, 4.0/4.75-mm, 4.0/4.80-mm threaded, and 4.0-mm cp titanium tap-in cylindrical Vent-Plant implants (Fig 22–5,Q,R). Once the implant has integrated, the central healing screw is removed; the bone that has healed to and over the healing washer

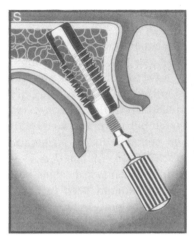

FIG 22–5 (cont.).
S, the removal of the central healing screw, during second-stage abutment connection surgery, leaving the Osseolock washer in place. Any bone which grows to and over the washer is allowed to remain undisturbed. The washer must be removed with certain abutments designed to interface with the external hex such as the fixed-angle Robutment abutment.

remains undisturbed (Fig 22–5,S). This eliminates the unnecessary crestal bone destruction sometimes associated with the removal of large one-piece cover screws and when widely flaring countersink burs are used. Worthington et al.[39] have stated, "It must be remembered, however, that the normal countersinking step often produces a radiographic appearance suggesting marginal bone loss and the radiographs must be interpreted with care." They also caution that, "Over-enthusiastic counter-sinking of the fixture at the time of installation may mean that no superior cortical bone plate is available for thread cutting and thus the initial stability of the fixture is diminished."[39]

The balance of the Vent-Plant implants have an Osseolock healing collar built in and only require a small healing screw during the passive healing period. Once the healing screw has been removed at the time of abutment connection, a Robutment abutment or solid abutment device is installed into the same threaded opening.

VENT-PLANT IMPLANT SURFACES

The Vent-Plant cp titanium–hydroxylapatite plasma-sprayed cylindrical implants are first coated with pure titanium by using techniques developed in the orthopedic coating industry. Plasma spraying is accomplished with a source of low interstitial ELI grade cp titanium microsphere powder refined from a high-vacuum plasma atomized process, rather than a source of titanium derived from a chemical reaction, as in titanium hydride. This cp titanium mesh is then plasma-sprayed with hydroxyapatite.

This eliminates possible surface contaminants such as aluminum and carbides during plasma spraying of the cp titanium mesh.[17] Experiments by Ducheyne et al.[40] show that aluminum is released in measurable quantities from porous-coated Ti-6Al-4V substrates, in which the coatings were cp titanium. Experimental results by Woodman et al.[41] have demonstrated that aluminum ions from Ti-6Al-4V implant substrates implanted in long bones showed continuously rising aluminum levels in the lung tissue of baboons. Albrektsson and Jacobsson[42] caution that more long-term data are necessary regarding the possible problems relating to aluminum contained in implanted materials, such as Ti-6Al-4V, unless it can be proved that the potentially neurotoxic aluminum ions taken up by the bloodstream do not cross the blood-brain barrier.

The surface of threaded Vent-Plant implants is prepared with a bonelike microstructure showing smooth granularity at the microstructural level.[17] The implants are then cleaned, passivated, and packaged by techniques which ensure pure titanium oxide on the surface of the implants.

All Vent-Plant implants are double-packaged and sterilized with gamma irradiation to eliminate possible surface contamination from the deposition of salts that may be present in steam autoclaves.

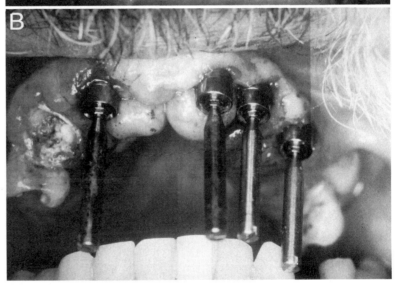

FIG 22–7.
A, direction indicators demonstrating the path of emergence of Vent-Plant implants in the angular bone of the anterior maxilla. **B,** locking ball-and-socket pivoting 25-degree universal Robutment abutment devices correct the unfavorable angulation of the implants.

straight versions in lengths of 2.5, 4.0, and 5.5 mm. Once the periabutment tissues have healed around straight or rotating Robutment abutments, they can be interchanged readily, without further surgical intervention. Vent-Plant, Osseolock, Robutment, and solid abutment devices are compatible with the Brånemark implant. Any abutment with the standard configuration can accept the following prosthetic adaptors (see Fig 22–2).

1. Four- and 3-mm machined standard fixed detachable cylinders with or without antirotational hex bases are available to accept flathead titanium alloy screws that resist breaking and loosening.

2. When resiliency is desired, especially while interposing rigid osseointegrated implants with periodontally involved teeth, the Vent-Plant resilient abutment can be used as a stress-breaking device.[17, 43] This system eliminates problems associated with bacterial proliferation and the periodic maintenance of plastic-type flexible inserts that are used within implants that require the removal of the abutment, as well as the prosthesis, to perform routine replacement. Acrylic burnout patterns form a

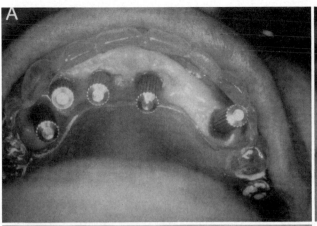

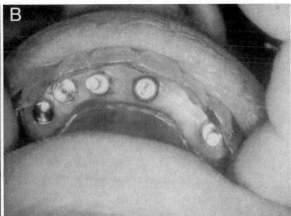

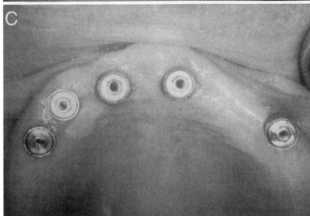

FIG 22–8.
A, a surgical-prosthetic template and direction indicators demonstrate the path of emergence of Brånemark implants in the angular bone of the anterior maxilla. The two fixtures in the midline region were placed with a lingual access technique designed to maximize the bone-to-implant interface. A functional compromise may have occurred if the final prosthesis had been fabricated on these fixtures. The fixture in the left canine region would have created a cosmetic compromise. **B,** three locking ball-and-socket pivoting 25-degree universal Robutment abutment devices correct the unfavorable angulation of these implants. **C,** final tissue reaction.

precise concavity to help sandwich a pink silicone rubber ring. The ring is sealed tightly between the concavity in the fixed detachable prosthesis and a titanium washer, which is placed upon a rotational Robutment abutment or a solid abutment device. A double-headed titanium alloy fixation screw, designed to resist loosening, secures into place the final resilient fixed detachable prosthesis. The ring is readily and easily replaceable during each preventive maintenance visit when the fixed detachable prosthesis is removed and replaced, leaving the transmucosal abutments undisturbed. Two hundred to 400 μm of movement have been measured, simulating the movement of the periodontal ligament, while maintaining the integrity of the implants and their transmucosal abutments.

3. Overdentures are accomplished by the use of O ring or magnetic keepers which are designed and engineered to thread directly into any abutment de-

vice and to be highly resistant to loosening or breaking (Figs 22–10,A,B and 22–11).

4. A crown and bridge adaptor converts standard abutments to receive cemented fixed partial prostheses.

The occlusal configuration of standard Vent-Plant transmucosal abutments is the same as Brånemark abutments. This allows compatibility of all Vent-Plant prosthetic components with Brånemark abutment components. Existing gold fixed detachable cylinders, screws, and prosthetic components are conversely compatible with standard Vent-Plant abutment components.

One- and 2-mm short abutments are available for close bite cases. These abutments along with the tapered minicap of the fixed-angle Robutment abutments accept the minicap configuration fixed detachable machined cylinder and crown and bridge adap-

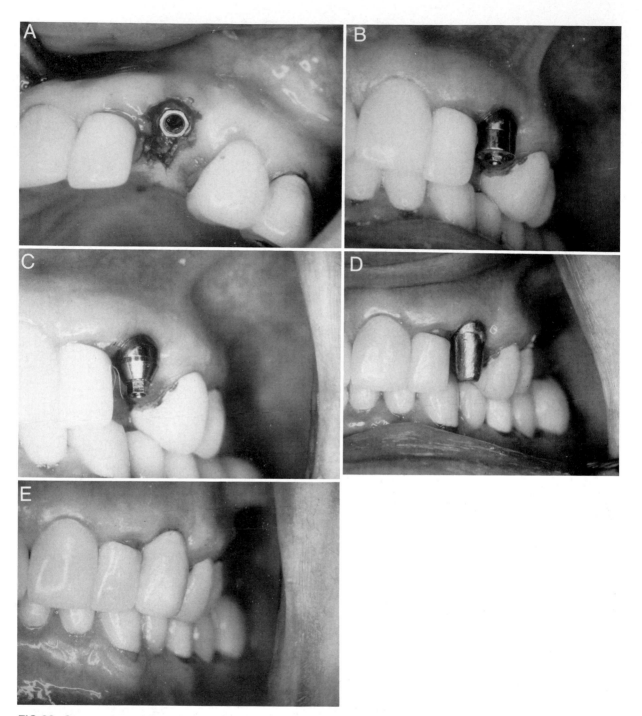

FIG 22–9.
A, exposure of an integrated 4.0/4.80-mm cancellous threaded external hex head implant placed at an extreme angle to avoid a severe external apical bony undercut. **B,** installation of a 30-degree fixed-angle abutment with a standard cap is not well suited in this case owing to thin tissue, close interocclusal clearance, and an implant that was not placed below the crest of bone. **C,** a 30-degree fixed-angle abutment with a mini cap is placed to correct the unfavorable angulation of the implant. **D,** a crown and bridge prosthetic adaptor was cemented and screwed into place. The assembly was prepared to accept a ceramometal crown. An alternative fixed detachable crown approach could have been accomplished with a mini cap cylinder and screw prosthetic adaptor. **E,** final restoration cemented in place.

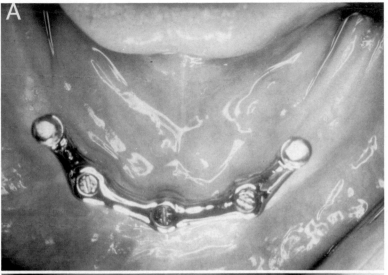

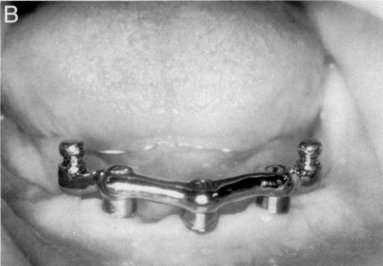

FIG 22–10.
A, occlusal view of an O ring bar, attached to three implants, utilized to support a mandibular overdenture. **B,** facial view of **A.**

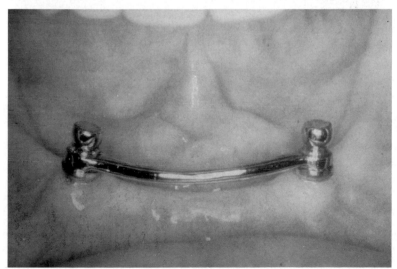

FIG 22–11.
Facial view of an O ring bar, attached to two 3.0/3.75-mm cortical threaded implants placed in thin symphyseal bone, utilized to support a mandibular overdenture.

tors. These abutments can be used on any external hex head implant without the Osseolock washer in place.

Three-millimeter narrow mini abutments have been designed for clinical cases where there is minimal room for adjacent abutments. These mini abutments are available in 1 and 2 mm heights and accept the mini configuration fixed detachable machined cylinder. These abutments can be used on all Vent-Plant implants through the use of the Osseolock washer in external hex head im-

plants or the built-in Osseolock collar in all other implants.

Direct-to-implant abutments are available for both external hex head implants and all other Vent-Plant implants with the built-in Osseolock collar. The direct abutments for external hex head implants have two versions: one with and the other without an antirotational female hex base. These abutments become part of the prosthesis and eliminate the abutment normally interposed between the implant and the prosthesis (see Fig 22–2).

FIG 22–12.
A, the initial stabilization and macroretention, established by the self-tapping 4.0/4.80-mm cancellous threaded implants, permit the use of the semisubmerged healing technique (connection of abutments at the time of first-stage surgery) in this right posterior mandible where there is no opposing occlusion. **B,** the left posterior mandible of the same patient shown in **A.** The semisubmerged technique eliminates the necessity for second-stage surgery in good quality and quantity of bone while allowing for a delayed loading protocol.

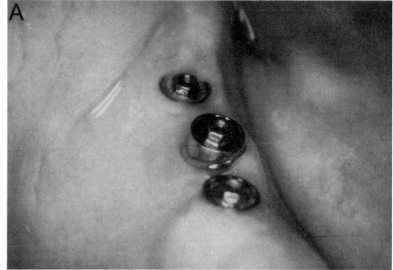

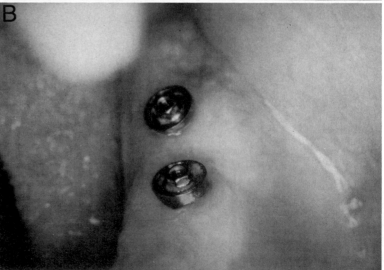

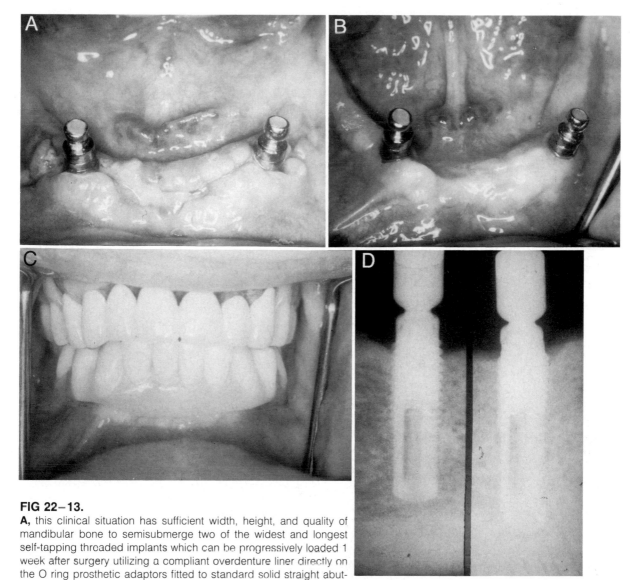

FIG 22–13.
A, this clinical situation has sufficient width, height, and quality of mandibular bone to semisubmerge two of the widest and longest self-tapping threaded implants which can be progressively loaded 1 week after surgery utilizing a compliant overdenture liner directly on the O ring prosthetic adaptors fitted to standard solid straight abutments. The delayed soft tissue healing is due to removal of several incisor teeth with large periapical cysts. **B,** occlusal view after 18 months in function. The O rings were installed in the denture after 6 weeks. **C,** facial view of the completed mandibular prosthesis. **D,** periapical radiographs of the implants after 18 months in function.

DISCUSSION

The definition of the term *osseointegration* seems to be changing as our scientific knowledge increases.[44, 45] The dynamics involved with the elimination of fibrous tissue at the human bone-to-implant interface is not yet fully understood.

The success of all Vent-Plant osseointegrated compatible implants is dependent upon gentle, intimate, and atraumatic insertion with maximum initial fixation in bone. The design and manufacturing techniques of the Vent-Plant implants allow these implants to be inserted into their respective osseous recipient sites and to establish good initial stability through creating the maximum quantity and quality of bone at the implant-to-bone interface. This initial

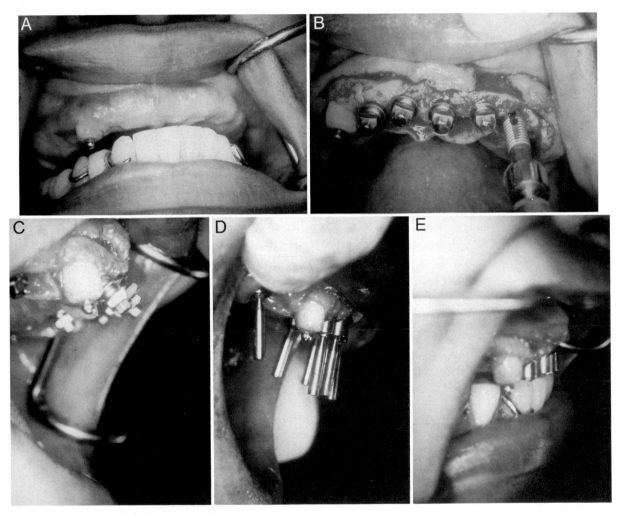

FIG 22–14.
A, this clinical situation has sufficient width, height, and quality of maxillary bone to semisubmerge the widest and longest self-tapping 4.0/4.80-mm cancellous threaded implants which can be progressively loaded from the day of surgery directly on the universal Robutment abutments utilized to correct the angle of emergence of the implants. **B,** handpiece self-tapping a 4.0/4.80-mm threaded implant into the 4.0-mm prepared bony crypt. **C,** the fixture mounts demonstrate the angle of emergence of these well-placed implants in this lateral view. **D,** abutments have been locked in place at appropriate angles to compensate for the angle of emergence of the implants and the orifice of the fixation screws as demonstrated by the guide pins which have been attached to the abutments. **E,** locked abutments with mucosal tissue reflected. *(Continued.)*

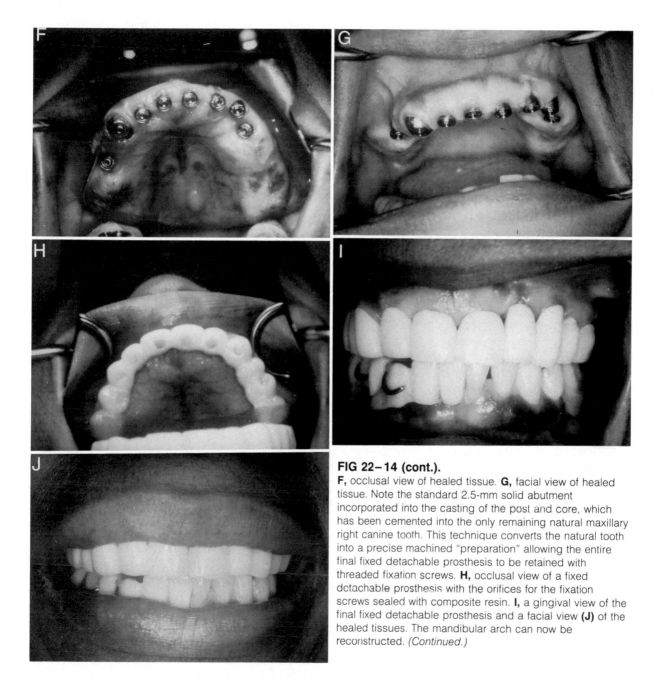

FIG 22–14 (cont.).

F, occlusal view of healed tissue. **G,** facial view of healed tissue. Note the standard 2.5-mm solid abutment incorporated into the casting of the post and core, which has been cemented into the only remaining natural maxillary right canine tooth. This technique converts the natural tooth into a precise machined "preparation" allowing the entire final fixed detachable prosthesis to be retained with threaded fixation screws. **H,** occlusal view of a fixed detachable prosthesis with the orifices for the fixation screws sealed with composite resin. **I,** a gingival view of the final fixed detachable prosthesis and a facial view **(J)** of the healed tissues. The mandibular arch can now be reconstructed. *(Continued.)*

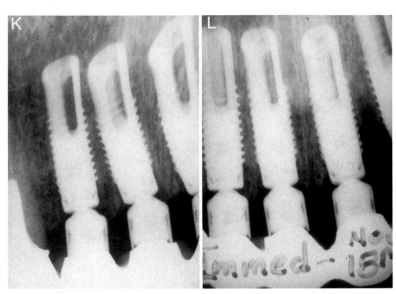

FIG 22–14 (cont.).
K, this patient has been functioning for a total of 18 months from the day of surgery culminating with this fixed detachable prosthesis without any loss of osseointegration or further loss of crestal bone as demonstrated in this periapical radiograph. **L,** an 18-month postoperative radiograph demonstrating another view. The abutments used in this case were of the original design which allowed 34 degrees of orientation due to a thinner neck in the ballfitting. The current design has a thicker neck and has been limited to a maximum 25 degrees of correction.

macroretention, in an atraumatically prepared bone site, coupled with aseptic surgical conditions, a clean passivated implant surface, appropriate healing protocol, and prosthetic reconstructive procedures are ultimately responsible for the long-term success and osseointegration of the implant. These factors are thought to encourage healing by primary intention and increase the rate of osseointegration by a direct proportion and decrease the amount of necessary healing time by an indirect proportion.[46]

Other tap-in cylindrical implants lack outwardly extending antirotational pillars and are very susceptible to spinning in the prepared socket. Other screw-type implants that utilize a separate bone-tapping insertion procedure may result in gaps at the bone-to-implant interface even with a well-done bone-tapping procedure.[17] Fibrous connective tissue can form in these gaps. The looser the texture of the cancellous core of bone, the more unlikely it will be to establish a properly tapped recipient site, resulting in poor initial stabilization. An oversized implant must then be inserted, crushing its way into bone. Whether by second choice or by first choice, the crushing of bone with threaded endosseous implants creates good initial stabilization but, soon after, the catabolic stage of healing creates a situation prone to the loosening of the implant and the formation of fibrous tissue. The fibrous tissue, which forms in either case, can be replaced by bone. This osseous healing usually occurs with delayed loading and protracted healing times, but in many cases the fibrous tissue is never replaced completely and bone creates an osseovariegated interface[46] comprised of diversified patches of both fibro-osseous and osseointegrated interfaces.

Because of the design and insertion techniques, some cylindrical implant mechanical resistance forces, especially those which resist torquing, are very low at the time of insertion or soon thereafter. Immediate loading of these types of root form or cylinder and screw-type implants can result in early implant loss, with severe stress concentration around the neck of the implant being transferred to the surrounding crestal bone.[47]

The initial stabilization and macroretention established by the self-tapping threaded Vent-Plant implants enhance the use of semisubmerged healing techniques and make possible the immediate insertion of implants directly into noninfected extraction sockets in selected cases (Figs 22–12,A,B; 22–13,A–D; 22–14,A–L, and 22–15,A–J).

The outwardly extending end-cutting pillars of the plasma-sprayed hydroxyapatite Vent-Plant tap-in implants establish excellent initial stabilization and antirotational macroretention.

Badly resorbed residual ridges and vital anatomic landmarks often necessitate the placement of implants at an unfavorable angle in order to optimize

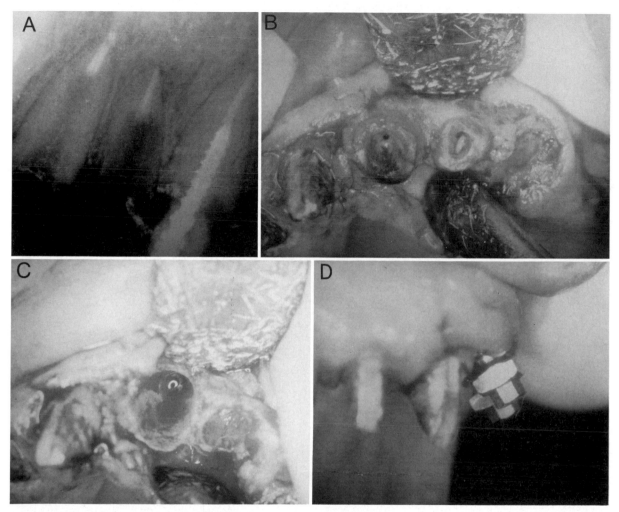

FIG 22–15.
A, periapical radiograph of the left central and lateral maxillary incisor teeth affected with nonrestorable caries. **B,** clinical view of nonrestorable teeth. **C,** extraction of the left central and lateral maxillary incisor teeth. **D,** lateral clinical view. The fixture mounts demonstrate the angles of emergence of these threaded implants placed into the prepared extraction sockets. *(Continued.)*

the bone-to-implant interface. Implants may emerge at atypical angles, creating functional and esthetic compromises. Robutment abutment devices have been suggested to compensate for angle-of-emergence problems.

Widely flaring countersink burs and the removal of large one-piece healing screws sometimes create excessive crestal bone destruction. The Osseolock collar has been suggested to help eliminate the collar on all but those implants designed for use in dense,

symphyseal bone. The countersunk preparations that are necessary for these collars act as a vertical seat in bone to prevent inadvertent loading by a mandibular denture through the mucoperiosteal tissue during the passive healing period. The narrow smooth Osseolock collar is more conducive to the preservation of thin crestal bone.

The Vent-Plant Osseointegrated Compatible Implant System[17] has incorporated these and other vital features with biological, biomechanical, and bioma-

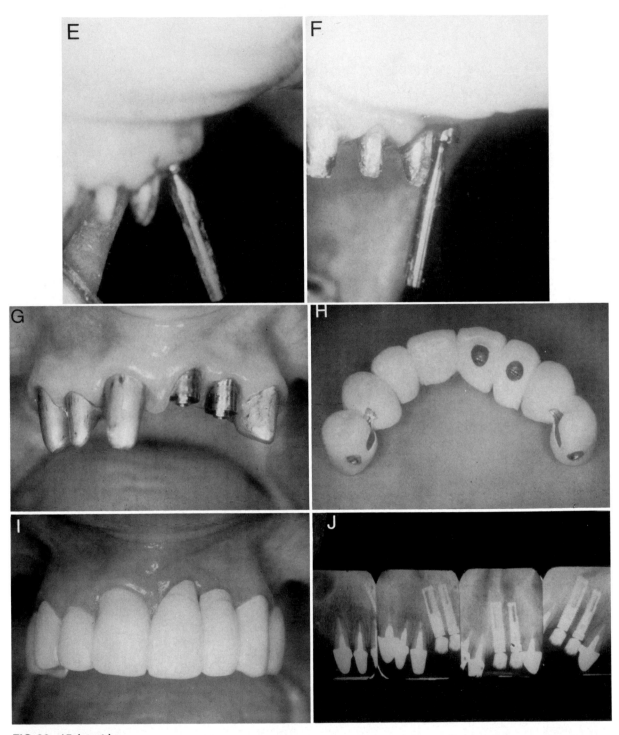

FIG 22–15 (cont.).
E, universal Robutment abutments placed immediately into the implants and lightly tightened. Guide pins are inserted into the abutments at a straight emergence. **F,** universal Robutment abutments compensating for the angle of emergence of the implants and locked into position. Guide pins inserted into the abutments demonstrate the new emergence angle. **G,** the healed mucosa around the abutments and the gold copings covering the natural teeth. **H,** palatal view of the final ceramometal fixed detachable prosthesis. **I,** facial view of the final prosthesis. **J,** 2-year postoperative periapical radiographs. The abutments used in this case were of the original design which allowed 34 degrees of orientation. The current design has a thicker neck and has been limited to a maximum 25 degrees of correction.

terial considerations. The system allows functional and esthetically pleasing prostheses to be fabricated by compensating for unfavorable emergence angles and lack of resiliency. The system is compatible with most existing instrumentation and has been designed for ease of surgery and insertion. Multiple designs provide the ability to compensate for a broad spectrum of indications and uses.

REFERENCES

1. Linkow LI: Intra-osseous implants utilized as fixed bridge abutments. *J Oral Implant Transplant Surg* 1964; 10:17–23.
2. Linkow LI: Metal implants assessed. *Dent Times* 1965; 9:6–7.
3. Linkow LI: Clinical evaluation of the various designed endosseous implants. *J Oral Implant Transplant Surg* 1966; 12:35–46.
4. Linkow LI: The age of endosseous implants. *Dent Concepts* 1966; 18:4–10.
5. Linkow LI: The radiographic role in endosseous implant interventions. *Chron Omaha Dent Soc* 1966; 29:304–311.
6. Linkow LI: Maxillary endosseous implants. *Dent Concepts* 1966; 10:14–23.
7. Linkow LI: The versatility of implant interventions. *Dent Concepts* 1966; 10:5–17.
8. Linkow LI: L'era degli impianti ossei. *Inform Odontostomat* 1966; 8:14–15.
9. Linkow LI: The era of endosseous implants. *JDC Dent Soc* 1967; 42:47.
10. Linkow LI: Prefabricated endosseous implant prostheses. *Dent Concepts* 1967; 10:3–11.
11. Linkow LI: Internally threaded endosseous implants. *Dent Concepts* 1967; 10:16–20.
12. Linkow LI: Atypical implantations for anatomically contraindicated situations. *Dent Concepts* 1967; 11:11–17.
13. Linkow LI: Histopathologic and radiologic studies on endosseous implants. *Dent Concepts* 1968; 11:3–13.
14. Linkow LI, Cherchève R: *Theories and Techniques of Oral Implantology,* vol 1. St Louis, CV Mosby Co, 1970.
15. Linkow LI, Cherchève R: *Theories and Techniques of Oral Implantology,* vol 2. St Louis, CV Mosby Co, 1970.
16. Linkow LI, Edelman AE: Intra-osseous pins and posts. US patent no. 3,499,222, March 10, 1970.
17. Linkow LI, Rinaldi AW: Evolution of the Vent-Plant Osseointegrated Compatible Implant System. *Int J Oral Maxillofac Implants* 1988; 3:109–122.
18. Linkow LI: Histopathologic and radiologic studies on endosseous implants. *Dent Concepts* 1968; 11:3–13.
19. Linkow LI: The endosseous blade: A new dimension in oral implantology. *Rev Trim Implant* 1968; 5:13–24.
20. Linkow LI, Martini J: Case report of the month—the value of dental tissues in the reconstruction of a cleft palate-lip-anodontic case with the aid of endosseous implants. *NY J Dent* 1969; 39:15–19.
21. Linkow LI: The status of oral implants. *Inform Odontostomat* 1969; 1.
22. Linkow LI: The endosseous blade—a progress report. *Prom Dent* 1969; 5:6–17.
23. Linkow LI: Mouth reconstruction for the edentulous maxilla using endosseous blades. *Dent Concepts* 1969; 12:3–21.
24. Linkow LI: The endosseous blade implant and its use in orthodontics. *Int J Orthodont* 1969; 18:149–154.
25. Linkow LI: Endosseous oral implantology: A 7 year progress report. *Dent Clin North Am* 1970; 14:185–200.
26. Linkow LI: Endosseous blade-vent implants: A two year report. *J Prosthet Dent* 1970; 23:441–449.
27. Linkow LI: Alloplastic implants, in Goldman HM, Forrest SP, Byrd DL, et al (eds): *Current Therapy in Dentistry.* St Louis, CV Mosby Co, 1968.
28. Linkow LI: Implants for edentulous arches, in Winkler S (ed): *Essentials of Complete Denture Prosthodontics.* Philadelphia, WB Saunders Co, 1979, pp 633–694.
29. Linkow LI: *Maxillary Implants.* North Haven, Conn, Glarus Publishing Co, 1978.
30. Linkow LI: *Mandibular Implants.* North Haven, Conn, Glarus Publishing Co, 1978.
31. Smithloff M, Fritz ME: Use of blade implants in a selected population of partially edentulous patients. *J Periodontal* 1982; 53:413–418.
32. Smithloff M, Fritz ME: The use of blade implants in a selected population of partially edentulous adults. *J Periodontal* 1976; 47:19–26.
33. Schnitman PA, Shulman LB: *Dental Implants: Benefits and Risk, an NIH-Harvard Consensus Development Conference.* DHHS Publ No (NIH)81–1531, 1980, pp 326–339.
34. Brånemark PI, Hansson BO, Adell R, et al: *Osseointegrated Implant in the Treatment of the Edentulous Jaw. Experience From a 10 Year Period.* Stockholm, Almqvist & Wiksell International, 1977.

35. Adell R, Lekholm U, Rockler B, et al: A 15-year study of osseointegrated implants in the treatment of the edentulous jaw. *Int J Oral Surg* 1981; 10:387–416.

36. Brånemark PI, Zarb GA, Albrektsson T: *Tissue-Integrated Prostheses*. Chicago, Quintessence Publishing Co, Inc, 1985.

37. Hahn H, Palich W: Preliminary evaluation of porous metal surfaced titanium for orthopaedic implants. *J Biomed Mater Res* 1970; 4:571.

38. Cook SD, Kay JF, Thomas KA, et al: Interface mechanics and histology of titanium and hydroxyapatite coated titanium for dental implant applications. *Int J Oral Maxillofac Implants* 1987; 2:15–22.

39. Worthington P, Bolender CL, Taylor TD: The Swedish system of osseointegrated implants: Problems and complications encountered during a 4-year trial period. *Int J Oral Maxillofac Implants* 1987; 2:77–84.

40. Ducheyne P, Healy K, Black J, et al: The effect of hydroxyapatite coatings on the metal ion release from porous titanium and cobalt-chromium alloys (abstracted). Presented at the 33rd Annual Meeting, Orthopaedic Research Society, San Francisco, Jan 19–22, 1987.

41. Woodman JL, Jacobs JJ, Galante JO, et al: Metal ion release titanium-based prosthetic segmental replacements of long bones in baboons: A long-term study. *J Orthop Res* 1984; 1:421.

42. Albrektsson T, Jacobsson, M: Bone-metal interface in osseointegration. *J Prosthet Dent* 1987; 57:597–607.

43. Rinaldi AW, Goldberger EB, Mingledorff EB, et al: Biomechanical considerations in implant prosthodontics. *J Prosthet Dent* 1983; 50:220–223.

44. Johansson C, Albrektsson T: Integration of screw implants in the rabbit: A 1-yr follow-up of removal torque of titanium implants. *Int J Oral Maxillofac Implants* 1987; 2:69–75.

45. Brånemark PI, Breine U, Lindstrom J, et al: Intraosseous anchorage of dental prostheses I. Experimental studies. *Scand J Plast Reconstr Surg* 1969; 3:81–93.

46. Linkow LI, Rinaldi AW, Weiss WW, et al: Factors influencing long-term implant success. *J Prosthet Dent* 1990; 63:64–73.

47. Kinni ME, Hokama SN, Caputo AA: Force transfer by osseointegration implant devices. *Int J Oral Maxillofac Implants* 1987; 2:11–14.

Chapter 23

The Nobelpharma Implant System

Barry M. Goldman, D.D.S., M.S.
Allen L. Sisk, D.D.S.

A major factor in elevating dental implants to their current level of popularity and respectability was the publication of the results of intensive, long-term research of the biological, physiologic, and mechanical aspects of the Nobelpharma implant system developed by Brånemark and colleagues. While many implant techniques and designs have been utilized in the management of edentulous patients, none have been more extensively scientifically researched and documented than the pure titanium threaded fixture used in the Nobelpharma implant system. Implant success, which with this system means osseointegration, depends upon implant material, design, and finish; the status of the bone receiving the implant; surgical technique; and finally, prosthodontic technique and maintenance by meticulous oral hygiene. In order to achieve osseointegration of an implant, the factors that are most important surgically are atraumatic, aseptic insertion, and undisturbed bone healing. Surgery is performed in such a way that rapid bone healing without extensive remodeling can take place.

PATIENT SELECTION AND INSTRUMENT PREPARATION

Implants are used only in carefully selected patients. Included in criteria for patient selection are appropriate anatomic factors, including jaw relationship, ridge height, cortical bone thickness, quality of trabecular bone and attached gingiva or mucosa, and a thoroughly evaluated and prepared patient. These factors are described in detail in Chapter 7. The Nobelpharma implant procedures for insertion and for abutment connection may be carried out in a hospital setting using general anesthesia, or in an office setting with sedation or local anesthesia. Whatever the locale, the surgical suite must be maintained with strict adherence to aseptic techniques.

Prior to the surgical procedure for placement of implants, the patient is prepared and draped appropriately for an intraoral surgical procedure. The patient's face is scrubbed with a suitable surgical disinfectant such as povidone-iodine, and the inside of the patient's mouth is prepared using a 10% povidone-iodine solution or a 0.12% chlorhexidine solution. Following preparation of the face and mouth, sterile drapes are placed covering the patient's hair, chest, nose, and eyes. An adhesive plastic surgical drape may also be applied to further isolate the surgical field. Surgeon and assistants then don appropriate surgical attire, including sterile gowns and gloves. The handpiece control unit is covered with a nonadhesive, transparent, sterile surgical drape so that controls will be visible and accessible to the surgical team. The electric motors and cords for the two handpieces are sterilized using ethylene oxide, or

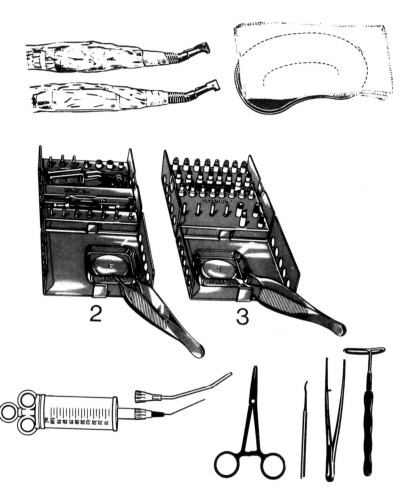

FIG 23–1.
The handpieces are covered with sterile sleeves. The second *(2)* and third *(3)* set of instruments are used for fixture site preparation and installation. (From Brånemark PI, Zarb G, Albretksson T: *Tissue-Integrated Prostheses—Osteointegration in Clinical Dentistry*. Chicago, Quintessence Publishing Co, Inc, 1987. Used by permission.)

they may be covered with sterile cloth, plastic, or paper sleeves (Fig 23–1). The two contra-angle handpieces are connected, but before connection are carefully cleaned with gauze sponges to remove excess oil. The motors and attached handpieces are then run for a few minutes with the heads held downward to eliminate excess oil, and wiped again with dry gauze sponges. There are three sets of instruments used in the surgical procedure; these three instrument sets should remain separated. The initial set of instruments is used at the flap reflection stage (Fig 23–2), the second set during bone preparation, and the third set for insertion of the implants (see Fig 23–1). Implant data are provided in Table 23–1 and the three surgical procedure instrument sets are included in kit no. SDIB 100.

SURGICAL PROCEDURE

Implant Insertion

Mandible

Inferior alveolar blocks are given bilaterally. In addition, local anesthetic is infiltrated in the area between the mental foramina. Long-acting local anesthetics are useful in postoperative pain control.

An incision is made in the depth of the buccal vestibule between the canine areas, and a lingually based mucoperiosteal flap is carefully reflected to expose the crest of the alveolar ridge (Fig 23–3). Using blunt dissection, the mental nerves are next identified as they exit from the mental foramina. The incision is then extended posteriorly to allow the entire anterior alveolar ridge to be visualized. Any

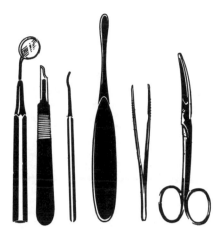

FIG 23–2.
The first set of instruments is used for reflection of the flaps. (From Brånemark PI, Zarb G, Albretksson T: *Tissue-Integrated Prostheses—Osteointegration in Clinical Dentistry*. Chicago, Quintessence Publishing Co, Inc, 1987. Used by permission.)

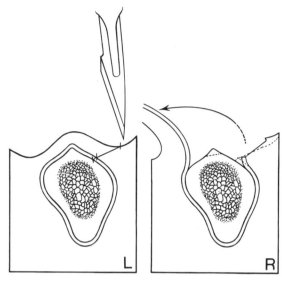

FIG 23–3.
(L) Lingually based mucoperiosteal flap with incision in the buccal sulcus. (R) Thin or sharp areas of crestal bone are removed. (From Brånemark PI, Zarb G, Albretksson T: *Tissue-Integrated Prostheses—Osteointegration in Clinical Dentistry*. Chicago, Quintessence Publishing Co, Inc, 1987. Used by permission.)

thin, sharp areas of crestal bone are removed, and implant sites are selected and the drilling procedure is begun (see Fig 23–3).

The implant sites are selected with due regard to the local anatomy and the planned prosthodontic restoration. For restoration with a fixed prosthesis, a minimum of four sites, and preferably five or six sites, local anatomy permitting, are selected. The implants should be spaced at least one fixture diameter (3.5 mm) apart, so that the centers of adjacent sites are no closer than 7 mm. For restoration with an overdenture, fewer, more widely spaced fixture sites are chosen. Two, three, or four fixtures may be used for overdentures, in accordance with the prosthodontist's plan. The entries of the fixture sites are marked with the guide drill and the high-speed (maximum 2,000 rpm) handpiece (Fig 23–4). Copious irrigation with saline solution is applied while drilling,

TABLE 23–1.
The Nobelpharma Implant System

Product name	Nobelpharma implant (Brånemark implant)	
Manufacturer	Nobelpharma AB, Göteborg, Sweden	
Supplier	Nobelpharma USA Inc.	
	5101 South Keeler Avenue	
	Chicago, IL 60632-4287	
	(800) 347-3500	
Material	Commercially pure (cp) titanium	
Cost	Fixture, abutment, and abutment screw, Gold alloy cylinder and gold screw $380 (approx)	
Instrument kits	DEC 500 Drilling equipment	$6,689
	SDIB 100 Fixture installation set	$4,937
	SDIB 200 Abutment connection set	$1,904
	DIC 300 Prosthetic instrument set	$989

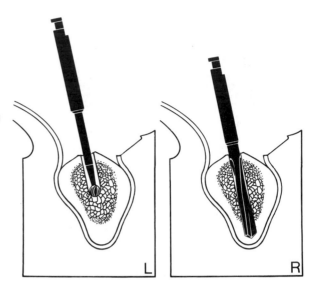

FIG 23–4.
Guide drill begins the preparation. *(L)* Small twist drill used to final depth of fixture site *(R)*. (From Brånemark Pl, Zarb G, Albretksson T: *Tissue-Integrated Prostheses— Osteointegration in Clinical Dentistry.* Chicago, Quintessence Publishing Co, Inc, 1987. Used by permission.)

and during drilling the bur is moved up and down to allow saline to reach all cutting edges of the bur. The guide drill is used to penetrate through the superior cortical plate of bone. A small spiral drill, which is marked to indicate appropriate depths, is used for preparation to the final depth of the fixture site (see Fig 23–4). When multiple implants are to be used to support a fixed prosthesis, it is recommended that the site closest to the midline be prepared first, with

its direction carefully established in relation to the maxilla. A direction indicator is placed into this initial site (Fig 23–5), and the other surgical sites are prepared with the small twist drill. Direction indicators are used to achieve parallelism, by installing them step by step in the prepared sites.

A pilot drill is used to enlarge the marginal opening of the sites. Preparations are made to the depth indicated on the pilot drill (Fig 23–6). A large

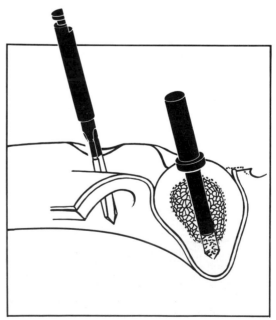

FIG 23–5.
The midline site is prepared first, a direction indicator is placed, and the most distal site is drilled parallel to it. (From Brånemark Pl, Zarb G, Albretksson T: *Tissue-Integrated Prostheses—Osteointegration in Clinical Dentistry.* Chicago, Quintessence Publishing Co, Inc, 1987. Used by permission.)

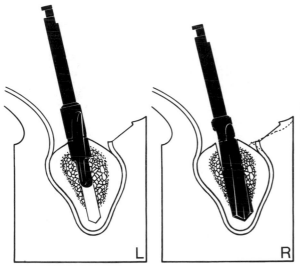

FIG 23-6.
(L) Pilot drill used to depth guide mark. *(R)* Large (3 mm) twist drill used to final depth of site. (From Brånemark Pl, Zarb G, Albretksson T: *Tissue-Integrated Prostheses— Osteointegration in Clinical Dentistry.* Chicago, Quintessence Publishing Co, Inc, 1987. Used by permission.)

twist drill (3.0 mm diameter) is next used, together with direction indicators, to prepare the fixture sites to their final depth (see Fig 23-6). If the mandibular bone is very dense, a slightly larger twist drill (3.15 mm diameter) is used. The entries to each site are prepared with a countersink (Fig 23-7). The goal in countersinking is to achieve complete insertion of the cover screw, and also to maintain implant

threads in the superior cortical plate. Excessive countersinking may reduce initial stability; in situations where the implant will not also penetrate into the inferior cortical plate, limited use of the countersink is recommended.

The next steps of the surgical procedure are performed using the third instrument set (the titanium fixture set), and the slow-speed contra-angle hand-

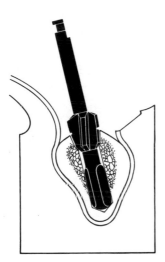

FIG 23-7.
Countersink bur used to prepare marginal compact layer of bone. (From Brånemark Pl, Zarb G, Albretksson T: *Tissue-Integrated Prostheses—Osteointegration in Clinical Dentistry.* Chicago, Quintessence Publishing Co, Inc, 1987. Used by permission.)

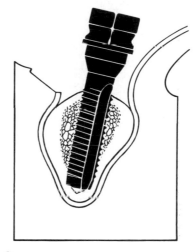

FIG 23-8.
Titanium tap prepares threads to full depth of fixture site. (From Brånemark Pl, Zarb G, Albretksson T: *Tissue-Integrated Prostheses—Osteointegration in Clinical Dentistry.* Chicago, Quintessence Publishing Co, Inc, 1987. Used by permission.)

piece (15–20 rpm). It is very important that the taps and implants used in this stage of the procedure not be touched with anything other than titanium-tipped forceps. Using the titanium tap, the implant sites are threaded to the full length of the implant to be used (Fig 23–8). Care must be taken to ensure that the tap does not continue to turn once it reaches the bottom of the preparation, as this will strip the bone threads. The tap is removed by reversing the direction of rotation of the handpiece. The site is allowed to fill with blood; this is not removed before placement of the implant.

The implant, which is attached to a fixture mount, is inserted by rotating it into the threaded site with the slow-speed handpiece. (Fig 23–9). No irrigation is used until the horizontal canal in the implant is well into the site; copious saline irrigation is then used. The implant is inserted until the handpiece stops. If significant resistance is encountered, the fixture wrench is used for final tightening. The fixture wrench is also used to check all implants for final tightness. Once the implant is tightly screwed into the recipient site, the fixture mount is removed with a screwdriver; an open end wrench is used on the square part of the fixture mount to apply countertorque and to prevent torque force from being applied to the implant itself. Parallelism can be maintained by inserting threaded direction indicators into the implants (Fig 23–10).

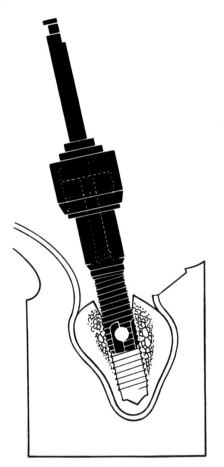

FIG 23–9.
Installation of implant with its attached fixture mount is done at 15 to 20 rpm, with no irrigation until the horizontal canal is totally within the threaded site. (From Brånemark PI, Zarb G, Albretksson T: *Tissue-Integrated Prostheses—Osteointegration in Clinical Dentistry.* Chicago, Quintessence Publishing Co, Inc, 1987. Used by permission.)

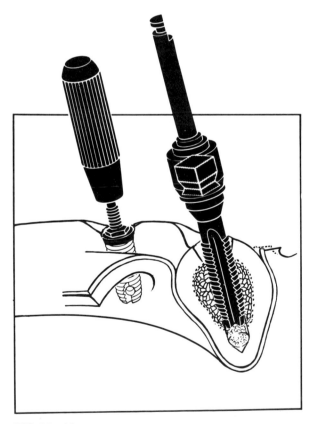

FIG 23–10.
Direction indicator placed into first fixture aids in parallel placement of succeeding implants. (From Brånemark PI, Zarb G, Albretksson T: *Tissue-Integrated Prostheses—Osteointegration in Clinical Dentistry.* Chicago, Quintessence Publishing Co, Inc, 1987. Used by permission.)

Cover screws are placed on each implant with the aid of the handpiece-driven screw inserter (Fig 23–11). If countersinking was not possible because of a thin superior cortical plate of bone, an internal cover screw may be used to minimize the pressure placed on the mucoperiosteal flap. Cover screws should be tightened manually to ensure seating.

After all implants and cover screws have been placed, the surgical sites are thoroughly debrided. The flap is replaced and sutured with horizontal mattress sutures of a nonresorbable material (Fig 23–12). It is important that the sutures not lie directly over the cover screws, and that the sutures penetrate through periosteum on both margins of the incision. A moist gauze pressure dressing is placed

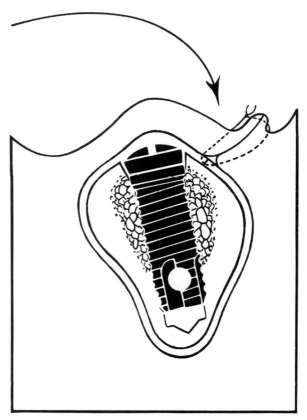

FIG 23–12.
Flap adaptation with mattress sutures through the periosteum. (From Brånemark PI, Zarb G, Albretksson T: *Tissue-Integrated Prostheses—Osteointegration in Clinical Dentistry.* Chicago, Quintessence Publishing Co, Inc, 1987. Used by permission.)

over the area, and the patient is instructed to maintain pressure for at least an hour (Fig 23–13). Sutures are removed 1 week later. The mandibular denture should not be inserted for at least 2 weeks. Before the denture is inserted, it should be generously relieved in the area corresponding to the implant placement, and relined with a soft tissue conditioner (Fig 23–14). Healing time after placement of implants in the mandible should never be less than 3 months.

Maxilla

Placement of implants in the maxilla is not recommended for the surgeon who has limited experience with the Nobelpharma implant system. At least 20 mandibular implant procedures should be com-

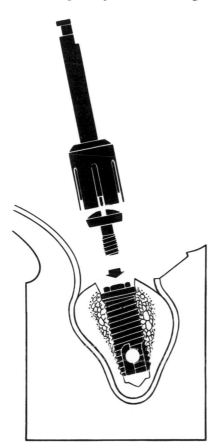

FIG 23–11.
Placement of a cover screw using the handpiece insertion tool. (From Brånemark PI, Zarb G, Albretksson T: *Tissue-Integrated Prostheses—Osteointegration in Clinical Dentistry.* Chicago, Quintessence Publishing Co, Inc, 1987. Used by permission.)

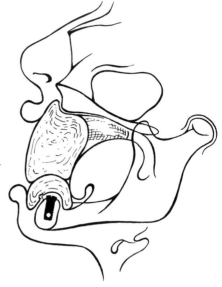

FIG 23–13.
Large gauze packs used to maintain compression of the operative site. (From Brånemark Pl, Zarb G, Albretksson T: *Tissue-Integrated Prostheses—Osteointegration in Clinical Dentistry.* Chicago, Quintessence Publishing Co, Inc, 1987. Used by permission.)

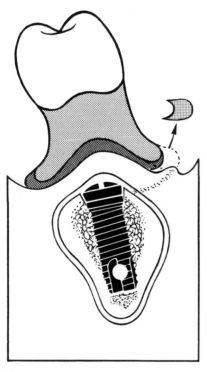

FIG 23–14.
Mandibular denture shortened and relieved for placement of tissue conditioner liner during healing. (From Brånemark Pl, Zarb G, Albretksson T: *Tissue-Integrated Prostheses—Osteointegration in Clinical Dentistry.* Chicago, Quintessence Publishing Co, Inc, 1987. Used by permission.)

pleted before the surgeon attempts the first maxillary implant. The maxilla differs from the mandible in shape, resorption pattern, density of bone, and other anatomic features such as the maxillary sinuses and nasal fossae. These factors are discussed in detail in Chapter 6. Implant insertion in the maxilla is significantly more difficult than placement of implants in the anterior mandible.

Access to the maxillary alveolar ridge is achieved with a palatally based mucoperiosteal flap, created by making a horizontal incision in the depth of the buccal sulcus from the first molar area on one side to the first molar area on the opposite side. Following flap reflection, the maxillary anatomy should be assessed carefully. In particular, the level of the piriform rim, the anterior extensions of the maxillary sinuses, and the lateral expansion of the incisive canal should be determined (Fig 23–15). For a fixed prosthesis, at least four implants should be placed, with the longest fixtures that the canine struts permit.

The preparation of recipient sites and the insertion of implants are performed using techniques similar to those previously described for the mandible, with the following modifications. When using the small- and large-diameter twist drills, the layer of compact bone in the nasal floor or the floor of the maxillary sinus may be deliberately perforated to allow the implant to be more stable. The mucoperios-

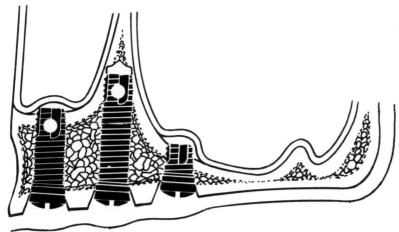

FIG 23–15.
Placement of implants of various lengths in the maxilla requires careful assessment of nasal floor level, maxillary sinus extension, and strut of bone between the two cavities. Longer fixtures usually are possible in the canine struts. (From Brånemark PI, Zarb G, Albretksson T: *Tissue-Integrated Prostheses— Osteointegration in Clinical Dentistry.* Chicago, Quintessence Publishing Co, Inc, 1987. Used by permission.)

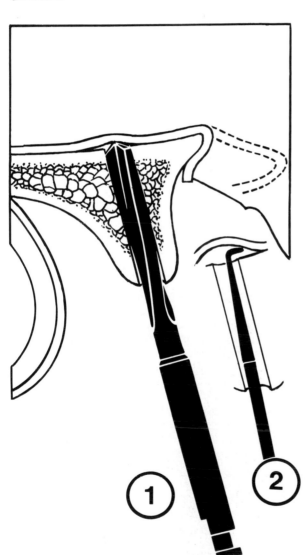

FIG 23–16.
Site preparation with small twist drill *(1)* perforates nasal cavity or maxillary sinus compact bone layer. Elevation of mucoperiosteum with a bent dissector or curette *(2)*. (From Brånemark PI, Zarb G, Albretksson T: *Tissue-Integrated Prostheses—Osteointegration in Clinical Dentistry.* Chicago, Quintessence Publishing Co, Inc, 1987. Used by permission.)

teum in these areas should not be penetrated (Fig 23–16). Any unnecessary countersinking should also be avoided in order that initial stability of the implant can be achieved. If the bone is noted to be extremely soft, only the coronal portion of the recipient site should be tapped; the apical portion of the site will be threaded by the self-tapping end of the implant. Internal cover screws are usually necessary secondary to the limited amount of countersinking that is possible in the maxilla. Healing time in the maxilla should be at least 6 months before abutment connection.

Abutment Connection

The soft tissue overlying the implants is infiltrated with local anesthetic. The mouth is disinfected using 10% povidone-iodine or 0.12% chlorhexidine solution. The cover screws are located by palpation and probing (Fig 23–17,A). A small incision, ap-

FIG 23–17.
A, location of cover screw with probe. **B,** initial incision. **C,** margins retracted to visualize cover screw. **D,** coring tissue with tissue punch. **E,** removing cover screw. **F,** removing bony and fibrous overgrowth with cover screw mill. (From Brånemark PI, Zarb G, Albretksson T: *Tissue-Integrated Prostheses— Osteointegration in Clinical Dentistry.* Chicago, Quintessence Publishing Co, Inc, 1987. Used by permission.)

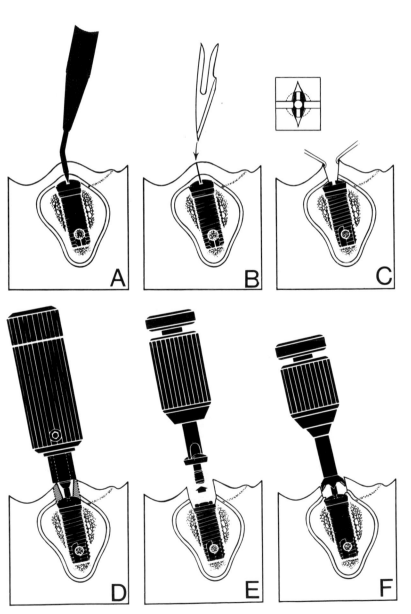

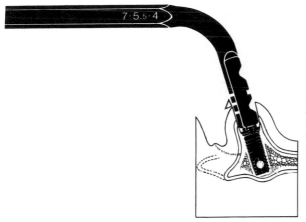

FIG 23–18.
Use of abutment probe discloses need for 5.5-mm abutment in this example. (From Brånemark PI, Zarb G, Albretksson T: *Tissue-Integrated Prostheses— Osteointegration in Clinical Dentistry.* Chicago, Quintessence Publishing Co, Inc, 1987. Used by permission.)

proximately 0.5 cm long, is made over each of the cover screws, and the incision is widened to allow the cover screw to be seen (Fig 23–17,B,C). The tissue punch is inserted into the central hole of the cover screw and is pressed or rotated to remove overlying gingival or mucosal tissue. The cover screw is then removed with a screwdriver. On occasion, bone will have proliferated over the top of the cover screw. This bone may be removed using a hand instrument or with the cover screw mill. Any soft tissue that has grown between the cover screw and the implant must also be removed (Fig 23–17,D–F).

An abutment collar of appropriate length is selected. This is done by measuring the distance from the top of the implant to the top of the surrounding soft tissue using the graded abutment probe (Fig 23–18). The top of the abutment cylinder should be approximately 2 mm above the tissue in the mandible and 1 mm above the tissue in the maxilla, with slightly longer abutments recommended in the areas of the mental foramina in the mandible. With the assistant reflecting the margins of the incision away from the implant, the abutment cylinder and screw assembly is inserted and screwed into the implant until it contacts the hexagonal implant head (Fig 23–19,A). The abutment cylinder is then loosened slightly until it can rotate freely. The cylinder is grasped with the abutment clamp, rotated slightly, and pressed apically until the abutment cylinder engages the hexagonal head of the fixture (Fig 23–19,B). The abutment screw is then further tightened (Fig 23–19,C). The gingival incisions are closed with nonresorbable sutures to closely adapt the wound edges to the abutment cylinder. Healing caps are screwed onto the abutments (Fig 23–19,D). A periodontal pack is placed between and over the healing caps to compress the gingiva into place. The healing caps, periodontal pack, and sutures are removed 1 week later, and the area thoroughly cleaned.

PROSTHODONTIC PROCEDURE

Early Care and Interim Prosthesis

Clinical experience dictates that the submerged period of healing time after fixture placement is 3 to 6 months, with the longer period usually recommended for the maxilla. This waiting period is often difficult for the patient, especially once he has had the implant fixtures surgically placed. Most patients are managed by providing an interim prosthesis for function and cosmetic appearance. This can be achieved by placement of a substantial thickness of an elastomeric tissue conditioner in the preexisting prosthesis and replacement of the tissue conditioner on a regular basis. The operator must first decide if the present prosthesis is adequate to accomplish the desired interim function. Factors to consider are:

- Esthetics
- Integrity and strength of the existing prosthesis
- Thickness of the prosthesis for adequate tissue conditioner

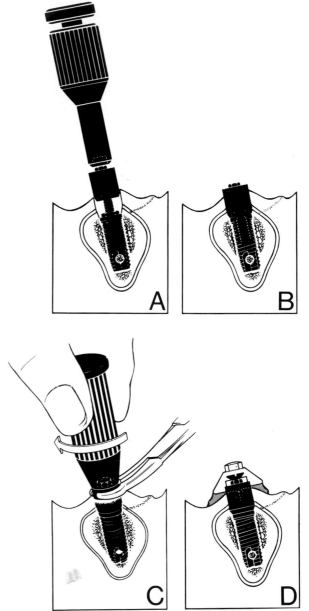

FIG 23–19.
A, abutment and screw placement into fixture. **B,** final position of abutment correctly seated on the hexagonal portion of the fixture. **C,** abutment clamp pushes apically for hex portion to engage. The clamp is then used to apply countertorque while tightening the screw with the hex wrench. **D,** gingival tissues are sutured and periodontal dressing is placed around the healing cap. (From Brånemark PI, Zarb G, Albretksson T: *Tissue-Integrated Prostheses—Osteointegration in Clinical Dentistry.* Chicago, Quintessence Publishing Co, Inc, 1987. Used by permission.)

- Accuracy and stability of the occlusion
- Patient acceptance of the existing prosthesis.

If the existing prosthesis is inadequate or unserviceable for any reason, the dentist should consider the fabrication of an interim prosthesis as the first choice. In many cases, this is the best alternative considering the factors of time, expense, and desired functional results during the transitional healing period. Often, when the existing prosthesis is used, it is difficult to salvage it once multiple changes of the tissue conditioner lining have been made. The fabrication of a new interim prosthesis has the added benefit of providing the dentist with a convenient means of making desirable changes to the occlusion, vertical dimension, and esthetics in a trial fashion. We have found that this approach leads to better patient acceptance of the definitive implant prosthesis.

It is imperative to maintain close follow-up of an interim prosthesis after implant placement. The borders of the denture must be shortened and rounded to avoid pressure on the healing tissue flaps. The internal surface is relieved 2 to 3 mm for placement of an adequate thickness of a soft, resilient tissue conditioner material such as Lynal* (see Fig 23–14). The patient is scheduled for frequent appointments to relieve any sharp, rough edges or hardened areas of the liner. The liner should be replaced as needed during the submerged phase of healing.

Prosthodontic Care After Abutment Connection

After the abutment connection by the surgeon, the patient is seen in 1 week by the surgeon and prosthodontist. At this visit the surgical pack, healing caps, and sutures are removed. The area is debrided and cleaned gently. If the flap integrity is good, preliminary impressions are made with alginate in stock trays modified with periphery wax. This appointment provides a good opportunity for the clinician to examine the panoramic radiograph to confirm that all of the abutment cylinders are completely seated on the fixtures with no visible space between the abutment and the fixture. Corrections should be made if any of the abutment cylinders are not seated.

If primary tissue closure is not evident, a fresh surgical pack is placed around the healing caps. Many surgeons who perform the Nobelpharma implant procedure prefer that the patient refrain from prosthesis wear for the first 7 to 14 days after abutment connection, until sutures are removed and flap integrity is assured.

The patient is placed on an oral hygiene program which becomes more aggressive as the healing progresses. This program should include a soft

toothbrush, interproximal brush, rubber tip, superfloss, and gauze strips or gauze tape. Some operators prescribe a chemical antiplaque rinse, such as chlorhexidine, as an adjunct. Meticulous plaque control is emphasized at all visits.

At the second appointment, usually 2 weeks postoperatively, the healing caps and the second surgical pack are removed. The abutment cylinder surfaces are cleaned with plastic scalers to remove any adherent debris or particles of surgical pack. The abutment screws are checked for tightness with the torque screwdriver.

Final Impression Procedure

The cast obtained from the preliminary impression is blocked out with a column of wax over the abutments to allow space for the transfer copings (Fig 23–20). This cast must include the usual landmarks for a complete denture impression, such as the residual arch structures, the retromolar pads, in addition to the abutment cylinders. A custom tray is formed with self-cure acrylic resin and is made with an open top over the column of wax.

The desired transfer copings are selected and are placed on the abutment cylinders, and the long guide pins are tightened with a torque screwdriver. Square impression copings are used when space permits, as the square copings offer precise positioning and retention in the impression material. A figure-of-eight type of scaffold is tied around the cylinders with dental floss tape to act as a matrix to support acrylic resin. Duralay* resin or impression plaster is brushed around the cylinders and between each cylinder to link the copings together (see Fig 23–21). The resin should be kept off the gingival tissues. The tray is relieved to assure complete seating (Fig 23–22), and the peripheral borders are shortened where indicated or extended with modeling compound. The impression material of choice, usually polyether or polyvinyl siloxane, is mixed, syringed around the abutments, and loaded into the custom tray, using the wax cover in the open top to contain the material. The tray is seated to place, and the tops

*Lynal, L.D. Caulk Division, Dentsply International, Milford, Del.

*Duralay, Reliance Dental Manufacturing Co., Worth, Ill.

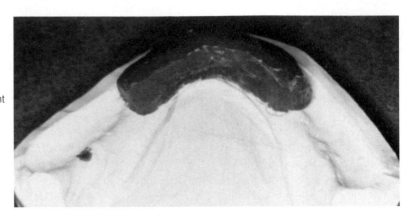

FIG 23–20.
Vertical wax column over the abutment area of the preliminary cast to form a custom tray with anterior window.

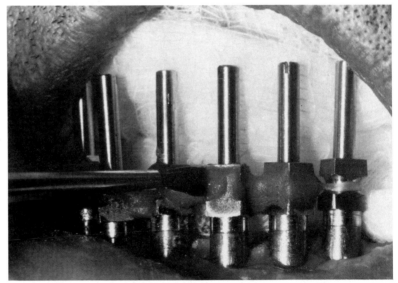

FIG 23–21.
Square impression copings linked together with resin applied over dental floss matrix.

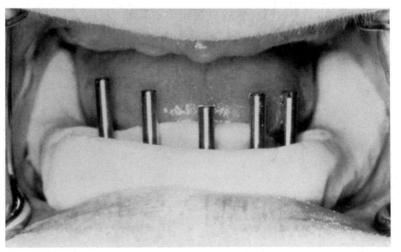

FIG 23–22.
Custom tray adjusted and seated over impression coping linkage.

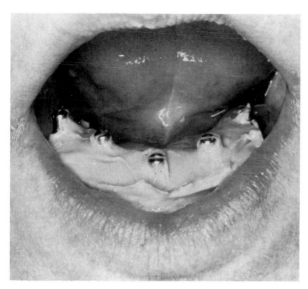

FIG 23–23.
Wax lid in tray window is removed after impression sets to expose tops of the guide pins.

of the guide pins are exposed by wiping with a finger or by contacting the wax lid (Fig 23–23).

Once the impression material is set, the guide pins are unscrewed, the tray is removed, and the impression is examined for completeness and accuracy. If impression material extends over any coping edge onto its internal surface, the operator should assume that the coping was not seated and should recover the coping assembly from the impression. The cop-

ing that was not fully seated should be sectioned free from the acrylic resin matrix, retightened with the torque screwdriver, and secured into the matrix by brush application of additional Duralay resin. Then the impression is repeated.

Normally, the patient's previous prosthesis or interim prosthesis can be successfully returned by hollowing out the implant area and relining the prosthesis with tissue conditioner over the abutment cylinders. In some instances, this is not feasible and another interim prosthesis may be made using the teeth from the original prosthesis directly in the mouth[1] or on the new working cast. Another alternative is for the patient to accept a short period with no prosthesis while the definitive one is completed.

Brass laboratory analogs are placed on each coping with guide pins tightened by the torque screwdriver (Fig 23–24). The impression is boxed and poured in a high-strength, improved dental stone. The resultant master cast is used to fabricate the final prosthesis.

Maxillomandibular Relationship Records

Appropriate wax relief is applied around the brass abutment analogs on the master cast. Short guide pins or gold alloy cylinders are placed on three abutments, and self-cure resin is adapted to form a trial record base. Wax occlusion rims are formed on the trial base. The incorporation of guide pins or

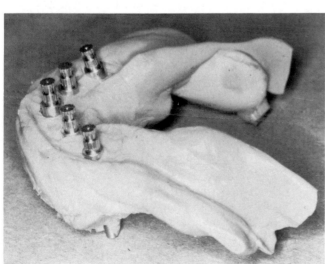

FIG 23–24.
Brass abutment analogs are placed on impression copings with guide pins.

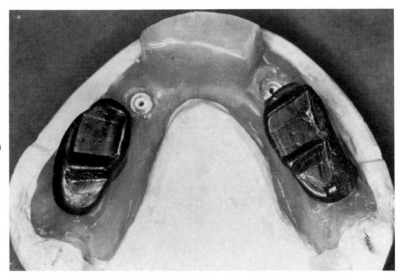

FIG 23–25.
Gold cylinders in trial base improve stability for maxillomandibular registration records.

gold cylinders in the trial base markedly improves the stability of the base to allow accurate jaw relation recordings (Fig 23–25). Normal anatomic, physiologic, and esthetic principles are employed by the clinician to establish the tentative occlusal plane, lip support, vertical dimension, and interocclusal distance. A face-bow transfer is used to mount the maxillary cast. A centric relation record is then made on the trial bases, and the master casts are mounted in a suitable articulator.

Trial Setup of Teeth and Patient Try-in

For the fixed type of full-arch prosthesis supported by four to six implants, a trial setup and patient try-in is necessary before the cast framework is made. For the clip-bar overdenture retained by two to four implants, the patient try-in is desirable but not mandatory prior to making the cast bar.

Acrylic resin or composite resin teeth are normally selected for the artificial teeth, because of the ease of modifying the resin in limited spaces adjacent to the abutments, and because of the relative

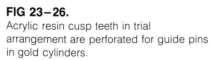
FIG 23–26.
Acrylic resin cusp teeth in trial arrangement are perforated for guide pins in gold cylinders.

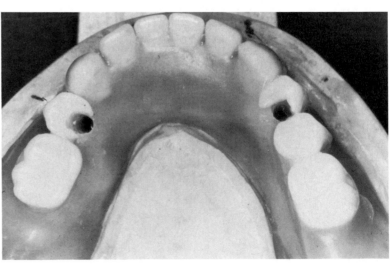

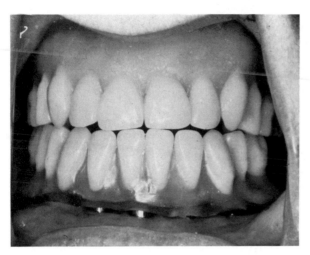

FIG 23–27.
Trial arrangement in mouth for evaluation of occlusion, vertical dimension, esthetics, and phonetics.

shock absorbance of resin compared to porcelain. The denture teeth are arranged according to the guidelines provided by the operator via the wax rims and by markings placed on the casts. If a guide pin in the trial base interferes with the desired position of a tooth, the tooth should be relieved or perforated, with the best esthetic result in mind (Fig 23–26). The choice of posterior occlusal scheme is somewhat controversial in the current literature. We prefer a bilateral balanced occlusion with a shallow incisal

guidance. This may be achieved with cusp teeth adjusted to balance with the minimal incisal guide angle, or with a lingualized scheme of balanced occlusion.[2]

The length of the posterior cantilever distal to the last implant abutment is decided at this time. Since it is known that the maximum load per implant may reach one-and-a-half to two times the applied load with moderately long cantilevers, the clinician must be deliberate in his choice of cantilever extensions.[3] Some of the factors to consider in this decision are:

1. The number of fixtures
2. The length of the fixtures
3. The character of the bony support, i.e., maxilla vs. mandible
4. The rigidity and design of the cast superstructure

Although there are no definitive rules for cantilever extension, a common guideline is not to exceed 16 mm from the most distal abutment in the mandibular arch and no more than 12 mm in the maxilla.

During the try-in appointment, the usual factors of denture esthetics, occlusion, and vertical dimension are assessed in the mouth and altered if needed (Fig 23–27). It is essential to verify the articulator mounting by making a new centric jaw relation

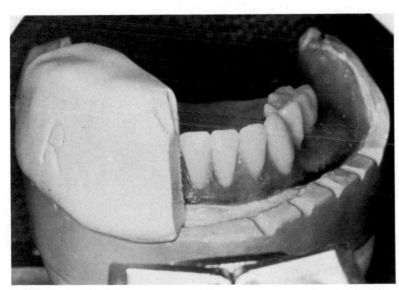

FIG 23–28.
First half of stone index made on notched land area of cast to preserve tooth position.

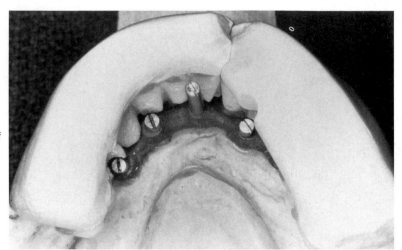

FIG 23–29.
Stone matrix with teeth is placed on cast to aid in wax-up of framework and relief of teeth.

record in the mouth and verifying the hinge position of the articulator with this record. This critical appointment should not be considered final until the patient is pleased with the cosmetic result.

LABORATORY PROCEDURES

The tooth position in the final setup is preserved by making a stone or silicone index of the facial and occlusal surfaces of the teeth on the master cast (Fig 23–28). The index is used to reposition the teeth ac-

curately during the fabrication of the cast framework and to replace the teeth on the framework later.

After the acrylic resin base and the wax are removed, gold alloy cylinders are screwed into place on the brass analogs with short guide pins. The cylinders are connected with a small framework of Duralay resin, using the stone matrix with the denture teeth as an aid in forming the bar (Fig 23–29). The final wax-up is formed with inlay wax over the resin bar to achieve the various aspects of bulk for strength, retention areas for the teeth, adequate embrasures for hygiene, finish lines, and esthetics.

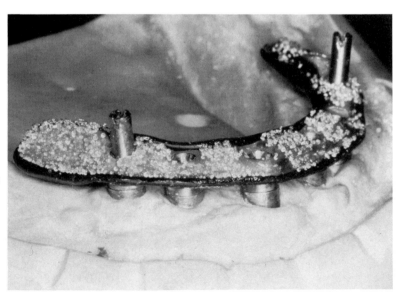

FIG 23–30.
Wax-up is formed over gold cylinders linked with acrylic resin. Wax loops, retention beads, and continuous finish lines are added. Adequate connector height in cantilever extensions and open embrasures are mandatory.

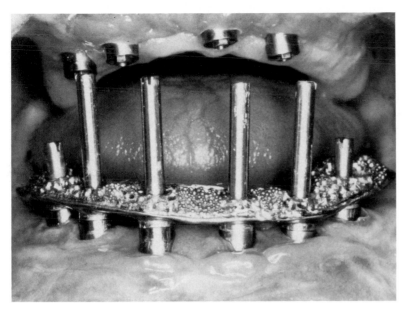

FIG 23–31.
Trial placement of cast framework in mouth to verify accurate, passive fit and open embrasures.

With the denture teeth secured in the index, it is replaced on the cast to perform the final modifications of the wax-up and the teeth for the screw access holes (Fig 23–30). The wax-up is sprued, invested, and cast in silver palladium, gold palladium, or extrahard gold alloy. The casting should be tried in the patient's mouth to verify a precise, passive, and stable fit (Fig 23–31). The framework is sectioned if the fit is not passive and soldered to achieve this necessary accuracy.

The index is used again to replace the teeth on the casting with baseplate wax (Fig 23–32), and the prosthesis is tried in the mouth to verify the occlusion and esthetics for the final time (Fig 23–33). If satisfactory, the prosthesis is invested, and heat-cured acrylic resin is processed to unite the teeth to the framework. The occlusion is carefully adjusted on the articulator in the centric and eccentric positions.

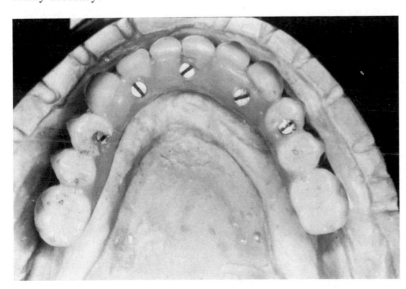

FIG 23–32.
Denture teeth are replaced on cast framework with base-plate wax for final try-in procedure. Access chambers are maintained with short guide pins.

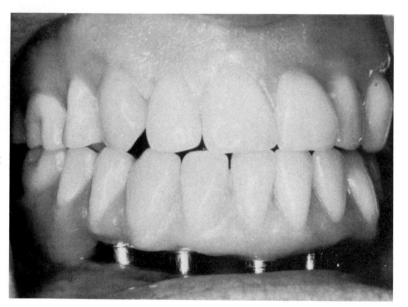

FIG 23–33.
Final wax try-in of arrangement on cast framework to verify all factors and patient acceptance.

PATIENT PLACEMENT

The completed prosthesis is placed on the abutments in the mouth and tested for a passive fit. The gold screws are tightened alternately with the torque screwdriver. The occlusion is checked in the centric and eccentric positions and adjusted as needed to achieve the desired occlusal scheme. An articulator remount procedure is desirable to perfect the occlusion. All gingival embrasure spaces are evaluated for the patient's access for hygiene aids, such as proximal brushes and superfloss (see Fig 23–33). The patient is educated in the critical areas of plaque control, masticatory function, speech, and appearance.

Once all adjustments and the final polishing have been accomplished, the screws are checked again with the torque screwdriver. A bit of gutta-percha is placed over the screwheads and a cotton pel-

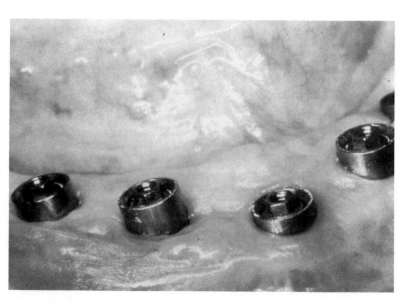

FIG 23–34.
Removal of prosthesis at 1 year post-insertion to assess osteointegration and periodontal health. Plaque control would be easier if the shortest abutment in the midline had been replaced with a longer one.

let, and finally temporary cement is used to seal the access holes. Most clinicians maintain some type of provisional material in the screw chambers for a brief period ranging from 2 weeks to 1 month, depending on patient hygiene, occlusal modifications, or esthetic needs. Once the clinician and the patient are satisfied with the results, the screwheads are again protected with gutta-percha, and the chambers may be sealed with light-cured resin. The patient should be recalled at regular intervals in accordance with the adequacy of his plaque control or his liability for periodontal problems. In the first year, 3-month recalls are recommended for most patients. Many authorities recommend that the prosthesis be unscrewed and removed by the dentist at annual intervals to permit thorough plaque removal and to evaluate the osseointegration of each fixture separately (Fig 23–34). The retrievability of the screw-anchored prosthesis is an advantage that permits this type of periodontal maintenance or any needed modification, such as an implant failure or abutment screw fracture.

SINGLE TOOTH ABUTMENT

Other abutments that are available to improve the esthetics of the implant-supported restoration are the UCLA abutment developed by John Beumer and the Brånemark single-tooth abutment (or Jemt single tooth abutment) developed by Torsten Jemt.

In the UCLA abutment system, a plastic pattern is used to replace the gold cylinder, and the completed prosthesis is seated directly on the implant fixture. The plastic pattern has the hexagonal shape at the base, a 0.5-mm shoulder, a short gingival collar, and a long waxing sleeve for the center screw. Thus the restoration may be made with porcelain extended subgingivally, for maximum esthetics. It is reported that gold alloys contacting titanium should not result in electrolytic problems in the mouth.[4]

The Brånemark single-tooth abutment differs from the UCLA abutment in its manufacture and laboratory technique. Manufactured of titanium, it is available in various gingival collar lengths from 1 to 5 mm. It has a 1-mm shoulder at the base and an external hexagonal shape above the gingival collar to prevent rotation of the cast portion of the final restoration. After soft tissue healing, the clinician measures sulcus depth from the top of the fixture to the free gingival margin. This dimension is used to select the gingival collar length of the abutment, normally 1 to 2 mm subgingivally.[5]

The primary clinical difference between the Brånemark abutment and the UCLA abutment is that titanium contacts the fixture at the bone level and that the subgingival collar is primarily titanium. Thus the clinician has the option of choice of the material, as this question has not yet been resolved by research.

Single Tooth Abutments for Malaligned Implants

The use of these abutments can be helpful in solving the problem of improper implant angulation or alignment, which may occur when surgical placement is done without the aid of proper diagnostic steps such as diagnostic casts, wax-ups, and surgical stents. In cases of poor angulation of the fixtures, the screw-access channel may emerge through the facial surface, incisal edge, or buccal cusp, thus compromising function or appearance of the final prosthesis, or both.

Lewis et al. described the use of the UCLA abutment to overcome moderate or severe angulation problems.[6] This abutment provides at least 3 mm additional space incisogingivally by connection to the fixture at the osseous crest level. This extra space will allow the making of a larger screw opening, which can be placed entirely on the lingual surface of an anterior restoration for acceptable function and esthetics. The lingual opening can then be restored with light-cured composite resin.

For severe angulation problems, the standard use of the single tooth abutment may not suffice, as the screw-access opening might emerge in areas that are unacceptable. In such cases, the clinician should make an impression with the Nobelpharma impression coping to secure a working cast with implant fixture analogs. This cast will allow the fabrication of a fixed interim prosthesis, which will aid in determining the best solution of the problem. One possible solution may be the use of individual UCLA abutments to fabricate telescopic copings to support and retain an overlay casting that can be cemented on the abutment telescopic copings. These copings must be designed with grooves and a precision taper with maximum parallelism of all copings to be used for the overlay casting. It is necessary to use a milling machine to accomplish the necessary accuracy and precision.[6] Cementation of the superstructure should be done with a provisional cement to allow retrievability of all segments of the prosthesis. Permanent cementation is never indicated.

CONCLUSION

The Nobelpharma implant system, when performed using a strict surgical placement protocol and meticulous prosthodontics, has demonstrated consistently positive and highly predictable results (Fig 23–35). As with all implant systems, the clinical success of the Nobelpharma implant is highly technique-sensitive.

Osseointegration, defined as direct structural and functional connection between ordered, living bone and the surface of a load-carrying implant,[7] depends upon a surgical technique that minimizes thermal changes in bone. Studies indicate that heat in excess of 47°C causes local bone necrosis which will result in interposition of connective tissue between implant

and bone.[8] In order to have bone healing around any implant, surgical trauma must be controlled to avoid elevating bone temperature above this resorption threshold. Premature loading of the implant also may result in lack of osseointegration.[9] Surgical techniques to minimize trauma—gentle handling of soft tissues to maintain osteogenic capability of the periosteal tissues, constant cooling of bone, appropriate drill geometry and speed, and careful tapping of the implant recipient site—are all crucial if osseointegration is to occur. After insertion, the implant is left unloaded for a minimum of 3 to 6 months, since even minor movements inhibit osteogenesis and may result in failure. Long-term data indicate that the Nobelpharma implant system is highly predictable provided that the recommended protocol for manufacture, sterilization, surgical placement, prosthodontic management, and oral hygiene is followed.

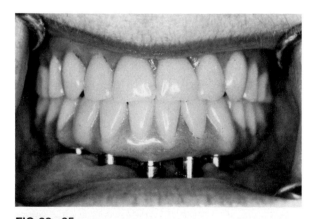

FIG 23–35.
Five-year follow-up of the patient shown in earlier figures illustrates predictable clinical success with minimal radiographic or periodontal changes.

REFERENCES

1. Parel S: Modifications of existing prosthesis with osseointegrated implants. *J Prosthet Dent* 1986; 56:61–65.
2. Parr G, Loft G: The occlusal spectrum for complete dentures. *The Compendium* 1982; 3:241–252.
3. Skalak R: Biomechanical considerations in osseointegrated prostheses. *J Prosthet Dent* 1983; 49:843–848.
4. Nilner K, Lekholm U: On electric current creation in patients treated with osseointegrated dental bridges. *Swed Dent J* (Suppl) 1985; 25:85–92.
5. Jemt T: Modified single and short span restorations supported by osseointegrated fixtures in the partially endentulous jaw. *J Prosthet Dent* 1986; 55:243–248.
6. Lewis S, Avera S, Engelman M, et al: The restoration of improperly inclined osseointegrated implants. *Int J Oral Maxillofac Implants* 1989; 4:147–152.
7. Brånemark PI, Zarb G, Albretksson T: *Tissue-Integrated Prostheses—Osseointegration in Clinical Dentistry.* Chicago, Quintessence Publishing Co, Inc, 1987.
8. Eriksson AR, Albretksson T: Temperature threshold levels for heat-induced bone tissue injury: A vital-microscopic study in the rabbit. *J Prosthet Dent* 1983; 50:101–107.
9. Albretksson T: Direct bone anchorage of dental implants. *J Prosthet Dent* 1985; 50:255–261.

Chapter 24

The Core-Vent Implant System

Carl E. Misch, D.D.S., M.D.S

The goal of modern dentistry is to predictably return a patient's teeth to normal contour, comfort, function, esthetics, and health, regardless of the degree of disease, trauma, injury, or disorder. Dental implants are often required to support prostheses to reach this goal in the partially or completely edentulous patient. Since the anatomic, psychologic, and financial variations are unlimited in implant candidates, many treatment alternatives are required to satisfy these conditions. The Core-Vent implant system provides a wide range of implant designs and prosthodontic options to the restoring dentist (Fig 24–1).

This chapter presents an overview of the Core-Vent implant system, which consists of five cylinder or root form and two plate or blade form designs (Table 24–1). A description of each implant, patient evaluation, surgical procedures, prosthetic considerations, and a discussion of advantages and disadvantages are presented.

THE IMPLANT SYSTEM

The Core-Vent implant is a two-stage implant that combines the advantages of a hollow vented cylinder in the apical portion with those of flat-based self-tapping threads in the superior portion. Developed by Gerald Niznik in 1982,[1] it is manufactured from titanium alloy (Ti-6A1-4V), which exhibits 60% better tensile strength compared to commercially pure titanium.[1] The Core-Vent implant is pro-

vided in four manufactured lengths of 16, 13, 10.5, and 8.0 mm (Fig 24–2). The smooth neck offers the option of placing the implant level with bone or 1 mm above it, allowing further length variation. The Core-Vent implant is available in three diameters. Unlike most implants, it is referred to by the measurements of the nonthreaded cylindrical portion, respectively 3.5, 4.5, and 5.5 mm, because these correspond to the size of the trephine drill used during the surgical procedure. The outside thread diameter of the implant, 4.3, 5.3, or 6.3 mm, is the dimension used to select the implant once the ridge width is determined.

The Screw-Vent implant is provided in four lengths of 16, 13, 10, and 7 mm, and one diameter, 3.75 mm (Fig 24–3). It is 0.55 mm narrower than the smallest Core-Vent implant. It is made of commercially pure titanium (99.82%) as its solid design does not require the stronger alloy. It is very similar to the Nobelpharma implant and Swede-Vent in thread design, material, and dimensions, but differs in four respects. It is threaded to the apex, hence is self-tapping, although a hand tap is provided. The neck dimension approximates the thread diameter, so countersinking with a larger-diameter bur is not necessary. The implant may be connected to the abutment with an internally threaded straight screw, or with a hex hole for a cemented angled or straight abutment for prosthodontic flexibility. The surface of the Screw-Vent is acid-etched to eliminate metal contaminants.

The Micro-Vent implant is the third cylinder or

TABLE 24–1.

The Core-Vent Implant System

Product name	The Core-Vent Implant Systems
Supplier	Core-Vent Corporation
	14821 Ventura Boulevard
	Suite 420
	Encino, CA 91436
	(818) 783–1517
	800–551–3838
Material composition	Titanium alloy (Ti-6Al-4V)
	Core-Vent
	Micro-Vent
	Swede-Vent
	cp Titanium
	Screw-Vent
	SUB-Vent
	Hydroxylapatite-coated
	Micro-Vent
	Bio-Vent
	Swede-Vent
	SUB-Vent
Approximate costs	Implants
	Core-Vent and Screw-Vent $135
	Swede-Vent $115
	Micro-Vent and Bio-Vent $160
	SUB-Vent $130
Armamentarium	Core-Vent starter system kit $1475 (6 implants)
	$2,325 (10 implants)
	Micro-Vent implant $2,375 (includes 10 implants)
	complete system
	Electric motor, physiologic $1,260
	dispenser, irrigation
	handpiece

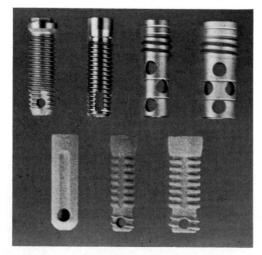

FIG 24–1.
The Core-Vent system offers a wide range of different designs for endosseous implants.

root form shape implant (see Fig 24–4). Manufactured of titanium alloy, it has a hydroxylapatite coating. It is provided in two diameters, 3.25 and 4.25 mm, and in four lengths, 16, 13, 10, and 7 mm with either a hex-thread central hole for a threaded abutment connection or a hex hole for a cemented abutment connection (Fig 24–4). This implant presents parallel rings with a vertical antirotation slot, three apical threads, and an apical vent for bone ingrowth. The neck widens 0.25 mm from the fluted body, and any abutment of the Screw-Vent system is accepted by the Micro-Vent. The surface area of the smallest Micro-Vent is about 25% less than the Core-Vent implant. Therefore, it cannot withstand the same load, and either support from additional implants or decreased load should be considered with this implant.

The Swede-Vent implant is the fourth root-

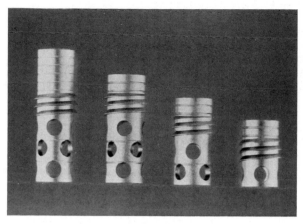

FIG 24–2.
The Core-Vent implant is provided in four lengths—16, 13, 10.5, and 8.0 mm—and two diameters—3.5 and 4.5 mm.

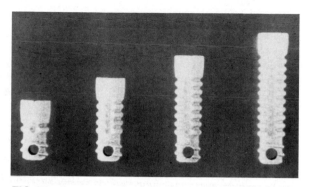

FIG 24–4.
The Micro-Vent implant has a hydroxylapatite coating and is provided in four lengths—16, 13, 10, and 7 mm—and diameters of 3.2 and 4.2 mm.

shaped implant manufactured of titanium (Fig 24–5). It is a direct copy of the Nobelpharma implant in fixture design; however it is acid-etched after machining. The Swede-Vent is provided in 3.75 and 4.0 mm diameters, and in lengths of 7, 10, 13, 15, and 18 mm (see Fig 24–5). The Swede-Vent uses internally cooled drills, and a fixture mount is not required. Instead, a hex hand or engine drill allows the bone tap and implant to be inserted with instrumentation similar to other root forms of the Core-Vent system. The prosthodontic abutments are versatile, enabling the operator to cope with angulation or esthetic considerations.

The Bio-Vent is the newest addition to the Core-Vent system (Fig 24–6). This bullet-shaped implant is similar in design to the hydroxylapatite IMZ implant of Interpore, or the Integral implant of Calcitek. The major differences of the Bio-Vent are vertical antirotation slots and an apical hole and apex depression which helps ensure complete seating of the implant even in the presence of intraosseous blood at surgery and rigid integration in the presence of horizontal forces. The design may have its main indication in the maxilla. This implant is provided in similar dimensions as the Screw-Vent. All the prosthodontic abutments of the Core-Vent system can be used in the Bio-Vent implant.

The SUB-Vent (*S*ubmergible *U*niversal *B*lade-Vent) implant is a plate or blade form implant available in two widths, 1.2 and 2.4 mm, and two

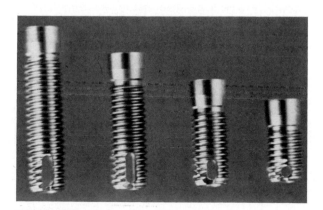

FIG 24–3.
The titanium Screw-Vent implant has four lengths: 16, 13, 10, and 7 mm and is 3.75 mm in diameter.

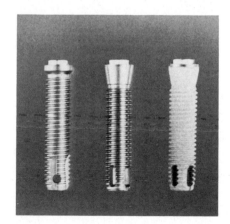

FIG 24–5.
The Swede-Vent implant is acid etched after the machining process and may be hydroxylapatite coated. The lengths offered are 18, 15, 13, 10, and 7 mm.

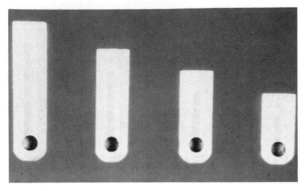

FIG 24–6.
The Bio-Vent implant is bullet shaped and hydroxylapatite coated. It has a vertical slot and an apical hole. It is offered in four lengths: 16, 13, 10, and 7 mm.

lengths, 26 and 34 mm, each 14 mm high (Fig 24–7). The grid form body and buttress post of the implant were modified from earlier designs of Driskell and James and are made of commercially pure titanium which allows bending of the body and neck. It can be modified into almost any shape because of the small grid pattern in the body of the implant. Two prosthodontic abutments are available for attachment to the bendable post. A tapered titanium abutment for conventional fixed partial denture procedures is the most frequently used blade abutment. A castable plastic sheath for fabrication of a

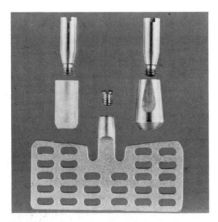

FIG 24–7.
The SUB-Vent implant is available in three lengths: 18, 26, and 34 mm; each is 14 mm high and there are two widths: 1.2 and 2.4 mm. It has a grid pattern and a buttress anchor design. Two abutment posts are available for this implant.

fixed–detachable prosthesis, which permits versatility similar to the cylinder implant, is also available.

PATIENT EVALUATION

The first requirement of implant dentistry is to determine the type of prosthesis that will obtain optimal results and satisfy the needs and desires of the patient. This may range from a completely fixed prosthesis to a prosthesis with primarily soft tissue support. Once the final prosthesis is defined, the number and location of abutments necessary to satisfy prosthodontic requirements can be determined. The primary determinant in selecting the type, number, and location of the implant abutment is the amount of available bone.

The available bone for endosteal implants is measured in width, length, height, and trajectory. The following classification of available bone for implant type selection can be used. Division A has abundant bone and is ideal for root form implants. Division B has adequate bone and offers the option of restoration with blade form implants or osteoplasty or augmentation to change the category to division A. When available bone is inadequate for predictable endosteal implant placement, it is placed in division C. The implant dentist must choose between augmentation to change the division, a subperiosteal implant placed upon the bone, or endosteal implants with an elevated risk of failure. The edentulous ridge with basal bone loss resulting in a completely flat maxilla or pencil-thin mandible is placed in division D. I recommend that these ridges be treated with augmentation to improve the category of bone before implant placement.

The width of bone is the most important of these factors in selecting implants from the Core-Vent system.[2] The bone should be 1 mm or more wider than the implant. For example, for a ridge 7.3 mm or greater in width, a 5.5-mm Core-Vent implant (with an external thread diameter of 6.3 mm) should be placed. An edentulous ridge 4.25 mm wide should receive a Micro-Vent implant that is 3.25 mm wide.

The use of the widest possible implant offers five advantages to endosteal implants. First, an optimal utilization of available bone reduces stress at the implant-bone interface. A larger implant has greater surface area to load the bone. In addition, the larger implant has a thicker abutment post, hence less risk for long-term fracture of metal at the perimucosal site. The larger the abutment post, the better the esthetic result of the crown on the implant, especially in the anterior region. The larger abutment post also offers a greater cement surface area or abutment screw for the prosthesis.

The length of the implant selected should also employ the greatest vertical dimension of available bone, without encroaching on opposing landmarks. These landmarks may be the mental foramen or canal, the inferior border of the mandible, the nares, the maxillary sinus, or the adjacent roots. The minimum required available bone height is approximately 8 to 10 mm.

The length of available edentulous bone must be greater for a narrower width. If a SUB-Vent implant is inserted in 3.2 mm of bone width, for example, then at least 15 mm of bone length is necessary to ensure sufficient surface area for predictable support. An optimum result is achieved with maximum use of available bone. Therefore, the greater the length of edentulous ridge, or the more teeth missing, the greater the number of implants to be inserted.

The trajectory of bone is the fourth consideration for endosteal implants. The angulation of the prosthodontic abutment with the implant body should not exceed 30 degrees. The Core-Vent system provides straight preformed abutment posts. If this is not satisfactory for the planned prosthesis, the abutment post may be cast and individualized to the other implants or natural abutments. This has proved advantageous, especially in the maxilla.

The solid Screw-Vent or Micro-Vent implant is indicated over the hollow-cylinder Core-Vent implant in two situations. The first is related to the width or length of the edentulous ridge. The Screw-Vent and Micro-Vent implants are, respectively, 0.55 and 1.1 mm narrower than the smallest Core-Vent implant, and therefore can be placed in ridges of smaller dimensions. Although more clinical situations require a smaller implant because of width, mesiodistal length can also be a factor. For example, when single tooth implants are used for the maxillary lateral incisor, the span between the natural teeth of-

ten favors a narrower implant. This same reason may indicate a Screw-Vent implant when desired between the mental foramen and canine in the mandible or maxillary sinus and anterior tooth in the maxilla when mesiodistal dimension is a limiting factor. The smaller-diameter Screw-Vent will allow placement of five implants in a 31-mm-long ridge with 2 mm between each implant and the adjacent teeth or mandibular nerves. This same 31-mm ridge length will accept four 3.5-mm Core-Vents. Hence, in this case, greater implant bone surface area is achieved with the Screw-Vent.

The second indication for the smaller Screw-Vent or Micro-Vent implant is related to the solid screw or post design. If the inferior border of the mandible, maxillary sinus, or nares is perforated with the hollow-cylinder Core-Vent, the core may fill in with fibrous tissue rather than bone. The solid screw can seal the penetration and allow bone formation around the body of the implant. The hollow-cylinder Core-Vent bone preparation is most difficult in thick cortical bone at the apical portion. The solid spade drill preparation of the solid implant designs will be less likely to burn very dense bone.

The Micro-Vent implant offers the advantages of a solid design, similar to the Screw-Vent. In addition, it is the narrowest cylinder-form implant available in the system. The implant also has a hydroxylapatite coating which may enhance the bone-implant surface area despite its small diameter. The larger-size Micro-Vent (4.2 mm) proves very useful in sinus elevation procedures in conjunction with implant placement, since it is tapped into position. Also, when teeth have long clinical crowns and an adjacent implant is being placed, threading the implant into position is difficult. The Micro-Vent may be tapped completely into position and eliminates the threading process.

SURGICAL PROCEDURES

The Core-Vent implant system instrumentation is similar regardless of the cylinder form implant selected. An internally cooled series of spade drills is used to prepare the bone. Titanium hex tools and a rachet wrench help thread the implants into position.

A press-fit polysulfone healing cap, or threaded healing insert is used within the implants during the submerged healing period.

All cylindrical implants of the Core-Vent system are designed to be submergible under the periosteum during healing periods ranging from 3 to 8 months. The surgical protocols for all implants of the Core-Vent system require the use of slow-speed cutting instruments with external and internal irrigation. With the cylindrical Core-Vent, Screw-Vent, and Micro-Vent implants, the mandatory immediate congruency is accomplished by precisely matching the diameter of the drill to that of the implant. With all threaded implants, immediate fixation is accomplished with self-tapping threads, although bone taps are available for the Core-Vent, Screw-Vent, and Swede-

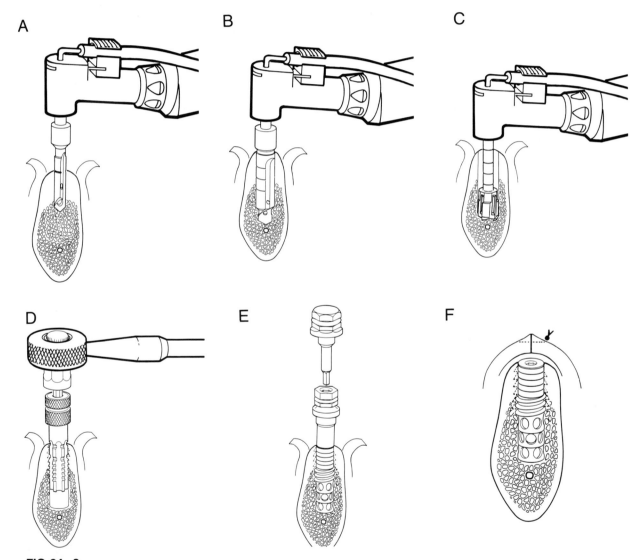

FIG 24–8.
A, the Core-Vent implant surgery begins with a initial trephine drill, which corresponds to the width of the selected implant. This is referred to as stage I implant preparation. **B,** the trephine bur of the proper size is then used. **C,** a trephine drill prepares a bone core at the apical portion of the implant site. This is referred to as stage II of the implant preparation. **D,** a bone tap may be used in dense bone. **E,** a diagram of the threaded implant placed into position. **F,** the final placement and tissue approximation over the implant. The drill is internally cooled.

Vent implants for their placement in dense bone.

Each implant has its own specific cutting instrument with gauge lines matching the four lengths for depth control (Fig 24–8). A magnified (25%) schematic is provided for each of the five cylindrical implants to allow approximate width and length selection by superimposing the transparency over the radiograph. Corresponding charts are provided to correlate the selected length with the appropriate gauge lines. Surgical techniques in the mandible should include the visualization of the mandibular foramen to verify the measurements taken with the grids.

Core-Vent Surgical Protocol

The Core-Vent preparation is accomplished with a combination of spade and trephine drills that leave a bone core at the base of the receptor site, fitting in the hollow-vented inferior aspect of the implant (see Fig 24–8,A–D). Optionally, spade drills can be used to the full depth of the preparation prior to final sizing with the trephine instruments. This minimizes heat generation in the dense bone of the symphysis, and speeds the surgical procedure but eliminates the bone core if the spade drill is used to the full depth of the corresponding implant. While the retention of the bone core is preferable theoretically, its removal does not seem to affect the final result (see Fig 24–8,E and F).[3] I prefer this technique. The greater the width of the Core-Vent implant, the greater the amount of bone core allowed to remain in the bone site. Hence, the 5.5-mm implant uses the spade drill for only stage I, or the initial preparation.

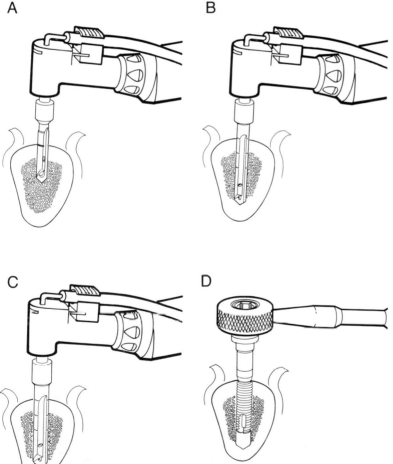

A

B

C

D

FIG 24–9.
A, a schematic of the Screw-Vent surgical procedure for a 16-mm implant. A 2-mm pilot drill starts the bone preparation. **B,** a 2.5-mm internally cooled drill is used to the gauge line that corresponds to the implant length desired. **C,** a 3.2-mm internally cooled drill prepares the final bone site. **D,** the Screw-Vent implant may be self-tapping or placed after a bone tap has been used.

Screw-Vent Surgical Protocol

The Screw-Vent implant matches the design of the Nobelpharma implant and the Swede-Vent with the four exceptions previously noted. Internally irrigated spade drills are available in two diameters to provide for sequential enlargement of the bone site. While the implant is self-tapping, an optional bone tap is recommended for use in the dense bone of the edentulous symphysis (Fig 24–9,A–D).

Micro-Vent Surgical Protocol

The Micro-Vent implant, available in 3.25 and 4.25 mm diameters, was designed to facilitate a simplified tap-in surgical placement while assuring immediate fixation. Its 3 mm of threads in the apical end engage the bone in the specially prepared surgical site while its 0.25-mm-wider neck slightly expands the crest. The body of the implant consists of a series of flutes or round ledges for added surface area under occlusal loading. This design overcomes the potential problem inherent to tap-in implants where the surgical site is prepared either too small, resulting in incomplete seating, or too large, resulting in a loose initial fit. The Micro-Vent internally irrigated spade drill is stepped down at its end to create a smaller apical diameter of the bone preparation for engagement of the threads (Fig 24–10,A and B). This drill design also allows sequential cutting with only one drill. In slightly less than 4.3-mm ridges, an optional bone expansion technique is recommended using a 2.4-mm spade drill for initial preparation. The 3.25-mm Micro-Vent is tapped in until it meets resistance and then screwed to the full depth of the preparation; the threads seat the implant while the body and wider neck progressively expand the bone (Fig 24–11,A and B).

The SUB-Vent Surgical Protocol

The SUB-Vent submergible blade implant follows surgical principles essential to achieving osseointegration. Because of the inherent design of blade implants (narrow and long), the simplified and reproducible surgical procedure of matching the diameter of the drill to the diameter of the cylindrical implant is not possible, and the procedure is more operator-dependent. The SUB-Vent provides a series of slow-speed, internally irrigated saws, graduated in diameter and width for initiation of the bone channel. Whether these saws are used or not, the final preparation of the site is accomplished with a slow- or moderate-speed tapered fissure bur. The implant may require bending of its body to fit the implant site, which follows the curve of the arch, enhancing lateral stability to the implant, but making it more operator-dependent. If necessary, the SUB-vent can be modified to various designs with actual size and

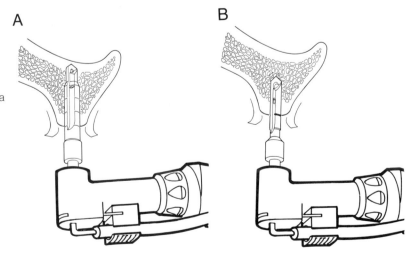

FIG 24–10.
A, the Micro-Vent implant begins with a 2-mm pilot drill for initial bone penetration (maxillary preparation diagrammed). **B,** a 3.2- or 4.2-mm spade drill is used for final bone preparation. This drill is internally cooled.

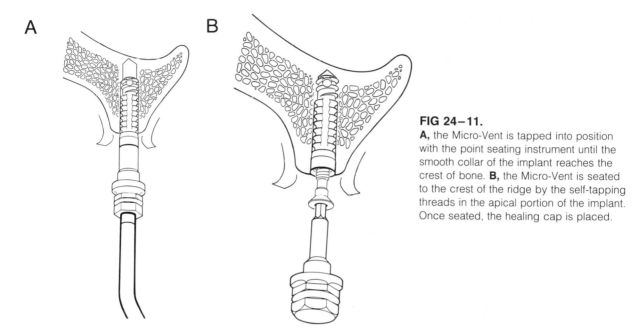

FIG 24–11.
A, the Micro-Vent is tapped into position with the point seating instrument until the smooth collar of the implant reaches the crest of bone. **B,** the Micro-Vent is seated to the crest of the ridge by the self-tapping threads in the apical portion of the implant. Once seated, the healing cap is placed.

magnified schematics provided to assist the procedure. The neck of the implant can be bent to accommodate for angulation prior to the seating of the implant into the bone channel. Immediate fixation is accomplished by wedging of the implant against the bone.

Healing

To achieve osseointegration, the implant is allowed to remain out of function for 3 to 8 months. Suturing tissue over the head of the implant is not essential to obtain rigid osseous fixation as long as movement at the implant-bone interface does not occur.[4] The longer healing period is recommended for the more cancellous bone found in the maxilla.[5]

Once the implant is integrated with bone, the prosthodontic abutment post is added. Rigid osseous fixation is determined clinically by the lack of mobility, the demonstration of a ringing sound on tapping with a mirror handle, and complete comfort on loading of the implant. This condition is accompanied by the absence of radiographic peri-implant radiolucency. If, after uncovering the implant, it is found to have any mobility, it should be considered for removal.

PROSTHETIC APPLICATIONS

The Core-Vent system of osseointegrated implants offers 12 threaded and ten cemented prosthetic abutment options to achieve the esthetic and functional goals of restorative dentistry. The type of connection to the implant controls the prosthetic result to a great extent. All five cylindrical implants of the Core-Vent system discussed in this chapter are designed with hex holes for threading of the implant into position. Implants can be ordered with the hex portion extending the full length of the hole to accept cemented abutments or with internal threading below 2 mm of a hex hole (called hex threads) to accept both cemented and threaded abutments.

Fixed Prosthetics

Four abutments are designed for fixed prosthetic applications, with several common features. All are tapered and provide a straight emergence profile (flush-fitting) from the implant onto the abutment without narrowing of the neck, allowing extension of the margin of the restoration subgingivally if necessary. Two of the abutments are designed for cementation.

The plastic coping insert (Fig 24–12) is made from castable acrylic and can be modified either directly in the mouth or indirectly, by a transfer system of analogs, on the working cast. This is the most versatile of the crown and bridge abutments and is usually indicated in the maxillary arch because of the angulation requirements of the available bone. The custom-cast post can be fabricated in semiprecious alloy or a type 4 gold alloy.

The titanium coping insert (see Fig 24–12) provides 4 degrees of taper on three sides and 9 degrees of taper on the fourth side. It is used when the implant is placed in almost perfect angulation compared to the adjacent abutments. The primary area of indication is the mandibular arch. Even then, angulation from lingual to labial, dictated by the mylohyoid fossa in the posterior, may contraindicate this abutment.

The third insert used for crown and bridge applications is the titanium threaded insert (see Fig 24–12). It connects to a threaded implant and therefore does not offer the option to bend or modify the post for parallelism. It can be used for retention of fixed-detachable prostheses with a fixation screw. If a threaded implant was placed and the 7-degree taper is not adequate for parallelism, a plastic coping insert is available for fabrication of cast posts into threaded implants.

Fixed-Detachable Prosthetics

Four different attachments of the Core-Vent system enable the practitioner to design a fixed-removable prosthesis. These attachments can be used with internally threaded implants for support of fixed bridges retained by fixation screws. This is ideally suited for the symphysis of the edentulous mandible where parallelism usually is not a problem. Even if angulation is not within the 7 degrees on all the inserts, the framework can be fabricated to rest on top of the inserts with the screws being independently placed, eliminating the concern of parallelism.

The titanium screw insert-overdenture (Fig 24–13) and the titanium straight insert have a straight-walled head on a bendable, cemented, or threaded post. The cemented insert allows a great deal of versatility since it can be bent slightly to prevent encroachment on soft tissue or to direct the screw through the occlusal aspect of the prosthesis. Both inserts can be used to splint implants with an overdenture bar (Figs 24–14 and 24–15) in either arch or to support a lower fixed-detachable prosthesis where esthetics is not an issue, since metal is ex-

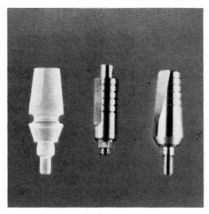

FIG 24–12.
The Core-Vent system offers several options for the implant prosthesis. A cemented post may be used for a conventional cemented prosthesis. The titanium coping insert *(right)* and the plastic coping insert *(left)* for custom posts, if angulation is required, and a two-piece titanium sleeve for custom threaded post abutments *(center)*.

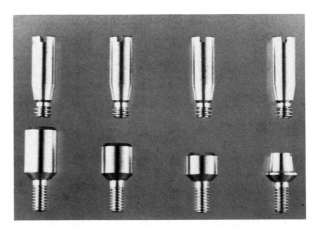

FIG 24–13.
A fixed/detachable prosthesis may be fabricated with the use of two different Core-Vent attachments. The titanium straight insert *(first to third inserts from left)* threaded post. The titanium screw insert/fixed is similar to the previous two, except for its tapered head *(right insert)*.

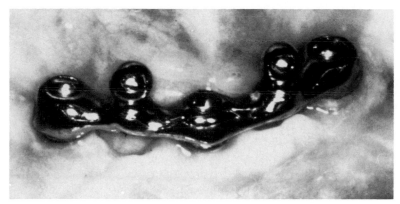

FIG 24–14.
Three fixed/detachable posts splinted together with an O ring bar for an overdenture.

posed. Parallelism is not a concern, since with this abutment the framework rests on top of the straight posts. In addition, this insert may be combined with a resilient O ring to hold the overdenture bar, thus creating a stress breaker between the bar and the implants (Fig 24–16).

The titanium screw insert/fixed (see Fig 24–13) is similar to the titanium screw insert-overdenture except for its tapered head. It therefore accommodates for parallelism, and the prosthesis may conceal the metal post for esthetics. It is ideally suited for minimal bone loss, and when the prosthesis is designed to appear similar to a fixed prosthesis on nat-

ural teeth. The abutment post may be slightly bent, provided it is less than 15 degrees.

A cemented magnet adaptor can be used to retain tissue-supported overdentures. Two or three abutments in the symphysis with magnet adaptors provides an effective and economical solution to lower denture problems.

Complete Edentulous Prosthodontic Options

The complete edentulous arch may benefit from several treatment options with the Core-Vent system, depending on the needs and desires of the patient. A

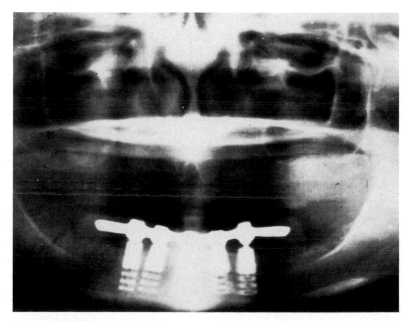

FIG 24–15.
Five Core-Vent implants with a fixed/detachable hybrid prosthesis.

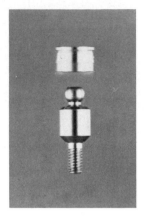

FIG 24–16.
The Core-Vent system also provides an O ring attachment that may be used as an independent abutment.

fixed prosthesis similar to a 12-unit conventional fixed partial denture can be fabricated. A fixed hybrid prosthesis, which is a combination of acrylic denture teeth and metal framework, may be cantilevered off anterior implants or connected to anterior and posterior root or blade forms (Fig 24–17,A–D). Usually five or more implants are necessary.

An implant-supported overdenture retained by attachments or connecting bars may also be fabricated for the completely edentulous patient. Decreased available bone, parafunctional habits, improved maintenance procedures, and cost are several factors which may influence this choice. Four to five endosteal implants are usually needed for this prosthodontic approach.

An overdenture, soft tissue–borne posteriorly, and implant-supported anteriorly, is often selected. This is indicated when a cost-effective and uncomplicated prosthodontic approach is desired. Two to three anterior cylinder form implants are needed for this treatment plan (see Fig 24–15).

Partially Edentulous Prosthodontic Options

The partially edentulous patient without adequate natural teeth support for a fixed prosthesis may also benefit from the Core-Vent system. Rigid osseous fixed implants exhibit no mobility. Therefore, the prosthesis connected to these implants should be designed to be rigid. When implants are splinted to teeth, several options are available to improve their rigidity. The periodontal membrane of a healthy, natural tooth is 0.15 to 0.3 mm wide. Since this fibrous membrane is confined in a narrow space, vertical mobility is minimal, approximately 0.028 mm. Splinting of "nonmobile" posterior teeth further enhances the rigidity of the prosthodontic abutments. Therefore most fixed prostheses connected to natural teeth should have two nonmobile adjacent teeth splinted together. An absence of lateral contacts on the posterior implant prosthesis during mandibular excursions lessens the concern for lateral movement of teeth or prostheses against the implants. However, anterior teeth are more mobile than posterior teeth, and lateral contacts occur in excursions. Anterior teeth may move 0.11 mm or more. Therefore, cross-arch splinting to prevent the movement of anterior natural abutments may be needed for additional support of the implant-tooth prosthesis.

Another procedure in prosthodontic reconstruction is to add enough implant abutments so that the natural teeth are not required for additional support. For example, the Core-Vent system may be used to replace a single tooth, or more than one implant may replace additional teeth. The teeth may be added to the prosthesis, but act as living pontics. Usually two endosteal implants are needed for each two to three units of fixed prosthesis in the maxilla, and every three units of fixed prosthetics in the mandible to allow independent support. This eliminates the concern of further treatment requirements for the natural teeth.

There is never absolute immobility of the implant prosthodontic system. The modulus of elasticity of titanium is approximately five times that of cortical bone. The trabecular bone around the implant reflects strain relative to the stress applied. The prosthodontic mesostructure also possesses strain, as does the superstructure itself. Hence, the stomatognathic and prosthodontic systems respond to forces with strain related to the force per area or the stress applied. The principle to keep in mind, however, is to limit the modulus of elasticity for implant prostheses. The exception to this rule is a full-arch prosthesis in the mandible where posterior implants are used. Flexure of the mandible may range up to 1.2 mm and requires a stress equalizer anterior to the

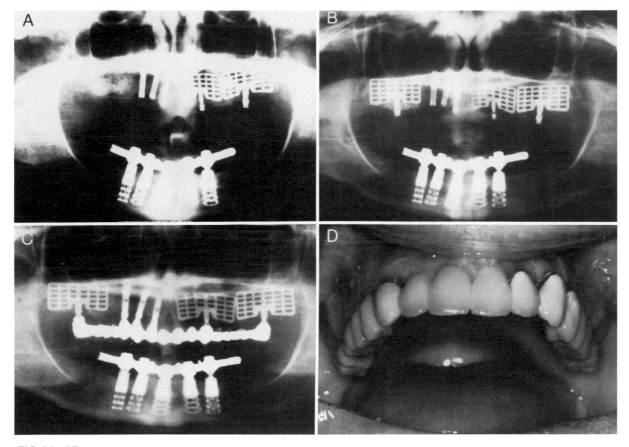

FIG 24–17.
A, the radiograph shows a hybrid fixed/detachable prosthesis in the mandible (5 years' duration) and SUB-Vent implants in the maxilla with three Micro-Vent implants in the right premaxilla. This patient had bilateral sinus elevation and subantral augmentation with demineralized bone and tricalcium phosphate ceramic. **B,** SUB-Vent implant placed into grafted sinus. **C,** final radiograph of fixed prostheses on SUB-Vents and Micro-Vents in maxilla and Core-Vents in mandible. **D,** maxillary fixed prosthesis in place.

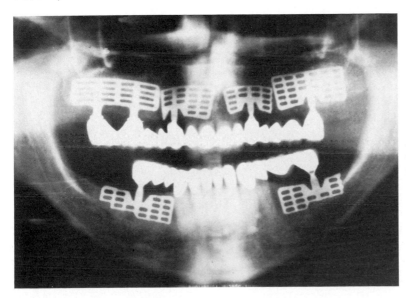

FIG 24–18.
A 4 year postoperative radiograph of fixed cemented prostheses in the maxilla and mandible using SUB-Vent implants.

mental foramina to allow for lateral medial movement in the molar region (Figs 24–18 and 24–19).

DISCUSSION

Studies on primates and dogs have shown that Core-Vent implants at the light microscopic level demonstrate osseointegration of the implants either unloaded or in various periods of clinical function.[6, 7] Niznick evaluated a Core-Vent implant removed after 2 years of function in a patient (removed for psychological reasons) and confirmed rigid osseous fixation at the light microscopic level.[8]

Clinical success with any endosteal cylinder form implant system depends upon its ability to achieve osseointegration on a highly consistent basis and to maintain function. The first factor is dependent upon simplified surgical procedures allowing a large number of practitioners, with various levels of training and skill, to consistently follow the surgical protocols described. The second factor is dependent upon the size and design of the implant which determine its surface area available to transmit occlusal loading to the bone in a physiologic manner. Lubar and Katin presented 100 consecutively inserted Core-Vent implants (3.0–4.5-year follow-up) with 94% achieving and maintaining osseointegration.[9] Laskin compiled data from five independent clini-

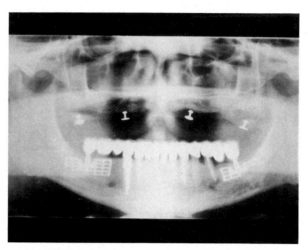

FIG 24–19.
A combination of SUB-Vent and root form implants restore the partially edentulous mandible with a fixed prosthesis and precision attachment. Intramucosal inserts are placed in the maxillary removable prosthesis. (Implants inserted and restored with Craig Misch, D.D.S.).

cians, showing that 96.6% of 609 implants achieved osseointegration.[10] English[11] surveyed 2,500 Core-Vent system users with 672 reporting on 15,150 implants. Overall success was 93.5% with one third of the dentists who placed 20 to 100 implants reporting zero to 1 failures. Of those implants reported as failures, 50% occurred in the first 10 implants placed by the individual practitioners.[11] Clinicians from our

TABLE 24–2.

Core-Vent 5-Year Clinical Study: 3–64 Months' Observation Period (Median 26.7 Months), 1,605 Implants Consecutively Placed and Uncovered

Investigators	Maxillary Implants				Mandibular Implants			
	Inserted	Follow-up	Removed	Success (%)*	Inserted	Follow-up	Removed	Success (%)*
R. Luber 9–64 mo (median 41 mo)	69	65	4	93.9	144	135	9	03.3
D. Patrick 5–57 mo (median 32 mo)	139	137	4	87.1	212	207	3	98.5
A. Buchs 4–41 mo (median 19 mo)	204	204	6	97.1	387	355	7	98.0
J. Zosky 3–50 mo (median 15 mo)	216	195	9	95.4	234	226	12	94.7
Compiled results	628	601	23	96.2	977	923	29	96.7
*Success is defined as osseointegration.								

TABLE 24–3.

Core-Vent 5-Year Clinical Study: Partially Edentulous Patients, 3–64 Months' Observation Period, 826 Implants Consecutively Placed and Uncovered

Months	Anterior Mandible (92 Implants With Follow-up)				Posterior Mandible (367 Implants With Follow-up)			
	Failed to Integrate— Removed	Failed in Function— Removed	Osseoin- tegrated— Retained	Success (%)*	Failed to Integrate— Removed	Failed in Function— Removed	Osseoin- tegrated— Retained	Success (%)*
3–6	2	0	90	97.8	4	1	362	98.6
7–12	0	0	90	97.8	5	0	359	97.8
13–18	0	0	90	97.8	0	0	357	97.3
19–24	0	0	90	97.8	0	0	357	97.3
24–64	0	0	90	97.8	0	0	357	97.3

Total mandibular implants installed	475
Total mandibular implants with follow-up	459
Total mandibular implants removed	12
Total mandibular implant success rate	97.4%
Mandibular implants lost after 1 year in function	0

*Success is defined as osseointegration.

group report a survival rate of more than 95% for Core-Vent system implants placed from 1983 to 1988 (Tables 24–2, 24–3, 24–4).

SUMMARY

The Core-Vent implant system consists of many different submergible endosteal implants. These im-plants vary in width and design. The Core-Vent im-plant is a hollow cylinder with vents in the apical portion, and a threaded superior part. This implant design has been in clinical use since 1982. Its suc-cess rate is reported to be approximately 94%, with 50% of the failures occurring in the first ten implants placed by individual practitioners.

The Micro-Vent has parallel rings with an apical thread, and is coated with hydroxylapatite. The solid

TABLE 24–4.

Core-Vent 5-Year Clinical Study: Partially Edentulous Patients, 3–64 Months' Observation Period, 826 Implants Consecutively Placed and Uncovered

Months	Anterior Maxilla (174 Implants With Follow-up)				Posterior Maxilla (168 Implants With Follow-up)			
	Failed to Integrate— Removed	Failed in Function— Removed	Osseoin- tegrated— Retained	Success (%)*	Failed to Integrate— Removed	Failed in Function— Removed	Osseoin- tegrated— Retained	Success (%)*
3–6	0	0	174	100	1	0	167	99.4
7–12	2	2	172	98.8	0	1	166	98.8
13–18	0	0	170	97.7	0	1	165	98.2
19–24	0	0	170	97.7	0	0	165	98.2
24–64	0	0	170	97.75	0	0	165	98.2

Total maxillary implants installed	351
Total maxillary implants with follow-up	342
Total maxillary implants removed	7
Total maxillary implant success rate	97.9%
Maxillary implants lost after 1 year in function	0.03%

*Success is defined as osseointegration.

screw-type implants have several indications where the hollow-cylinder Core-Vent cannot be used.

The SUB-Vent blade implant is designed for the narrow edentulous ridge.

The strength of the Core-Vent system is (1) eight different widths are provided for utilization of available bone, and (2) 12 threaded and ten cemented abutment posts are used for the optional type of prosthodontic restoration. This provides a wide range of treatment plans to satisfy the patient's needs and desires.

REFERENCES

1. Niznick GA: Endosseous dental implant system for overdenture retention, crown and bridge support. United States Patent No. 4,431,416 filed April 29, 1982.
2. Misch CE: Available bone influences prosthodontic treatments. *Dentistry Today* 1988; 7:44,75.
3. Lum L, Beirne OR: Viability of the retained bone core in the core-vent dental implants. *J Oral Maxillofac Surg* 1986; 44:341–345.
4. Misch CE: Osteointegration and the submerged blade-vent implant. *J Houston District Dent Soc,* January 1988; pp 12–16.
5. Misch CE: Bone character: Second vital implant criteria. *Dentistry Today* 1988; 7:39–40.
6. Boyne PJ, Scheer PM: Comparison of interface osteointegration of different designs of intraosseous implants. *J Dent Res* 1988; 67(spec issue):182.
7. Beirne OR, Lum LB, Dillinges M, et al: Osseointegration of Biotes and Core-Vent implants in non-human primates. *J Dent Res* 1988; 67(spec issue):182.
8. Niznick GA: Osseointegration—an idea whose time has come. *Destinations/Dental Issue* summer 1986; 10.
9. Lubar R, Katin R: Two year clinical results with core-vent implants (abstracted). Presented at the First International Congress on Preprosthetic Surgery, Palm Springs, Calif, May 1985.
10. Laskin D: Survey of core-vent system (abstracted). Presented to the American Association of Oral and Maxillofacial Surgery, New Orleans, Feb 1986.
11. English C: Results of survey of 2500 core-vent system users (abstracted). Presented at the Second International Symposium on Preprosthetic Surgery, Palm Springs, Calif, May 14–16, 1987.

Chapter 25

The IMZ-Interpore Osteointegrated Implant System

Charles A. Babbush, D.D.S., M.Sc.D.
Axel Kirsch, D.D.S.

The Intramobile cylinder (IMZ) two-stage osteointe-grated implant system (Table 25–1) with an in-tramobile element (IME) was developed by Dr. Axel Kirsch over 17 years ago in Stuttgart, Germany[1] (Fig 25–1). He developed this implant system in re-sponse to his patient population analysis which was 80% partially edentulous and 20% totally edentu-lous. He believed that in order to reconstruct the ma-jority of his patients with a fixed prosthesis, as they requested, and splint a rigidly ankylosed osteointe-grated implant to a natural tooth unit with its suspen-sory mobile periodontal ligament, a device for stress absorption and stress distribution in conjunction with the implant would be required. If a rigid fixed pros-thesis were placed between a natural tooth unit (with its flexibility) and an ankylosed implant with no shock-absorbing element, one of several, if not all, of the following detrimental events could take place: (1) flexure of the metal substructure could result in fracture of the veneer surfaces; (2) bone could resorb around the implant, the natural tooth, or both; (3) the cement that secures the rigid cast appliance to the natural tooth has a high modulus of elasticity, and the cement bond could fail; (4) eventually micro-movement of the retainer on the natural tooth could create continuous microtrauma resulting in complica-tions to the natural tooth (teeth); and (5) solder joints could fail related to the micromovement.

It has been demonstrated in many situations that a shock-absorbing element that can significantly re-duce the stress transmission to the implant and sur-rounding, supporting bone results in an improved long-term implant performance.[2] The implant shock-absorbing mechanism, IME, reacts to applied forces in a manner similar to the natural dentition[3] (Fig 25–2). The various advantages of an IME when a prosthesis is connected to an osteointegrated implant and a natural tooth have been reported.[2] A cylindri-cal implant configuration combined with a spherical apical area and a viscoelastic IME provides for the transfer of occlusal forces evenly to the bone-implant interface.

The level of stress at the bone-implant interface can be controlled by the shock-absorbing element. This element can be designed to simulate the func-tion of the periodontal ligament similarly as the overloading of a natural tooth is partially moderated by proprioceptive control through the periodontal ligament and its nerve receptors.

The IME is made from polyoxymethylene (Del rin) which was introduced in 1960 by E.I. du Pont de Nemours & Co., Inc. It has been used in both the cardiovascular and orthopedic fields for many years. It is used where clinical situations require strength, rigidity, fatigue, wear resistance, toughness, and elasticity.[4]

Extensive testing was conducted by an indepen-dent testing laboratory to identify possible dimen-

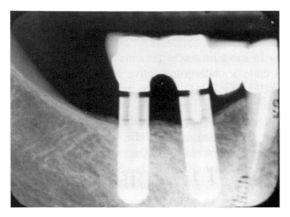

FIG 25–4.
Unilateral free-end reconstruction with IMZ implants.

Bilateral Free-End

This indication can be used whenever the patient is reconstructed in either the maxilla or mandible in both the right and left quadrants (Fig 25–5).

Wide Edentulous Span

An implant can be used in either arch to support a long-span edentulous area between two natural abutments. The implant serves as an intermediary pier to support a fixed-removable prosthesis (Fig 25–6).

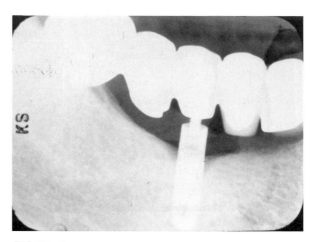

FIG 25–6.
Wide edentulous span using an IMZ implant as an intermediary pier.

Additional Abutment

Single or multiple implants can be used in conjunction with other residual natural dentition in either jaw. In the judgment of the clinician, this reconstruction is not possible with fixed-removable appliances without the use of implants. Most commonly, this indication is used in edentulous areas of either arch to support periodontally involved teeth that are judged to be salvageable (Fig 25–7).

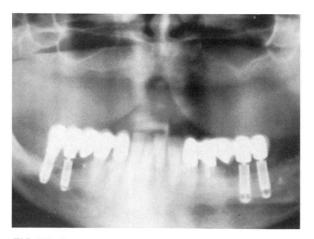

FIG 25–5.
Bilateral free-end reconstruction with IMZ implants.

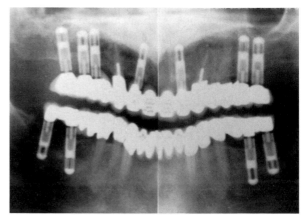

FIG 25–7.
Full arch reconstruction using implants.

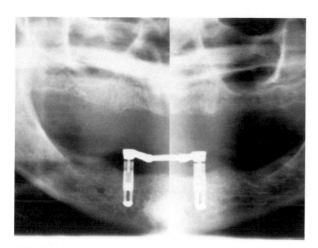

FIG 25–8.
IMZ implants in anterior mandible with an IMZ connector bar for restoration with an overdenture utilizing internal clip fixation.

Fully Edentulous Arch

Implants can be used to reconstruct a totally edentulous maxillary or mandibular arch. This form of reconstruction involves one of several restorative designs. One design is the two-implant, connector bar–overdenture with an internal clip fixation (Fig 25–8). The second design is the three- or four-implant custom-designed connector bar–overdenture with internal clip fixation (Fig 25–9). The third design employs five to eight implants with a screw-on

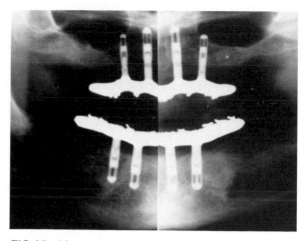

FIG 25–10.
Full-arch reconstruction, eight IMZ implants with a screw-on denture which is totally supported by implants.

type of denture which is totally implant-supported (Fig 25–10). The final restorative option utilizes five to ten implants with fixed-cast removable bridgework (Fig 25–11).

PRESURGICAL EVALUATION

Once the patient has been screened medically and dentally as an acceptable candidate for implant

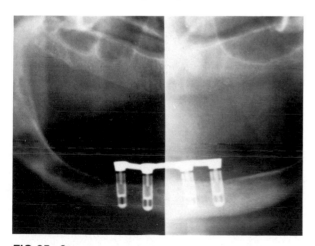

FIG 25–9.
Full-arch reconstruction, four IMZ implants, custom bar–overdenture, internal clip fixation.

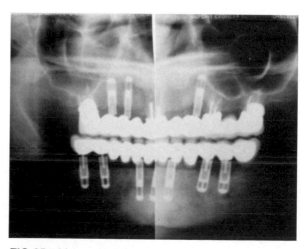

FIG 25–11.
Full-arch reconstruction, ten IMZ implants with fixed-removable cast appliances.

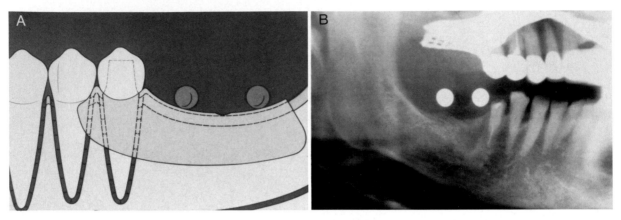

FIG 25–12.
A, an acrylic resin splint containing 5 mm stainless steel markers is placed in the oral cavity presurgically and **B,** a panoramic radiograph is obtained. The vertical measurement determined from the radiograph can be used to calculate radiographic distortion.

reconstruction, appropriate dental diagnostic aids should be utilized.

Radiographs

Definitive analysis of the intended implant site cannot be carried out with periapical films exclusively. The panoramic radiograph provides a more accurate determination of available alveolar and residual bone as well as the borders of adjacent vital structures such as the mandibular canal, maxillary sinus, nasal cavity, etc.[9] Additionally, lateral head films and occlusal radiographs are also useful. In those cases where sufficient quantities of bone are in question, a computed tomograph (CT) scan or Dentascan procedure should be considered.*[10, 11]

Study Cast

Study casts should be obtained for each patient and mounted on semiadjustable articulators. This diagnostic tool provides the ability to evaluate arch form and relationships as well as the adjacent and opposing dentition. In this manner, the selection of the appropriate number and position of the implants can be determined. If necessary, a diagnostic wax-up of the intended reconstruction can be carried out to determine the above.

*General Electric CT Division, Milwaukee.

Acrylic Measurement, Surgical Splint

To assist in determining the vertical dimensions of residual bone, radiographs are taken using a clear acrylic resin template with 5-mm stainless steel radiographic markers located mesial and distal to the intended implant site.* The template is placed in the oral cavity and a panoramic radiograph is taken (Fig 25–12). The dimension of the marker image on the radiograph is measured vertically. This is compared to the marker's known dimension. The distortion factor of the radiographic markers is then used to determine the actual vertical bone dimension at the implant site. Implant location is transferred from the diagnostic cast to the patient's mouth by means of a perforation in the diagnostic template used at stage I surgery. The same template is used at the stage II surgical procedure to locate the mucosa-covered, osteointegrated implant.[1]

IMZ IMPLANT SYSTEM

The implant is supplied in two diameters, 3.3 and 4.0 mm. The 3.3 mm diameter has lengths of 8, 10, 13, and 15 mm. The 4.0 mm diameter has lengths of 8, 11, 13, and 15 mm. Design characteristics of the IMZ implant system that are pertinent to

*Implant Support Systems, Irvine, Calif.

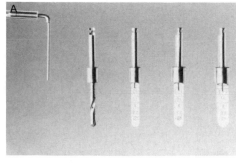
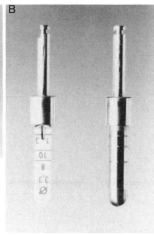

FIG 25–13.
A, the drill set, composed of precision internally and externally irrigated drill points. **B,** the cannon burs are flat on one side and demarcated corresponding to the lengths of the implants in the system.

long-term success include a commercially pure (cp) titanium cylinder that is coated with titanium plasma spray. The coronal 2 mm of the implant body is not coated and is highly polished. Research has documented that cp titanium is an effective biocompatible material for endosseous dental implants.[12, 13] The plasma spray coating is a very fine-grain titanium powder applied to the cp titanium cylinder in an argon environment under extremely high temperature, pressure, and velocity. The purpose of this surface preparation is to increase the surface area of the implant sixfold which in turn enhances the initial press-fit fixation and improves osteointegration when compared with a smooth-surface implant body.[14–20]

A set of six internally and externally irrigated precision drills has been designed for atraumatic preparation of the osseous receptor site (Fig 25–13). With this set of drills of increasing diameter, thermal and mechanical trauma is reduced to biological tolerances of the osseous structures.[21] They provide a precision friction fit between the osseous walls and the walls of the titanium cylinder. The drills must be used in an appropriate drill-motor system. The system must be a latch-type, low-speed contra-angle configuration. A range of three speeds must be available: 0 to 20 rpm for the screwdriver bur to insert and remove the various component parts of the implant system, a 500-rpm range for the externally irrigated pilot and round countersinking bur, and 1,500 rpm for the series of internally irrigated burs. The drill system must provide a forward and reverse

mode, an irrigation system to deliver sterile irrigants, and finally the handpieces, motors, and tubings should be designed for autoclavable sterilization.

All prosthetic reconstructions must be designed to be removable over the implant unit to permit direct access for postoperative evaluation, hygiene, troubleshooting, and the changing of the IME on an annual basis (Fig 25–14). Two occlusal fastening screws of 11 and 17 mm are used for this purpose. The transmucosal implant extension (TIE) is a cp titanium, highly polished collar which extends the implant cylinder at stage II through the mucoperiosteal tissues into the oral environment. From stage II on-

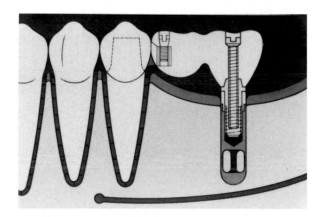

FIG 25–14.
The prosthesis fabricated over the implant unit must be a fixed-removable design. An occlusal fastening screw and precision attachment are used to facilitate removal of this segment.

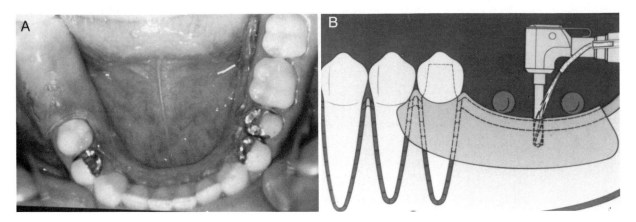

FIG 25–15.
A, a surgical splint with a hole prepared over the exact point of implant placement. **B,** a pilot drill is used to penetrate the hole, through the mucoperiosteum and into the bone.

ward the TIE must be used with all other component parts: the second-phase sealing screw, the impression post, and the IME. The TIE, because of its highly polished finish, allows healthy adaptation of the gingiva as well as allowing the IME to be in a supragingival position, accessible for oral hygiene and replacement.

TWO-STAGE IMPLANTATION PROCEDURE

A stress-free healing period of 90 to 120 days, during which the implant cylinder is totally immobilized, is a major factor in the success of this implant.

This healing period is the time between stage I surgical insertion and stage II reopening and fabrication of the prosthesis.

Stage I

The patient is placed under appropriate anesthesia. Local anesthesia is always used in addition to intravenous anesthesia or even, in some cases, general anesthesia. The previously prepared measurement–surgical splint with holes through the acrylic over the intended receptor site is placed into the mouth. The 1-mm pilot drill, used at 500 rpm, penetrates the hole in the splint down through the mucoperiosteal tissues into the underlying bone. This procedure des-

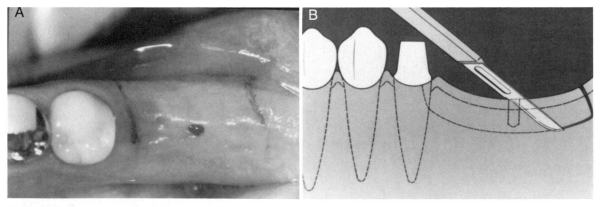

FIG 25–16.
A and **B,** the incision is usually made at the mucogingival junction. A full-thickness mucoperiosteal reflection, with a lingual hinge, provides visualization of the width and direction of the alveolar bone.

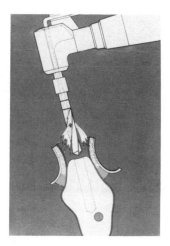

FIG 25–17.
An internally irrigated twist drill is used to achieve proper depth and preparation of the receptor site.

ignates a marked position for the final osseous receptor site (Fig 25–15).

The surgical splint is removed from the oral cavity. The incision is usually created in a labiobuccal version with a lingual hinge (Fig 25–16). The flap is a full-thickness mucoperiosteal reflection off of the crest of the edentulous site. In order to create a self-retained flap, a 3-0 silk suture is placed into the flap and tied cross-arch to the residual dentition. The pilot hole is easily identified.

The remaining drills are used in sequence, without skipping a size, to achieve a congruent precision receptor site. The internal irrigation spiral drill with a diameter of 2 mm and indicator marks at 8, 11, 13,

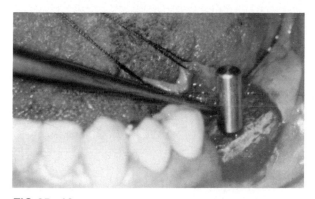

FIG 25–18.
Paralleling pins are inserted after the internal irrigated twist drill is used, to determine axial direction and relative parallelism.

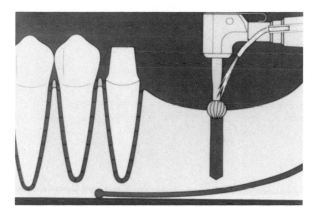

FIG 25–19.
An externally irrigated round drill is used to create a depression in the ridge crest for use as a purchase point for the rounded end of the cannon burs.

and 15 mm is used to establish the correct implant receptor site depth. The stem of the paralleling pin is the same diameter as the spiral bur; it is inserted into the bone site at this time. This procedure is done to obtain optimal axial direction and parallelism between multiple implants and adjacent or opposing dentition (Figs 25–17 and 25–18).

The 2.5-mm-diameter rose drill (round), which is externally irrigated, is used to obtain a 2- to 3-mm-deep countersink at the receptor site which provides a positive seat for the rounded end of the cannon burs (Fig 25–19). This receptor site prevents skipping and sliding of these specialized burs which could traumatize the adjacent soft tissue or result in an oversized receptor site. The specially designed internally irrigated cannon burs are used in increasing diameters of 2.8, 3.3, and 4.0 mm to match the final size of the implant length (8, 11, 13, and 15 mm) and width that was indicated for this site (Fig 25–20). Once the receptor site preparation has been completed, the correct depth can be verified with the depth gauges* (3.3 and 4.0 mm diameters) marked with the corresponding implant lengths.

Once the receptor site is completed, the appropriate-size implant vial is removed from the inventory by the circulating assistant. The plastic seal is removed, the cap is unscrewed, and the internal sterile vial containing the implant surgical stage I components is emptied onto the sterile instrument tray.

*Implant Support Systems, Irvine, Calif.

FIG 25–20.
Internally irrigated cannon burs are used in sequence (2.8, 3.3, and 4.0 mL) until the appropriate-size receptor site is achieved.

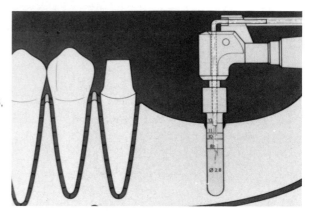

The surgeon removes the cap of the internal sterile vial which is positioned over the top of the surgical inserting head which is screwed into the implant body. It is carried (the cap, inserting head, implant) to the bony receptor site by the plastic cap and inserted initially into the bony site. It is advanced with finger pressure, which will usually achieve a two-thirds insertion. The plastic handle is tilted and will automatically disengage. The implant seating instrument is superimposed over the surgical inserting head and gently tapped with the surgical mallet until the implant is in its final position (Fig 25–21). The implant is considered to be in its final position when 0.5 mm of the upper polished implant collar is above the superiormost aspect of the residual bone.

The surgical inserting head is removed using the reduction gear contra-angle with the accompanying handpiece screwdriver bur in the reverse mode. The internal aspect of the implant is irrigated and dried (Fig 25–22). Medication (Corticosporin) is placed into the upper chamber to create a watertight seal and to act as a lubricant so removal is easier at stage II. The titanium sealing screw is removed from the cap of the sterile vial, picked up with sterile surgical forceps, and carried to the implant cylinder. It is placed in the cylinder and tightened to its final position (Fig 25–23).

Rentention sutures are cut, releasing the flap. The flap is repositioned and sutured with suture material and design of choice (Fig 25–24). If the patient has or wants to wear his or her removable ap-

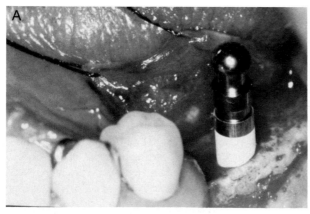
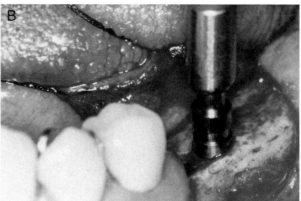

FIG 25–21.
The implant is tapped to its final position with the inserting instrument and surgical mallet.

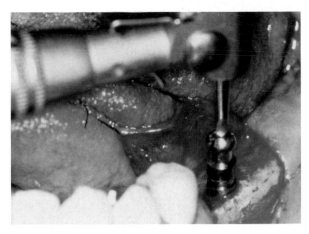

FIG 25–22.
The surgical inserting head is removed and the inner aspect of the implant is dried.

pliance, it should be vigorously relieved and relined with a soft tissue conditioning material (Viscogel*).

Stage II

After a minimum of 3 to 4 months of stress-free healing, the patient returns for the surgical reentry. Local anesthesia is administered. The original surgical splint is placed into the oral cavity. The submerged implant is located by passing an explorer through the hole in the splint and puncturing the soft tissue, which now creates a point of orientation (Fig 25–25). The tissue overlying the submerged implant is removed using a wire-loop electrosurgical tip. A light paintbrushing motion is used until the translucence of the implant is seen. Care must be taken so that the tip is not held against the implant for any prolonged period. An appropriate size tissue punch (3.5 or 4.0 mm) is used to remove the remaining residual soft tissue (Fig 25–26). The healing screw is removed. The implant cleaning instrument is wrapped with cotton soaked with 3% hydrogen peroxide and used to clean the internal aspect of the implant. It is then dried and the TIE and second-phase sealing screw are inserted into the implant body (Fig 25–27).

If the patient is using a temporary prosthesis, it

*Dentsply Ltd., Surrey, England.

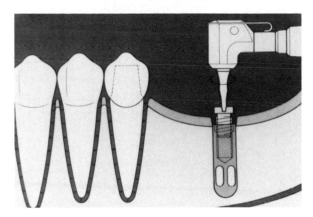

FIG 25–23.
The titanium sealing screw is secured into the implant.

is relieved to now fit over the second-phase screw projection, and relined with soft tissue conditioner (Fig 25–28).

PROSTHETIC PHASE

The TIE is used with all supragingival component parts once the implant has been extended into the oral environment, i.e., the impression post, second-stage healing screw, and IME. Often the making of the final impression can be carried out simultaneously with the implant recovery. This is particularly the case with fixed partial prosthetic fabrications where the tissue contour around the immediate

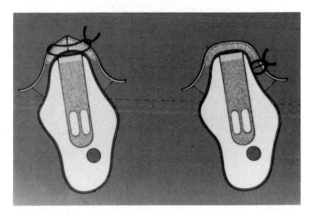

FIG 25–24.
The mucoperiosteal flap is repositioned and sutured.

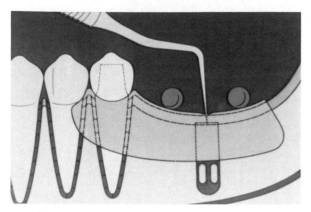

FIG 25–25.
Stage II surgery—the original surgical splint is placed over the implant site and an explorer perforates the soft tissue via the hole in the splint, identifying the implant location.

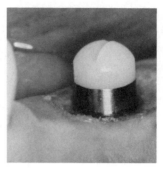

FIG 25–27.
The transmucosal implant extension and second-phase sealing screw are placed.

periphery of the implant is not critical to the final design of the prosthesis. When an impression is not obtained in this manner, the patient will utilize the second-phase sealing screw and TIE.

Three impression post sizes are available with a TIE of corresponding size. One fits the 3.3-mm implant and two are designed for the 4-mm implant. Of the 4-mm posts, one is 2 mm high and the other is 4 mm high. The latter is designed for the management of patients with thick overlying soft tissues. The sec-

ond-phase sealing screw is removed from the implant body along with the TIE. The TIE is removed from the second-phase sealing screw and placed over the threaded end of the selected impression post. One end of the TIE is smaller in diameter than the other. This smaller end portion is designed to fit within the contours of the implant body and should therefore face the threaded end of the impression post. The TIE has a passive fit over the impression post and may fall off when the post is inverted to be screwed into the implant. To prevent this, a small amount of water-soluble lubricant is placed on the threads of the post. The superior portion of the impression post is now inserted into the seating instrument, carried to the implant, and screwed into position in the implant body. After the first few threads

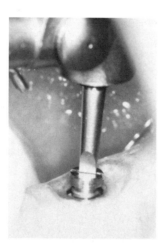

FIG 25–26.
The sealing screw is uncovered with an appropriate-size tissue punch after the superficial tissue is removed with a wire electrosurgical tip. The sealing screw is removed with the screwdriver instrument.

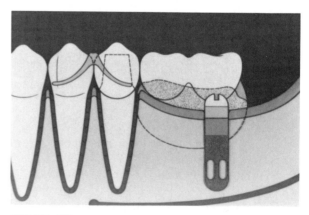

FIG 25–28.
The existing prosthesis is relieved and relined to fit over the dome.

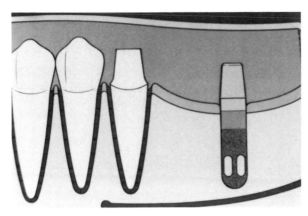

FIG 25–29.
The impression post is placed using the transmucosal implant extension and the impression is obtained using conventional techniques.

of the impression post have been engaged, the TIE is pushed down with a small instrument to ensure that the countersunk lip is properly seated to the implant body. Failure to seat the TIE properly could result in its damage as the impression post is tightened into place (Fig 25–29).

Impression Making

The use of retraction cord around the impression posts is contraindicated. Impression making is conventional and no special procedures other than those normal to accepted prosthetic techniques need be taken. As with any other abutment or critical area of the impression, impression material is injected carefully around the impression post so that no voids appear in the final impression. Any deficiency in the quality of the impression around the impression posts may result in an unstable post during the pouring of the master cast, which will create an inaccurate representation of the implant location or angulation (Fig 25–30). With the impression post instrument, the impression post and TIE are unscrewed from the implant body. The TIE is separated from the post and repositioned over the second-phase sealing screw. The screw and TIE combination are repositioned in the implant body and tightened firmly with the hand screwdriver. The patient may continue functioning with the existing prosthesis while the final prosthesis is being fabricated.

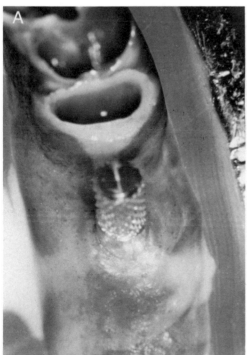

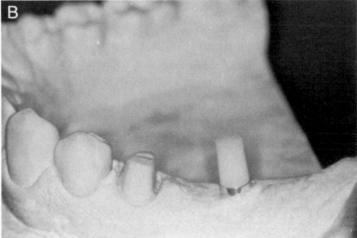

FIG 25–30.
A, the impression post is removed from the implant and screwed into the dowel pin (implant analog). **B,** the combined impression post–dowel pin is inserted into the impression and the master cast is poured.

Pouring the Impression

The IMZ dowel pin (implant analog) of appropriate-size diameter (3.3 or 4.0 mm) is screwed onto the impression post, and the post–dowel pin assembly is repositioned in the final impression. Care must be exercised to not allow the impression post to move from its positive seat in the impression material when the impression is vibrated and poured with stone. This stability can be secured by placing a small drop of cyanoacrylate cement (Superglue) at the interface of the dowel pin and the impression material. With the impression post–dowel pin assembly firmly fixed, the impression may be poured in a conventional manner (see Fig 25–30).

Laboratory Intramobile Element (IME Analog)

Following the intraoral registration of maxillomandibular jaw relationships, the master casts are mounted on a semiadjustable articulator utilizing a face-bow transfer. The impression post is unscrewed from the dowel pin and discarded. The metal laboratory analog of the IME is inserted into the dowel pin and tightened firmly into position (Fig 25–31). Careful and complete seating is important to prevent damage to the laboratory IME and to ensure accurate representation of the final position of the clinical IME.

Coronal Fixation Screw and Frame Waxing

The IME is replaced annually, and therefore all prostheses are designed to be retrievable. A fixed-removable appliance is also advantageous for routine recall evaluations, prophylaxis, or the treatment of potential complications or failure. Titanium occlusal fastening screws are available in 11 and 17 mm lengths for prosthesis fixation. The selected screw is inserted into the laboratory IME and the articulator closed to verify adequate vertical dimension to the opposing occlusal table to accommodate its length. If not, the length of the screw is reduced by cutting the threaded end with a silicone carbide separating disk until, when threaded completely into the labora-

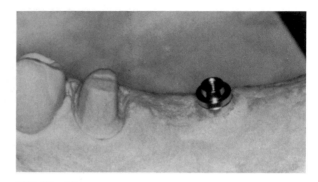

FIG 25–31.
The metal laboratory analog of the intramobile element is inserted into the dowel pin.

tory IME, the screwhead is approximately 1 mm out of occlusion with the opposing surface when the articulator is closed. This is particularly important if the screw opposes a centric occlusion stop cusp.

Intimate adaptation of the final casting to the occlusal fixation screw is essential for proper retention of the prosthesis to the implant. All beveled seats at the base of the screwhead and those on the superior surface of the IME must be replicated in exact detail. This is readily accomplished with the use of prefabricated, precision-machined, plastic sleeves that adapt over the fixation screw prior to initiating the construction of the wax pattern (Fig 25–32). The plastic pattern will burn out during the wax elimination process leaving a mold cavity of accurate proportions. Since each fixation screw must be adjusted to the individual interocclusal distance and crown height, the plastic waxing sleeve must also be adjusted for alignment. A section cut from the center of the sleeve is removed to reduce its overall length to an appropriate dimension. The two remaining ends may then be luted back together without compromise of the critical seats on each end of the precision pattern. Once placed back on the coronal screw, the fabrication of the wax framework pattern is completed incorporating the sleeve into the final pattern.

FIXED RESTORATIVE DESIGN

Because the IMZ implant system was designed to be splinted to adjacent natural tooth units via its

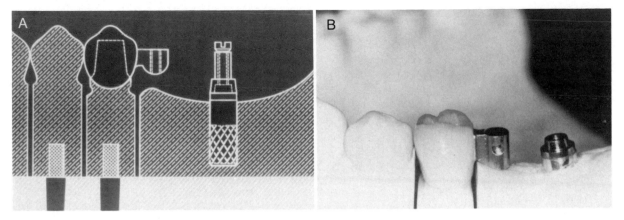

FIG 25–32.
A, the occlusal fastening screw is adjusted for the opposing occlusal table with a minimum 1.0-mm clearance. **B,** the prefabricated, precision-machined plastic waxing sleeve is adjusted to the screw length.

IME, it is possible and desirable to fabricate a fixed-removable prosthesis. Since the retrievability of that portion of the restoration connected to the implant is essential, attachments to natural abutments are always indicated. Modalities for attachment must be carefully evaluated. Whenever possible, and particularly in edentulous spans of over 10 mm, precision attachments are preferred. The T-Bloc* and the 'TS' screw type in an extracoronal block are two of the more advantageous examples of this type of attachment. For shorter edentulous spans, a pin and tube type of design such as the Stabilized Cylinder* can be used. This castable design incorporates a locking tube and pin accompanied by matching parallel walls or guiding planes that resist lateral distortion. This type of attachment can only be utilized when the implant is distal to natural abutments. In this configuration the natural anterior component of force will seat the male pin into the intracoronal female under function. Natural abutments posterior to the implant will always require an attachment with some locking mechanism such as a screw. Without the mechanism, the anterior component of force would have a tendency to lift the male pin from the female under function, compromising the connection of the individual portions of the restoration (Fig 25–33).

*Implant Support Systems, Irvine, Calif.

Framework Try-In

Once the framework has been completed and before veneering, the casting should be tried on the actual implants and natural abutments. Because of the compressibility of the clinical polyoxymethylene (POM) IME, the try-in should be conducted on the metal laboratory IMEs. Discrepancies between the fit of the casting on the cast and in the oral cavity can be easily discerned. If the try-in were conducted on the POM-IME it would be possible, through tightening of the coronal fixation screw, to exert enough force and stress on the POM-IME to draw it up against a distorted framework making it appear to fit properly. If this were done and the restoration carried to completion, the excessive continual tensile loads on the IME would cause its premature failure when subjected to functional loading.

INSERTION OF THE FINAL PROSTHESIS

The second-phase sealing screw, along with the TIE, is removed from the implant and the internal aspect of the implant body is cleaned using the cleaning instrument, cotton, and 3% hydrogen peroxide. The clinical POM-IME is fitted to the end of the IME insertion instrument, the TIE is placed over the threaded end of the IME, and the IME is

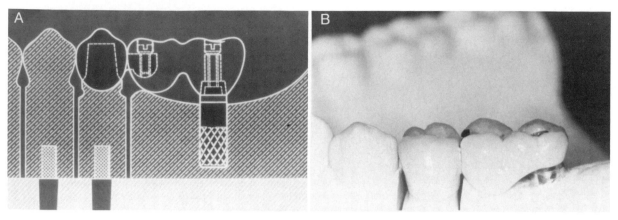

FIG 25–33.
A and **B,** the final prosthesis consists of a removal unit over the implant. It incorporates a rigid precision attachment distal to the adjacent natural abutment and an occlusal fastening screw.

threaded into the implant (Fig 25–34). If the restoration includes a natural tooth abutment, the corresponding crown is cemented on this abutment using normal procedures and materials. The removable portion of the restoration is then positioned over the implant, seating the precision attachment components together and the implant-borne pontic on top of the IME. The titanium fastening screw is seated through the prosthesis and tightened firmly with the hand screwdriver. If screws have been used with a precision attachment, they are tightened into position. Refinement of the prosthesis involves verification and adjustment of any occlusal discrepancies, removing, reglazing, and replacing the restoration if necessary. For esthetic reasons it may be desirable to

cover the occlusal fastening screw. Should this be the case, the slot in the screwhead is covered with Dycal* or gutta-percha. Light-cured resin may then be placed over the countersunk screw (Fig 25–35).

Careful patient selection, critical diagnosis, thorough preoperative treatment planning, precise surgical and prosthetic techniques, as well as patient education and motivation, are important factors in the long-term success of the IMZ implant system (Fig 25–36).

The IMZ implant system has been used in Europe for many years and in North America since 1985.

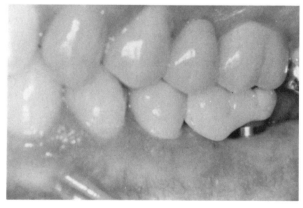

FIG 25–35.
Buccal view of completed distal free-end reconstruction.

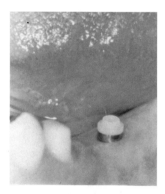

FIG 25–34.
The intramobile element is placed into the implant and tightened into position.

*L.D. Caulk Co., Milford, Del.

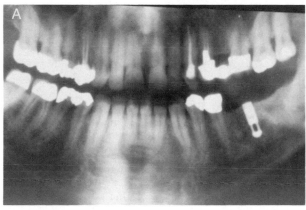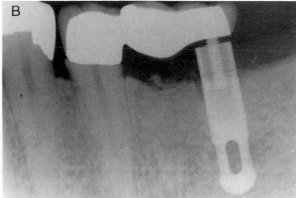

FIG 25–36.
A, immediate postinsertion radiograph. **B,** 5-year postreconstruction radiograph.

As of this writing, Kirsch has placed over 4,269 implants in 1,806 patients. Only 99 implants have been removed, with a resultant 97.6% survival rate. (Of the 4,269 implants in 1,806 patients, 10.9% have been lost to follow-up.) One of us (C.A.B.) has placed 561 implants with only 14 removals over a 3-year period— a 97% survival rate. (All of these patients have been followed on an annual basis.) Others have reported 802 implants, with 13 removals and 7 lost to follow-up over a 4-year period, a 98.38% survival rate.

REFERENCES

1. Babbush C, Kirsch A, Mentag P, et al: Intramobile cylinder (IMZ) two-stage osteointegrated implant system with the intramobile element (IME): Part I. Its rationale and procedure for use. *Int J Oral Maxillofac Implants* 1987; 2:203–216.
2. Fuhrmann G, Kirsch A, Sauer G, et al: Strength and elastic properties of various stress absorbing elements in IMZ implants (in German). *Dtsch Zahnarztl Z* 1983; 38:123–125.
3. Benzing U, Weber H, Geis-Gerstorfer J, et al: The mechanical load on IMZ implants. Fundamental problems of measurement technique and data collection (in German). *Zeitschrift fur Zahnaerztliche Implantologie* 1987; 3:858–861.
4. *Interpore IMZ Technique Manual.* Irvine, Calif, Interpore International.
5. *Fatigue Testing of Polyacetyl Intramobile Element in Axial Compression,* Irvine, Calif, Analytical Service Center, American Hospital Supply Corp, February 1987.
6. *Report on the Geometric, Mechanical, Physical, and Chemical Characteristics of Exchanged TME's.* Irvine, Calif, Analytical Service Center, American Hospital Supply Corp, March 1987.
7. *IMZ Two-Stage Osteointegration Endosseous Implant System.* Submitted to American Dental Association, Council on Dental Materials, Instruments, and Equipment Acceptance Program for Endosseous Implants. Irvine, Calif, Interpore International, March 1987.
8. Babbush CA: *Surgical Atlas of Dental Implant Techniques.* Philadelphia, WB Saunders Co., 1980.
9. Babbush CA, Kirsch A, Mentag P, et al: The IMZ endosseous two-phase osteointegration implant system. *Alpha Omegan* 1987; 80:52–61.
10. Schwartz MS, Rothman SLG, Rhodes ML, et al: Computed tomography: Part I. Preoperative assessment of the mandible for endosseous implant surgery. *Int J Oral Maxillofac Implants* 1987; 2:137–141.
11. Schwartz MS, Rothman SLG, Rhodes ML, et al: Computed tomography: Part II. Preoperative assessment of the maxilla for endosseous implant surgery. *Int J Oral Maxillofac Implants* 1987; 2:143–148.
12. Weiss, CM: Tissue integration of dental endosseous implants: Description and comparative analysis of the fibro-osseous integration and osseous integration systems. *J Oral Implantol* 1986; 12:169–214.
13. Brånemark P-I: Osseointegration and its experimental background. *J Prosthet Dent* 1983; 50:399–410.
14. Kirsch A, Donath K: A histologic evaluation of various titanium implant surface textures in animals (in

German). *Fortschrifte der Zahnaertliche Implantologie* 1984; 1:35–40.

15. Babbush CA, Kent JN, Misiek DJ: Titanium plasma-sprayed (TPS) screw implants for the reconstruction of the edentulous mandible. *J Oral Maxillofac Surg* 1986; 44:274.

16. Babbush CA, Kent JN, Salon JM: A solution for the problematic atrophic mandible: The titanium plasma spray (TPS) screw implant system. *Geriodontics* 1986; 2:16–23.

17. Babbush CA: Mandibular subperiosteal, endosteal blade-vents, titanium plasma spray and endosteal hollow-cylinder systems for maxillofacial reconstruction, in Fonseca RJ, Davis WH: *Reconstructive Preprosthetic Oral and Maxillofacial Surgery,* Philadelphia, WB Saunders Co, 1986, pp 245–281.

18. Schroeder A, van der Zypen E, Stich H, et al.: The reactions of bone, connective tissue, and epithelium to endosteal implants with titanium-sprayed surfaces. *J Maxillofac Surg* 1981; 9:15–25.

19. Schroeder A, Pohler O, Sutter F: Tissue reaction to a titanium hollow-cylinder implant with titanium sprayed layer surface. *Schweiz Monatsschr Zahnheilkd* 1976; 86:713–727.

20. Erickson RA, Adell R: Temperatures during drilling for the placement of implants using the osseointegration technique. *J Oral Maxillofac Surg* 1986; 44:4–7.

21. d'Hoedt B, Nay Th, Mohlmann H, et al: The use of an infrared technique to measure temperature during bone preparation for dental implants (in German). *Zeitschrift fur Zahnaerztliche Implantologie* 1987; 3:123–130.

Chapter 26

The Steri-Oss Implant System

Jack A. Hahn, D.D.S.

SYSTEM OVERVIEW

The Steri-Oss implant system by Denar Corporation incorporates a two-stage implant made of 99.5% commercially pure titanium. The screw-shape implant is designed to achieve osseointegration and long-term success, building on the scientific studies conducted in Sweden over a 20-year period.

The implant is supplied precleaned and sterile in a no-touch double-aseptic transfer package. This enables implant placement without the danger of contamination of the critical titanium oxide surface of the implant.

The surgical system is designed for maximum simplicity and efficiency of the surgical team. The system utilizes a high-torque low-speed handpiece with a sterile irrigation system. The internally irrigated titanium nitride–coated cutting instruments are contained in a surgical tray.

The versatility of the five types of prosthetic attachments allows flexibility in treatment planning and prosthetic construction ranging from overdenture retention to single tooth replacement to full-arch fixed and fixed-removable restorations (Table 26–1).

IMPLANTS

The root form implants are available in three different diameters (Fig 26–1), identified by color codes on the outside of the package:

The 3.8-mm miniseries (color-coded white) has

a 2-mm-long straight polished neck and is available in lengths of 8, 10, and 12 mm. This series is indicated where bone height is limited and for general use where ridge width will not likely result in post-surgical bone resorption.

The 3.5-mm series (color-coded red) and the 4.0-mm series (color-coded blue) have a 4.5-mm-long tapered neck, with the uppermost 2 mm polished. These series are available in lengths of 12, 16, and 20 mm. The 3.5-mm and 4.0-mm series are indicated where uneven ridge shape will cause a portion of the neck to be exposed when the implant is placed.

The implant design has three different areas:

The highly polished periodontal neck is designed to enable long-term maintenance of the soft tissue around the implants. The tight fit of the neck into the prepared implant site prevents the invasion of soft tissue during the healing phase. The internal threads in the neck accept a wide range of standard prosthetic attachments.

The screw-shape body achieves immediate rigid fixation in the bone at the time of placement. The thread design (Fig 26–2) distributes vertical occlusal loads uniformly throughout the bone, while maximizing the volume of bone between the threads. Acid etching of the surface results in an extremely clean uniformly textured surface. Scanning auger microscopy, used for thin-film analysis and routinely used to inspect the implant surfaces, shows the implants to be clean and free of contaminants, an important aspect for achieving osseointegration.

TABLE 26–1.

The Steri-Oss Implant System

Product name	Denar Steri-Oss implant system
Manufacturer/supplier	Denar Corporation
	901 East Cerritos Avenue
	Anaheim, CA 92805
	1-800-854-9316
	(714) 776-9000
Material composition	
Implants	CP Titanium
Prosthetic attachments (heads)	Titanium alloy (Ti-6Al-4V)
Approximate cost	Steri-Oss root form implants, all sizes $145
	Steri-Oss blade form implants $145
	Prosthodontic starter kit
	Prosthodontic instrumentation and manual only, no abutments $200

The self-threading implant tip allows the implant to be screwed into soft bone such as the maxilla, without tapping, to maximize the initial fixation at the time of placement.

The company also manufactures a Steri-Oss blade and plate form implant.

SURGICAL SYSTEM

Each system contains an implant organizer, which displays the implant packages and helps the staff maintain inventory levels; a surgical kit; hand-piece system; surgical manual; and prosthetic manual (Fig 26–3).

Specially designed slow-speed, high-torque handpiece systems are available with either air-powered or electric-powered control units. The speed range of the air system is 0 to 200 rpm and of the electric system is 20 to 300 rpm. Each system utilizes a self-contained sterile irrigation delivery system (see Fig 26–3).

The surgical kit contains internally irrigated, titanium nitride–coated surgical burs. The surgical burs are color-coded by size to correspond to the im-

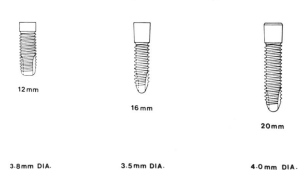

3.8mm DIA.   3.5mm DIA.   4.0mm DIA.

FIG 26–1.
The Steri-Oss root form first-stage endosteal implants are available in 3.5- and 4.0-mm-diameter implants in lengths of 12, 16, and 20 mm. The 3.8-mm-diameter miniseries implant for limited bone situations is available in lengths of 8, 10, and 12 mm.

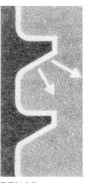

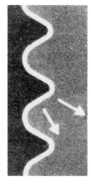

DENAR
THREAD DESIGN

OTHER LEADING
IMPLANT THREAD DESIGNS

FIG 26–2.
Diagram depicting the design of the Denar root form threads *(left panel),* which provide good force distribution and maximize volume of bone between threads. Other implant thread designs are shown in *center* and *right panels.*

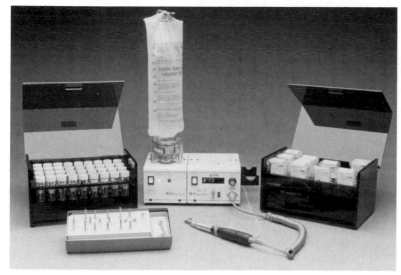

FIG 26–3.
The Steri-Oss complete surgical implant system armamentarium.

plant size being placed, thereby reducing confusion in the operating room. Each bur is clearly marked with depth reference lines for easy placement of the implant even with the crest of the ridge (Fig 26–4). A description of each bur follows:

Pilot drills—The anterior pilot drill is marked for implant lengths of 12, 14, 16, and 20 mm and the posterior drill marked for lengths of 8, 10, and 12 mm (see Fig 26–4). The diameter of the pilot drills is 2 mm.

Sizing drills—The 3.8-mm series anterior drill is marked for implant lengths of 12, 14, and 16 mm and the posterior drills marked for lengths of 8, 10,

and 12 mm. The 3.5- and 4.0-mm series anterior drills are marked for implant lengths of 12, 16, and 20 mm and the posterior drills are marked for lengths of 12 and 16 mm (see Fig 26–4).

Counterbores—There is one counterbore for each series of implant. The top edge of the cutting flutes is the depth reference mark for each counterbore (see Fig 26–4).

Thread formers—The 3.8-mm series anterior thread formers are marked for implant lengths of 12, 14, and 16 mm and the posterior thread formers are marked for lengths of 8, 10, and 12 mm. The 3.5- and 4.0-mm series anterior thread formers are marked for implant lengths of 12, 16, and 20 mm and the posterior thread formers are marked for lengths of 12 and 16 mm. The last thread on each thread former is the reference line for the shortest implant for that thread former (see Fig 26–4).

PROSTHETIC ATTACHMENTS

The Steri-Oss prosthetic attachments are standardized to fit the entire range of implants. The five different prosthetic attachments include coronal screws and telescoping abutments for fixed removable bridgework; full-arch reconstructions and tissue bars for overdenture retention; fixed abutments for single tooth replacements, fixed bridges, and full-

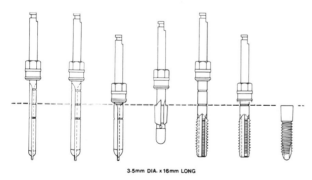

3.5mm DIA. x 16mm LONG

FIG 26–4.
The Steri-Oss surgical inserting instruments. *From left to right,* pilot drill, anterior sizing drill, posterior sizing drill, counterbore, anterior thread former, posterior thread former, and implant for comparison.

arch fixed restorations; O ring and magnetic attachments for overdenture retention.

Each attachment is available in two lengths which, when combined with the 4-mm tissue abutment, allow 2-mm adjustments in abutment length.

The abutments are made of titanium alloy (Ti-6Al-4V) for superior strength and each component which is designed to pass through the soft tissue is highly polished. The 3.8 mm diameter of the abutments matches the superior diameter of each of the implants, eliminating any overhang or undercuts which can make cleaning around the abutment-to-implant junction difficult.

PATIENT SELECTION

Implant candidates are patients for whom conventional prosthetic restorative dentistry is of no avail. The decision whether the patient who could benefit from an implant or implants can have the procedure would depend largely on his or her existing medical and psychological conditions and habits.

From a medical standpoint, any preexisting or existing condition that would interfere with hard and soft tissue healing would contraindicate the placement of implants. Psychological disorders or the patient's lack of appreciation for the implant benefits might contraindicate the use of implants in a treatment plan. Habits such as chronic smoking, frequent alcohol consumption, nail or pencil biting, tobacco chewing, or bruxism may also contraindicate implant placement.

Careful evaluation of both medical and psychological conditions should be considered before deciding on implant surgery. Blood studies as well as physician consultations should be performed prior to implant surgery. If it is determined the patient can have and will benefit from a dental implant, then it should be performed on an informed patient who is in complete understanding of the benefits and associated risks. The patient must be educated and motivated to care for the implant(s) and associated prosthetic reconstruction.

TREATMENT PLANNING

The Steri-Oss implant may be used freestanding for single tooth replacement, as a pier abutment for long-span bridge construction, as a distal abutment for a fixed bridge, or in series (two or more) for fixed detachable prosthetic reconstructions.

Clinical observation should consist of noting the condition and position of existing teeth, periodontal support, occlusal relationship, and temporomandibular joint condition. In the edentulous area, height and width of the ridge, soft tissue architecture, and mesiodistal span should be noted. In some instances it may be necessary to graft tissue where implants are to be placed and there is an insufficient zone of attached tissue. Radiographic examination should include bone height, density, location of the maxillary sinus, the inferior alveolar canal, and the mental foramen.

Mounted study models and diagnostic wax-ups of the case should be made to identify implant locations. Surgical stents made from the study models and diagnostic wax-up are extremely helpful in aiding the surgeon place the implants in the proper location and angulation for optimal prosthetic reconstruction.

IMPLANT PLACEMENT

Surgical Preparation

Sterile technique must be used during the surgical procedure. It is recommended that the implant team consist of at least three persons: clinician, surgical assistant, and nonsterile circulating assistant. The clinician and surgical assistant should be gowned, masked, and wear talcum-free sterile gloves. All equipment that will be touched by the sterile members of the team must be sterilized or draped with sterilized covers.

The implants require no preparation. The implants are left in the double-aseptic packaging until actual time of placement. This will minimize the problem of the implant package being opened and the implant not being used because of an unforeseen change in treatment.

Patient Preparation

Infiltration anesthesia (bucco-lingual) is used to completely anesthetize the surgical site. As an adjunct in more extensive procedures, the clinician may want to use intravenous sedation or oral premedication along with local anesthetics.

Surgical Procedure

After the patient is anesthesized, a sharp incision of appropriate design is made. The incision should be longer than the span that the implants will cover.

The tissue is reflected from the ridge with a sharp periosteal elevator to expose the lingual and buccal or labial dimension of the bone. All tissue tags should be removed from the ridge to ensure that no soft tissue is incorporated in the bone preparation.

If the crestal ridge is sharp or spiny, it should be flattened so the buccolingual width is at least 5.5 mm. The height of usable bone remaining must be at least 9 mm from vital structures.

The crestal cortical bone is penetrated with either a no. 6 round bur or 1.5-mm twist drill in a slow-speed handpiece or a 700XXL bur in a high-speed handpiece (Fig 26–5). Copious sterile external irrigation should be used during this procedure. In some instances where the bone is extremely dense, it may be necessary to prepare the site to the final depth with the twist drill or the 700XXL bur.

Care should be taken to ensure that the angulation of the drill is parallel to the lingual and buccal cortical plates. If there is a severe undercut to the lingual plate it should be noted to prevent perforation.

The drill or bur should be aligned such that the implants will be parallel to adjacent roots and the succeeding implant(s) will be parallel to the first. Bone preparation should allow the implants to be spaced at least 4 mm apart (8 mm center to center) and at least 2 mm or more from the inferior alveolar ridge and mental foramen. To be safe, at least 5 mm distance should be allowed anterior to the foramen.

The implant site is next drilled to final depth with the 2-mm internally irrigated pilot drill utilizing a high-torque slow-speed handpiece. The internally irrigated drills require a specific drilling technique to prevent clogging of the fluid pathway and to maintain the flow of irrigation. The bone is drilled for

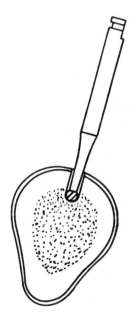

FIG 26–5.
Pilot hole through cortical bone being created with a no. 6 round bur.

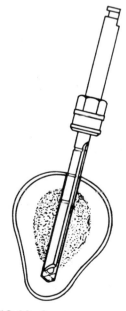

FIG 26–6.
Pilot drill cutting initial channel.

a period of 2 to 3 seconds, the drill removed from the bone entirely, and the bone chips washed away. This method is followed until the desired depth reference line is even with the crest of the ridge (Fig 26–6).

A parallel pin is placed in the prepared pilot hole and the operator proceeds to the next site. The pilot drill is aligned parallel to the pin when available bone permits and the next hole(s) is drilled.

The implant site is next enlarged with the appropriate sizing drill (corresponding to the implant size being placed) utilizing the same drilling technique (Fig 26–7). Small corrections in alignment of the holes may be made at this time if required.

The superior portion of the drill site is next prepared with the counterbore to accept the neck portion of the implant. This prepares the bone so there is an exact adaptation at the neck of the implant to ensure prevention of soft tissue invagination.

The pilot of the counterbore is placed in the drilled site and, utilizing the same technique as before, the hole is drilled until the tops of the flutes of

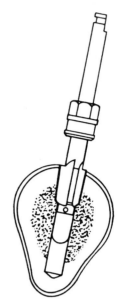

FIG 26–8.
Counterbore drill preparing the implant neck site.

the counterbore are even with the crest of the ridge (Fig 26–8).

When inserting an implant into dense bone, it is necessary to thread the implant site with a thread former. If the bone is soft or spongy, this step should be omitted and the implant threaded directly into the site as it is prepared at this point.

Threading should be done at extremely slow speed (20–50 rpm). The tip of the thread former is placed into the prepared implant site. Firm pressure is applied and rotation of the thread former is begun. When the threads engage, the thread former is fed without pressure.

The hole is threaded to the corresponding depth reference line and stopped (Fig 26–9). The handpiece is switched into the reverse mode and *the thread former is backed out*. The thread former must not be pulled from the socket.

Should the handpiece stall in extremely dense bone, the latch is disengaged from the thread former and the handpiece is removed. The ratchet and adaptor are engaged onto the hex hub on the thread former and the threading operation is completed. The ratchet is turned over and the thread former is unscrewed from the bone.

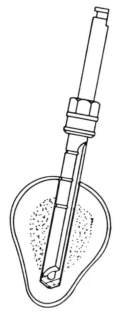

FIG 26–7.
Sizing drill developing the channel to correct depth and width.

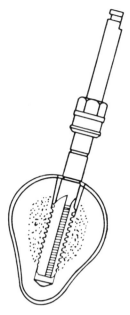

FIG 26–9.
Tapping the channel with the thread former.

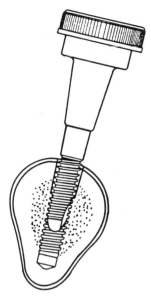

FIG 26–10.
Inserting the implant in the surgical site with the sterile plastic implant carrier.

Implant Placement

The scrub nurse opens the outer vial of the implant package and places the inner sterile vial onto a sterile field. The plastic seal on the inner vial is removed and the implant is withdrawn by the white plastic carrier. Care should be taken not to touch or contaminate the implant.

The tip of the implant is placed into the prepared site and the implant is screwed into place utilizing the plastic carrier. The implant will become very firm when the neck portion is seated (Fig 26–10). The implant should not be overtightened; overtightening in the bone can cause pressure necrosis. The plastic carrier is detached from the implant by flexing it buccolingually. An explorer is used to remove the small plastic residue that attached the carrier to the implant and usually is left in the internal threads.

The hex wrench in the surgical kit may be used with the hand knob or ratchet to tighten the implant into place if the implant cannot be screwed into place with the plastic carrier.

The label is removed from the carrier and the

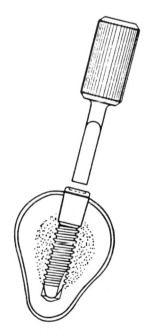

FIG 26–11.
Trial seating of the implant with the hex wrench and insertion of the healing collar with the screwdriver.

plastic healing collar is removed. The tip of the screwdriver is placed into the slot in the healing collar and the healing collar is screwed into the implant (Fig 26–11). Titanium healing collars (packaged separately) are also available as an alternative to the plastic healing collar.

The soft tissue should be sutured to obtain complete closure over the bone and implants. Interrupted suturing is preferred using .003 polyglactin 910 (Vicryl) as the material of choice. To avoid tearing tissue, the needle should be passed through one flap with a 2.5-mm bite, the suture pulled through, then the needle passed through the second flap and the two flaps pulled together and the suture tied.

After the soft tissue is sutured, the patient's existing appliance is relieved and relined with a soft reline material. Any forces that could cause movement of the implants during the healing phase must be avoided. Radiographs may be taken at this time as a final check.

Postoperative Management

The patient is instructed to place ice to the outside of the face over the surgical area for the first 24 hours: 10 minutes on, 10 minutes off. A soft diet is recommended for at least 2 weeks. The patient should be placed on antibiotics for 7 days starting on the day of surgery. Penicillin (500 mg doses three times a day) is the antibiotic of choice. If the patient is allergic to penicillin, erythromycin or tetracycline may be substituted. Vicodin may be prescribed for discomfort for the first few days, followed by a less potent analgesic. It is also recommended that the patient be placed on a nonsteroidal anti-inflammatory drug such as ibuprofen (Motrin), 800 mg on the morning of the procedure and continued for the next 2 days.

The patient is appointed to return to the office 10 days postoperative for suture removal. At that time the tissues should be closed with absence of swelling or exudate at the surgery site. The soft liner in the provisional appliance must be checked and may be changed periodically over the healing period.

The patient should be seen at least once a month until the implants are uncovered and loaded.

IMPLANT EXPOSURE

Healing time for the implants should be a minimum of 3 to 4 months in the mandible and 6 months in the maxilla. Healing time should be adjusted on an individual basis depending on the patient's age, healing capacity, and the quality of bone.

After the tissue is anesthetized, a sharp probe is used to locate the implants. If a surgical stent was used for surgery, it can be used to locate the implants. The implants may be exposed either by making an incision or by using a 4-mm tissue punch, which makes a very clean round hole through the tissue.

The tissue above the implant(s) is cut away to expose the healing screw. The healing collar is removed and any tissue or bone above the implant must be dry and free of debris. Flushing the implant with sterile saline solution and use of hemostatic agents will aid in preparing the site for the abutment placement. Care should be taken that no material is left under the soft tissue.

One of several abutments may be placed in the implant at this time. The abutments are all packaged individually and are sterile. The abutments are:

Polysulfane temporary healing abutment—This 3-mm-tall plastic abutment is designed to be placed in the implant during the healing phase before final abutment placement. This abutment is typically placed by the surgeon who is referring the patient to a restorative dentist (Fig 26–12).

Tissue abutment—This 4-mm-tall titanium alloy abutment is used as an extension of the implant. It is screwed into the implant and has an internally threaded hole that accepts all the prosthetic attachments in the system. During the healing phase it should be plugged with either a healing screw or temporary healing abutment (see Fig 26–12).

Restorative abutment—Any of the permanent abutments—fixed telescoping, O ring, or magnetic—may be placed at this time and the patient's appliance relined to accommodate it on a temporary basis until final reconstruction.

PROSTHETIC RECONSTRUCTION

The Steri-Oss system comes with a complete, illustrated step-by-step prosthetic manual for the dentist and laboratory technician. A summary of the prosthetic attachments and their uses follows.

The *4-mm tissue abutment* is used as an extension of the implant through the soft tissue (see Fig 26–12). The tissue abutment screws into the implant and accepts all the attachments, both threaded and cemented. Adjustments of 2 mm in abutment lengths can be achieved by combining the different-length abutments with the tissue abutment. For example, a 3-mm O ring attachment is used for tissue thickness up to 2 mm. The 1-mm O ring attachment may be combined with the tissue abutment to accommodate tissue up to 4 mm thick, etc. The same can be accomplished with the different abutment systems.

The *transfer pin* is used to transfer implant location to a laboratory model (Fig 26–13). The transfer pin is screwed into either the tissue abutment or directly into the implant. After an impression is made, the transfer pin is unscrewed from the tissue abutment or implant. An implant analog is screwed onto the transfer pin and the transfer pin inserted back into the impression and the stone model poured.

The transfer pins are used to make transfers when working with coronal screws, O ring attachments, and castable abutments.

Coronal screws are available in 5.5 mm and 12 mm lengths (see Fig 26–12). Coronal screws are commonly used for constructing tissue bars for overdentures, full-arch fixed-removable bridgework, and fixed-removable bridgework.

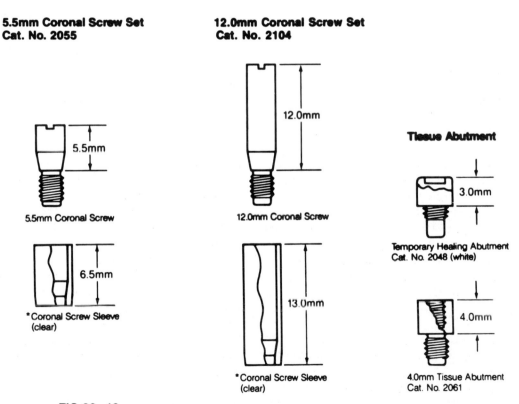

**5.5mm Coronal Screw Set
Cat. No. 2055**

5.5mm
5.5mm Coronal Screw

6.5mm
*Coronal Screw Sleeve (clear)

**12.0mm Coronal Screw Set
Cat. No. 2104**

12.0mm
12.0mm Coronal Screw

13.0mm
*Coronal Screw Sleeve (clear)

Tissue Abutment

3.0mm
Temporary Healing Abutment
Cat. No. 2048 (white)

4.0mm
4.0mm Tissue Abutment
Cat. No. 2061

FIG 26–12.
Prosthetic abutments: the coronal screw system abutments and tissue abutments.

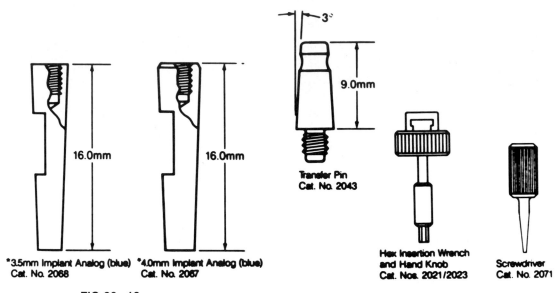

FIG 26–13.
Prosthetic transfer pins, implant analogs for impression casts, and instrumentation.

Coronal screws are most often used in conjunction with the 4-mm tissue abutment, but can also be affixed directly to the implants. Each screw comes with a matching plastic sleeve used as a burnout pattern and incorporated into the wax-up of the prosthetic superstructure (see Fig 26–12). The sleeves mate to the tissue abutments or implants with a flat surface; therefore, nonparallel implants may be restored without correcting for path of insertion.

In the laboratory, coronal screws and sleeves are attached to the analogs in the model and the bar or framework waxed. The finished bar or bridgework is placed on the implants and the screws inserted and screwed tight. In the case where the sleeve is placed through the tissue directly onto the implant, the superior portion must be sealed with a composite material.

Telescoping abutments are available in 5.5 mm and 7.5 mm lengths (Fig 26–14). Each abutment comes with a transfer coping, plastic laboratory coping, and coping screw. The abutments have an 18-degree taper which allows for misalignment between implants.

Telescoping abutments are most commonly used as distal abutments and for short-span (two to three units) fixed-removable bridges. The abutments are screwed into place with the telescoping abutment wrench. The transfer copings are then placed onto the abutments and an impression made which retains the transfer copings when removed. Telescoping abutment analogs and implant analogs are screwed together and inserted into the impression and the model poured. A plastic coping is attached to the analog with a laboratory coping screw and the framework is waxed. The finished bridgework is attached to the telescoping abutment with the small coping screw.

Fixed abutments are available in 7- and 9-mm screw-in style, 7-mm straight cement-in, 15- and 20-degree cement-in, and a plastic castable abutment (Fig 26–15).

Fixed abutments are used for single tooth replacements, short- and long-span bridges, and full-arch reconstructions. The angled abutments are especially useful when restoring the anterior maxilla. The abutments may be modified in length before affixing to the implants. Once placed in the mouth, they may be additionally modified for path of insertion and margins. Standard impressions are made and the models poured up in hard diestone. The bridgework is made directly from the stone models. The finished bridgework is then cemented into place on the abutments.

Castable abutments are modified by the labora-

**5.5 mm Telescoping Abutment Set
Cat. No. 2050**

**7.5mm Telescoping Abutment Set
Cat. No. 2051**

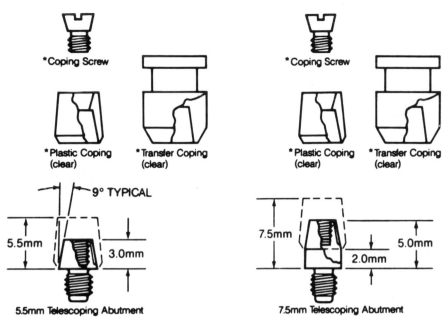

FIG 26–14.
Prosthetic telescoping abutment set components for second-stage reconstruction.

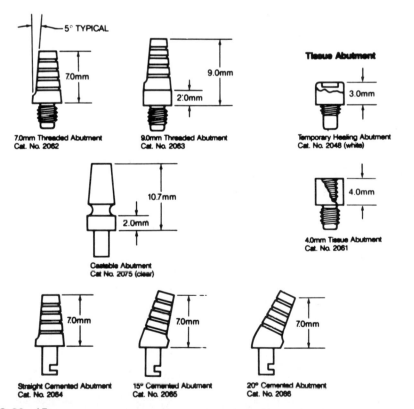

FIG 26–15.
Prosthetic fixed attachment and angled head abutments for second-stage reconstruction.

TABLE 26–2.

Steri-Oss Clinical Implant Study: Age Distribution of Patients

Age Group (yr)	Male	Female
14–20	3	0
21–30	2	2
31–40	8	8
41–50	6	12
51–60	20	23
61–70	13	20
71–80	6	7
81–90	0	1
	58	73

tory and cast with either a precious or semiprecious material having a minimum 60,000 psi yield strength. The abutments are cemented into the implant and impressions are made.

O ring attachments are available in 1 mm and 3 mm lengths. The attachments are utilized with two or more implants for overdenture retention and have the advantage of being resilient in all planes of motion. The abutments are screwed into the implants with at least 1 mm of the base protruding above the tissue. A gold-plated stainless steel ring, which retains the O ring, is processed into the denture either in the laboratory or at chairside with cold-cure acrylic. When O rings are to be processed into the denture in the laboratory, transfer pins are utilized for taking the impression and making the model as described previously.

Magnetic attachments (Shiner magnet) are available in a stainless steel keeper screw and a keeper screw affixed to a 2-mm titanium alloy base. The Shiner magnet has a unique spherical magnet assembly in a threaded plastic housing. The magnet is free to rotate in the housing in response to denture movement, thereby keeping the magnet in contact with the keeper screw. Magnets are utilized with two or more implants for overdenture retention. Magnets add very little lateral retention to a denture; therefore, the denture must have adequate flanges to prevent sliding. The magnets may be either processed into the denture in the laboratory or at chairside with cold-cure acrylic. The magnet set contains an impression piece, model piece, and processing piece. The impression pieces index into the keepers in the implants and are picked up in the impression. The model pieces are inserted into the impression and the model is poured. The processing pieces are placed on the model and processed into the denture. When the denture is complete, the processing pieces are unscrewed and the magnets are screwed into place.

The magnets may also be processed into the denture at chairside by making a direct pickup from the keepers. The processing pieces are inserted into the indexing holes in the keepers and the denture is relieved to fit over the processing pieces. Cold-cure acrylic is placed into the denture and the denture fitted into place over the implants. When the acrylic has cured, the processing pieces are unscrewed from the denture and the magnets are screwed into place.

DISCUSSION

The Steri-Oss implant system provides a two-stage root form endosteal implant system that is adaptable to many intraoral situations and provides a wide series of prosthetic options. The implants are

TABLE 26–3.

Steri-Oss Clinical Implant Study: Evaluation of Root Form Implants

	Inserted	Arches	Exposed	Removed	Success Rate*
Maxilla	233	73	232	4	98.3%
Mandible	237	64	233	14	94.0%
Total	470	137	465	18	96.1%

*Implants not yet exposed were not counted in the success rate calculations.

TABLE 26–4.

Steri-Oss Clinical Implant Study: Evaluation of Blade Form Implants

	Inserted	Arches	Exposed	Removed	Success Rate
Maxilla	15	9	15	0	100.0%
Mandible	35	26	35	0	100.0%
Total	50	35	50	0	100.0%

made of commercially pure titanium and utilize the basic implant research principles and clinical data emanating from the Brånemark-led Swedish implant research teams. The prosthetic attachments or second-stage superstructures (heads) are composed of titanium alloy (Ti-6Al-4V) for maximum strength and compatibility with the first-stage endosteal portion.

We have recently completed a 3½-year clinical study with this implant system. The study included 131 patients of which 97 patients received root form Steri-Oss implants and 7 patients received Steri-Oss blade implants. Twenty-seven patients received both blade and root form implants. The age distribution of the patients is shown in Table 26–2.

The success rates for the root form implants are shown in Table 26–3 and the success rates for the blade form implants are shown in Table 26–4.

Chapter 27

The Integral Implant System

Dennis G. Smiler, D.D.S., M.Sc.D.

THE IMPLANT

The Integral biointegrated dental implant system is designed for use in totally edentulous mandibles or maxillae or as a terminal or intermediary abutment for fixed or removable bridgework. The Integral implant system uses a two-stage implantation process to ensure complete bone fixation prior to loading.

The implant is cylindrical and is coated with dense hydroxylapatite (Calcitite) (Fig 27–1). The implants are 3.25 and 4.0 mm in diameter with lengths of 8, 10, 13, and 15 mm. The central core is titanium alloy and a titanium alloy healing screw covers the coronal portion of the implant during the osseous biointegration healing stage. Packaging in sterile vials ensures a clean noncontaminated implant surface that is not touched during the surgical phase of implant placement.

The system offers the clinician a wide selection of interchangeable threaded attachments to allow for maximum flexibility of prosthetic restoration (Table 27–1). This versatility makes the system suited for restoration of both the edentulous and partially edentulous mandible or maxilla. Threaded prosthetic abutment components include posts for cemented fixed restorations, abutments for fixed-removable prosthetics, a coronal screw system for nonparallel implant placement, and magnetic Zest anchor, ball, and O ring attachments.

Proper selection of implant material and design affects not only the transfer of mechanical forces to the implant-tissue interface but also the prediction of long-term success of the implant system. The cylindrical design of the implant provides more favorable stress distribution than conical, blade forms, or basket-type designs. In photoelastic analysis of single tooth implants, Mohammed and co-workers concluded that an endosseous implant with a smooth cylindrical shape has maximum mechanical compatibility with bone.[1] During the past decade, there have been many different types of implants offered to the practitioner; some have proved to be successful, others not. The causes of failure or success include criteria relating not only to the design of the implant, stress and strength calculations, and surface characteristics but also to the lack of osseous integration resulting from bone resorption under excessive compressive loads during physiologic masticatory function.

PATIENT CONSIDERATION AND SELECTION

Prior to diagnosis and treatment planning, the clinician must evaluate the patient from a medical and dental point of view. A careful history and physical examination will often apprise the dentist of the prognosis before surgery is begun. This evaluation should include factors relating to (a) psychological evaluation, (b) medical and laboratory tests, (c) dental, periodontal, and occlusal evaluation, and (d) oral hygiene.

Prosthetic evaluation is essential before placing

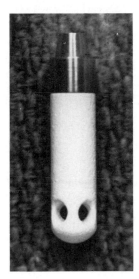

FIG 27–1.
The Integral biointegrated dental implant.

the implants. Dental models should be mounted and a trial setup accomplished; this will provide information on the ideal placement of teeth, vertical dimension, and interocclusal distance. In some quadrant implant restorative situations, and certainly in full-arch cases, this trial setup can be taken to the mouth for patient preliminary approval. From this trial setup, surgical stents are constructed and used as an aid for ideal placement of the implant.

Selection of proper implant size is crucial to the long-term success of the implant. It is desirable to utilize the maximum implant length possible, without encroachment on anatomic structures, for greatest stability of the overlying prosthesis. Available bone and the position of the anatomic structures ultimately defines the size of the implant to be used and its location in the arch. For example, if the width of the crestal bone is 3 mm wide, the clinician cannot place a 4-mm-wide cylindrical implant. If the mandibular canal is positioned 10 mm from the crest of the bone, the clinician cannot place a 13-mm-long implant.

The key to implant success is availability of sufficient bone.[2] The implant must be supported by bone to function. The clinician is obliged to consider the quantity, quality, and morphology of bone as well as the anatomic structures. Anatomic landmarks of the mandible and maxilla are relatively few. With the aid of diagnostic models, panographic and periapical radiographs, computed tomography (CT) scanning techniques, and tomograms, these landmarks can be defined. Accurate measurements from these diagnostic techniques allow for proper implant length selection to avoid the maxillary sinus space, the floor of the nose, the mandibular canal, or perforation of the inferior aspect of the mandible.

In the mandible the clinician needs to know the position of the mylohyoid line and the lingual depression of the inferior border. In the anterior region the position of the genial tubercles and the direction

TABLE 27–1.
The Integral Implant System

Product name	The Integral biointegrated dental implant
	The Integral SD biointegrated dental implant
Manufacturer/supplier	Calcitek
	2320 Faraday Avenue
	Carlsbad, CA 92208
	1-800-854-7019
	in California: 1-800-542-6019
Material composition	Titanium alloy coated with Calcitite brand of dense
	hydroxylapatite on the implant body
Approximate cost	Integral implant $185
	Integral SD implant $185
	Titanium healing screw $40
	Abutment heads $40–$50
Surgical instrumentation kit for Integral or Integral SD implants, without any implants	$575

of bone resorption will aid in proper angulation of implant placement. Of paramount importance is the position of the mandibular canal and nerve. This nerve continues forward a few millimeters anteriorly to the canal before it exits. If the implant is placed too close to the foramen or canal, permanent nerve damage may result.

Bone resorption patterns in the maxilla often leave acute undercuts, depressions, and dehiscences in bone. The cortical plates in the maxilla are thinner than in the mandible, and the bone is more porous. The width of bone between the palatal and labiobuccal cortices is often thin. The position of the sinus in relation to the crestal bone often gives rise to insufficient height of bone to permit implant anchorage in bone. Advanced surgical techniques utilizing the increased bone-to-implant bonding strength of the implant and particulate hydroxylapatite grafting can overcome this problematic situation.

INSTRUMENTATION

Pilot Drill.—The pilot drill is 1.5 mm in diameter and is 8 mm from the tip of the drill to the end of the flutes (Fig 27–2). This drill is used to establish correct direction, parallelism, and initial length of the drilling site. This drill is used with external irrigation and drilling speed of approximately 800 to 1,000 rpm.

Rosette Bur.—The rosette bur is placed over the site made with the pilot drill (see Fig 27–2). At slow speed (600–800 rpm) and with external irrigation the bur is drilled only to the equator of the bur. This provides a circular indentation or dimple in the bone to accommodate the tip of the intermediate spade drill and the final spade drill.

Intermediate Spade Drill.—The intermediate spade drill is 3 mm in diameter and has markings to indicate depths of 8, 10, 13, and 15 mm (Fig 27–3). The central irrigation port at the top of the drill receives the internal irrigation needle. The flutes are designed to irrigate the bone during drilling and carry debris upward. This drill is run at speeds of 600 to 850 rpm with high torque and internal irrigation. Drilling should be with a straight up-and-down pumping motion and a duration of no more than 5 to 10 seconds at a time.

Spade Drill.—The final spade drill comes in four lengths, 8, 10, 13, and 15 mm, by 4 mm in diameter (Fig 27–4). This drill allows for internal irrigation and is designed to run at high torque speeds of 600 to 850 rpm. The drill is inserted into the site after the intermediate spade drill and with light pressure is carried to the entire depth of the drill. No attempt should be made to continue drilling once the drill has been completely seated in the bone. Drilling should be with a straight up-and-down pumping mo-

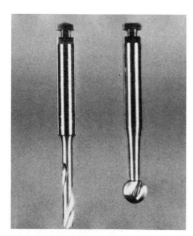

FIG 27–2.
The pilot drill *(left)* and the rosette bur *(right)*.

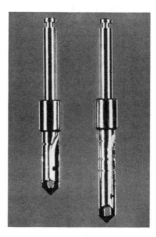

FIG 27–3.
Intermediate spade drills—10 mm *(left)* and 15 mm *(right)*.

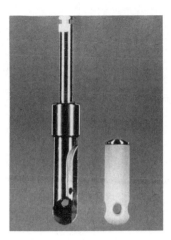

FIG 27–4.
The spade drill demonstrated against an Integral implant with healing screw in place.

tion and a duration of no more than 5 to 10 seconds at a time.

Parallel Pins.—Parallel pins are used to establish parallelism and draw between implants and the natural teeth (Fig 27–5). One end of the pin fits into the site prepared with the pilot drill. Insertion into the pilot drill site will provide a reference guide for the placement of further implants.

The opposite end of the parallel pin is 3 mm in diameter and can be seated into the hole drilled with the intermediate spade drill. This provides final angulation guides before the final drilling stage.

Try-In Guide.—The implant try-in guide is slightly smaller in diameter than the final spade drill. It is marked in lengths of 8, 10, 13, and 15 mm to provide depth guidance before insertion of the implant.

Implant.—Integral implant bodies are available in four lengths. The implant bodies are provided in a double-wrapped sterile transfer system ready for immediate implantation with the titanium healing screws attached (Fig 27–6). The plastic handle is twisted to remove the implant from the vial and to place it into the prepared bone site. The plastic handle is then moved mesiodistally to remove it, leaving the implant in the bone.

Tapper.—The tapper is placed so that the plastic nylon portion is on the titanium healing screw of the implant body. With gentle tapping the implant is seated flush or slightly below the bone level.

Temporary Gingival Cuff.—The titanium temporary gingival cuff is provided in lengths of 5, 7, and 10 mm. After osseous biointegration healing, the implant is located and the titanium healing screw is removed. Following irrigation of the threads, the temporary gingival cuff can be placed. Gingival healing adapts to the cuff in approximately 2 to 3 weeks. At this time the cuff can be removed and the final prosthetic abutment head placed.

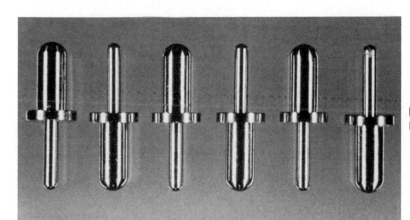

FIG 27–5.
Integral parallel pins.

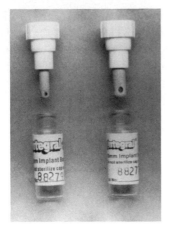

FIG 27–6.
The Integral implant attached to the transfer handle after removal from the sterile packaging container.

SURGICAL PROCEDURE

The biocompatibility of implant materials like titanium or hydroxylapatite is so firmly established that it is not considered to be a significant factor in endosseous implant failure.[3–6] Poor surgical planning, technique, patient selection, and infection are usually the problem in failure of implants prior to prosthetic loading.

What is needed is a surgical protocol that will avoid rejection on a cellular and subcellular level and a method to promote wound healing.[7] The simplified surgical procedure used when placing the implant greatly reduces the risk of bone trauma, provides an excellent environment for bone modeling and repair, and ultimately provides a biointegrated implant.

Heat is the enemy when drills are used to prepare the implant site so there must be a reduction in cutting pressure to avoid heat buildup in the bone.[8, 9] In addition, coolants should be applied during the drilling cycle to reduce temperature increases. Bone temperatures above 47°C will produce protein coagulation, cell necrosis, and resultant fibrous connective tissue, not bone. With the Integral surgical procedure bone is cooled during the staged drilling phase by internal irrigation. The design of the drill simultaneously removes the cutting debris while irrigating the drill-bone interface.

Sufficient thickness of alveolar bone must be present. Ample ridge width is more favorable than a knife-edge ridge. Width of bone should allow a minimum of 0.5 to 1.0 mm between the outer edge of the implant and the outer cortex.

In the maxilla the vertical dimension should ideally allow 2 mm between the implant and the floor of the nose or sinus. However, mucosal lift procedures with or without placement of hydroxylapatite can improve this relationship. The antral floor or nasal mucosa can be surgically elevated to accommodate the implant without perforating the membranes.

An antibiotic of choice is given to the patient at least 2 hours prior to surgery and continued for 10 days postoperatively. A soft diet is necessary and the patient is either restricted from wearing any denture or the prosthesis is relieved and relined with a soft material. During the 3 to 4 months' healing period in the maxilla and mandible, the implants are not loaded.

As in any surgery, it is important that the implantation procedure be aseptic. All instruments should be clean and sterile. Integral surgical instruments must be sterilized prior to use. The surgery for implant insertion and abutment connection can be performed in the office under local anesthesia, with or without intravenous sedation. Integral implants are provided sterile, in individual vials. Owing to the nature of the hydroxylapatite coating on the implant, special consideration is required for handling. Only powder-free gloved hands, or nonmetal instruments should be used to handle the implant.

Bone Preparation.—A mesiodistal incision is made along the buccal side of the alveolar crest through the mucoperiosteum and attached gingiva to the bone. An alternative incision can be placed laterally, and the mucoperiosteal layer elevated over the crest. This incision has the advantage of preserving the periosteum in the area over the implant. The incision should be long enough to permit adequate reflection without tearing the tissue and also provide a broad field of view.

Flap reflection should be minimal, but provide adequate exposure for visualization and drilling. It is important to preserve the subperiosteal osteogenic capacity of the flap for rapid healing. Spinous ridges or other bone irregularities should be removed using rongeurs, bone files, or alveolectomy burs. The flattest possible bone plateau should be created while keeping bone removal to a minimum to maintain the blood supply to cortical bone. A 4- to 6-mm space should be maintained between implants and adjacent natural teeth.

Pilot Drill.—The pilot drill is used to penetrate the dense ridge crest (Fig 27–7). This drill establishes the location and angle of the implant and should be prepared with the aid of a preprosthetic surgical splint as a guide. The drill is used with external irrigation down to the depth of the flutes, 8 mm.

Parallel Pins.—The small end of the parallel pin is inserted to check for parallelism and draw (Fig 27–8). The parallel pin is left in the first pilot hole while the operator moves on to the next preparation, referring to angularity and draw requirements established by the first implant site preparation, and proceeding in this way until all pilot holes are drilled.

Rosette Bur.—The rosette bur is used to create a dimple on the surface of the pilot hole to better ac-

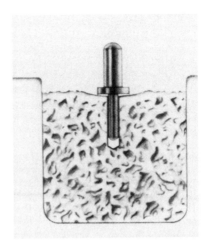

FIG 27–8.
The parallel pin in the pilot hole allows inspection for depth and angle of draw.

commodate the tip of the intermediate spade drill. As with the pilot drill, use of the rosette bur is done with slow speed, high torque, and copious irrigation.

Intermediate Spade Drill.—The intermediate spade drill is internally irrigated and designed to

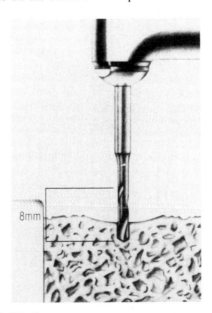

FIG 27–7.
The pilot drill creating an 8-mm-deep initial socket.

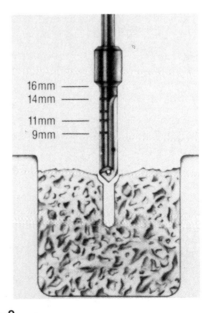

FIG 27–9.
The intermediate spade drill creates the bone channel to the predetermined depth.

make a channel of proper depth as indicated by concentric rings marked on the drill (Fig 27–9).

Parallel Pin.—The larger portion of the parallel pin is placed in the hole (Fig 27–10). Minor correction to obtain proper alignment can be made at this drilling stage with the intermediate spade drill.

Final Spade Drill.—The full-diameter implant matching spade drill is used to complete the implant site preparation (Fig 27–11). Each drill has a diameter and length that corresponds to a special Integral implant. Their length, however, is 1 mm longer than the corresponding implant body to allow seating of the implant below the alveolar crest. This drill is designed for internal irrigation and should be used with copious amounts of sterile water, at low speed and high torque. The final drilling in a straight up-and-down motion will create the ideal receptor site for the implant.

Implant Body Try-In Guide.—The implant body try-in guide is placed into the prepared osseous site to check for depth (Fig 27–12). If the hole is not deep enough, proper length can be created by drilling again with the final spade drill. The bone site is checked again with the try-in guide before selecting and seating the implant.

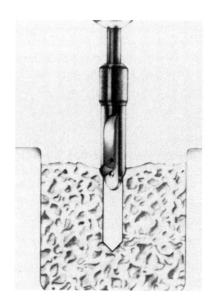

FIG 27–11.
The final spade drill completes the implant site preparation.

Implant Placement.—After irrigation of the receptor site with sterile water, the implant is removed from its sterile vial using the plastic cap. The implant is inserted into the bone and with gentle pressure fitted until the healing screw is flush or 1 mm below the bone margin (Fig 27–13).

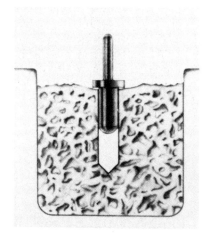

FIG 27–10.
The parallel pin used to check an angle of draw after the channel is completed.

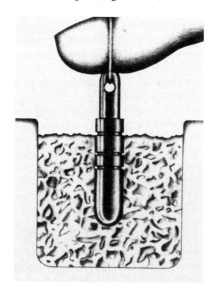

FIG 27–12.
The implant body try-in guide allows evaluation of the surgical site for depth and width prior to implant placement.

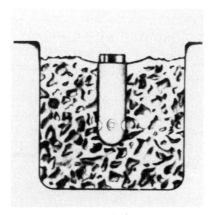

FIG 27–13.
The implant is properly seated when the implant sits level with or 1 mm below the alveolar bone crest.

Final seating can be accomplished using gentle tapping with a rubber mallet and the tapper.

Closure.—The mucoperiosteal flap should be carefully repositioned for maximum tissue adaptation, and then sutured.

Postoperative Care.—Procedures that must be strictly adhered to are those that contribute to fixation and biointegration of the implant to bone. These include: (1) maintenance of osseous margins around the surgical preparation, gentle surgical technique, continuous irrigation, and low-speed and high-torque drilling procedures; (2) preservation of subperiosteal osteogenic capacity by the avoidance of overstripping of the periosteum; (3) close adaptation of the periosteal bony margins to the implant; (4) firm stabilization of the submerged implant in bone during the healing cycle; (5) adequate healing time; and (6) no immediate loading when the implant is uncovered and the second-phase prosthetic abutment is attached.

The patient should be instructed to follow a routine postsurgery regimen, including cold packs for the initial 24 hours. The antibiotic is continued for 10 days postoperatively. Analgesics are prescribed as needed.

Sutures may be removed after 1 week. It is suggested that any removable prosthesis resting on the implant be adequately relieved and relined using a soft tissue conditioner reline material.

A first-stage healing period of approximately 3 to 4 months is recommended. It is important that the implants be left unloaded during the healing period to allow for optimum rigid biointegration and bone interfacing to the hydroxylapatite-coated body. The patient should be seen periodically until the prosthesis is seated to monitor proper healing of the soft and hard tissues.

DISCUSSION

One of the critical factors affecting long-term success of implants is the interaction at the biomaterial-tissue interface. Many of the clinical problems of implant failure can be attributed to the instability of the implant-bone interface under continual masticatory function.[10] The biomaterial used for an implant is an important factor that may influence the tissue interface that forms after implantation.

An ideal surface for an implant would be one that would perform as if it were equivalent to the host tissue, maintain a stable interface between implant surface and bone or gingiva, have an implant surface for bone bonding (biointegration), provide increased shear strength of the implant-bone interface, be nontoxic, and produce no inflammatory reactions.

Hydroxylapatite ceramic is an ideal implant material because it makes up the bulk of our skeleton. Evidence from electron microscopic studies reveals that biological apatite can be deposited directly on the surface of hydroxylapatite implants.[11] There is a narrow amorphous zone similar and perhaps identical to natural bone-cementing substance. Although the hydroxylapatite coating does not induce bone to grow, it provides a matrix suitable for deposition of new bone. The soft tissue fibroblast and gingival cells have been shown to attach and adhere to the surface of the hydroxylapatite, so that the interface has essentially the same appearance as the epithelium–natural tooth interface.

The healing at the interface with hydroxylapatite is faster than that seen with titanium. Immediately after insertion into bone the surface is coated with a blood clot to which epithelium and connective tissue cells attach. Within 3 months collagen fibers interface directly to the implant and epithelial cells adhere to the surface. The first contact of new bone with apatite in dogs can be found at 5 days. Within 10 days the area of bone formation enlarges until the surface is covered with new bone. By 60 days bone tissue and bone crystallization on the apatite are almost the same as those of normal bone.[12]

Hydroxylapatite ceramic may be the ideal implant material because it performs as if it were equivalent to the host tissue.[13] The strength of bone-to-implant interface with hydroxylapatite ensures a tight union with hard tissues. When tested to failure, the implants do not fracture or fail at the interface because the strength of the hydroxylapatite-bone bond is greater than that of bone or the ceramic material.[12] The ceramic surface provides attachment sites for collagen fibers, which favors osteoblastic activity over fibroblastic activity. It appears that the result is a chemical bond that exists at the bone-ceramic interface.[11] Fibrous encapsulation may occur, however, if there is relative movement between bone and the implant during the initial healing phase. Ogiso and colleagues have shown that apatite implants protruding through the gingiva adhere to connective and epithelial tissues as do natural teeth.[14] After loading for 8 months in dogs, the gingival sulcus surrounding the implant was shallow with no infrabony pockets and the tensile adhesive strength between the hydroxylapatite and mandibular compact bone was more than 150 kg/cm^2. This may be the reason that epithelial downgrowth has never been reported for perimucosal apatite implants, even if they are implanted with a loose fit. This suggests a natural compatibility between hydroxylapatite ceramics and connective and epithelial tissues.

Clinical success is the most important consideration with respect to selection of a particular biomaterial, design, and treatment plan. Mechanical force transfer from implant to bone must be kept within physiologic limits to ensure clinical success for the implant and the prosthesis it supports. Sufficient numbers of implants must be placed so loads will be within physiologic limits. Cook and co-workers showed *in vivo* that with hydroxylapatite-coated implants in dogs, the interfacial shear strength was five to eight times greater in bone attachment strength than on smooth titanium metal implants.[12] The hydroxylapatite-coated implant displayed bone growth and mineralization directly on the implant surface. In addition, the coating thicknesses as a function of implantation time showed that the coating remained at approximately 50 μm. Testing the interfacial tensile and shear strength of the hydroxylapatite coating on metals demonstrated a strong adherence of the coating to the metal even after extended aging periods in agitated Ringer's solution.

SUMMARY

Until now various dental implants have been screwed or malleted into living bone. Most have required mechanical retention to secure the implant to living bone.[15, 16] It would be better to devise an artificial system that could be intrinsically incorporated into the human system without resorting to screws, flutes, holes, or vents for mechanical retention and adaptation. The Integral system combines contemporary implant research and the most advanced principles of biomaterials engineering to provide such a system. It is a clinically proven two-stage system that is biointegrated into bone and allows for a wide variety of fixed or removable prosthetic applications.[12, 13, 17] The basic biologic profile of hydroxylapatite ceramic materials include:

1. Lack of local or systemic toxicity.
2. Lack of inflammation or foreign body reaction.
3. Absence of intervening fibrous tissue between bone and implant.
4. Ability to directly interface to bone by what may be natural bone cementing mechanisms.

The advantages of the hydroxylapatite coating and the Integral implant system are:

1. A true biochemical biologic union between bone and hydroxylapatite.
2. Healing is more rapid with bone growth

covering a greater percentage of the implant surface.

3. Periosteum will intimately grow to the surface of the hydroxylapatite coating.
4. There is resistance to epithelial downgrowth.
5. Hydroxylapatite-coated implants under continual loading will maintain rigidity in bone by continual remodeling of supporting bone.
6. A simplified surgical procedure.
7. Versatile prosthetic applications can be carried out.

REFERENCES

1. Mohammed H, Atmaram GH, Schoen FJ: Dental implant design: A critical review. *J Oral Implantol* 1979; 8:393.
2. Ling RSM: Observations on the fixation of implants to the bony skeleton. *Clin Orthop* 1968; 210:80–96.
3. Hench LL: Special report: The interfacial behavior of biomaterials. *J Biomed Mater Res* 1980; 14:803–811.
4. Boretos WJ: *Contemporary Biomaterials: Materials and Host Response, Clinical Application, New Technology and Legal Aspects*. Parkridge, NJ, Noyes Publications, 1984.
5. Cook SD, Kay JF: Variables affecting the interface strength of hydroxylapatite implant surfaces. *Trans 12th Ann Meeting Soc Biomater* 1986; 14.
6. Jarcho M: Biomaterial aspects of calcium phosphate: Properties and applications. *Dent Clin North Am* 1986; 30:25–47.
7. Urist MR: *Fundamental and Clinical Bone Physiology*. Philadelphia, JB Lippincott Co, 1980.
8. Eriksson RA, Albrektsson T: The effect of heat on bone regeneration: An experimental study in the rabbit. *J Oral Maxillofac Surg* 1984; 42:705–711.
9. Matthews L, Hirsch C: Temperature measured in human cortical bone when drilling. *J Bone Joint Surg [Am]* 1972; 54:297–308.
10. Brunski J, Moccia A: The influence of functional use of endosseous dental implants on the interface. *J Dent Res* 1979; 58:1953–1969.
11. Jarcho M: Calcium phosphate ceramics as hard tissue prosthetics. *Clin Orthop* 1981; 157:259–278.
12. Cook SD, Kay JF, Thomas KA, et al: Interface mechanics and histology of titanium and hydroxylapatite-coated titanium for dental implant applications. *Int J Oral Maxillofac Implants* 1987; 2:15–22.
13. Block MS, Kent JN, Kay JF: Evaluation of hydroxylapatite-coated titanium dental implants in dogs. *J Oral Maxillofac Surg* 1987; 45:601–607.
14. Ogiso M, Kaneda H, Arasaki J, et al: Epithelial attachment and bone tissue formation on the surface of hydroxlyapatite ceramics (abstracted). Presented at First World Biomaterials Congress, Baden, Austria, May 1980.
15. Linkow LI, Chercheve R: *Theories and Techniques of Oral Implantology*. St Louis, CV Mosby Co, 1970.
16. Albrektsson T: Direct bone anchorage of dental implants. *J Prosthet Dent* 1983; 50:255–261.
17. Block MS, Finger IM, Fontenot MG, et al: Loaded hydroxylapatite-coated and grit-blasted titanium implants in dogs. *Int J Oral Maxillofac Implants* 1989; 4:219–225.

PART III

Clinical Considerations of Implant Management

Chapter 28

Practical Implant Prosthodontics

Glenn E. Minsley, D.M.D.
David L. Koth, D.D.S., M.S.

Today there are many functional and acceptable implant systems on the market. Each of these systems has its own unique prosthodontic technology. It is not the purpose of this chapter to deal with each one of these systems in any detail. Rather, an attempt is made to describe in generic terms important prosthetic principles that may apply to each system.

The chapter provides important details concerning partially edentulous and fully edentulous mouths where implants may be used alone as support or in combination with natural abutment teeth. The chapter presents functional considerations, criteria for diagnostic evaluation and treatment planning, and has specific suggestions for partial edentia to include single tooth replacement, fixed partial prostheses with natural tooth abutments, fixed partial prostheses without natural tooth abutments, and the fully edentulous mouth in terms of overdentures and the fixed-removable prosthesis.

FUNCTIONAL CONSIDERATIONS

If the implants have been placed with the proper surgical technique, and in the proper location, they are ready for prosthetic application. The prosthetic reconstruction may well determine the success or failure of the implants, and prosthetic design must take into account the anchorage of the implant in bone as well as the attachment of the prosthesis to the implant. It is generally accepted that the less tissue space there is between the radicular portion of the implant and the bone investing the implant, the greater the chances that the implant will be a long-term success.[1, 2] In order to maintain this narrow dimension of tissue between implant and bone, it is important to note that bone needs a low stimulus in order to constantly remodel. This stimulus must occur during the dynamics of mastication and be maintained during physiologic limits.[3] In other words, what occurs functionally after prosthesis placement will influence the integrity of the bone-implant interface. A dental implant with a minimal amount of tissue interposed between it and bone can function but cannot physiologically adapt to situations.[4] Some authors have suggested that the application of physiologic functional loading will increase the stability of the bone-implant interface.[5-7] Furthermore, they suggest that if there is functional overload of either magnitude or direction of force, the nature of the interface will change from bone to fibrous tissue. Consequently, the healthy maintenance of the tissue interface between implant and bone depends on interactions between the bone, the implant, and the prosthesis. The restoring dentist has the responsibility to control the force generated to the dental implant through the prosthesis and thus influence the implant tissue interface.

There are two distinctly different prosthetic problems to consider when transferring force to bone. One could be called a composite system in which a tooth and an implant will each function as an abutment for a fixed bridge. The second would be called a single system where the entire support mechanism for the prosthesis are implants.

It has been suggested that because an endosteal implant is rigid in bone, that the torque transmitted to the bone through the implant is greater than that transmitted through a natural tooth which is cushioned by its periodontal ligament.[8] In the composite system each support unit, that is, the implant and the natural tooth, has a different modulus of elasticity.[9, 10] These rigid and nonrigid systems are connected by a prosthesis.

In the single system the entire support mechanism for the prosthesis are the implants. Therefore, the supporting system of the prosthesis has the same modulus of elasticity. When a fixed prosthesis is placed in conjunction with the composite system, essentially a rigid beam is placed between two supporting structures. This beam, under functional load, may become a lever. At one end, it is anchored to a tooth that is capable of lateral and intrusive movements and at the other end it is anchored to an endosseous implant that is relatively immovable. Some authors have suggested that the application of a vertical load to the tooth at one end of the lever will intrude the tooth into a socket. The load at the other end, the implant, will not cause intrusion because of the lack of movement in a vertical direction by the implant. Therefore, the implant will comply to the load by bending.[4, 11, 12] Others have suggested that torsional stresses set up within the implant head-neck connection may elicit a stress transfer from the implant to bone resulting in a breakdown of the implant-bone interface.[13, 14]

Assuming that this stress may cause destruction to bone, it should therefore be absorbed somehow, other than by the bone. This may be accomplished in the form of nonrigid connectors, veneering the metal substructure with a superstructure of a low modulus of elasticity, or the use of an implant insert which would absorb some of the shock or allow for movement. In any event, it is important to remember that the inevitable consequence of excessive compressive stress on bone is osteoclastic activity and bone resorption.[3]

In the single support system, the lack of like movement between abutments is not important be-

cause all of the abutments are dental implants. However, it has been suggested that the material covering this substructure should be of a low modulus of elasticity in order to absorb the forces of mastication.[2, 8]

DIAGNOSTIC EVALUATION AND TREATMENT PLANNING

Prosthetic considerations begin prior to surgical placement of any implant. At the initial consultation visit, a detailed medical history is acquired from the patient. Patients having a negative history for any systemic disease would be considered as acceptable candidates for dental implant procedures. Patients having a history of slight or moderate systemic disease that is well controlled and does not interfere to any significant extent with the patient's normal physiologic function could also be considered acceptable for implants.[15]

There are systemic diseases which should be considered as major risks for implant procedures and would preclude a patient as an acceptable candidate: major cardiovascular disorders respiratory disorders, malignant disease and associated radiotherapy or chemotherapy, uncontrolled diabetes, hematologic disorders, and psychological disorders.[15] In addition, patients with extreme unrealistic expectations should also be viewed as poor candidates in their acceptance of this therapy.[16]

Diagnostic dental information should be obtained during the initial visit. This information is gathered from a clinical examination of the oral cavity and paraoral structures, radiographs, and photographs. Radiographs should include a panoramic radiograph, lateral cephalometric radiograph, and occlusal films. Periapical radiographs are made, if necessary, to gain further detail of areas of consideration.[17] Computed tomography (CT) scans providing three-dimensional views are helpful but probably not practical for every candidate because of the high cost of this procedure.

Preoperative study casts should be obtained from impressions of the patient's maxillary and mandibular arches and mounted on a suitable articulator using a face-bow at an acceptable vertical dimension of occlusion. Placement of prosthetic teeth and a wax try-in of this arrangement should be performed with the patient to verify esthetics, phonetics, and occlusion. It also provides another diagnostic tool for determining the placement of the implants.

Adequate height and width of the bone in the arch is needed for the placement of the implants. The density of the bone should be suitable for the particular implant system chosen for treatment. There should be an adequate ratio of cortical bone to cancellous bone to provide initial stabilization of the implant at the time of placement as well as excellent adaptation and final stabilization of the implant with the resultant surrounding bone that regenerates during the brief healing period. A predominance of one type of bone over the other will either compromise the initial stabilization of the implant or delay the length of the healing period.[18]

The soft tissues of the arch should be firm, keratinized tissues. However, it has been documented that when implants are placed in unkeratinized mucosal tissues, these tissues have responded well provided that meticulous oral hygiene was maintained around the implants.[19] This response has also been observed clinically by us. Pendulous tissues present in a potential implant site should be trimmed during the surgical placement of the implant or prior to prosthodontic procedures.[17] Any high muscle attachment present in a potential implant site should be eliminated prior to surgical placement of the implant.

Interarch skeletal relationships should be noted prior to surgical implantation. Severe Angle Class II or Class III relationships could present problems, especially in edentulous patients, owing to discrepancies between the centers of the denture-bearing regions. These discrepancies could place unfavorable stress on the implants as well as on the tissues of the opposing arch. The possibility of orthognathic surgery should be considered to obtain a more normal Class I arch relationship prior to implant therapy.[17, 18]

Interarch distance must be observed to be sure that the placement of implants does not infringe on the interocclusal distance or the occlusal plane of the subsequent prosthesis in its relation to both arches.

Placement of prosthetic teeth and a wax try-in of this arrangement should be performed with the patient to verify esthetics, phonetics, and occlusion. It also provides another diagnostic tool for determining the placement of the implants. Once these determinations have been verified, a clear surgical stent can be prepared from the articulated case to aid in the exact surgical placement of the implants.

PROSTHODONTIC APPLICATIONS

There are basic considerations which should be noted in the design for each method of prosthodontic reconstruction.

Single Tooth Replacement

There are no data indicating the longevity of a prosthodontic restoration retained by a single implant for replacement of a missing individual tooth. Therefore, the guidelines for this design of single tooth replacement can only be general. The single tooth implant may be an alternative when replacement of a single tooth would involve preparation of unrestored teeth adjacent to the edentulous space. The maintenance of a plaque-free dental implant and proper functional forces are the paramount considerations in this situation.

In function, a single tooth implant should be in centric contact with equal pressure with the rest of the teeth. The single tooth implant should not be the only contact in function during eccentric movements so that it would bear the entire load while causing disocclusion of the other teeth in the mouth. An example of this would be a canine tooth. Group function should be the occlusal design during eccentric mandibular movement toward the functioning side in order to distribute the occlusal force to a number of anterior and posterior teeth and minimize lateral stress on the canine implant.

The faciolingual and mesiodistal dimensions of the perimucosal portion of most implants are less than those of the natural tooth root. In the best of situations, a crown which is over a dental implant should taper to fit the implant leaving at least 1 mm of the implant exposed above the tissue. Obviously, in the anterior portion of the mouth, this would leave a very unesthetic situation. A common problem in the use of dental implants in esthetically important areas is the need for compromise to access for the maintenance of a plaque-free implant surface. A common alternative is to design a crown that is similar in configuration to a modified ridge lap pontic (Fig 28–1,A and B). The more pieces of hardware that are necessary to attach the crown to the implant, the more difficult the situation becomes. Single tooth posterior implants do not create as difficult a problem as anterior teeth from an occlusal or esthetic perspective.

Fixed Prostheses

The determination of the maxillomandibular relationship to use as a reference position during treatment is of primary importance in controlling occlusal stress to the components of the implant system. Maximum intercuspation must occur at a maxillomandibular position that results in harmonious function with the muscles of mastication and temporomandibular joints.

An analysis of a patient's existing occlusion is needed to identify various occlusal problems including occlusal plane irregularities, functional and nonfunctional interferences, deflective occlusal contacts, and perhaps the necessity of altering the vertical dimension of occlusion. These conditions require careful planning if occlusal stress is to be kept at a minimum. It is imperative that preoperative casts be mounted in a correct maxillomandibular relationship and that adequate diagnostic procedures be carried out on these casts including the establishment of

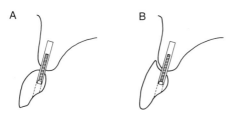

FIG 28–1.
A, a schematic mesial view of contours of a central incisor arranged for optimal oral hygiene. This would likely be unesthetic. **B,** a schematic mesial view of contours of a central incisor arranged for optimal esthetics and oral hygiene access. The facial aspect should be concave only in one plane.

proper curves and planes of occlusion. Diagnostic waxing is performed to verify the accuracy and practicality of these corrections.

Once the maxillomandibular position for treatment is determined, the primary occlusal consideration is to provide simultaneous bilateral posterior occlusal contact in that position. This results in stabilization of this position and becomes a reference position for tooth- and condyle-guided lateral mandibular movements.

In general, it is thought that it is desirable to have posterior teeth disocclude during eccentric mandibular movements. However, if an implant is involved in this disocclusion, then it may be proper that the guidance be placed into group function.

The edentulous area may be restored utilizing a natural tooth or teeth as an abutment in combination with an implant (composite system), or the prosthesis may be completely supported by implants (single system). When a natural tooth is used as an abutment, it is necessary to consider the implications and solutions as mentioned previously in this chapter in the discussion of composite systems. Consideration of one of these items not only may result in a more favorable stress distribution throughout the appliance implant system but will allow for retrievability of the prosthesis. If an implant-associated problem occurs, the restoration connected to the implant may be removed without jeopardizing the restoration as a whole, part of which is attached to the natural tooth.

Regardless of whether a composite or single system is the option, consideration must be given to proper maintenance of a plaque-free environment at the perimucosal area of the implant. The abutment crown contours must be designed so the patient will have easy access to these areas and the pontic design must leave adequate embrasure areas for the use of oral hygiene aids (Fig 28–2,A and B). If esthetics is a compelling consideration, then pontics and abutment crowns should be designed to have tissue contours as in the application of the single crown (Figs 28–1 and 28–3). Proper pontic designs are described in several textbooks.[20, 21]

Occlusal loading for an entirely implant-supported prosthesis (single system) should be designed so there is equal stress distribution. This can be accomplished by using rigid fixed partial dentures with

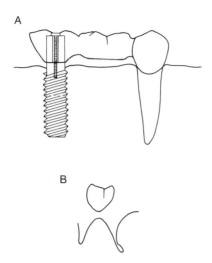

FIG 28-2.
A, a schematic facial view of a mandibular fixed partial denture illustrating ideal proximal contours for access for oral hygiene procedures. **B,** a schematic mesial view of a cross section through the pontic area illustrating ideal contours and tissue relationships. The distance from the ridge facing the side of the pontic to the ridge tissue should be 2 to 3 mm.

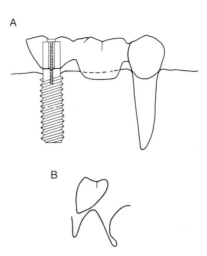

FIG 28-3.
A, a schematic facial view of a fixed partial denture illustrating an acceptable compromise for esthetics. **B,** a schematic mesial view of a cross section through the pontic area of an esthetically arranged mandibular fixed partial denture. Note that the pontic does not contact tissue.

equal distribution of centric contacts. If the prosthesis is involved with eccentric tooth guidance, the guidance should be as shallow as possible.[22]

Overdentures

Overdentures have been used with a wide variety of implant systems including blade implants and the osseointegrated implants. The overdenture provides additional retention and stability over a conventional denture. Overdentures usually involve the incorporation of various attachment systems when they are used with implants. Yet the patient can remove the prosthesis at any time.

Overdentures can be used with most of the implant systems presently available. There are numerous attachment systems commercially available that can be used to retain an overdenture. Two methods are used most commonly to provide retention for overdentures: bar attachments and magnets.

Bar Attachments

There are two groups of bar attachments: bar units and bar joints. Both types provide retention for

an overdenture while splinting the abutments. The bar unit provides rigid fixation while the bar joint provides rotational, resilient, or combined movement to the overdenture.[23] Both types could be used with implants. However, it appears that the more popular type used with implant-retained overdentures is the bar joint system. The bar joint systems traditionally used with natural teeth can be used with the various implant systems. Some implant systems have their own bar joint components specifically manufactured for use with that particular system.

In bar joint systems the overdenture is supported in part by the mucosal tissues of the ridges. Thus, it is important that the borders of the overdenture be properly extended to provide stability and retention present with conventional dentures in addition to the retention and stability provided by the attachment system. The principle of the bar joint system is to provide retention of the overdenture against vertical dislodging forces. When the overdenture is functionally loaded during occlusion, there is a shared distribution of the occlusal forces between the mucosa and the bar joint.[24] Rotational movements of the overdenture in the frontal and sagittal planes are permitted by the rotation of the sleeve about the bar. However, these movements are guided by the bar joint system eliminating any excessive, undesirable movements against the mucosal tissues.[24]

The guidelines involved in the fabrication of an overdenture for natural teeth using the bar joint system can be applied for bar joint systems with implants. In most cases, the bar is placed in the anterior region. The bar should be placed directly over or slightly lingual to the crest of the ridge in a straight, horizontal alignment. In the anterior region, the bar should be perpendicular to a line bisecting the angle formed by the posterior alveolar ridges (Fig 28–4).[24, 25] While the arch form (i.e., V-shaped arch) may limit the use of the bar joint system depending on the position of the remaining natural teeth, the flexibility in the placement of the implant fixtures could allow for satisfactory alignment of the bar. Even so, there may be situations where the bar cannot be aligned adequately, negating the use of a bar attachment. In these cases, the use of individual abutments to retain an overdenture with or without some other attachment system (i.e., magnets) would be feasible.

There should be at least 2 mm of space existing between the inferior surface of the bar and the gingival tissues of the alveolar ridge (see Fig 28–4). However, it has been stated that there is no disad-

vantage to having the bar in direct pressure-free contact with the ridge as long as regular oral hygiene is maintained by the patient.[24]

Certain bar joint systems, such as the original Dolder system,* contain a prefabricated gold alloy bar which is sectioned to the appropriate length and soldered to the abutment copings with a solder that is compatible with both the bar and the copings. However, the majority of the bar joint systems presently available have plastic bar forms. They can be easily adjusted to fulfill the desired form and can be waxed to the copings. The entire assembly can then be cast as a single unit with a metal alloy designated by the manufacturer as being compatible with the copings. The tedious technical aspects involved with soldering are eliminated with this process.

Metal or nylon sleeves can be used with these bar joint systems. The flanges of the sleeve flex over the bar when the overdenture is seated to provide the retention for the system. The metal sleeves are adjustable to allow for flexibility in controlling the degree of retention. However, they can be difficult to replace or repair. The nylon sleeves are not adjustable but can be replaced easily.[26] Specific technical aspects concerning the fabrication of the bar joint system with various implant systems are covered elsewhere in this book.

Magnets

Magnetically retained overdentures have become very popular with the various implant systems. Magnets have been used successfully for years with natural teeth to retain overdentures.[27, 28] Owing to their strong attractive force, they possess great resistance to vertical dislodging forces. However, they have little resistance to lateral forces and can be easily moved in a horizontal vector thus providing an inherently stress-relieved system as less lateral force is transmitted to the abutments.[29] The majority of the force is directed apically along the long axis of the abutment. Owing to the stress-breaking component inherent in this system, it can be used with implants, natural teeth, or combinations of both abutments.[29] In addition, the system is technically easier to use

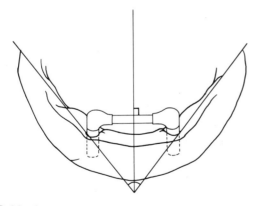

FIG 28–4.
Schematic view illustrating the position of a bar joint attached to two implants. The bar should be centered over or slightly lingual to the crest of the ridge. It should be in horizontal alignment and be perpendicular to a line bisecting the angle formed by two lines paralleling the crests of the posterior ridges. (Adapted from Dolder E, Durrer G: *The Bar-Joint Denture.* Lombard, Ill, Quintessence Publishing Co, Inc, 1978, p. 41. Used by permission.)

*Attachments International, Inc. San Mateo, Calif.

and repair as compared to other attachment systems.

The system basically consists of a magnet and a keeper. Earlier types of magnets used over the years included ferrite and alnico magnets. However, the samarium-cobalt and the neodymium-iron-boron magnets have become the more popular magnets over the last 20 years. Owing to their unique crystalline structure, the strength of the rare earth magnets are 20 to 50 times greater per unit volume than the strongest ferrite or alnico magnet.[28] In addition, they can be machined to small sizes without loss of magnetic strength.[28] The magnetic strength ranges from 250 to 1,000 gs. They are available in either open-field systems or closed-field systems. The closed-field system provides more efficient use of the magnetic strength by using both poles of the magnet compared to the open-field system which uses only one pole of the magnet (Fig 28–5).[30]

The magnetic system also contains a metal plate known as a keeper. This keeper is usually attached to the abutment and is made from a ferromagnetic alloy to allow for attraction by the magnet. Various ferromagnetic alloys can be used such as palladium-cobalt (containing more than 50% palladium content) or stainless steel.[29]

Magnets can be used with virtually any implant system. If the implant does not have a prefabricated keeper screw or coping for that system, a customized coping must be made from a ferromagnetic alloy. There are a number of implant systems that contain prefabricated keepers in the form of copings or screws that attach directly to the implant fixture. It is recommended that all keepers be cemented, even if there is an additional retentive mechanism existing in the keeper (i.e., threads), to provide a primary form of retention for some keepers and as a barrier between the two dissimilar metals of the implant and the keeper. This barrier will protect the implant from any electrogalvanic reaction that might cause corrosion of the implant.[29] However, one report indicated no evidence of any galvanic action between the dissimilar metals when the keeper was in direct contact with the implant.[30]

A sufficient number of magnets should be used to provide at least 400 to 1,000 g of magnetic strength for the overdenture. This amount of retention is required to adequately resist vertical displacement of the overdenture in the oral cavity (Fig 28–6,A,B).[28]

Fixed-Removable Prosthesis

The fixed-removable prosthesis resembles a flangeless denture that is retained solely by several osseointegrated implants. This retention is obtained by the use of screws positioned into the prosthesis and threaded into the internal aspect of the implants. In most cases, the implants are present in the anterior region of the mandible or maxilla. The anterior portion of the prosthesis is secured to the implant fixtures with screws. The posterior portions of the prosthesis are cantilevered from the distal abutment implants (Fig 28–7). There is no contact between the prosthesis and the tissues of the alveolar ridge.

The original design of the fixed-removable prosthesis was developed by Swedish investigators using the two-stage endosseous implant system developed by Brånemark. The prosthesis consisted of a gold alloy framework attached to the copings of the implant. Acrylic resin denture teeth were arranged on the framework and secured with acrylic resin.[31] Later modifications of this design were developed at the University of Toronto. This design incorporated changes in the structure of the framework as well as

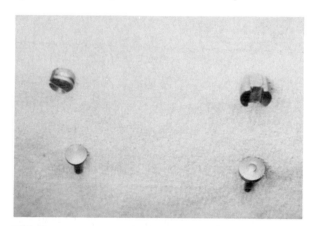

FIG 28–5.
Neodymium-iron-boron *(left)* and samarium-cobalt magnets (Jackson magnets, Solid State Innovations, Mt. Airy, N.C.) with their respective keepers. The keepers shown are for use with natural tooth roots. However, they can be adapted and incorporated as customized keepers for those implant systems that do not have prefabricated keepers.

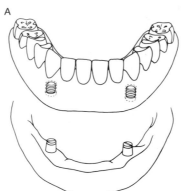

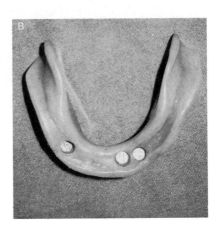

FIG 28–6.
Schematic view illustrating an overdenture with two magnets and a mandible with corresponding implant abutments. At least two magnets should be used to provide the minimum amount of magnetic strength for retention of the overdenture. **B,** however, additional magnets can be used to provide as much retention as desired.

the use of less expensive metal alloys with similar physical properties as the gold alloys.[32] Although this design was developed with the Bråanemark implant system, it should be adaptable with any similar two-stage endosseous implant system. The fixed-removable prosthesis represents a unique aspect of prosthodontic reconstruction for edentulous arches. General considerations are presented in this chapter.

Since the implants are situated in the anterior region, the posterior sections of the framework are cantilevered from the anterior portion of the framework. The length, height, and width of the cantilever are crucial in minimizing the amount of deformation of the prosthesis. According to Glantz, the amount of deformation of the cantilever is directly proportional to the cube of the length and inversely proportional to the width and the cube of the height of the

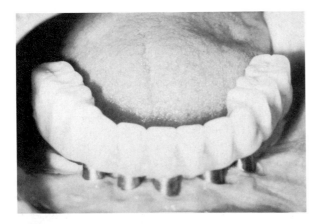

FIG 28–7.
A fixed-removable prosthesis supported by five implants.

cantilever.[33] In addition, there is a direct relation between the amount of deformation and the force of the occlusion (loading force) as well as an inverse relation with the modulus of elasticity of the material to be used for the framework. This relationship can be expressed in the following equation:

$$D = F \times L^3 \times constant / E \times W \times H^3$$

where D is the amount of deformation, F is the force of occlusion, L, W, and H are the length, width, and height of the cantilever, respectively, and E is the modulus of elasticity of the material. Therefore, the length of the cantilever should be minimized while maximizing the height and width of the cantilever. It is recommended that the cantilever should not exceed 20 mm in length using five or more abutments. If four abutments are used, the cantilever should not exceed 15 mm in length.[34] Other studies have shown that the length of the cantilever should be limited to the premolar region and that the length of the extension should be shorter in the maxillary arch as opposed to the mandibular arch because there is less cortical bone present in the maxilla.[35] The fixed-removable prosthesis should not be used with three or fewer abutments. In addition, the height and width of the cantilever should be in proportion to the height and diameter of the copings. The junction of the cantilever and the distal abutment should be provided with added height and width as this area is the primary stress point in relation to the cantilever (Fig 28–8,A and B). Insufficient bulk of material at this point could lead to fracture of the cantilever.

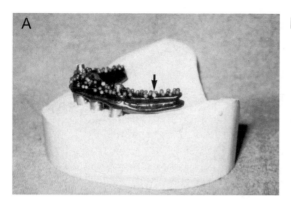

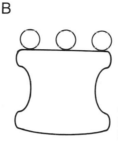

FIG 28–8.
A, lateral view of waxed framework for the fixed-removable prosthesis prior to spruing and casting procedures. The cantilever is 20 mm in length from the distal abutment. The cantilever is shaped in an I-beam design *(arrow)*. Additional bulk is provided around the junction of the distal abutment and the cantilever. There is approximately 1 to 2 mm of space between the crest of the mandibular ridge and the inferior surface of the cantilever. Beads have been added to provide additional retention for the acrylic resin. **B,** schematic cross-sectional view illustrating the I-beam design of the cantilever at the *arrow*.

The cantilever should have an I-beam design to increase the rigidity of this area.[32] There should be about 1 to 2 mm of space between the inferior border of the cantilever and the alveolar ridge to allow for adequate oral hygiene. Any large distance in this area could lead to escape of air during phonation, impairing proper speech. The anterior section should have discrete finish lines.

The literature reports casting the framework in type IV gold or precious metal alloys such as silver-palladium alloy.[32, 36] The decision on the type of metal alloy for casting should depend in part on the composition of the copings being incorporated in the framework. For example, the Brånemark system copings contain palladium as part of the composition of the alloy. Although the Swedish system recommended the use of a type IV alloy, it has been demonstrated that silver-palladium alloy bonds well with the copings due to the compatibility of the palladium between the coping and the casting alloy.[32] Those implant systems which use prefabricated plastic copings can cast the entire framework in any appropriate alloy (type IV gold, silver palladium, cobalt-chromium). It is recommended that the metal alloy possess sufficient yield strength (>300 MPa) and modulus of elasticity (>80,000 MPa) to prevent deformation and fracturing of the cantilevers. The framework can be waxed and cast in sections and soldered together following trial insertion in the oral cavity. It can also be waxed and cast as one unit.

Following casting of the framework, a trial insertion is performed in the oral cavity. There should not be any evidence of instability in the seating of the framework on the abutment posts. The framework should be attached to the abutment posts without any binding of the screws as they are threaded into the abutments. The patient should not experience any discomfort during the attachment of the framework to the abutments. There should be intimate contact between the copings and the abutment posts (Fig 28–9). If there is any evidence of inaccuracy in the seating of the framework, the framework should be sectioned and reattached to the abutment posts, luted together, and later soldered in the conventional manner. This procedure also applies if the framework was cast in sections. Once the framework appears to be accurate, occlusal force should be applied to the cantilever sections. One method, used by us, is to have the patient occlude on an orangewood stick placed between the cantilever and the opposing arch (Fig 28–10). The stick should be placed initially at the proximal portion of the cantilever and slowly moved distally as the patient continues to occlude repeatedly to determine if there is any extreme flexure of the mandible due to the rigidity of the system.[37] Flexure of the mandible can be determined clinically if the patient experiences discomfort either around the distal abutments or in the body of the mandible as the occluding force approaches the distal portion of the cantilever. The particular point of the cantilever where discomfort is first noted by the patient is marked and the cantilever is shortened until it is proximal to that point.

Following this procedure, the prosthetic teeth

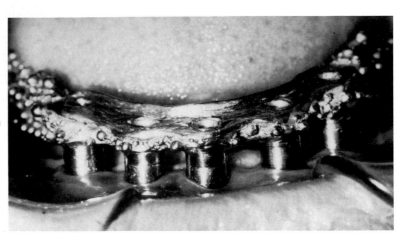

FIG 28–9.
Framework attached to the abutment posts. Note the intimate contact between the copings embedded within the framework and the abutment posts.

are arranged and the trial prosthesis is inserted intraorally for verification of esthetics and occlusion. The use of posterior prosthetic teeth with minimal inclinations is recommended to minimize any lateral forces on the cantilevers during excursive movements. Acrylic resin prosthetic teeth should be used to absorb the shock of occlusal force. The prosthesis is then processed and finished using conventional methods of removable prosthodontics.

DISCUSSION

Only after careful attention to the functional considerations and a meticulous diagnostic evalua-

tion, which should include all considerations previously described in this chapter, should a decision be made regarding a specific restoration.

If the decision is to restore form and function with fixed prosthetics, it is necessary to define whether the support will be via a single or composite system. The design characteristics of the prosthesis will be different for each system and must include considerations such as movement of natural abutment teeth versus the immobility of a rigid implant, esthetics, phonetics, and occlusal load.

In the fixed prosthesis it is important that design considerations include access for adequate plaque control at the perimucosal area of the dental implant. This is especially difficult to accomplish in esthetically important areas.

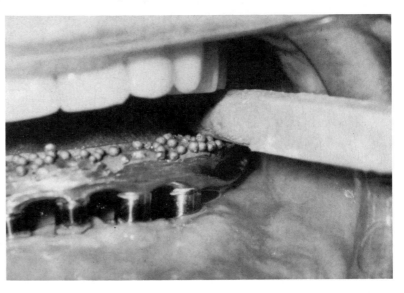

FIG 28–10.
Patient occluding on an orangewood stick placed between the opposing dentition and the cantilever to determine any clinical evidence of flexure of the mandible.

The use of dental implants for single tooth replacement is undocumented regarding long-term success rate and at this time dental implants should be used with caution in regard to this situation.

There are a variety of factors that will influence the indications for an overdenture, fixed prosthesis, or a fixed-removable prosthesis. The selection of the overdenture for implant prosthodontic reconstruction depends on several factors. One factor is the amount of bone resorption that has occurred in the arch. The presence of minimal height and width of the remaining bone, except in isolated areas, would prevent placement of a sufficient number of implants to adequately retain a fixed prosthesis. However, the existence of isolated areas with sufficient bone to allow for placement of one, two, or three implants would allow for the use of an overdenture.

In our opinion, the lack of sufficient cortical bone in the maxilla as opposed to the mandible does not allow the maxillary arch to be amenable to the full extension of the cantilever posteriorly for a fixed-removable prosthesis, thereby limiting the extent of occlusion and masticatory efficiency. This problem would be alleviated with the use of an overdenture. Severe resorption of the maxillary arch anteriorly might create unfavorable cantilever forces with a fixed prosthesis in order to provide adequate facial support, esthetics, and occlusion. An overdenture would be indicated in this situation.[38] Overdentures may be used in situations where the arrangement of the implant fixtures is unfavorable for retaining a fixed prosthesis.[38] Fixtures that have been positioned with excessive inclinations that may compromise esthetics or hygiene for a fixed prosthesis could be used with an overdenture.

The use of a fixed prosthesis retained by implants in the maxillary arch may cause difficulty during speech owing to an excessive escape of air through the spaces present between the fixtures. This problem can be resolved with the use of an overdenture.

Implant-retained overdentures have been used in the oral rehabilitation of patients with acquired or congenital defects of the maxilla and mandible. Other factors, such as cost and patient acceptance, play a role in the selection process.

There are several factors that favor a fixed-removable prosthesis. There are instances where severe resorption exists in the arch. Usually in the mandible, a minimal amount of posterior residual ridge remains and the labial and buccal muscle attachments are continuous with those of the floor of the mouth. In this situation, an overdenture may not be adequate because of the lack of sufficient ridge and vestibular depth for retention, support, and stability. Extensive surgical augmentation and vestibuloplasty would be required to improve the ridge form before the placement of an overdenture. The existence of minimal height in the posterior regions of the arch may preclude placing implants for a fixed prosthesis. However, anteriorly, there usually exists sufficient remaining bone for the placement of an adequate number of implants to retain a fixed-removable prosthesis.

Other factors include the patient's ability to adapt to a removable prosthesis. Some patients may not adapt psychologically to the wearing of a removable prosthesis while others may not have the neuromuscular coordination needed to retain a removable prosthesis. In these patients, a fixed-removable prosthesis may be indicated.

SUMMARY

Sound basic principles of prosthodontics need to be retained throughout the fabrication of the prosthesis. It is important that this philosophy begin with a thorough history and examination to determine the medical status of the patient as well as the dental deficiencies that exist and the resulting problems experienced by the patient. This knowledge is mandatory in determining the best possible treatment that can be offered to the patient.

This philosophy is probably more important with implants because of the rigidity of the system. Accuracy is imperative. Otherwise, the system may fail.

REFERENCES

1. Brånemark PI, Hansson B, Adell R, et al: *Osseointegrated Implants*. Stockholm, Almquist & Wiksell International, 1977.

2. Zarb GA, Albrektsson T: Nature of implant attachments, in Brånemark PI, Zarb GA, Albrektsson T (eds): *Tissue-Integrated Prostheses: Osseointegration in Clinical Dentistry*. Chicago, Quintessence Publishing Co, Inc, 1985, pp 89–97.

3. Smiler DG: Evaluation and treatment planning. *J Calif Dent Assoc* 1987; 15:35–41.

4. Weiss C: Tissue integration of dental implants: Description and analysis of the fibro-osseous integration and osseous integration systems. *J Oral Implantol* 1986; 12:169–214.

5. Roberts E, Smith RK, Zilberman Y, et al: Osseous adaption to continuous loading of rigid endosseous implants. *Am J Orthod* 1984; 86:95–111.

6. Dahl G: Mechanical considerations on dental implants. *J Oral Implantol* 1981; 9:310–315.

7. Forde TH: *The Principles and Practices of Oral Dynamics*. New York, Exposition Press, Inc, 1964, pp 265–273.

8. Skalak R: Biomechanical considerations in osseointegrated prosthesis. *J Prosthet Dent* 1983; 49:843–848.

9. Dahl G: The importance of the modulus of elasticity and the rigid connection of dental implants. *J Oral Implantol* 1981; 9:427–429.

10. McKinney R, Lemons J: *The Dental Implant: Clinical and Biologic Response of Oral Tissues*. Littleton, Mass, PSG Publishing Co, 1985.

11. Albrektsson T: Direct bone anchorage of dental implants. *J Prosthet Dent* 1983; 50:255–261.

12. Albrektsson T, Brånemark PI: Osseointegrated titanium implant requirements for ensuring a long lasting, direct bone to implant anchorage in man. *Acta Orthop Scand* 1981; 52:155–170.

13. Lemons JE: Surface conditions for surgical implant and biocompatibility. *J Oral Implantol* 1977; 7:362–374.

14. Boretos WJ: *Contemporary Biomaterials: Materials and Host Response, Clinical Applications, New Technology and Legal Aspects*. Parkridge, NJ, Noyes Publications, 1984, p 260.

15. Babbush CR: Selection of the implant candidate, in Hardin JF (ed): *Clark's Clinical Dentistry*, vol 5. Philadelphia, JB Lippincott, 1990, chap 47.

16. Blomberg S: Psychological response, in Brånemark PI, Zarb GA, Albrektsson T (eds): *Tissue-Integrated Prostheses: Osseointegration in Clinical Dentistry*. Chicago, Quintessence Publishing Co, Inc, 1985 pp 165–174.

17. Laney WR: Selecting edentulous patients for tissue-integrated prostheses. *Int J Oral Maxillofac Implants* 1986; 1:129–138.

18. Desjardins RP: Tissue-integrated prostheses for edentulous patients with normal and abnormal jaw relationships. *J Prosthet Dent* 1988; 59:180–187.

19. Adell R, Lekholm U, Rockler B, et al: A 15-year study of osseointegrated implants in the treatment of the edentulous jaw. *Int J Oral Surg* 1981; 10:387–416.

20. Dinga PD: Pontics for fixed prosthodontics, in Malone WFP, Tylman DD (eds): *Tylmans Theory and Practice of Fixed Prosthodontics*, ed 7. St Louis, CV Mosby Co, 1978, pp 274–290.

21. Keough BE, Kay HB, Rosenberg MM, et al: Periodontal prosthetics: Prosthetic management of the patient with advanced periodontal disease, in Hardin JF (ed): *Clark's Clinical Dentistry*, vol 5. Philadelphia, JB Lippincott, 1990, chap 41.

22. Schulte JK, Peterson TA: Occlusal and prosthetic considerations. *J Calif Dent Assoc* 1987; 15(10):64–72.

23. Mensor MC Jr: Attachments for the overdenture, in Brewer AA, Morrow RM (eds): *Overdentures* St. Louis, CV Mosby Co, 1980, pp 240–251.

24. Dolder EJ, Durrer GT: *The Bar-Joint Denture*. Chicago, Quintessence Publishing Co, Inc, 1978.

25. Preiskel HW: *Precision Attachments in Dentistry*. St. Louis, CV Mosby Co, 1979, pp 211–212.

26. Staubli PE, Haechler WH: The bar retained dental prostheses. *Trends Techniques* 1988; 5:26–31.

27. Gillings BRD: Magnetic retention for the overdenture, in Brewer AA, Morrow RM (eds): *Overdentures*. St. Louis, CV Mosby Co, 1980, pp 376–397.

28. Jackson TR, Healey KW: Rare earth magnetic attachments: The state of the art in removable prosthodontics. *Quintessence Int* 1987; 18:41–51.

29. Sendax VI: Magnetic retention system for implant prosthodontics. *J Oral Implantol* 1987; 13:128–155.

30. Jackson TR: The application of rare earth magnetic retention to osseointegrated implants. *Int J Oral Maxillofac Implants* 1986; 1:81–92.

31. Zarb GA, Jansson T: Prosthodontic procedures, in Brånemark PI, Zarb G, Albrektsson T (eds): *Tissue-Integrated Prostheses: Osseointegration in Clinical Dentistry*. Chicago, Quintessence Publishing Co, Inc, 1985, pp 241–282.

32. Cox J, Zarb G: Alternative prosthodontic superstructure designs. *Swed Dent J [Suppl]* 1985; 28:71–75.

33. Glantz PO: Aspects of prosthodontic design, in Brånemark PI, Zarb G, Albrektsson T (eds): *Tissue-Integrated Prostheses: Osseointegration in Clinical Dentistry*. Chicago, Quintessence Publishing Co, Inc, 1985, pp 329–332.

34. Bergman GF, Taylor RL: *Laboratory Technique for*

the Brånemark Osseointegrated Implant System. Chicago, Austenal Dental and Northwestern University, 1987, p 21.

35. Haraldson T: A photoelastic study of some biomechanical factors affecting the anchorage of osseointegrated implants in the jaw. *Scand J Plast Reconstr Surg* 1980; 14:209–214.

36. Zarb G, Symington JM: Osseointegrated dental im-

plants: Preliminary report on a replication study. *J Prosthet Dent* 1983; 50:271–276.

37. Finger IM, Guerra LR: Prosthetic considerations in reconstructive implantology. *Dent Clin North Am* 1986; 30:69–83.

38. Parel SM, Holt R, Brånemark PI, Tjellstrom A: Osseointegration and facial prosthetics. *Int J Oral Maxillofac Implants* 1986; 1:27–29.

Chapter 29

Clinical Evaluation Tools for Implant Performance

Ralph V. McKinney, Jr., D.D.S., Ph.D.
David L. Koth, D.D.S., M.S.
David E. Steflik, M.A., Ed.D.

One of the most important aspects of clinical management of implant patients is the evaluation of the implant treatment in relation to time. Most patients are recalled by the managing dentist for observation and prophylaxis service on a scheduled basis. These return visits usually also include updated radiographs. But beyond the radiographs and the empiric clinical observation by the dentist, little is done to accurately record clinical data that may be accumulated for a prognostic overview for that patient, or provide a retrospective review of a series of implants of given materials and designs.

The use of dental implants for patient treatment without the adequate use of clinical parameters to assess performance is one of the features that has in some cases alienated the mainstream dental profession from dentists practicing implantology.[1] Another factor has been the sales promotion of dental implants by proprietary companies without scientific clinical data to back up their claims.[2] Also, many of these industrial companies are owned or controlled by dentists who are advocating their particular type of implant or system.

Much of that has changed now with the first National Institutes of Health (NIH) consensus conference on dental implants in 1978 (cosponsored by Harvard University), which focused attention on this field and suggested standards for clinical performance.[3] The recently completed 1988 second NIH consensus conference solidified the position of implantology as a full-fledged dental treatment modality and outlined in broad terms directions for the future.[4] It is rather unusual to have two federal conferences within a decade on the same subject and so substantiates the importance of this field within dentistry. (A. Rizzo, D.D.S., personal communication, February 1989).

Also contributing to the increased requirement for clinical evaluation is that the American Dental Association Council on Dental Materials, Instruments, and Equipment and the US Food and Drug Administration have issued guidelines that detail the criteria and type of data that are needed to allow these agencies to approve implant devices (either provisionally or fully) for acceptable use in human patients.[5, 6] In these litigious times, these are important considerations.

PRACTICAL CLINICAL EVALUATION CRITERIA

The dentist in implant practice needs a rapid and reproducible method to evaluate the health of dental implants in his or her patients when they return for recall or treatment. This evaluation must be simple, concise, and quick because the dentist does not want to be saddled with minute data collection and the filling out of forms.[7]

Although it would be nice to collect load cell biting force data and periodontometer mobility data, these procedures are complicated and time-consuming and thus are not performed in the practical clinical situation. The evaluation data to be collected must be simple to gather and must be able to be performed by the dentist in his treatment of the patient.

CLINICAL EVALUATION TOOLS

The patient has basically two questions regarding implant(s) and associated bridgework: Will it function comfortably? and, How long will it remain serviceable in my jaws?

The first question can be answered by the patient himself. If the implant is comfortable and he can chew, then the treatment must be successful. But beyond that patients must rely on the skill and knowledge of the dentist to evaluate their implant treatment. In order to do this the dentist must have a set of evaluation criteria that are based on more than just an empiric impression and a panographic radiograph. The dentist must have an established set of evaluatory guidelines that he or she can use to measure qualitative and quantitative data about the implant.

PURPOSE

The purpose of this chapter is to present simple qualitative and quantitative evaluation indices that can be performed easily and with a minimum of time by the clinician in order to achieve standardized information that will permit statistical comparison between implants in different recipients as well as comparisons between different materials and designs.

GENERAL EVALUATION CRITERIA

Generally, evaluation in the clinical setting is based on three criteria: the peri-implant gingival

health, the peri-implant bone health, and the subjective comments of the patient as to service and function. (Table 29–1).

THE EVALUATION TOOLS

The Gingival (Bleeding) Index

The presence of inflammation in the free gingival margin and attached gingiva can be quantitated by employing a modification of the gingival indices of Loe and Silness.[8, 9] The index scale is rated as 0, 1, 2, or 3 based on the bleeding response to gentle 1- to 2-mm-deep circumferential periodontal probing (Table 29–2). Since bleeding is an end result of gingival inflammation, it directly conveys the status of the gingival health. Some dentists have difficulty determining between 0 or 1, but careful inspection will usually reveal the subtle loss of tissue stippling (a rating of 1) that occurs in early gingivitis (see Table 29–2). A periodontal probe or blunt explorer should be used for the evaluation procedure.

TABLE 29–1.

Endosteal Dental Implant Evaluation Criteria: General Principles and Evaluatory Indices

Requirement	Evaluation Tool
I. Assessment of periimplant gingival health	
Gingival inflammation	Gingival bleeding index
Gingival sulcus depth	Periodontal probe index
Sulcular fluid volume production	Sulcular fluid volume index
Oral hygiene assessment	Plaque and calculus index
Professional assessment of overall gingival health	Dentist's subjective evaluation index
	Patient comfort index
II. Assessment of periimplant bone health	
Bone physiologic health	Radiographic index
Stability of implant in situ	Mobility index
Professional assessment of overall bone health	Dentist's subjective evaluation index
	Patient comfort index
III. Assessment of comfort and function	
Patient comfort	Patient comfort index
Physiologic function	Patient comfort index
	Dentist's subjective evaluation index
	Radiographic index

TABLE 29-2.

Gingival Bleeding Index*

Index	Clinical Presentation
0	Gingiva of normal color and stippling; no bleeding on probing
1	Gingiva of normal color and stippling with slight hyperemia; no bleeding on probing
3	Gingiva markedly red and edematous, with spontaneous bleeding on finger pressure

*Modified from Loe H, Silness J: *Acta Odontol Scand* 1963; 21:533–551, and Silness J, Loe H: *Acta Odontol Scand* 1964; 22:121–135.

Periodontal Probe (Sulcus Depth) Index

Gingival sulcus depth should be measured and recorded using a standardized 0.7-mm-thick periodontal probe. Ideally, a force of 17 to 30 g should be used in measuring sulcus depth. The measurements should be taken from each of the four quadrants around an implant as recommended by the NIH-Harvard consensus conference[10]; however, in reality this is not always practical because of the presence of fixed bridgework on the implant. As a minimum, buccal and lingual sulcus depths should be recorded. It should also be noted that some endosteal implant designs, such as those with shoulders, do not lend themselves to this assessment. Furthermore, a number of clinicians and scientists believe that probing may be damaging to the biological seal around the implant and thus the sulcus is better left unmeasured. We recommend probing not be initiated prior to 3 months post-insertion.

The Sulcular Fluid Volume Index

It has been well documented that the gingival sulcular (or crevicular) fluid volume and character are associated with periodontal health status. Investigators have shown that the volume and protein character of the sulcular fluid indicate the presence or absence of inflammation in the gingiva and can serve as a diagnostic aid in determining the relative presence of periodontal disease.[11] One of the problems associated with sulcular fluid assessment has been the lack of simple standardized methods for accurate, repeatable evaluation of the sulcular contents.

Previously, sulcular fluid volume assessment required the creation of customized filter measuring strips and employment of the biochemical nenhydrin assay technique, not a procedure for the routine dental office. Golub and Kleinberg[12] have developed an electronic instrument, called a Periotron,* that allows quantitation of the volume of sulcular fluid absorbed using a supplier-provided standardized strip of filter paper. The original design instrument used a two-strip method. The standardized filter strip is placed in the gingival sulcus, which has been isolated with a cotton roll, for 30 seconds to drain the ambient fluid contents. This strip is removed and discarded, and the sulcus is allowed to refill for exactly 27 seconds (a timer is part of the Periotron). At 27 seconds a new strip is placed in the sulcus for 3 seconds. The strip is then removed and immediately inserted between the electronic sensing electrodes of the Periotron. The instrument measures the amount of fluid picked up in the filter strip and provides a lighted electronic (LED) display of an arbitrary numeric value for the liquid volume.

An improved Periotron instrument has been developed with more sensitivity and a simplified one-strip method. With this newer device the tooth is isolated, the gingiva is gently air-dried, and a standardized strip is inserted in the sulcus for 10 seconds and then removed and placed in the instrument-sensing electrodes. The investigators have established biological interpretations for the arbitrary scale that indicate the presence or absence of inflammation in the periodontium (Table 29–3). The accuracy of the Periotron and the interpretation of the readout values have been validated by an independent investigation.[13] Filter strip readings should be taken from the buccal and lingual sulci of the implant and control teeth if possible. Scores of 5 to 10 or below indicate good gingival health.

The Plaque and Calculus Index

A combined plaque and calculus index is used to evaluate qualitatively the amount of oral deposits on the implant and adjacent teeth, if present (Table

---

*Available from IDE Interstate, 1500 New Horizon Blvd., Amityville, NY 11701.

TABLE 29–3.

Crevicular Fluid Volume Index*

Periotron Index	Periodontal Health Status
	Two-strip method (60 sec)
0–10	No inflammation; tissues essentially normal
11–20	Slight-to-mild inflammation
21–40	Moderate inflammation
>40	Severe inflammation
	One-strip method (10 sec)
0–5	No inflammation
6–10	Slight-to-mild inflammation
11–25	Moderate inflammation
>25	Severe inflammation

*Modified from index data as suggested by Golub LM, Kleinberg I: *Oral Sci Rev* 1976; 8:49–61, and IDE Interstate, 1500 Horizon Blvd, Amityville, NY 11701.

29–4). For control purposes, when an adjacent abutment tooth and a nonrestored tooth are present with endosteal implants, they are evaluated using the same criteria. The advantage of using a numerically scored plaque index is that it allows for averaging, mean determination, and statistical analysis of the collected data over a period of time. It must be emphasized that the evaluation is directed solely at the supragingival (within 2 mm of the free gingival margin) or subgingival accumulation of soft or mineralized deposits, not the total surface area of the implant or tooth. In this manner a better relationship between the deposits and the status of gingival health

TABLE 29–4.

Plaque and Calculus Index for Endosteal Implants and Natural Teeth

Index	Clinical Impression
0	No plaque can be scraped off; no calculus
1	Plaque can be scraped off but it is not visible to the clinician; or supragingival calculus extending no more than 1 mm below the free gingival margin
2	Visible plaque within the gingival sulcus or on the tooth and gingival margin; or subgingival calculus extending more than 1 mm into the sulcus; or moderate amounts of supragingival and subgingival calculus
3	Heavy accumulation of plaque within the sulcus or on the tooth and gingival margin; or heavy accumulation of supragingival calculus

is established. The plaque index of Silness and Loe[9] and the calculus index from Ramfjord[14] are both scored on a basis of 0 to 3. The highest reading, soft or hard deposits, is recorded for the evaluation period. This index is not a serviceability-failure determinant but is an indicator of peri-implant gingival health and allows statistical correlation with other peri-implant gingival health indices.

The Mobility Index

A mobility index for endosteal implants was developed from Wasserman and co-workers' modification of the Miller index.[15] To assess mobility the clinician places a blunt wooden dowel against the implant, or implant-supported prosthesis, and makes a clinical judgment of mobility, as well as checking to see if the implant is rotatable or depressible. Based on the dentist's perception of the amount of movement, a quantifiable index number is assigned (Table 29–5).

One feature of endosseous implants when they are used as fixed prosthesis abutments is that the mobility of the implant or abutment teeth alone cannot be judged; rather the mobility of the fixed bridge as a unit is being judged. Thus, a score of 2 or less is considered clinically acceptable when a fixed bridge is cemented to the implant; 1.0 or less is the standard for single implants.

For subperiosteal implants, the mobility determination is primarily one of looking for evidence of vertical or depressible movement at any one or more of the transmucosal implant posts. This is evaluated

TABLE 29–5.

The Mobility Index*

Index	Clinical Impression
0	No mobility
1	Slight buccolingual mobility, ≤ than 0.5 mm
2	Slight buccolingual mobility, >0.5 mm but <1.0 mm
3	Mobility >0.5 mm in buccolingual and mesiodistal directions
4	Depressible

*Modified from Wasserman BH, Geiger AM, Turgeon LR: *J Periodontol* 1973, 44.572–578.

again by using a wooden dowel placed on the occlusal surface of the prosthesis attached to the implant.

The Radiographic Index

A radiographic index is used to assess the health of the jaw bone associated with the implant. Since it is difficult to "grade" radiographs on a numeric basis because of the many variables, such as cone angulation and the results of bone surgery, a plus-minus score is used for assessment. For endosseous implants four critical zones between implant and bone and abutment teeth and bone are examined. These critical zones are (1) the cervical or neck area of the implant, (2) the radicular area of the implant, (3) the periodontal ligament space of the nearest natural abutment tooth, and (4) infrabony pocket formation, if present. All ratings should be made by comparing current evaluatory radiographs with baseline radiographs. Both panographic and periapical radiographs can be used for evaluation. The baseline and evaluation periapical radiographs can be mounted in 2- × 2-in. frames and compared side by side on a screen using dual slide projectors. Any implant receiving negative ratings in more than two of the four zones is given an overall failure rating for the radiographic index. Detailed analyses of the radiographic evaluation areas are as follows:

1. The cervical or neck area: The level of alveolar bone at the cervical area of the implant at evaluation should be compared with the bone level in radiographs taken at baseline. If the bone shows apical migration, or has developed very indistinct margins, it is rated as negative. If the bone level has essentially not changed and has distinct margins, it is rated as positive. There may be a surgical defect created during the operative procedure; thus baseline radiographs are important. If the implant employs a collar or shoulder in its design, this structure should not be used as a reference point.

2. The implant radicular area: The radicular (root) implant-bone interface should be studied. If a radiolucent area is present at baseline between bone and implant, and this area has become wider or has indistinct margins at recall, this area is treated as negative. If the peri-implant bony margins are distinct and the radiolucent zone is unchanged, narrower, or does not exist, this area is rated as positive.

3. The abutment periodontal ligament space: When the implant supports a fixed prosthesis and the periodontal ligament space of the nearest natural abutment is widened, as compared with the baseline radiograph, then the implant is not considered to be acting as a proper abutment and this area is rated as negative. No change in the natural abutment periodontal ligament space is rated as positive. For single implants this evaluation is eliminated.

4. Infrabony pocket formation: If there is radiographic evidence of infrabony pocket formation when compared with the baseline view, the implant is rated as negative; no change is rated as positive.

An example of how the radiograph index may be scored for one or several implants is shown in Table 29–6.

TABLE 29–6.

Scoring of the Radiographic Index*

Implant No.	Area Evaluated				=	Overall Rating
	Neck	Root	PDL Space	Bony Pocket		
1	+	+	+	−	=	+
2	+	−	−	−	=	−
3	−	+	+	+	=	+
4	+	−	+	−	=	+
5	+	+	NA	−	=	+

PDL = periodontal ligament; NA = not available.
*Example of determination of overall ratings based on plus or minus values from the four areas rated.

The Patient Comfort Index

The patient comfort index is used to record the patient's perception about the performance of his implant(s) and attached prosthesis if present. Included in the questions should be limitations of function, pain, looseness, or any unusual reactions. If the patient is comfortable and can function with the implant, the index is rated as positive. If the patient relates pain, loss of function, or other complications, the implant is rated as negative.

Controls

An evaluation employing quantitative measurements such as these must be balanced by the assessment of controls. For endosteal implants, control teeth should be selected for evaluation. For implants that serve as abutments for fixed prostheses, controls should include a natural abutment tooth and an unrestored tooth, preferably in the same quadrant.

MINIMAL STANDARDS FOR CLINICAL SERVICEABILITY

All implantologists want to achieve longitudinal serviceability for the implants they place. As a judge of the potential continued service or failure of an implant, the evaluation tools detailed here will provide the clinician a guide to continued service and, when comparing previously recorded data, indicate potential problems or biological reactions that may predict potential failure.

One of the advantages to evaluating implants in terms of numeric values is that it allows both retrospective comparisons and determination of continued success of the implant. To judge an implant successful, or *serviceable,* a more correct term, we have developed a set of minimum standard values from our controlled clinical study experiences which we believe will provide the individual practitioner with a guide for qualitative service judgment. These minimum standards for the seven chairside-monitored implant indices are shown in Table 29–7. We have found good predictability with these values for the measurements taken.

TABLE 29–7.

Minimal Standards for Implant Clinical Serviceability*

Index	Accepted Index Standards
Gingival bleeding	1.0 or less, or if > 1 but <2, no greater a difference between implant and control than 0.5 unit
Gingival sulcular fluid volume	10 units or less (two-strip method) 5 units or less (one-strip method)
Gingival sulcus depth†	No minimum, but must not vary more than 3 mm between implant and control
Mobility	2.0 or less with cemented prosthesis; 1.0 or less if freestanding implant
Plaque and calculus	No minimum but must not vary more than 0.5 unit between implant and control
Radiographic bone	Two positive ratings
Patient comfort	Positive rating

*Overall clinical standards: To be rated as meeting minimal clinical standards the implant must achieve acceptable ratings in five of the seven measured indices.
†Index may be eliminated if design of implant precludes measuring or if in the judgment of the clinician measurement may have destructive potential to the biological seal.

We believe that the use of these standards allows an implant to be considered clinically functional (successful) if it meets the minimum standards in five of the seven categories (see Table 29–7).

Further, the use of numeric values for the standards also allows the measuring data to be statistically analyzed. How to carry out this process is covered in Chapter 37.

CONCLUSIONS

The ultimate goal of treatment with implants is to achieve an extended period of acceptable serviceability. To define this biological acceptability in terms of clinical practice, the clinician must be prepared to chart and measure this biological performance as defined in this chapter. This allows the implant to be cross-evaluated at recall against previously recorded data, and thus sound judgments can be made for the patient as to prognosis and future service. It has been the purpose of this chapter to detail the simple evaluation indices that should be standard procedure in every implant practice.

REFERENCES

1. James RA: Dental implants—moving into the mainstream. *J Calif Dent Assoc* 1984; 6:22–25.
2. James RA: The dental implant-tissue interface: Sales hype, hoopla and facts. *J Calif Dent Assoc* 1986; 14:57–61.
3. Schnitman PA, Schulman LB (eds): *Dental Implants: Benefit and Risk. An NIH-Harvard Consensus Development Conference.* Bethesda, Md, US Department of Health and Human Services Publication No (NIH) 81-1531, 1980.
4. National Institutes of Health: National Institutes of Health Consensus Development Statement: Dental implants. *J Am Dent Assoc* 1988; 117:509–513.
5. Association Reports: Expansion of the acceptance program for dental materials, instruments, and equipment: Endosseous implants. *J Am Dent Assoc* 1981; 102:350.
6. US Department of Health and Human Services, Food and Drug Administration: *Guidance for the Arrangement and Content of a Premarket Approval (PMA) Application for an Endosseous Implant for Prosthetic (Draft).* Silver Springs, Md, DHHS, Food and Drug Administration, September 1988.
7. McKinney RV Jr, Lemons JE (eds): *The Dental Implant: Clinical and Biological Response of Oral Tissues.* Littleton, Mass, PSG Publishing Co, 1985, pp 129–130.
8. Loe H, Silness J: Periodontal disease in pregnancy: I. Prevalence and serverity. *Acta Odontol Scand* 1963; 21:533–551.
9. Silness J, Loe H: Periodontal disease in pregnancy: II. Correlation between oral hygiene and periodontal condition. *Acta Odontol Scand* 1964; 22:121–135.
10. Recommendations, in Schnitman PA, Shulman LB (eds): *Dental Implants: Benefit and Risk: An NIH-Harvard Consensus Development Conference.* Bethesda, Md, US Department of Health and Human Services Publication No (NIH) 81-1531, 1980, pp 326–339.
11. Rudin HJ, Overdiek HF, Rateischak KH: Correlation between sulcus fluid rate and clinical and histological inflammation of the gingiva. *Helv Odontol Acta* 1970; 14:21–26.
12. Golub LM, Kleinberg I: Gingival crevicular fluid: A new diagnostic aid in managing the periodontal patient. *Oral Sci Rev* 1976; 8:49–61.
13. Garnick JJ, Pearson R, Harrell D: The evaluation of the Periotron. *J Periodontol* 1979; 50:424–426.
14. Ramfjord SP: Indices for prevalence and incidence of periodontal disease. *J Periodontol* 1959; 30–59.
15. Wasserman BH, Geiger AM, Turgeon LR: Relationship of occlusion and periodontal disease: VII. Mobility. *J Periodontol* 1973; 44:572–578.

Chapter 30

Prosthetic Laboratory Relationships for Endosteal Implants

Gregory R. Parr, D.D.S.
L. Kirk Gardner, D.D.S.

In the 1990s implant dentistry is an exciting place to be, both for the dentist and for the dental laboratory. It can easily be said that it is impossible for the dentist to do excellent implant dentistry without the association of an excellent dental laboratory. Unfortunately, two trends which have their roots in dental educational decisions made years ago have come back to haunt implant dentistry. These are:

1. Dental schools have been increasing the curricular emphasis on the basic sciences and the medical and behavioral aspects of dental care to the detriment of the laboratory aspects of prosthodontic restorations. Prosthodontists have complained about this direction in dental education for years, with little effect. The result, however, is that a graduating dentist knows little about the technical and laboratory procedures involved in routine prosthodontics, not to speak of the more sophisticated procedures for dental implants. His or her ability to coordinate complex laboratory sequences and to supervise the sophisticated technical aspects of implant dentistry is severely compromised.

2. The second trend is for the dentist, pressured by economics and the dictates of practice management, to delegate to trained auxiliary personnel all procedures which he or she does not legally need to perform. While this in and of itself is not necessarily bad, it may lead the inexperienced practitioner to neglect some important and required aspects of his laboratory obligations and to delegate them to the laboratory technician. The technician, not wishing to alienate his dentist-supplier, does the best he can with the information given to him. The result is often a marginally successful or an outright unsuccessful case. I emphasize the words "trained auxiliary personnel" and discuss this aspect of the training and education of the laboratory technician later.

The partnership between the implant dentist and the dental laboratory is one of shared responsibilities and mutual understanding. It evolves from a degree of interdependence which must be based on trust, respect, and, above all, communication if a high-quality final product is to be produced. Indeed, the dentist is utterly dependent upon the integrity and competence of the laboratory. It should always be remembered that the technician produces that part of the restoration which the patient is most interested in and that the dental laboratory can make the dentist look very good or very, very bad!

This chapter discusses the various aspects of this relationship from the point of view of the dental implantologist and dental laboratory technician with the goal of improving the understanding and communication involved in this necessary partnership.

THE DIAGNOSTIC WAX-UP

In the development of the treatment plan by the dentist and the work plan by the dental laboratory it is often good to begin with a visualization of the end product and to work backward from that point. This is accomplished via a diagnostic mounting of the patient's models and a diagnostic wax-up of the final case. In most prosthetic training programs this diagnostic wax-up is done by the dentist. In practice, however, this time-consuming procedure, if it is done at all, is often delegated to the laboratory technician. This will accomplish its aim if the technician and dentist communicate closely during the procedure to ensure that both understand what the final product and the limiting factors will be. By using this procedure the technician will become involved in the case at a much earlier point and the dentist and technician will be taking advantage of both right- and left-brained forms of communication.[1] The essentials of this procedure are:

1. The diagnostic casts are usually mounted in the centric relation position for the purposes of occlusal analysis and mock occlusal equilibration. Partially edentulous implant patients often present with extruded, tilted, rotated, and otherwise malpositioned teeth which are not recognized until this point. Neglecting these aspects of the treatment plan may lead to implant failure due to improper implant loading.

2. The location and orientation of the occlusal plane must be considered. It is desirable to generate occlusal curves that are as shallow as possible so that the destabilizing forces introduced by steeper curves are controlled and limited. The use of an occlusal template, as advocated by Heartwell and Rahn,[2] is a rapid and simple method to accomplish this end. The amount of tooth reduction needed and the necessity of periodontic procedures for crown lengthening, endodontic procedures due to projected pulp exposures, and restorative procedures to restore occlusal morphology will be disclosed. Properly selected denture teeth can be set on trial denture bases in the edentulous areas and, if desired, tried in the mouth. At this time the dentist will begin to visualize the end point of his final occlusal scheme.

3. The esthetics and arrangement of the anterior teeth should be considered. These are often the prime considerations for the patient and should be held in high regard by the dentist and laboratory, but not to the neglect of other important mechanical factors.

4. The incisal guidance and control of excursive movements are important also for the control of esthetics and mechanics. Perhaps the patient's esthetic desires are not compatible with the occlusal scheme that will provide the best mechanical loading of the implants. If this is the case, modifications can be made and discussed with the patient to reach a compromise that will satisfy esthetic considerations and promote denture stability.

5. Alternative treatment plans can be developed at this time for use in case of implant failure.

The importance and usefulness of the diagnostic wax-up procedure does not end with the completion of this exercise. Rather, it serves as the point of departure for the laboratory and the dentist. The laboratory, having the end point visualized, can estimate the time involved in the completion of the case and the subsequent cost to the dentist. The dentist can use the diagnostic wax-up for several procedures:

1. The dentist can place round metal shot in the wax-up in areas where he or she wishes to locate the implants.[3] Radiographs taken of the patient with the diagnostic wax-up in place orally will enable the dentist to estimate the magnification of the radiographs, locate the implants mesiodistally, and determine with greater accuracy the length of the implants to be placed and their relationship to the occlusal units or to important limiting anatomic structures. A suitable measuring device can be used to measure the buccolingual width of the ridge in the area of potential implantation and combined with probing of oral tissue depths to roughly define the width of bone available in the area under consideration.

2. With the above information, the dentist can design a surgical template that will aid the surgeon in locating the implants where they will provide the most mechanical, esthetic, and functional advantage.

3. Temporary and provisional restorations can be designed and fabricated so that esthetic or func-

tional problems can be worked out well before the implants are placed.

4. The plan of treatment can now be completed, including the often neglected laboratory steps. The generation of this protocol to control and coordinate both the clinical and the laboratory phases of the patient's implant care will aid the dentist in breaking down the complexities of the case into smaller units and to formulate the written instructions and information that will be supplied to the technician. It will also allow the dentist to determine the points at which the technician's procedures are checked for quality control purposes.

These diagnostic procedures have been a part of many prosthodontic teaching programs for years. They have been a valuable teaching tool. With both the age of the average prosthodontic patient and the complexity of his care increasing, the need for the development of a protocol that integrates the laboratory steps into the dental treatment plan has moved out of the ivory tower and has become a necessity for the practitioner. The procedure will aid the practitioner in controlling the complexity of the case to keep it within his capabilities and those of the dental laboratory he works with.

THE DENTIST'S OBLIGATIONS

With the end point of the case visualized and the treatment protocol in mind the dentist can sequence the patient's care and begin the treatment with his obligations well in view.

The patient should be free of dental disease and dedicated to excellent oral hygiene before the implant procedure is begun. Good preparations must be accomplished allowing for parallelism of abutments and implants with good occlusal and facial clearance and a balanced occlusal plane. Full-arch master casts should be made and mounted on an articulator selected to meet the complexity of the final restoration. The articulator should be properly adjusted and a custom incisal guide table provided when appropriate. Stable dies, fully seated into the master cast, with margins properly trimmed, marked, and protected, should be provided. Instructions should be

given for the thickness of relief desired under the final casting as well as the metal to be used. As a general rule, it is best to avoid the use of base metals over titanium dental implants. Although titanium is a metal that can be coupled (placed in contact) with other metals without fear of corrosion,[4] more reactive metals may be caused to corrode at the marginal areas leading to peri-implant problems. Such a reaction could lead to a long-term implant failure and might bring both the dentist and the laboratory into legal confrontation. Type IV dental gold is an excellent choice for this application.

The type of occlusal anatomy and eccentric excursive controls have already been visualized with the diagnostic wax-up, making the written work authorization less complicated. The frequent use of the telephone to review and reinforce what has been written is a valuable adjunct. We prefer to generate the functional occlusal units, especially in nonesthetic areas, in metal rather than porcelain. There are several reasons for this:

1. Less occlusal reduction is necessary with metal occlusals, which makes the procedure kinder to the abutment teeth. It is certainly desirable to avoid additional complications (in an already lengthy and complicated treatment plan) from teeth injured by additional reduction for occlusal porcelain.

2. Porcelain occlusals, in most dental laboratories and dental offices, are generated by firing, grinding, and glazing. While this procedure can be used effectively, a greater degree of accuracy can be accomplished with hand-waxed metal occlusal surfaces.

3. Abrasion of opposing dental units, if the porcelain occlusal surface looses its glaze, is a real long-term problem which is best avoided by providing metal occlusal surfaces.

This is not to say that fixed units with porcelain occlusals may not be the restoration of choice in selected cases where esthetic demands are severe.

The shape and form of the esthetic units have also been visualized and discussed. Any modifications desired by the patient following his experience with the provisional restorations should be made known to the technician, preferably with the use of models as well as written instructions that leave no room for misinterpretation. The dentist needs to supply the shade of the porcelain veneer. It is not appropriate for the dentist to place this responsibility on the laboratory as this, once again, could later become a matter of legal contention.

Previously agreed-upon checkpoints should be observed. The difficulty of doing this with an offsite laboratory is well recognized. The necessity, especially in the early stages of the technical procedures, should also be recognized. Checks should be made on the articulator as well as in the patient's mouth. Magnification and good lighting are important. Notation of the check procedures accomplished should be made in the patient's chart for legal purposes to establish the standard of care.

THE DENTAL LABORATORY'S OBLIGATIONS

By incorporating the diagnostic wax-up into the implant procedure the dental technician's responsibilities no longer begin and end with the articulated dies supplied by the dentist. The technician instead is involved much earlier in the procedure and can much more easily visualize the desired end product. This makes the technician's job of understanding the written work authorization much easier. It does not make the job of following it any easier. Few dentists appreciate the true complexities of the dental laboratory industry and the burden of knowledge, experience, and integrity which the reputable full-service dental laboratory carries.

Naturally, the laboratory has the obligation to handle all models, dies, and other diagnostic adjuncts with the utmost care. A thorough knowledge of the articulator used and the design of the substructure, including the occlusal and axial surfaces, is mandatory. Knowledge of the biological implications of pontic form and margin design is essential. An applied knowledge of dental materials, especially as to how they relate to the implant and the metal used for the reconstruction, can have important long-term effects.

Lastly, and not of least importance, the laboratory must be well versed with the implant system being used. Laboratory staff should have a thorough knowledge of the components of the implant system which have been designed to make the manufacturing procedure more accurate and cost-effective. Laboratory analogs, plastic waxing sleeves, prefabricated copings, and a myriad of other components are available for many systems. Multiply these by the 28 or more endosseous implant systems available on the US market today and you have but a small estimate of the knowledge required by the laboratory staff which the dentist has selected to provide this service.

THE WRITTEN WORK AUTHORIZATION

In times past the written work authorization was the only form of communication between the dentist and the laboratory technician. It is still a valuable form of communication and is adequate for uncomplicated prosthodontic cases. It also remains the accepted legal form of communication. Two copies of the laboratory work authorization should be made, one retained by the dentist for legal purposes and for reference when conferring with the laboratory by telephone. The written work authorization takes advantage of the left side of the dentist's and technician's brain. This side of the brain processes information which deals with the linguistic and organizational aspects of dentistry. Although not yet proven, one might expect dentists to be more left-brained in their thought, organization, and communication.

The written work authorization should no longer be the only form of communication. Diagrams, photographs and diagnostic models, of the type described earlier, take advantage of the right-sided aspects of the brain. This side deals with creative, artistic, and spatial information. One might expect this to be more the domain of the technician, although many of the more creative and imaginative dentists undoubtedly have also been right-brained.

By taking advantage of both of these aspects of communication and information processing, the dentist and technician can together achieve the best possible result.

DENTAL LABORATORY EDUCATION

There are four routes that laboratory technicians take during their training.

1. By far the largest number of dental laboratory technicians are trained by the apprentice method. They begin their careers performing simple and relatively unimportant tasks in the laboratory and gradually build their expertise to include more complicated and more important procedures. They supplement this training with short continuing education courses which are mostly presented by the manufacturers and suppliers of the products that the technicians use. The dentist should be aware that although he may have done a few of the laboratory procedures he will be using, the technician has done hundreds of the procedures and can easily be called the more expert partner in the laboratory relationship.

2. Many laboratory technicians are graduates of dental laboratory technology training programs in schools or colleges. They usually receive an associate's degree in dental technology. All of these programs have varying requirements, curricula, and length of study. Few include implants.

3. The armed forces provide dental laboratory technicians with a program in the basic sciences followed by applied dental technology. After this training the technician is assigned to a dental laboratory unit and increases his or her knowledge with on-the-job experience as well as short refresher and update courses.

4. The last avenue for training, and the one taken by the fewest people, is the technician who is trained by the dentist in an in-house dental laboratory.

The training and experience of the individual laboratory technician is highly variable. The American Dental Association recognizes the education and qualifications of the dental laboratory technician with its certification program. To date, however, little material on dental implants is part of the certification examination. There is little state or national regulation of the dental laboratory trade. The progress made by the industry in the past is probably in large part owing to this lack of regulation. It remains, however, that it is difficult for the dentist to decide upon a laboratory and the dentist would be well advised to know the laboratory well before he sends implant cases to it for service. It is in this light that the earlier admonition concerning "trained auxiliary personnel" should be considered. The dentist has the ultimate responsibility for the final result. He can delegate nonbiological aspects of the case to people he believes are competent to handle them, but in the end he is the judge of their competence. If the dentist himself is not well versed in the laboratory procedures in question, how can he judge the competence of the laboratory?

CONCLUSION

The dental laboratory industry manufactures its products with technology that is very crude when compared to the sophisticated techniques used elsewhere in manufacturing. In spite of this burden, beautiful and functional restorations are produced on a daily basis which serve our patients for many years. The dental implant industry is developing at a rapid rate, making it critically important for both dentists and dental laboratory technicians to participate actively in available educational activities. The dentist should encourage his dental societies and organizations to take a more active part in this educational process and to make courses available to the dental laboratory technician at an affordable price and convenient location.

REFERENCES

1. Edwards B: *Drawing on the Right Side of the Brain.* Los Angeles, JP Tarcher, Inc, 1979.
2. Heartwell CM, Rahn AO: *Syllabus of Complete Dentures.* ed 4. Philadelphia, Lea & Febiger, 1986.
3. Engelman MJ, Sorensen JA, Moy P: Optimum placement of osseointegrated implants. *J Prosthet Dent* 1988; 59:467–473.
4. Parr G, Gardner LK, Toth RW: Titanium: The mystery metal of implant dentistry. *J Prosthet Dent* 1985; 54:410–413.

Chapter 31

Oral Hygiene Protocol for Implant Patients

Philip J. Hanes, D.D.S., M.S.
W. Gregory Long, D.M.D., M.S.

The short-term success of the endosseous dental implant has been made possible by the implantologist's incorporation of surgical techniques that do not cause irreparable tissue damage[1] and by the use of implant materials and devices that possess optimal biomechanical and chemical properties.[2-5] Their long-term success, however, will most likely be patient-dependent, reflecting the patient's ability and willingness to control etiologic factors responsible for the onset and progression of "peri-implantitis." The purpose of this chapter is to present a plausible model for the pathogenesis of "peri-implantitis," to discuss the role of dental plaque in this regard, and to describe the armamentarium and techniques that patients may use to control the accumulation of bacterial deposits on implant fixtures and prostheses. In addition, recommendations are made for the dentist and the dental hygienist regarding the instrumentation of the implant for the purpose of plaque and calculus removal, and the characteristics of a maintenance program designed for the dental implant patient.

THE PATHOGENESIS OF "PERI-IMPLANTITIS"

As described in Chapter 9, fundamental differences exist between the natural tooth and a dental implant with respect to their relationship to the supporting tissues. For example, connective tissue fiber attachment does not occur to the dental implant as it does to cementum on the root of a tooth. Instead, suprabony connective tissue fibers are oriented parallel to the implant surface[6, 7] (Fig 31–1). In addition, supporting bone can be directly apposed against the implant.[4, 8, 9] These anatomic differences seem to correspond with differences in functional characteristics. In regard to their relationship with the epithelium, there appears to be a "biological seal" between the dental implant and the epithelium which is similar in structure[3, 10, 11] and function[12] to the junctional epithelium of the natural tooth. The relative resistance of these two anatomic systems to breakdown, however, is unclear.

The primary etiologic factor associated with the onset and progression of periodontal disease is bacterial plaque.[13] Bacterial and chemical components are present in dental plaque (for a review, see Socransky[14]) which have the ability to initiate the periodontal inflammatory lesion by inducing changes in the junctional epithelium[15, 16] and by providing the chemotactic stimulus for various inflammatory cells.[17-19] A direct relationship between the accumulation of dental plaque and the onset and progression of gingivitis has been well established.[13, 20-22] Hence, the periodontal inflammatory lesion has been termed a "plaque-induced" lesion.

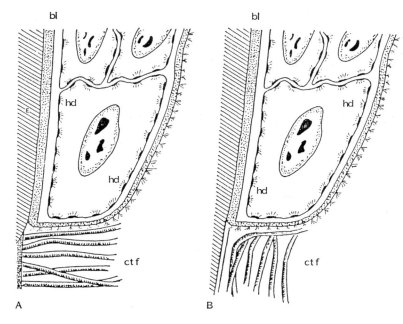

FIG 31–1.
A diagrammatic comparison of the relationship between the supporting tissues and a natural tooth **(A)** or a dental implant **(B)**. Cells of the junctional epithelium form a biological seal to both the natural tooth and the dental implant, which is maintained by an attachment apparatus consisting of a basal lamina *(bl)* between the epithelial cell and the tooth or implant, and intracellular hemidesmosomes *(hd)*. Apical to the junctional epithelium, connective tissue fibers *(ctf)* are oriented perpendicular to the root of a natural tooth, and insert into cementum on the root surface. Fibers adjacent to the dental implant, however, are oriented parallel to the surface and do not attach to the implant.

Although a direct relationship between the accumulation of bacterial deposits at the gingival margin and the development of "peri-implant gingivitis" has not been established, inflammatory, peri-implant disease is also assumed to be plaque-induced. This assumption is based on three factors:

1. A biological seal, similar in structure to the junctional epithelium, has been described in association with titanium,[3, 10] vitreous carbon,[23, 24] single-crystal sapphire,[11] and apatite[25] implant surfaces. The similarity of this biological seal to the normal junctional epithelium suggests that it, too, would function to prevent the apical migration and penetration of bacterial plaque into the subjacent connective tissue.

2. Samples of bacterial plaque collected from the surface of dental implants are similar in content to those sampled from natural teeth,[26–28] suggesting similar pathogenic characteristics or virulence.

3. Following professional removal of plaque deposits and the initiation of an effective daily oral hygiene regimen, patients with peri-implant gingivitis can regain the health of their gingival tissue.

If one assumes that "peri-implantitis" is indeed a plaque-induced inflammatory disease, the pathogenesis of the disease will be similar to that described for the periodontal lesion (Fig 31–2). The prevention or control of "peri-implantitis" would therefore be dependent upon the successful control of plaque accumulation at the gingival margin.

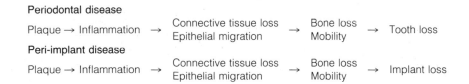

FIG 31–2.
The pathogenesis of peri-implant disease is similar to that described for periodontal disease, with the onset and progression of the disease associated with plaque accumulation at and below the gingival margin.

PLAQUE REGULATION BY THE PATIENT

In order to be successful, special plaque control programs must be designed for each patient in order to meet his or her specific needs. The criteria for success require flexibility and imagination on the part of the therapist in devising, prescribing, and instructing patients in methods of plaque regulation that are designed for the effective removal of plaque—given the patient's intraoral anatomy and prosthesis design, manual dexterity, and degree of motivation. In this section we describe the various instruments that can be prescribed for the daily removal of plaque deposits from the surface of dental implants, and the recommended use of these devices. This list is not intended to be all-inclusive, as other devices of similar design can often be substituted with good results. Furthermore, this list should not be interpreted as a complete oral hygiene prescription for each implant patient. In most cases, the oral hygiene program for a particular patient can be limited to three or four instruments, or even fewer. In each case, the protocol should be kept as simple as possible, because more complex requirements usually result in poor compliance.

The Plaque Control Program for the Dental Implant Patient

The effectiveness of a patient's self-performed plaque control program is dependent upon three factors:

1. The patient must be motivated to comply with all aspects of the plaque control program.
2. The patient must be instructed in the proper use of all prescribed plaque control devices, until proficient in their use.
3. The plaque control instrument prescribed for a patient must be appropriate for his or her specific anatomic characteristics.

The patient's willingness to comply with treatment recommendations, including a prescribed plaque control regimen, should be carefully evaluated before dental implants are considered as a treatment option. A patient's unwillingness to recognize and accept responsibility for daily, effective oral hygiene practices will put the long-term health of the tissues supporting the implant at risk, and makes that patient a poor candidate for a dental implant. On the other hand, once a patient has demonstrated a willingness to participate in and comply with treatment recommendations, it is the responsibility of the practitioner to devise a plaque control program using an armamentarium that is effective for that patient, and to instruct the patient in the proper implementation of that program.

Armamentarium and Application

The plaque control regimen designed for the dental implant patient should allow the patient to routinely remove plaque deposits from the facial, lingual, and interproximal surfaces of the implant fixture, as well as from the undersurface or mucosal surface of the implant-supported prosthesis.

Facial Surfaces.—The facial surfaces of the dental implant and the implant-supported prosthesis can often be effectively cleaned by using a toothbrush with soft, end-rounded nylon bristles no more than 10 mm in length. The best results are obtained with a small-head toothbrush with the table of bristle tufts no more than 25 mm in length. Brushes with three rows of bristle tufts are generally more effective than four-row brushes due to their better adaptation to the limited amount of space between the base of the prosthesis and the soft tissue (Fig 31–3). The total width of the brush table should be approximately 6 mm (Fig 31–4). In some instances, the space between the base of the prosthesis and the soft tissue is severely limited and will not accommodate a conventional three-row brush as described above. In these cases, an alternative approach is the use of a single-tufted brush with either a flat or point-trimmed tuft of bristles (Fig 31–5).

Lingual Surfaces.—The lingual surfaces of the dental implant fixtures and the implant-supported prosthesis are often quite difficult for patients to maintain plaque-free, owing to the bulk of the prosthesis and to interference from the mobile, soft tissue

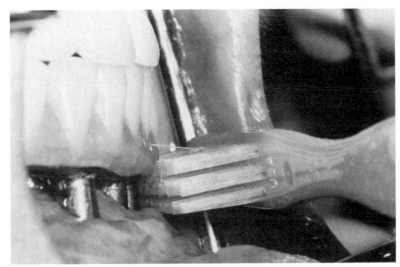

FIG 31–3.
The selection of a proper toothbrush for the patient with an implant-supported dental prosthesis should take into consideration the distance between the base of the prosthesis and the soft tissue. In most cases, brushes with three or fewer rows of bristles are most easily adapted on the facial surfaces.

in the floor of the mouth. Most patients are effective in their efforts, however, with the use of a single-tufted brush (Fig 31–6). In some instances, patients are unable to easily adapt this brush to the lingual surfaces owing to the straight configuration of the handle. In these cases, the brush can be modified by warming the handle over a flame or in hot water and then bending the handle below the brush to create an angle of approximately 135 degrees (see Fig 31–5).

Interproximal Surfaces.—The choice of a suitable instrument for the patient to use for the removal of plaque deposits from the interproximal surfaces

of the dental implant abutment is determined by the space available between the adjacent implant abutments and the natural teeth, as well as the distance from the base of the dental prosthesis to the soft tissue margin. When space allows, the most effective instrument for most patients is the interdental brush[29, 30] (Fig 31–7). These brushes are available in a variety of sizes and shapes ranging from approximately 3 to 6 mm in diameter. They are available on short, straight handles, or can be attached to longer handles which position the brushes at angles

FIG 31–4.
Recommended maximum dimensions of a toothbrush for the patient with an implant-supported dental prosthesis. If the distance from the base of the prosthesis to the soft tissue is severely limited, a brush of smaller size may be indicated.

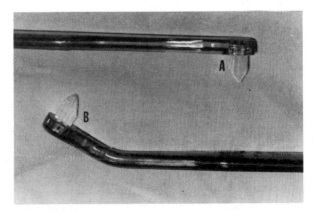

FIG 31–5.
The taper-cut, end tuft brush **(A).** These brushes are suitable for use on facial surfaces when the distance between the prosthesis and the soft tissue is limited, and on lingual surfaces. On the lingual surface, access can be facilitated by bending the handle as shown in **B.**

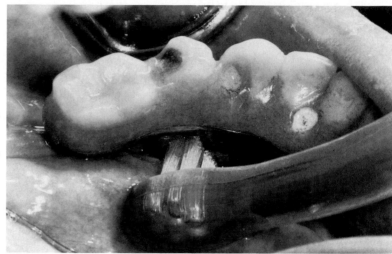

FIG 31–6.
The lingual surfaces of dental implant abutments can often be cleaned with a taper-cut end tuft brush. Access in this area can be improved by bending the handle of the brush as shown in Figure 31–5.

suitable for use in the posterior segments of the mouth (Fig 31–8).

Most interdental brushes are available with a plastic or polymer-coated wire core. These coated wire cores are better suited for use in patients with dental implants because they are less likely to scratch the metal surface of the implant or to cause a dissimilar-metal galvanic-type corrosion of the implant fixture (Fig 31–9).

In selecting the proper size of interdental brush, the brush that fills the interproximal space with moderate compression of the bristles will be the most effective. The brush should not be loose in the inter-proximal space, nor should it be so tight as to cause the patient discomfort when inserting it into the space. When possible, these brushes should be used from both facial and lingual approaches.

If adequate space is not available, alternatives to the interdental brush are various flosslike devices (Fig 31–10). The use of floss will usually require a threading device to allow the insertion of the floss under the prosthesis. A more convenient alternative to floss threaders, however, are devices such as Superfloss and Post-Care, which have a threading device incorporated into the floss (Fig 31–11).

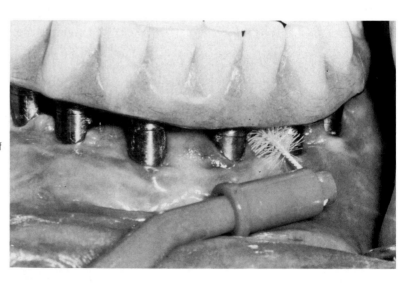

FIG 31–7.
Interproximal surfaces of dental implant abutments, as well as the tissue surface of the prosthesis, can often be cleaned with an interdental brush.

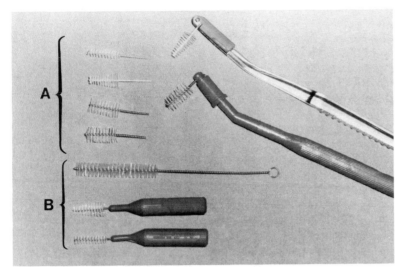

FIG 31–8.
Assorted interdental brushes. The longer handles with separate brush attachments **(A)** are necessary for use in the molar areas. Anterior to the second premolar region, the straight handle brushes **(B)** can be used.

The Mucosal Surface of the Prosthesis.—The removal of plaque from the mucosal or undersurface of the implant-supported prosthesis can often be accomplished with the interdental brushes as described above (see Fig 31–7). Other approaches are necessary, however, when minimal space is present between the prosthesis and the soft tissue margin. In this case, dental tape, Post-Care, Superfloss, gauze strips, or 0.25-in.-wide twill tape can be used[29, 30] (see Fig 31–11). The twill tape can be obtained from most fabric stores. The wider gauze strips or twill tape is the most effective of these alternatives, if the space permits their use (Fig 31–12).

Insertion of these materials under the prosthesis requires a threading device, and can usually be accomplished with a conventional floss threader. The exceptions to this, mentioned above, are Post-Care and Superfloss which have a stiff, threading end incorporated into the floss (see Fig 31–11). Inserting these materials under cantilevered extensions of the prosthesis can often be accomplished without the floss threader, however, by passing the floss or tape over and distal to the prosthesis, placing it in contact with the soft tissue, and then pulling the floss in an anterior direction passing under the prosthesis (see Fig 31–12). Patients should be instructed to use the floss or tape with a shoeshining motion moving in a buccolingual direction (Fig 31–13).

Instructing Patients in the Use of Plaque Control Devices

Equally important to the selection of appropriate instruments for a patient's plaque control regimen is thorough instruction in the use of these instruments. Merely dispensing a toothbrush and a spool of dental floss will rarely result in the effective use of these devices. Adequate instruction is necessary to facilitate effectiveness. In addition, the practitioner's willingness to devote office time to these instructions emphasizes the importance of the plaque control program to the patient and can reinforce compliance.

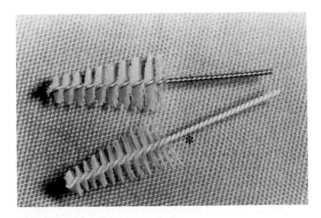

FIG 31–9.
Interdental brushes with a plastic or polymer-coated wire *(asterisk)* are best suited for removing plaque from the surface of a dental implant abutment. These coated wires are less likely to scratch the implant surface or to cause a dissimilar metal galvanic corrosion of the implant material.

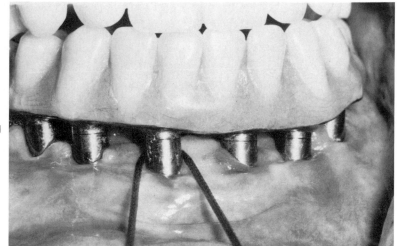

FIG 31–10.
Interproximal surfaces of the dental implant abutment can also be cleaned with flosslike devices.

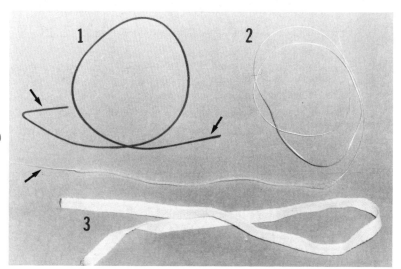

FIG 31–11.
Flosslike devices for dental plaque removal. Post-Care *(1)* and Superfloss *(2)* both have stiff, threading devices *(arrows)* incorporated into the ends of the floss. Twill tape *(3)*, 0.25 in. wide, can be obtained from most fabric stores.

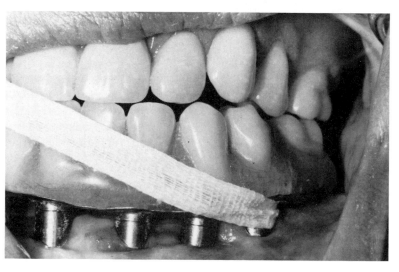

FIG 31–12.
Twill tape removes plaque effectively from the distal surface of a terminal abutment, and from the mucosal surface of the prosthesis.

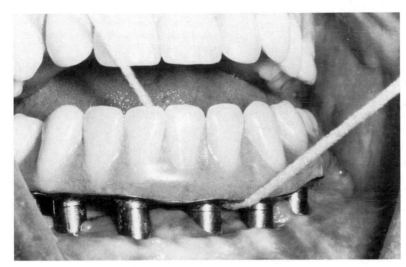

FIG 31–13.
Superfloss is useful for the removal of plaque from the mucosal surface of the prosthesis. A buccolingual, shoeshining motion is used with the floss.

Plaque control instructions should take place in a location that allows both practitioner instruction and patient demonstration. This usually requires either a hanging mirror over a sink, or a freestanding mirror on a bracket tray at the dental chair. Instruction should begin with the practitioner demonstrating the proper use of the instrument in the patient's mouth, followed by the patient demonstrating what he or she has been shown. This allows an evaluation of both the patient's understanding of the technique and instructions as well as his or her manual dexterity. A patient should be allowed to become proficient with one instrument before adding supplemental instruments to the plaque control program. If the patient has difficulty with the first instrument prescribed, other instruments may be added later, after a few days of practice has made the patient comfortable with the first device. Re-evaluation of a patient's plaque control practices should be made at frequent intervals until a consistent, effective level of plaque control is maintained.

Topical Antimicrobial Agents

Topical antimicrobial agents are intended for use as adjuncts to mechanical plaque removal, not as substitutes.[31] These agents, therefore, should be reserved for those patients for whom mechanical plaque removal has been ineffective. Although a number of so-called antiplaque rinses and dentifrices are marketed, only two have been able to show long-term clinical effectiveness in controlling plaque and gingivitis. These two agents are (1) 0.12% chlorhexidene gluconate (Peridex) and (2) a phenolic compound (Listerine).

Peridex is used as a 30-second rinse, twice a day, following routine mechanical plaque control procedures. Peridex has been reported to be very effective in long-term studies, reducing plaque by 55% and gingivitis by 45%.[32–34] The disadvantages of this agent include the cost, the requirement of a prescription, and side effects such as taste alterations and unsightly staining.

Listerine is available over the counter. It, too, is used in conjunction with normal plaque control practices as a twice-daily rinse. Listerine has also been shown to be effective in long-term clinical trials, reducing plaque by 25% and gingivitis by 29%.[35–37] Although reportedly less effective than Peridex in controlling plaque, it is not accompanied by the untoward side effects associated with Peridex.

REMOVING CALCULUS FROM DENTAL IMPLANT SURFACES

The maintenance care required for dental implant patients will include techniques of scaling and polishing to remove deposits of plaque, stain, and calculus. When employing these techniques, consideration must be given to the effects that such procedures may have on the chemical and surface characteristics of the dental implant. It has become apparent that instrumentation of titanium implant fixtures with ultrasonic scalers, air abrasive polishing devices, or metal instruments can scratch the metal surface[38, 39] perhaps making it more plaque-retentive. In addition, instrumentation of metallic implant surfaces with an instrument fabricated from a dissimilar metal may result in a galvanic-type corrosion of the implant surface.[40-42] For these reasons, it has been suggested that instrumentation of dental implant fixtures be accomplished with nonmetal instruments, Teflon-coated instruments, or instruments fabricated from a metal identical to that of the implant fixture.[29] The most readily available of these alternatives are the nonmetal scalers.

The effects of various polishing agents on the chemical and surface characteristics of the dental implant are not, as yet, fully recognized. Clinically, it is apparent that even the finest grade of prophylaxis paste can produce a visible alteration in the surface of a titanium fixture. The significance of this change, however, is unclear.

MAINTENANCE CARE FOR THE DENTAL IMPLANT PATIENT

Long-term clinical studies of treated periodontal patients have shown that reinforcement of plaque control practices and the professional removal of plaque and calculus deposits at regular 3-month intervals can prevent the further loss of periodontal attachment in most patients.[43-46] Although similar data are not available for dental implant patients, these studies of treated periodontal patients form the basis of most maintenance care programs designed for dental implant patients.

Based on these studies, it is generally agreed that patients with dental implants should be provided maintenance care at 3-month intervals. Each maintenance care appointment should include the following components:

1. The health of the peri-implant tissue should be evaluated using the criteria discussed in Chapters 3 and 30.

2. The patient's oral hygiene practices should be evaluated and reinstruction provided, as necessary.
3. All plaque and calculus deposits should be removed by scaling and polishing.
4. Restorative and prosthetic dental treatment should be reevaluated.

REFERENCES

1. Eriksson RA, Albrektsson T: The effect of heat on bone regeneration. *J Oral Maxillofac Surg* 1984; 42:701–711.
2. Klawitter JJ, Weinstein AM, Cooke FW: An evaluation of porous alumina ceramic implants. *J Dent Res* 1977; 56:768–775.
3. Schroeder A, Van Der Zypen E, Stich H: The reactions of bone, connective tissue, and epithelium to endosteal implants with titanium-sprayed surfaces. *J Oral Maxillofac Surg* 1981; 9:15–25.
4. Albrektsson T, Hansson HA, Ivarsson B: A comparative study of the interface zone between bone and various implant materials. *Trans Second World Congr Biomater* 1984; 7:84.
5. De Porter DA, Friedland B, Watson PA, et al: A clinical and radiographic assessment of a porous-surfaced, titanium alloy dental implant system in dogs. *J Dent Res* 1986; 65:1071–1077.
6. de Lange GL, de Putter C, de Groot K: Perimucosal dental implants: The relationship between sealing and fixation, in *Proceedings of the International Congress on Tissue Integration in Oral and Maxillofacial Reconstruction.* Brussels, Excerpta Medica, *Current Practice Series No 29,* 1985, pp 278–287.
7. Weiss CM: A comparative analysis of fibro-osteal and osteal integration and other variables that affect long-term bone maintenance around dental implants. *J Oral Implantol* 1987; 13:467–487.
8. Brånemark PI, Zarb G, Albrektsson T: *Tissue Integrated Prostheses: Osseointegration in Clinical Dentistry.* Chicago, Quintessence Publishing Co, Inc, 1985.
9. de Putter C, de Lange GL, de Groot K: Perimucosal dental implants of dense hydroxylapatite: Fixation in alveolar bone, in *Proceedings of the International Congress on Tissue Integration in Oral and Maxillofacial Reconstruction.* Brussels, Excerpta Medica, *Current Practice Series No 29,* 1985. pp 389–394.
10. Gould TR, Brunette DM, Westbury L: The attachment mechanism of epithelial cells to titanium *in vitro. J Periodont Res* 1981; 16:611–616.

11. McKinney RV, Steflik DE, Koth DL: Evidence for a junctional epithelial attachment to ceramic dental implants: A transmission electron microscopic study. *J Periodontol* 1985; 56:579–591.

12. James RA: Tissue response to dental implant devices, in Hardin JF (ed): *Clark's Clinical Dentistry,* vol 5. Philadelphia, JB Lippincott Co, 1990, chap 48.

13. Loe H, Theilade E, Jensen SB: Experimental gingivitis in man. *J Periodontol* 1965; 36:177–187.

14. Socransky SS: Relationship of bacteria to the etiology of periodontal disease. *J Dent Res* 1970; 49(suppl 2):203–222.

15. Thilander H: Epithelial changes in gingivitis—An electron microscopic study. *J Periodont Res* 1968; 3:303–312.

16. Freedman HL, Listgarten MA, Taichman NS: Electron microscopic features of chronically inflamed human gingiva. *J Periodont Res* 1968; 3: 313–327.

17. Jensen S, Theilade E, Jensen J: Influence of oral bacterial endotoxin on cell migration and phagocytic activity. *J Periodont Res* 1966; 1:129–140.

18. Baboolal R, Powell R: The effect of oral microbial endotoxins on rabbit leukocyte migration and phagocytosis, in Eastoe J, Picton D, Alexander A (eds): *The Prevention of Periodontal Disease.* London, Kimpton, 1971, pp 123–310.

19. Daly CG, Seymour GJ, Kieser JB: Bacterial endotoxin: A role in chronic inflammatory periodontal disease? *J Oral Pathol* 1980; 9:1–15.

20. Theilade E, Wright WH, Jensen SB, et al: Experimental gingivitis in man II. A longitudinal clinical and bacteriological investigation. *J Periodont Res* 1966; 1:1–13.

21. Loe H, Theilade E, Jensen SB, et al: Experimental gingivitis in man III. The influence of antibiotics on gingival plaque development. *J Periodont Res* 1967; 2:282–289.

22. Jensen SB, Loe H, Schiott CR, et al: Experimental gingivitis in man IV. Vancomycin induced changes in bacterial plaque composition as related to development of gingival inflammation. *J Periodont Res* 1968; 3:284–293.

23. Stallard RE, El Geneidy AK, Skerman HJ: Current research findings on the vitreous carbon tooth root replacement system. *Dtsch Zahnartzl Z* 1974; 29:746–748.

24. Skerman JH, El Geneidy AK, Stallard RE: Periodontal implications of the surface characteristics of dental implants in the area of the gingival junction. *J Periodontol* 1974; 45:731–738.

25. Jansen JA: Ultrastructural study of epithelial cell attachment to implant materials. *J Dent Res* 1985; 65:5.

26. Lekholm I, Ericsson R, Adell R: The condition of the soft tissues at tooth and fixture abutments supporting fixed bridges. A microbiological study. *J Clin Periodontol* 1986; 13:558–562.

27. Holt SR, Newman MG, Kratochvil F: The clinical and microbial characterization of peri-implant environment. *J Dent Res* 1986; 65(special issue): abstract No 703.

28. Sanz M, Newman MG, Holt SR: Microbiota associated with "sapphire" implants in partially edentulous patients. *J Dent Res* 1986; 65(special issue): abstract No 404.

29. Kraut R, Kuhar K, Shernoff A: Hydroxyapatite-coated dental implants used for the treatment of edentulous ridges. *Compend Cont Dent Educ* 1988; 9:405.

30. Balshi TJ: Hygiene maintenance procedures for patients treated with the tissue integrated prosthesis (osseointegration). *Quintessence Int* 1986; 17:95–102.

31. Ciancio SG: Use of mouth rinses for professional indications. *J Clin Periodontol* 1988; 15:520–523.

32. Bay LM: Effect of tooth brushing with different concentrations of chlorhexidene on the development of dental plaque and gingivitis. *J Dent Res* 1978; 57:181–185.

33. Lang NP, Hotz P, Graf H: Effects of supervised chlorhexidene mouth rinses in children. A longitudinal clinical trial. *J Periodont Res* 1982; 17:101–111.

34. Segreto VA, Collins EM, Beiswanger BB: A comparison of mouth rinses containing two concentrations of chlorhexidene. *J Periodont Res* 1986; 21(suppl 16):23–32.

35. Fornell J, Sundin Y, Lindhe J: Effect of Listerine on dental plaque and gingivitis. *Scand J Dent Res* 1975; 83:18–25.

36. Lamster IB, Alfano MC, Seiger MC: The effect of Listerine antiseptic on reduction of existing plaque and gingivitis. *Clin Prev Dent* 1983; 5:12–16.

37. Gordon JM, Lamster IB, Seiger MC: Efficacy of Listerine antiseptic in inhibiting the development of plaque and gingivitis. *J Clin Periodontol* 1985; 12:697–704.

38. Thomson-Neal D, Evans GH, Meffert RM: Effects of various prophylactic treatments on titanium, sapphire and hydroxyapatite-coated implants: An SEM study. *Int J Periodont Restor Dent* 1989; 9:301–311.

39. Parham PL Jr, Cobb CM, French AA, et al: Evaluation of titanium implant surfaces exposed to an air powder abrasive. *J Dent Res* 1988; 67(special issue): abstract No 1609.

40. Thompson N, Buchanan R, Lemons J: *In vitro* corrosion of Ti-6A1-4V and type 316L stainless steel when galvanically coupled with carbon. *J Biomed Mater Res* 1979; 13:35–42.

41. Lucas L, Bearden L, Lemons J: Ultrastructural examinations of *in vitro* and *in vivo* cells exposed to solutions of 316L stainless steel, ASTM STP 859, in Franker A, Griffin C (eds): *ASTM*. Philadelphia, American Society for Testing Materials, 1985, pp 208–221.

42. Van Orden AC: Corrosive responses of the interface tissue to 316 L stainless steel, titanium-based alloys and cobalt-based alloys, in McKinney RV Jr, Lemons JE (eds): *The Dental Implant: Clinical and Biological Response of Oral Tissues*. Littleton, Mass, PSG Publishing Co, 1985, pp 1–24.

43. Axelsson P, Lindhe J: The significance of maintenance care in the treatment of periodontal disease. *J Clin Periodontol* 1981; 8:281–290.

44. Ramfjord SP, Morrison EC, Burgett FG, et al: Oral hygiene and maintenance of periodontal support. *J Periodontol* 1982; 53:26–30.

45. Morrison EC, Ramfjord SP, Burgett FG, et al: The significance of gingivitis during the maintenance phase of periodontal treatment. *J Periodontol* 1982; 53:31–34.

46. Becker W, Becker B, Berg L: Periodontal treatment without maintenance. A retrospective study in 44 patients. *J Periodontol* 1984; 55:505–509.

Chapter 32

Dental Implant Practice Management

Alfred L. Heller, D.D.S., M.S.

Marketing has tremendous potential for building a successful dental implant practice. Yet it is probably the most misunderstood and misused tool in the profession. It is often looked upon with fear, apprehension, disdain, and mostly confusion. "Marketing" and "advertising" are terms we use as though they were interchangeable. They are not, but the confusion about the difference is why most dentists do not use either to their full advantage.

This chapter attempts to clear up that confusion—to give an understanding of marketing, why marketing can work for almost any dentist, and what it takes to make it work. I will present the most up-to-date views of marketing and public relations professionals who have studied the marketing challenges and opportunities that face dentists and implantologists. Those who read this and are willing to commit the time and effort to developing a marketing plan will find that it offers tremendous growth potential for their practices.

I caution, however, that before a marketing plan is developed, the practitioner needs to examine his or her personal life to ensure that all is in order. The dentist and implantologist who does not have a stable life will not be able to satisfy or retain the new patients that are attracted by these marketing efforts. In addition, looking at the matter in terms of the personal benefit that the dentist derives, a dental career will be fulfilling only if his or her personal life is fulfilling.

WHAT IS MARKETING?

If there is one thing that I have learned about marketing in my 21 years as an implantologist, it is that marketing, like dentistry, is both an art and a science. For most of us, marketing just doesn't seem to come naturally. It takes study, lots of thought, and hard work. On the plus side, though, anyone with the skills and intelligence to be a quality dentist or implantologist can also be a successful marketer, if he or she is willing to devote some time to developing the art and science of marketing!

My personal opinion is that most successful dentists make marketing a way of life. They realize that everything they do affects others, even what they consider the private matters of their personal lives. But think about it! Who would you rather do business with—the person who appears stable, happy, content with life, or the one who is distracted, diffuse, negative, "grumpy?" Our personal life is often the first place we should look to improve the marketing of our practice! If our personal lives are not stable, that will have a major impact (whether we like it or not, and whether we know it or not) on the two groups of people most important to the success of our practice: staff and patients.[1-3] Both of them look up to you. Both want to respect you. Both are supersensitive to what is going on in your personal life. You can fool some of the people all the time and all the people some of the time, but you can hardly ever fool your staff. They will be infected by any negative attitude you have and carry it to other staff

411

members and your patients. And don't kid yourself about the fact that your patients are very sensitive, also. When a patient senses that something is wrong, that you don't really have your mind on your work, he or she is going to have a hard time trusting you with one of the most vulnerable places on the body. So, if you have an unfulfilled, unstable life outside the office, even the greatest marketing plan in the world is only going to help your practice grow to a limited extent because you'll be fighting yourself in the process![4] You will be the biggest barrier to success. The first step on the road to success, then, is to get your life together. That may be easier said than done, but we have seen it done, and have helped it happen with dozens of people over the years.

POSTGRADUATE EDUCATION

The one aspect of implantology that just can't be stressed enough is education. Without it, you are at risk in a number of ways, and you'll only compound the risk by marketing. The training I speak of is much more than the typical "weekend wonder" courses put on by an implant manufacturer who spends 2 or 3 days explaining his system. This is simply inadequate! Implantology is very successful with the proper training. Without it, it is impossible! That applies to everyone—general dentist or specialist.

Surgical anatomy, tissue management, bone physiology, proper implant selection for available bone, sterile technique, proper implant placement— whether in or on bone, restoration techniques, patient management before and after implant placement—all are important. Conscious sedation (requiring a 2–4-hour appointment) plays a welcome role in helping the patient with the implant procedure, but this is also a skill acquired through education and training. And, of course, marketing skills are important to building a successful practice. No phase of the process can be slighted in favor of another because there is probably no other type of dentistry that requires the mastery of as many skills as does implant dentistry!

Postgraduate education is very much misunderstood these days. It should not be a 1, 2, or 3-day slide show of a certain technique or modality, but a true continuation of quality dental education. It should include sharing new, up-to-date ideas about a technique or modality, followed by hands-on training with a real patient (under proper supervision). Your patients and staff will benefit immensely from skills you learn by this method.

Dr. Roger Blackwell, marketing professor at Ohio State University and world-renowned marketing consultant to companies such as IBM, Ford, 3M, Johnson & Johnson, and The Limited stores tells us that there is a difference between marketing and advertising.[5] Advertising (or "selling," if you prefer) is "getting rid of what you have," while marketing is "having what you can get rid of." He says that if you haven't learned any new skills since dental school, then you must sell—get rid of what you have; but hands-on postgraduate education will give you the ability to have something—implants—that your patients want. It will put a spark into your dental practice that will attract patients who will appreciate your care, skill, and new-found abilities to help them in ways no one could before.

FIND SOMEONE TO FOLLOW

Something that I rank in the category of education, and would encourage anyone who wants to get into implantology to do, is to find a role model— someone who is willing to be a mentor—and to spend time with that person. It would be advisable to spend a lot of time because it will enable you to develop good habits that you might not otherwise pick up. It's a big commitment on your part and on theirs, but well worth it. Dr. L.D. Panky[6] was a role model for me. He generously shared his dental skills as well as his "life skills" with me. Throughout my career, whenever I realized that an area of my practice needed attention, I would take the initiative to seek out the best person I knew in that field and spend time with him or her. Many of the most truly successful people are willing to share their knowledge, because they know that in so doing, they learn and grow as well. The biblical principle of "the more you give, the more you get back" is as applicable to dentists as anyone else.

PERSONALITY—YOURS AND YOUR STAFF'S

Before you actually get started in marketing, give some thought to the type of personality that you have and that each of your staff members has. While there are personality studies that get much more detailed than we are able to in this chapter, let's use the two that most are familiar with: introvert and extrovert. Both are good. After all, God created each of us the way we are for a purpose and He wants us to use our personalities in our profession! The important thing to remember is this: whatever your personality or the personality of your staff members, it can be a positive factor in your marketing efforts. I would like you to consider everything I say about marketing and advertising in terms of your personality and the personalities of your staff. (For example, I suggest that you utilize every opportunity to speak to community groups about your practice. If you consider yourself to be an introvert, however, ask an extroverted member of your staff to do this instead. Have introverted members of your staff do marketing projects that are less "people-intensive" and extroverted members do those that are more people-intensive.)

WHAT IS MARKETING?

Before you do anything in the way of marketing, there is one other very important thing that must be done to help ensure that all your marketing and advertising efforts will be productive. It addresses the problem of dentists thinking like dentists, not like their patients. Ed Churchill, former executive director of the Midwest Implant Institute, explains it this way: "You must understand your patients' physical and psychological needs, and then design the attitudes, services, and communications of the practice to satisfy those needs so that patients get the benefit of all the dental services they need."[7] What is this? It's a very good definition of marketing! This process takes a lot of thought and planning, but without this crucial first step, I can guarantee you that your efforts will be a waste of time and money. Unfortunately, dentists often don't stick to their marketing

plans. It's a process that takes a lot of thought and planning. You must be prepared to commit yourself to it. By doing this you make it your plan; you'll have "ownership" in it and a lot more initiative to stick to it.

Kotler and Clarke[8] emphasize the role of the patient when they write that marketing "relies heavily on designing the organization's offering in terms of the target markets' needs and desires, and on using effective pricing, communication, and distribution to inform, motivate, and service the markets."

Allow me to give you an example of the whole concept of thinking like your patients. Let's say you have invested a great deal of money in a new office building with the most up-to-date operating room and equipment and decide to do a television commercial to show potential patients what you have to offer them. So you have a beautiful ad produced and air it on the evening news when you feel that the greatest number of your patients will see it. Then you go to your office and are very surprised when the phone doesn't ring off the hook with new patient inquiries. What happened? It may be that you didn't stop to consider your patients' psychological need to have personal contact with you; they didn't want "bricks and mortar," they wanted you—they wanted to know they were going to get personal attention. If this were the case with your patients, you would want to spend a little more time than you normally would in the initial visit. You might also be sure that your staff is sensitized to the need for projecting a warm, caring attitude to the patients. And, of course, any marketing you do should reflect these "personal touches" that make a visit to your office special.

Brown and Morley[9] make the point that the time your patient spends with you is not the only factor that determines your patient's overall impression of your practice. They point to at least six factors:

- The pre-visit phone call
- Arrival at your office
- The time they spend in the reception area and waiting room
- The time with you
- Departure from your office
- Contact after the visit

Carefully considering each of the above will help you view your practice as your patient does.

Another example of your patient's perspective deals with the physical needs of your patients. Let's say you decide to market your practice to the elderly in your community. What do you think their response would be if they find that they have to climb a lot of steps to get to your office door? Or if the only magazines they find in your reception room are *Ingenue* and *Seventeen?* Or if your receptionist just doesn't get along with older people? Remember to consider the physical and psychological needs of your patients before you put your marketing plan together! As you begin that process, you need to answer the question "Whom do I want to market to?" What age group should I concentrate my efforts on? Who can best use my services? Who can pay for my services?

INTERNAL VS. EXTERNAL MARKETING

It might help to think of marketing in terms of internal and external. While they are very different in many ways, they complement each other and there is a balance between them (Fig 32–1). Internal marketing is directed to your patients and their referrals. External marketing is directed to everyone else. These definitions enable us to communicate more effectively.

External

External marketing is what is commonly thought of as marketing because, for the most part, it is directed to potential, not existing, patients. While I believe that, as a rule of thumb, internal marketing is more effective and can improve the "return on investment" in external marketing, no one should ignore opportunities for external marketing.

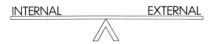

FIG 32–1.
The balanced components of marketing: internal and external factors.

What comes to mind first in external marketing is direct advertising of one sort or another. This can be an excellent way to market your practice, as long as you put it into proper perspective. Remember that over 85% of your new patients come from referrals from patients, other practitioners, and other specialists, according to an American Dental Association (ADA) study.[10] So you shouldn't spend all your time advertising at the expense of building your referral base. The *Yellow Pages* may be an excellent form of advertising for you, especially since it's a great aid in letting people know where you are located. But remember that, as with a newspaper ad or television commercial, they know that you have paid to reach them and that competent and incompetent practitioners alike can advertise. From this standpoint, a news article about your practice is much more meaningful since it has the effect of an unbiased, third-party endorsement. I would encourage you to contact a public relations firm if you are unsure of how to deal with the news media. Remember to make copies of favorable articles to display in your office and to send out to callers.

One great form of advertising and publicity that is often overlooked is the neighborhood newspaper. It is a very personal way to reach a targeted and promising audience. For reasons that go beyond convenience, people like to patronize their neighbors, so I consider it very advantageous to advertise locally. Personally, we like "institutional advertising" such as sponsorship in local high school football programs, concert programs, symphony programs, etc. It is relatively inexpensive, creates goodwill that money can't ordinarily buy, and it's effective. One final thought on newspaper advertising: the purpose is to inform, not sell. People often don't respond well to ads that are designed to get them in the door, but they do appreciate help in locating it!

Personal Involvement
Another way to market your practice is to get involved in the community. If your practice is in a small town or a tightly knit neighborhood in a larger city, place an ad in the high school football or basketball program, or help pay for the fourth of July fireworks display. Better yet, get personally involved in civic affairs. You'd be surprised how your name

gets out by doing that and you will feel a real sense of reward for helping others. Try helping out with a fund drive for one of your favorite charities. Or, if you are sports-minded, you may want to become involved in coaching Little League sports such as soccer, swimming, football, or baseball. When patients see how well you care for the needs of their children, they are more likely to trust you with their dental needs, as well.

Local church involvement will also put you in personal contact with people on a regular basis. Like almost any activity you engage in, the more people who get to know you, the more people you will get in your door. The main benefit, though, is the spiritual health you will personally derive from this, especially in terms of getting your personal life in order and keeping it that way.

Study Clubs

Study clubs offer a way to show your dental colleagues that you are incorporating implants into your dental practice. If you live in a large metropolitan area, the local dental society publication might be used to reach those interested in starting an implant study club. If your practice is in a smaller community, personal telephone calls work well. It would not be unusual for dentists in a 50-mile radius to participate.

Community Presentations

Everyone feels a little uncomfortable speaking to large numbers of people. That's natural. If you're able to do it, however, you ought to spend a few hours working up a standard speech about implantology to give to senior citizen groups, the Rotary, and other community groups. It's not that hard to do, and once you have prepared one, it will require only minor modification for each particular group. It gives you a chance to reach people you might not otherwise be able to reach, and to reach them in such a way that they feel they get to know you personally. When you put your speech together, be sure to include some interesting facts about implantology. An example would be that the ancient Mayan and Egyptian cultures experimented with them. Keep your program short and don't forget to interject some humor. Include some props that you can pass around,

such as photographs that show what you are talking about. If you are going to make a commitment to do this on a regular basis, have some slides produced that will help keep your audience's attention. Slides are commercially available that give you a "starter set" to mix with your own slides. This combination is very effective. Don't be dismayed if you don't know of particular groups that might be interested in your program. Your local chamber of commerce probably has a list of clubs that are eager to get outside speakers. Most civic clubs have a meeting chairman who is always looking for topics of interest. "What's New in Dentistry" is a catchy title for your presentation.

Internal Marketing

While external marketing is important, I believe that internal marketing is even more so. No matter how good your external marketing, you are still going to get a majority of your long-lasting patients from referrals.[10] At the top of the list of tools you have for internal marketing is your staff!

Staff

The attitude of your staff will have a tremendous impact on your patients and their attitude about your practice.[11] Even dentists with superb skills in implantology and the ability to relate to people can lose patients because of a staff member's attitude problem. Quite often you won't get a second chance, because you just won't hear from them again. According to *Businessgram*,[12] while dissatisfied customers usually don't complain about discourteous service, nine out of ten will never again buy from a company they feel offended them. And they will tell at least nine other people about the experience!

Your staff is the best internal marketing tool you have. A patient is much more likely to take a staff member into his or her confidence than to take you! The reason is simple: the patient identifies more closely with the staff person. Ask any physician— the nurse's directions are followed more closely than the doctor's!

Mark Pearce, writing for *Cincinnati Medicine*,[13] stated the challenge this way: "Marketing has to satisfy patient needs in an on-going and consistent way—the goal is to make each and every contact a patient has with you or your staff a positive experience."

A dental assistant or hygienist who has a positive attitude and is well trained in the techniques of marketing can lead the patient into inquiring about the benefits of dental implants. A hygienist, in casual conversation while cleaning a patient's teeth, can become a salesperson by asking, "Are you really happy with your existing flipper or partial denture?" Or, "Did you know that Dr. —— has been studying the newest advancements in dental implants?" Your assistants will do you, and themselves, a real favor if they make it a habit to always bring up the subject of implants when the patient is considering a replacement of missing natural dentition.

The staff member should also take advantage of any opportunity to show photographs or models to the patient before the doctor mentions the possibility of an implant. After laying this foundation, the patient perceives the doctor's approval of them as a candidate for an implant as a verification of what the trusted staff member had suggested. This can make a big difference in the patient's perception of what is happening. If you are the first person to suggest implants, often the patient's immediate response is negative because he or she knows you will benefit financially from the procedure. In addition, as Schmidt notes,[14] "When a doctor feels awkward proclaiming his expertise, staff can lend third party credibility to patient encounters."

Staff members must work with the doctor, not for the doctor. The dental team must have a true desire to help patients receive the best dental treatment possible. If it becomes obvious that a staff member cannot reflect and enhance your level of skill and patient care, he or she should seek employment elsewhere. If, on the other hand, staff members do enhance and complement your work, let them know you appreciate them. Remember—staff personnel leave for lack of praise, not lack of raise. The doctor must edify his productive staff members daily, in front of patients. This will have the added benefit of increasing the patient's confidence in your staff. Remember to reward your dedicated staff members financially as well. Pay them as if they were family, the way you would like to see your children be paid for doing the same work.

Get involved in the lives of your staff. Find out what activities their family members enjoy. Remember to ask how the "big game" went. The surest way to build loyalty from your staff and to help them be fulfilled in their work is to take a personal, but proper, interest in their private lives.

Thank-U-Gram

I've found that one of the most successful marketing tools I've ever used is what we call the THANK-U-GRAM (Fig 32–2). My staff selects a "patient of the day" and I write a short note on the THANK-U-GRAM to that patient, saying something like, "The staff and I have chosen you as the 'Patient of the Day!' We appreciate you very much and thank you for selecting our office for your dental needs." This small gesture means more to most patients than you can imagine! You can also send THANK-U-GRAMS to anyone who helps you throughout the day—the teller at the bank, the neighbor who took the Federal Express package for you, etc. It doesn't take much time but it really gets results. When was the last time you received a thank-you note? Do you remember how good it made you feel? Well, it will do the same for your patients! They will show it to their friends and family members, the people who are your future patients!

This simple internal marketing tool was instrumental in building a very large practice that averaged 52 new patient referrals per month over a 7-year period. Everyone needs to know he is appreciated. A THANK-U-GRAM is a personal way of letting him know that you and your staff think he is special.

The Telephone

I also call every implant patient on the evening of surgery to see how he or she is feeling. I do it because I really do care about them. They can't believe that someone cares enough to check on them. I don't really do it as a marketing tool, but it has brought in many new patients. Therein is the real secret of successful referral networking—just let people know that you care about them and that they are important to you.

Newsletter

Consider a newsletter. There is a certain pride that implant patients share. A newsletter, if done

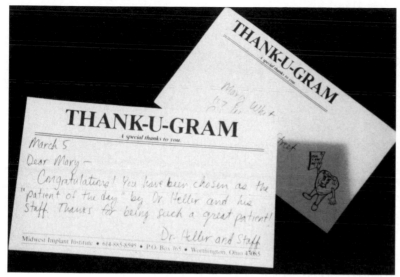

FIG 32–2.
The thank-u-gram that is sent to a special selected patient each day.

properly, can foster and spread that feeling and could really help someone who is "on the fence" about getting an implant to decide to go ahead with treatment. And you can use it to let patients know that you are getting extra training to advance your skills and to better meet their dental needs.

Do you realize how many mouths physicians look into? A newsletter directed to physicians can be a very effective marketing tool in building relationships between the physician and dentist. Physicians are often impressed with the new advancements of dentistry, especially in implantology.

Patient Photos

If you haven't already had slides and pictures made of patients before and after surgery, you should (Fig 32–3). It's one thing to tell prospective patients when you consult with them the first time that implants can have dramatic esthetic results, and it's another thing to be able to show them. The use of models is helpful, too. Videos are being used more and more and they provide a very impactful means of relaying patient testimonials. All of these devices are useful in that they allow the prospective patient to become personally involved in the decision process.

After you have built a group of implant patients who are satisfied with their treatment, they can become a resource for you. Have prospective patients call them and ask any questions they may have, such

as, How did the treatment go? How did you chew before and how do you chew now? and, Would you do it again? These people can be tremendously helpful because (1) they are satisfied patients, (2) they are credible because they have nothing to gain by telling them it was good if it wasn't, and (3) patients who are happy with their implants love to talk about them. Ask your satisfied patients if they would object to people calling them with a few questions. Explain to them that their testimony will help others enjoy the same benefits they are getting.

Patient Education Brochures

Patients need well-designed and easy-to-understand literature to educate them on the many different types of implants as well as why different types of implants are used in different situations (Fig 32–4). These brochures should include patient photos and comments. It's very reassuring for prospective patients to know that others are happy with their implants. Don't forget to include your name, address, and telephone number in block-sized letters!

The Cup

As a final note on internal marketing, we give a coffee cup to all implant patients. It is having a positive impact on our practice, and our patient referral base. The cup has a set of teeth and big smiling lips under the words, "Ask me why I'm smiling" (Fig 32–5,A). When the cup is filled with hot liquid, the

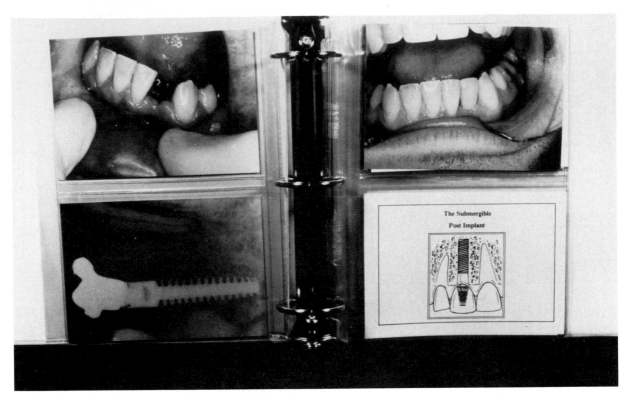

FIG 32–3.
Use of patient photographs and procedures (with permission) to help educate new implant patients in your practice.

FIG 32–4.
Implant literature oriented to the patients in your practice.

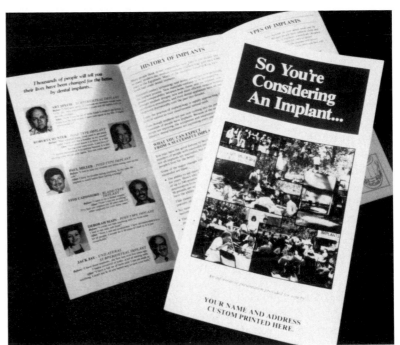

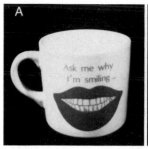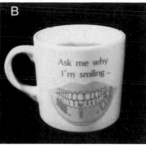

FIG 32–5.
A, coffee cup given to all implant patients. **B,** the coffee cup shown in **A** when filled with hot liquid reveals three implants in place with restorations. Note the blade root form and subperiosteal implants that appear.

lips fade away, revealing an illustration of three implants in place and restored—a blade, a post, and a unilateral "sub" (Fig 32–5,B). On the other side of the cup it says, "Smile courtesy of Dr. A.L. Heller." Patients love to show the cup to fellow workers, family, and friends. It sounds a little silly, but it really gets good results by bringing new patients into the office.

HAPPINESS IN LIFE = HAPPINESS IN DENTISTRY

Happiness is a word many of us use to describe a feeling we cannot define.[2, 3, 11] We send our children off to college and tell them we don't care what they do, we "just want them to be happy." We say that we were happy at one time, but not at another. We talk a lot about it, but just what is happiness? Are you happy reading this book? Were you happy driving to work today? How happy are we as individuals or as a profession? Our profession is high on the list of suicides, divorces, and heart attacks.[3] Are we happy?

As I noted earlier in this chapter, you cannot really separate happiness in life from happiness in dentistry. If we are not pleased with ourselves as individuals, we will not be pleased with our results in the dental office. Sooner or later, *our personal philosophy of life will become our professional philosophy* as well. And that will have a large and negative bearing on our patients and staff. We cannot separate

our philosophy of everyday living and moral standing from our philosophy, attitude, and demeanor in the office.

What is Your Philosophy of Life?

Since I can't know what your philosophy is, allow me to share the philosophy of someone I mentioned previously who greatly influenced me early in my dental career. This philosophy has a proven track record of producing excellent dental management skills in dealing with patients and staff. Most importantly, however, it has helped many people like you and me to really truly enjoy life each day and to put true meaning into our personal lives, the lives of our patients and staff, and especially the lives of our spouse and children. Read and re-read this philosophy and it will help you as it has many others.

Over 70 years ago, a Boston physician named Richard C. Cabot wrote a book entitled *What Men Live By*. Dr. Cabot explored the four elements of a balanced life: work, play, love, and worship. L.D. Panky used this philosophy to help thousands of dentists to find a way to balance life at home, the office, and in personal relationships with those who are truly important in our lives.

At the base of this philosophy is a simple truth: What kind of dentist would you like to entrust your mouth to, one wearing a mask and trying to present an image of happiness, or one whose balanced life is evident in every word and action?

There is a need in each of us to be the best we can with the talents we are given, to enjoy each day to its fullest, to have people in our lives that we care about and serve. Too much or too little of any of the four elements will eventually unbalance our lives. This in turn will:

- Destroy our sense of self-worth
- Keep us from enjoying life to the fullest
- Tear down the close relationships we have with spouse and children
- Keep us striving to find something that always seems to elude us.

But, with a balanced life of work, play, love, and worship, we can enjoy life as God intended us to.

Work

According to Cabot and Panky, a balanced life must have work that is challenging, real, and, for the most part, enjoyable. Of course, there are times in any career when the joy is just not there. But, overall, we should feel a sense of self-satisfaction and happiness.

William Davis, who wrote a book[6] about Panky, states that work should include:

- Enough of a challenge to call upon our powers of mastery
- Enough variety or enough predictability to suit our circumstances and temperament
- A realistic workload
- A chance to achieve, create, and see the fruits of our work
- A chance to be absorbed in the work
- Recognition and compensation for our work

How is your work life? Are you stimulated with new techniques and trends in dentistry or are you bored and feel "burned out?" Anyone can learn how to effectively market his or her dental practice, but the doctor who does not truly enjoy helping patients doesn't need the added patient load that marketing will bring. It will only bring additional stress.

Play

Play is our ability to get away from work, which helps us better enjoy it when we return. It involves enjoying our family members, our friends, and especially ourselves. For some, golf is the answer; for others, a good book; and yet others like some form of strenuous exercise. Effective play results in relaxation and renewed vigor.

Love

Love is probably the most misunderstood word in our vocabulary. Part of the confusion comes from the fact we have only one word for love in our language, whereas the Greeks had several. The Greek word *philos* means loving, as in brotherly love; *eros* means erotic or romantic love. Both of those are based on feelings and emotions. They had to coin a new word for the self-sacrificing love that Christ brought into the world: *agape*. This is love that may include an emotional feeling, but is not dependent upon it. Emotions are too fickle and too subject to change. Sometimes we feel like loving someone, sometimes we don't. But Christian love is different. It is love that exists due to the nature of its source, not its object. It is serving people even when the emotion is not there. The best definition I've ever heard is from my wife, Wanda: "Love is the giving of yourself without any thought of return." If we truly love our patients, our spouses, our children, our staff, and ourselves, we must learn to give without needing something in return.

Our staff and patients deserve our love, too. We must get out of our "comfort zone" and tell those close to us that we truly appreciate them, and, yes, that we love them.

Worship

Worship is necessary for a balanced life. Is it a part of your life? Do you start each day with your Creator? Do you pray when things are going well in your life, or just when things are in shambles? There is an old saying that there are no atheists in foxholes. If a child of ours has cancer, we call out to God for guidance, comfort, and understanding. When stress in our lives reaches a level we can't tolerate, we call out to God for peace of mind. But doesn't it make sense that God would want to be in our lives all the time? How would you feel if a friend only shared the terrible times with you, but never the joy? If we want to have a truly fulfilling relationship with God, if we want to have a truly fulfilling life, we need to include Him in the good times as well as the bad.

In the Old Testament book of Ecclesiastes 2:24–25, Solomon says, "There is nothing better for a man than to eat and drink and tell himself that his labor is good. This also I have seen, that it is from the hand of God. For who can eat and who can have enjoyment without Him?" This incredibly wise man, who had everything in abundance, acknowledges that man cannot have enjoyment without God and that man must tell himself that his work is good.

Worship could be the missing link in your

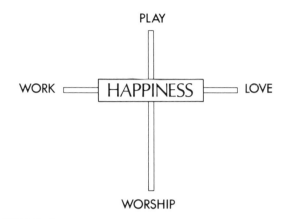

PLAY

WORK ——— HAPPINESS ——— LOVE

WORSHIP

FIG 32–6.
The ingredients of a balanced life needed to achieve a successful implant practice.

search for happiness and fulfillment. Have you been promising yourself that you will do it but keep procrastinating? Make the commitment today, and when you do it, be sure to take your family. You'll be amazed at the positive impact on your life. A relationship with God really enhances our relationship with the other people in our lives. I can say with confidence that no successful person will stay successful without a balanced life that includes worship (Fig 32–6).

DISCUSSION

Will Marketing Really Help My Practice?.— Yes! Developing and using good, sound marketing tools will bring patients into your dental office. Then you and your staff will have to use your God-given skills to bring those patients into your family of satisfied patients. But remember, you have a tremendous responsibility. There are lots of people who depend upon you: your family, your staff, and your patients. Think of all the people you will influence over the course of your career! It's especially important, then, to keep your life balanced. You yourself

can be a powerful marketing tool for your practice, but only if you have a balanced life style, and your daily habits inside and outside the office reflect it. If you can balance your life, you'll have much more than a productive practice; you'll have the kind of happiness that will be a blessing to everyone you touch in your life and career.

REFERENCES

1. Mandino O: *The Choice*. New York, Bantom Books, 1986.
2. Bland, G: *Success: The Glenn Bland Method*. Wheaton, Ill, Tyndale House Publishers, Inc, 1982.
3. Culligan MJ, Sedlacek K: *How to Avoid Stress Before It Kills You*. New York, Gramercy Publishing Co, 1980.
4. Swindoll C: *Living Above the Level of Mediocrity*. Waco, Tex, Word Books, 1987.
5. Engel JF, Blackwell RD, Miniard PW: *Consumer Behavior*. Chicago, Dryden Press, 1986.
6. Panky LD, Davis WJ: *A Philosophy of the Practice of Dentistry*. Toledo, Ohio, Medical College Press, 1980.
7. *Developing Your Own Personalized Marketing Strategy*, a 2 ½ day course taught at the Midwest Implant Institute; Ed Churchill, executive director.
8. Kotler P, Clarke RN: *Marketing for Health Care Organizations*. Englewood, NJ, Prentice Hall, Inc, 1987, p 5.
9. Brown SW, Morley AP Jr: *Marketing Strategies for Physicians*. Oradell, NJ, Medical Economics Books, 1986, p 102.
10. *Survey of Dental Practice*. Chicago, The American Dental Association, 1985.
11. Minirth FB, Meir PD: *Happiness Is a Choice*. Grand Rapids, Mich, Baker Book House, 1978.
12. *Businessgram*. Bowling Green, Ohio, April 1987, p 5.
13. Pearce: When do I start? *Cincinnati Medicine* Summer issue, 1985.
14. Schmidt D: Let your staff contribute to practice success. *Dental Economics* 1987; 77:76

Chapter 33

Clinical Management of Failing Implant Cases

Burton E. Balkin, D.M.D.

As dental implant techniques become more prolific in their use, it is essential that standardized methods be developed to provide procedures to treat deteriorating implant areas that may not be totally defective. The treatment is based upon the assumption that the initial implant procedures effectively provided a safe and effective implant, as well as a safe and effective implant prosthesis. Salvaging methods can enhance the longevity of implant procedures and provide an alternative means of solving problems other than the removal of the implants, which in many instances is unnecessary. This situation is not to be confused with a total implant failure indicating the necessity for an explant procedure. Unfortunately, current literature does not include corrective procedures relating to most implant techniques. The techniques outlined in this chapter are supported by my wide experience and by anecdotal evidence. Until such time as scientific long-term studies are supported and effected, the following information can be considered appropriate.

Dental implants that are starting to fail rarely do so without symptoms which the patient becomes aware of, or observations which the clinician notes during routine implant patient maintenance and recall visits. It should be observed that patients must be considered part of the therapy team in their responsibility to provide home care and seek regular professional recall appointments.[1] The patient should also be expected to question any symptoms, which

may include pain, foul taste, bleeding, drainage, swelling, mobility, loss of function (mastication), and changes in appearance. Any of these should initiate patient concern and the patient is advised to seek knowledgeable professional evaluation.

METHODS OF DIAGNOSIS

Methods of diagnosis include clinical observation, radiographic findings, microbiological testing,[2] and systemic considerations.

Clinical Observation

Tissue tone is most often an indicator of health or pathology present in the underlying tissues. Localized tissue inflammation around the pergingival site, or within 5 mm of the abutments, is not normal and often indicates loss of the biological seal[3] or alveolar bone loss, or both.

Infection with its resultant symptoms may or may not be related to underlying loss of bone support or loss of integration. Exudate from the pergingival site, or a nearby fistula, could indicate an underlying pathologic condition.

Probing pocket depth, although helpful in diagnosis, may not be possible owing to the shape of the implant or to the position of a fixed prosthesis. A deep gingival sulcus may also exist in a healthy stable implant with proper maintenance.[3] However, a deep probable area that bleeds profusely when probed bears further investigation.

Stability, or loss of stability of the implant abutments and prosthesis, as intended, indicates the state of health of the implant and the implant prosthesis. Cylindrical endosseous implants usually commence function with zero mobility assuming osteointegration. The abutments on these implants are either rigidly attached, or attached through a plastic device that allows slight movement, thus attempting to simulate the movement that occurs naturally in the periodontal membrane. Mobility in the abutment of an osteointegrated implant with rigid abutment design could indicate a loosened abutment attachment, a change in the integration of the bone to fibro-osteointegration, or loss of bone support for attachment of the implants, either full of partial.

Excess mobility of a prosthesis supported by an osteointegrated implant with a mobile element could indicate a loosening or wearing of the mobile element. It could also suggest a change in the integration of the bone to fibro-osteointegration, loss of bone support, or failure of integration of the implant, either full or partial. It must be determined whether mobility is mechanical or biological in origin, i.e., loose screw attachments, cement, or wear vs. loss of integration/attachment.

Blade or flat endosseous implants may commence function in either osteointegrated or fibro-osteointegrated capacity. If the implant started with zero mobility and movement of the prosthesis occurs, it should be determined whether or not this movement relates to the mechanical attachment, or whether the implant is biologically changed and is no longer osteointegrated. If the implant commenced functioning as a fibro-osteointegrated implant with slight mobility equal to that of a healthy periodontally supported tooth, or if it started in an osteointegrated state, and now has this type of movement and is functioning in a healthy manner, it may be allowed to remain in this state. If mobility has increased, it should then be determined whether or not the mobility is mechanical or biological. The differentiation of etiology of mobility in the prosthesis, the implant abutment, or the implant is necessary to determine the type and extent of appropriate treat-

ment. The treatment could vary from repair or replacement of mechanical components to surgical intervention or removal of the implant component.

Subperiosteal Implants.—Clinical observation of the mobility of the implant would determine whether or not the implant is setting on bone and maintaining its stability. It could also determine whether or not the implant can maintain its rigidity in light of possible bone changes that may have occurred since placement. This can be a determining factor as to whether or not the implant can be treated, modified, or should be removed.

Radiographic Findings

Radiographs can be useful in determining the extent of integration around the dental implant. Although this method of analysis cannot be relied upon as a thorough indicator of the status of the implant, it is an aid when there is a prosthesis which cannot be removed for evaluation of individual implants. Radiographs are also indicated where clinical pathology is present, and radiographic interpretation of the surrounding osseous structures can be of help in determining the extent of the degenerative process.

Various types of radiographs can be used, the most common being periapical radiographs. Panoramic radiographs are also useful because they can extend the areas covered, which cannot be achieved with periapical radiographs. Occlusal radiographs can reveal possible buccolingual changes.

Computed tomography (CT) scans are currently used to determine the extent of osseous breakdown in areas beyond those directly involved with the implant. The scans are generally disrupted by the presence of metal dental implants.

In examining radiographs one should observe the extent of osseous changes as to whether or not they partially surround the implant's perimeter, and the extent they follow from the occlusal to the apical end of the implant. With subperiosteal implants, which set on the surface of the bone, radiographic interpretation is of assistance in determining whether there is osseous stability or resorptive changes occurring beneath the bone surface of the residual ridges.

The presence of a fistula in the gingival area can

be traced with either gutta-percha or silver points, to determine if the source of origin is surrounding the implant, or from existing teeth.

Infection or pain are often attributed to dental implants with their subsequent removal, when in fact etiology is related not to the implant, but to natural teeth. A definite diagnosis should be established prior to considering explant procedures.

Culturing

Culturing may be used to determine the type or source of infection present, if it is felt that infection may be a problem involving the implant. If it is decided that the primary factor is infection, the type of organism is identified with drug sensitivity tests and the patient is then put on an appropriate medicinal regimen.

TREATMENT INTERVENTION

Following diagnostic procedures identifying the type of lesion, and the extent of the lesion in the bone and soft tissue surrounding the implant, appropriate treatment can begin.

Mild forms of a marginal gingivitis can be treated with scaling and curettage, and by improving home care with adequate plaque removal. Instruments used on the implants should be of materials that will not disturb the implant surface. This treatment often resolves potential complications of supraosseous soft tissue lesions when addressed early on.

Soft tissue problems often revolve around inadequate keratinized attached gingiva at the perigingival sites. This lack of adequate tissue is more easily corrected prior to implant insertion. However, if the problem exists, it may be corrected with soft tissue grafts to the site as necessary.

If the problems involve osseous tissues, a flap procedure may be indicated to expose the implant and the surrounding bone. This may be followed by open curettage to eliminate any soft tissue that has grown around the implant. One should also remove any hard calcareous deposits which may have formed on the implant. The surface of the implant should be thoroughly cleaned and irrigated. Should the lesion involve an area that is deemed beyond resolution by curettage of soft tissue from surrounding osseous areas, various augmentation materials may be utilized to fill in the defect. These range from resorbable hydroxylapatite, tricalcium phosphate, freeze-dried demineralized bone, or collagen. One may also utilize nonresorbable hydroxylapatite materials. Following the packing of the defect with these materials, the flaps should be repositioned and sutured tightly. The most effective methods utilized by me have been with resorbable hydroxylapatite.

A newer method of addressing peri-implant defects is to flap the area, remove all soft tissue from the osseous defects and around the implant, treat the surface of the implant to be certain it is free of foreign matter, and proceed with barrier-guided healing. This may be done utilizing any of the various augmentation materials mentioned previously, or with a complete blood clot. This region is then covered with a removable membrane or other barriers between the soft tissue and bone layer. Currently the most effective results are obtained by placing a membrane, repositioning the flap, and then suturing the tissue over the membrane. The membrane is allowed to remain for approximately 6 to 8 weeks, after which it is removed.

In the process of the open flap procedure, if the structure permits, sections of the implant could be removed without extracting the entire implant. However, if osseous breakdown occurs completely around the implant, and the implant has no support from the surrounding tissues, an explant procedure should follow. It may then be possible for the bone to fill in or to utilize bone-regenerative procedures, following which a new implant could be placed in the area.

Subperiosteal implants have remained stable for long-term duration. Studies, including those made recently, have indicated that subperiosteal implant results are often as favorable as any implant and more favorable than some. However, when subperiosteal implants do show resorptive changes between the implant frame and bone, it is often the posterior area. When this occurs, if the implant is basically stable and adequate tissue coverage remains, the bone could be augmented beneath it to prevent any movement. Should the implant be self-supporting, but totally cantilevered from the anterior area, the posterior segments could be removed with the anterior segments remaining firm. This can be done by flapping the region distal to the anterior posts; the frames can be sectioned, and the posterior segments dissected out. Revision of the superstructure is then necessary to provide tissue support for the posterior region with the anterior section able to yield over the implant upon function.

PROSTHESIS—OCCLUSION AND CONTOURS

In conjunction with the surgical approach, a view of the prosthesis has to be made to determine that the occlusion is nontraumatic and that the mechanical portions of the prosthesis are functioning adequately. Either may be primary etiologic factors and may have influenced the degenerative changes that have occurred. If present, they must be corrected.

If an explant procedure has taken place and the site has been allowed to fill in with new bone, then a new implant can be positioned, aligned in the previous site and with the existing prosthesis. It then may be adapted to the existing prosthesis with a minimum of modification of the prosthesis itself. This procedure is also often possible following loss of a natural tooth with an existing prosthesis, either tooth- or tooth implant–supported, thus maintaining the integrity and function of the prosthesis.

Often, owing to a prosthesis utilizing connecting bars intraorally, there can be hypertrophy of tissue beneath the bar and around the implant posts at the perigingival site. This may be trimmed back to provide a healthier environment, using a scalpel; if electrosurgery is used, caution must be taken to prevent contact with the surface of the implant or prosthesis.

It should again be noted that determination of the prosthetic function and load is vital in addressing problem implant cases. Changes often occur naturally in implant- and tooth-supported dentitions; however, implants often survive where adjacent teeth are lost and this puts excessive loads on the implants. This should be taken into consideration in the treatment of the remaining implants.

Dental implants have an inherent weakness in resisting lateral forces. Prostheses that do not avoid these stresses can compromise the implant support. Overloading functioning implants can possibly break down the integrated implant-bone status, indicating a need for evaluation and correction of occlusal forces. This enhances the survival of the implants according to the occlusal concepts utilized for the individual patient.

Prosthetic considerations such as crown contours to provide for adequate plaque removal, and narrow occlusal tables to minimize occlusal stresses, should be considered.

BACTERIOLOGIC CONSIDERATIONS

If it has been determined that infection is a possible etiologic factor, the area should be cultured prior to surgical intervention to determine the organisms present, either in higher concentration or beyond the extent of the normal oral flora. Drug sensitivity testing should then be performed on these organisms to determine appropriate medicinal therapy which could be administered alone or in conjunction with the surgical approaches described.

DISCUSSION

As implant dentistry has evolved into a more broadly based method of dental treatment, it has utilized specific instructions for various implant systems. As a result there has often developed a utilization of these systems without an overall broad-based knowledge as to those methods of treatment which might solve problems that can, and do occur with dental implants. Therefore, there appears to be a lack of information among many of the clinical practitioners of implant dentistry today, particularly those with short-term exposure to implant treatment, in the treatment of implant-related problems. All too often, the singular recourse to a problematic implant is removal. The concept of treating an implant problem, however, does not include treating an implant that exhibits a nonsalvageable state, or is in a state of total failure. This could include implants which display marked mobility, bleeding, exudate, or suppuration from the surrounding tissues, and the presence of radiographically demonstrable pathology.

In the modern history of dentistry there have been many concepts that address the treatment of soft tissue, bone, and prosthodontic problems. Although variations do apply to implant dentistry, many basic concepts of treating patients with a natural dentition do, in fact, apply to implant-restored patients, and should be considered and addressed rather than doing explant procedures. The attempt in this chapter is to address the methods of diagnosis to identify implant problems, and the methods of treatment that can be utilized. This treatment methodology could provide patients with an on-going state of health and function, and reverse destructive trends which may take place in implant-restored patients. With long-term exposure to implant treatment, methods of dealing with many problematic implant cases have evolved. As clinicians become more versatile and experienced in their implant-related treatment, it becomes more obvious that other methods, besides total removal, exist.

Various methods of correcting the implant structure, the osseous tissues, soft tissues, and implant prosthesis, if necessary, have been addressed. These methods, when applied to implant patients who have not passed beyond the salvageable level, can provide patients with continuous long-term use of their prostheses.

It should be observed that, as in other areas of dentistry, known scientific information should be applied to the clinical management of failing implant cases; to do less is not acceptable.

REFERENCES

1. National Institutes of Health Consensus Development Conference Statement on Dental Implants. June 13–15, 1988. *J Dent Educ* 12, 1988; 52.
2. Newman MG, Flemmig TF: Periodontal consideration of implants and implant associated microbiota. *J Dent Educ* 1988; 52:742.
3. McKinney RV Jr, Steflik DE, Koth DL: Evidence for a junctional epithelial attachment to ceramic dental implants. A transmission electron microscopic study. *J Periodontol* 1985; 56:579–591.

Chapter 34

Use of Polymeric, Ceramic, and Other Materials as Synthetic Bone in Implantology

Arthur Ashman, D.D.S.

We have seen the emergence of a new class of restorative materials in dentistry: synthetic bone. The magnitude of new uses and adaptability of these substitutes in solving old problems make this a welcome addition to the dentist's basic armamentarium.[1, 2]

The search for the "ideal" bone substitute material has been a goal of dental researchers for many years and many materials have been included in this search with varying degrees of success: autogenous[3, 4] and freeze-dried bone,[5, 6] allografts of plastic,[7] carbon,[8] and the apatite compounds.[9–12] The literature is abundant with cases utilizing all of these materials because negative results seem to surface with as much frequency as positive results. Some negative factors include resorption after successful placement, difficulty in handling, brittleness, difficulty in obtaining materials, questionable cadaver sources, and nonosteogenic induction. Many of these materials fall far short of the goal of being an ideal bone substitute (Table 34–1).

An ideal synthetic bone substitute should allow the dentist to *prevent* bone loss (e.g., post-extraction; Fig 34–1), as well as *restore* the bone lost by *trauma* (e.g., fracture), by *disease* (e.g., periodontal lesions), or by cancer. The development of such a synthetic bone substitute is the ultimate goal of a synthetic bone material.

THE IDEAL SYNTHETIC BONE MATERIAL

The most important characteristics of an ideal nonresorbable synthetic bone include that it be biologically compatible, act as a scaffold for new bone formation, be osteogenic, be radiopaque, be easy to use and handle, not support the growth of oral pathogens, be hydrophilic, can be provided in particulate and molded forms, be surface electrically active, microporous, and nonallergic, have a high compressive strength, and be easy to obtain.

PREVENTION AND RESTORATION

As previously stated, a synthetic bone substitute should be equally effective in bone as a *preventive,* as well as a *restorative* material. The reason for this is that the jaw bones are unique and following loss of teeth resorption and an eventual atrophy can leave as little as 2 to 3 mm of alveolar bone height.[13] This narrowing and loss of the edentulous alveolar ridge height post-extraction (as much as 40% to 60% in 2 years) is a dental certainty regardless of the age, sex, or health of the patient.[14]

Thus, as a preventive, a synthetic bone substitute should be able to prevent alveolar bone loss

TABLE 34–1.
Comparison of Available Synthetic Bone Materials

Ideal Characteristics of Synthetic Bone	HTR Polymer*	Calcitite† HA	Periograf Alveograf,‡ HA	OsteoGen§ HA	Interpore¶ HA	Synthograft‖ TCP	Cartilage	Cementum	Collagen	Plaster of Paris
Biologically compatible	++	++	++	++	++	++	++	++	++	+
Act as scaffold for new bones	++	0–+	0–+	++	++	+	+	0	+	+
Osteogenic	++	0–+	0	+	+	0–+	+	0	0	0
Radiopaque	++	++	++	++	++	++	+	+	0	++
Easy to handle	++	0	0	++	0	0	0	0	0	0
Nonsupporting of pathogens	++	0	0	++	0	0	0	0	0	0
Hydrophilic	++	0	0	++	0	0	0	0	0	+
Particulate or molded	++	+	+	+	+	0	0	0	0	0
Surface negative charge	++	0	0	+	0	0	0	0	0	0
Microporous	++	0	0	++	++	0	0	0	0	0
Easy to obtain	++	++	++	++	++	++	++	0	++	++
Nonallergic	+	++	++	++	++	++	++	0	+	++
Dental and medical uses	++	+	0	+	0	0	0	0	++	0
Graftable surface	++	0	0	0	0	0	0	0	+	0
Good matrix (carrier)	++	0	0	++	0	0	0	0	++	0
Strong (high CS)	++	++	++	+	0	+	0	0	0	+

HA = hydroxylapatite; HTR = hard tissue replacement; TCP = tricalcium phosphate. CS = compressive strength; 0 = no activity; + = moderate activity; ++ = strong activity.
*Plastic derivative (porous).
†Ceramic (nonporous).
‡Ceramic (nonporous).
§Nonceramic (porous; resorbable).
¶Ceramic (porous).
‖Ceramic (nonporous; nonresorbable).

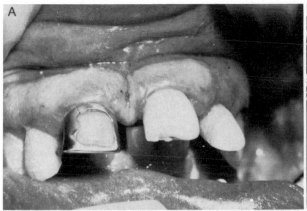

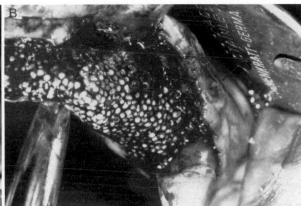

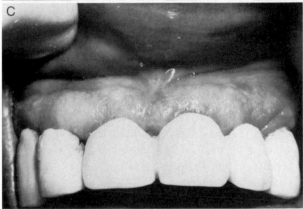

FIG 34–1.
A, this series demonstrates the use of a synthetic grafting material to prevent bone loss post-extraction and provide bone maintenance. This enables stabilization of the alveolar ridge for any future partial or full denture or any endosteal implant. Preoperative photograph shows the flaring of anterior teeth due to lack of bone support. **B,** HTR polymer injected into the extraction sockets. Note the cessation of bleeding as well as the ridge being augmented by building it up in height and width. **C,** temporary jacket crowns are inserted 3 months postoperatively. Note the health of the tissues.

post-extraction, prevent postextraction osteitis ("dry socket") and its complications (Fig 34–2), prevent the loss of alveolar bone proximal to extraction sites, and prevent alveolar bone loss after implant placement (Fig 34–3).

Again, in addition to being a preventive material, a clinically ideal synthetic bone substitute should function as a restorative material. It should be able to rebuild by ridge augmentation alveolar bone atrophy that has occurred as a result of longstanding tooth loss, help restore bone lost to periodontal disease, promote the formation of new bone, act as a scaffold for new bone, and restore, in conjunction with metal implants, *partially* atrophied jaw bones.

The purpose of this chapter is to examine most of the existing *synthetic* bone substitutes available today with an eye toward defining our criteria for their use in implantology and to give the dentist a background into this new emerging class of restorative materials. Krejci and colleagues have recently reviewed the current *osseous* grafting materials available to the dentist.[15]

SYNTHETIC BONE MATERIALS

Synthetic bone materials (nonosseous bone substitutes) may be classified into seven main categories: polymer derivatives, nonresorbable and porous; polymer derivatives, resorbable and nonporous; ceramic, nonporous and nonresorbable; ceramic, porous; ceramic, resorbable; nonceramic, resorbable; and plaster of Paris and silicones, which will not be discussed here.

Polymer Derivatives Nonresorbable and Porous

These compounds are composed primarily of polymeric materials that have been used clinically in

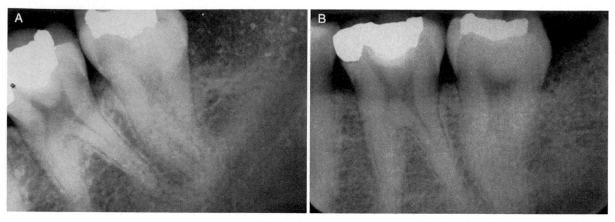

FIG 34–2.
A, these figures demonstrate the prevention of postextraction osteitis or dry socket. HTR polymer injected into the extraction site. Radiograph is 1 week post-operation. **B,** radiograph 3 years post-operation. Note the regeneration of bone adjacent to the second molar and complete fill-in around the socket of the third molar. No dry socket occurred because HTR polymer held the blood clot and did not allow it to break down. Note the prevention of bony breakdown adjacent to the second molar.

humans since the early 1930s in the field of orthopedic surgery. These nonresorbable microporous synthetic bone materials are unique and have little resemblance to the early methyl methacrylate forms. In recent years, various forms of these polymers have been used to fabricate contact lenses and lens implants, prosthetic heart valves, femoral head prostheses, orthopedic bone cements, root canal filling materials, implantable devices for the sustained re-

lease of medications, and in spinal fusion techniques.

Hard tissue replacement (HTR) polymer* is an example of this synthetic bone. It essentially combines a polymethyl methacrylate core with polyhydroxylethyl methacrylate (PHEMA) in a process that

*HTR Sciences, Division of US Surgical Corp., Norwalk, Conn.

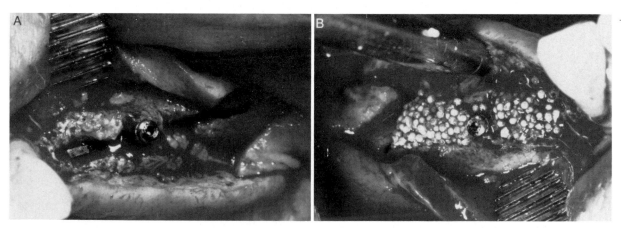

FIG 34–3.
Prevention of alveolar bone loss after implant placement as a result of the osteotomy necessary for the implant placement. **A,** a blade implant is inserted to the height of the alveolar bone. Anatomic considerations prevented it from being placed deeper in the bone. **B,** HTR polymer is placed into the osteotomy site and around the neck of the implant. Note the cessation of bleeding. In essence this is a modified ridge augmentation at the same time the implant is placed.

results in a biocompatible composite *without* the addition of catalysts, inducers, or impurities.[16] Its interface with bone is a calcium graft, which is on its outermost layer and in its micropores. Its inner core plastics do not interface with the bone, but aid in imparting essential properties to the material. HTR polymer is strong, not brittle, even though microporous. It is hydrophilic, extremely easy to use, does not get washed away by bone bleeding, biocompatible, radiopaque, and possesses a bone-inductive negative electric charge (A. Salkind, written communication, 1982). HTR polymer comes in particulate (granular), as well as molded forms, is easily trimmed, osteogenic, and handles well clinically. It gives the practitioner the technology to exactly replicate any hard tissue part in the body, e.g., the alveolar ridge, tooth root, cheek, or chin, at chairside or in the operating room in 10 to 15 minutes.[17] The ability of HTR polymer to aid in fracture repair, replace diseased bone, replace bone lost by periodontal disease,[18] prevent alveolar postextraction bone loss, eliminate postextraction osteitis (dry socket),[14] and prevent proximal bone loss post-extraction around retained teeth make this synthetic bone material impressive as to the variety of applications in the practice of dentistry.[17]

HTR polymer's wide application with dental implants include its usage before, during, and after implant placement: before, to build up an alveolar ridge prior to implant placement (see Fig 34–4); during, as an immediate replacement after extraction in conjunction with cylinder or blade placement (see Figs 34–5, 34–6, 34–7); and after, for repairs necessitated by bony breakdown around an implant (see Fig 34–4).

In a 2½-year survey conducted in over 647 clinical cases, postoperative infections did not occur, because HTR polymer does not promote the growth of pathogens.[19] A recent study revealed that HTR polymer forms a fibroblastic cellular attachment to tissue

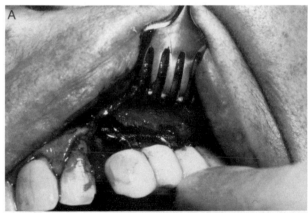
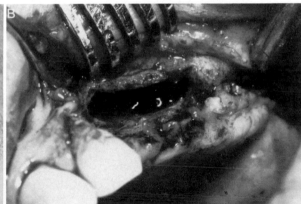
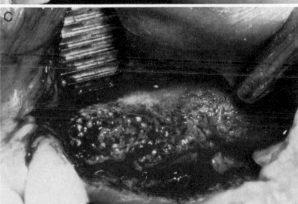

FIG 34–4.
These figures demonstrate the use of HTR polymer before the placement of a new implant. In this case, an existing implant caused severe bony breakdown. New alveolar bone regenerated after insertion of synthetic bone and 6 months later a blade implant was inserted into the newly regenerated bone. **A,** failing implant preoperative picture. **B,** the implant is removed and the tissue thoroughly curetted. Note the complete saucerization and cylindrical loss of bone around the previous implant which was in place for 16 years. **C,** 6 months after HTR polymer was placed into the defect the tissue is opened. Note the new alveolar bone. Subsequently a blade implant was placed in this ridge.

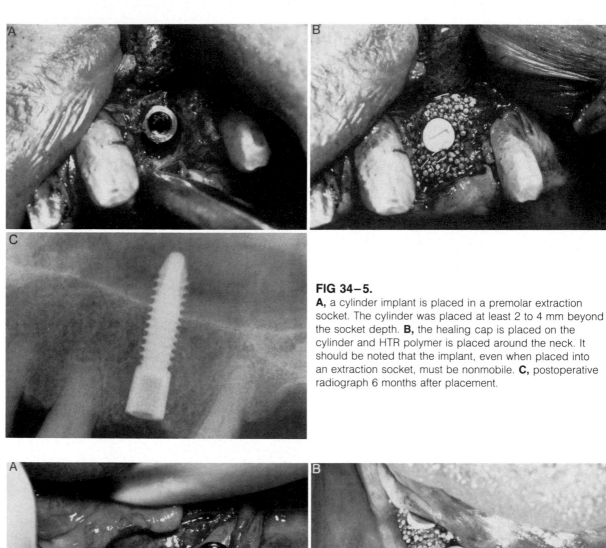

FIG 34–5.
A, a cylinder implant is placed in a premolar extraction socket. The cylinder was placed at least 2 to 4 mm beyond the socket depth. **B,** the healing cap is placed on the cylinder and HTR polymer is placed around the neck. It should be noted that the implant, even when placed into an extraction socket, must be nonmobile. **C,** postoperative radiograph 6 months after placement.

FIG 34–6.
A, implant cylinders placed to maximum depth. Note collars still exposed. **B,** ridge augmentation with HTR polymer around the neck as well as in adjacent bone. Note healing collars on the implants.

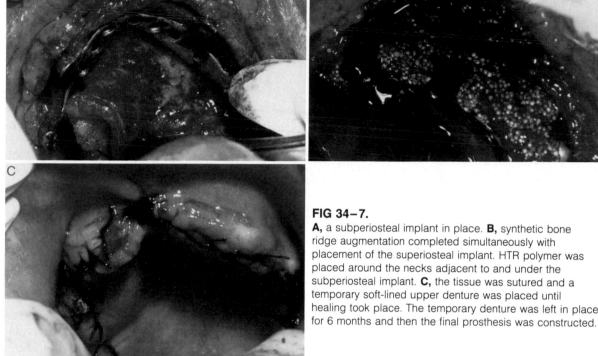
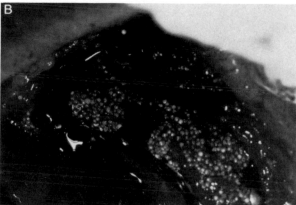

FIG 34–7.
A, a subperiosteal implant in place. **B,** synthetic bone ridge augmentation completed simultaneously with placement of the superiosteal implant. HTR polymer was placed around the necks adjacent to and under the subperiosteal implant. **C,** the tissue was sutured and a temporary soft-lined upper denture was placed until healing took place. The temporary denture was left in place for 6 months and then the final prosthesis was constructed.

rather than an encapsulation as seen in hydroxylapatite.[20] A recent periodontal study has shown, in human bone block specimens, histologic evidence of new attachment, osteogenesis, and cementogenesis in host tissues adjacent to the graft particles.[21]

HTR polymer is currently one of the best synthetic bone substitute materials available (see Table 34–1) and has also been used in a variety of nondental procedures, such as spinal fusions, bone filler in orthopedic reconstructive surgery, and augmentation for nose, chin, and cheek.

Eight university-based human clinical studies started in 1986 covering many applications of HTR polymer will be completed in 1991. The preliminary results are promising.[22]

Resorbable and Nonporous

These polymers, which are primarily based on lactic and glycolic acid compounds, are reported as both osteogenic and resorbable after placement.[23]

These materials are available in various forms that the practitioner can cut to fit a particular need during surgery. Polylactic polyglycolic granules have been used primarily in third molar extraction sites to assist in maintaining the clot and to generate new bone and have been in common use for years under such names as Gelfoam and Surgicel.[24]

Ceramic and Nonceramic Derivatives (Nonporous, Porous, Resorbable, Nonresorbable)

Hydroxylapatite is probably the most tested and studied material to date as a ceramic and nonceramic bone substitute material. Its biocompatibility has been successfully demonstrated in many animal systems.[25–27] Its nonresorbability, as well as its resorbability, are also well-known.[28] These properties depend upon the density and crystallinity of the material, as well as local environmental factors.[28]

Hydroxylapatite has been the subject of numerous investigations as to its osteogenic potential. It has been shown that when it is used in areas where host bone is found, bone can deposit on its nonporous *surface* by osteoconduction.[23, 28] However, individual particle areas surrounded by thick fibrous encapsulation have also been noted frequently, especially in areas not in direct opposition to bone. It appears, then, that hydroxylapatite may act only as a space filler in certain local situations and thus possesses little or no osteogenic potential.[29, 30] De Groot and co-workers have stated that the biomechanical properties of sintered hydroxylapatite are poor in terms of osteoinduction.[31]

Hydroxylapatite is a generic term for a form of calcium phosphate material. It is the principle inorganic component of bone and teeth. There are many different forms, rendering the material either nonresorbable or resorbable.[23] In 1985, a resorbable form was introduced into dentistry* but since hydroxylapatite is not osteogenic, one author has questioned its scientific value.[23]

Placement of hydroxylapatite coatings on endosteal and subperiosteal implants has created a whole new series of various implant offerings by manufacturers.[32] The theory behind this innovation is that this coated surface will increase the surface adhesion to bone. Concern has been voiced that, in the event of gingival recession around a hydroxylapatite-coated implant, there may be long-term periodontal maintenance problems.[23] Initial results seem promising, but it is too soon for final judgments.

Various forms of hydroxylapatite (Calcitite†, Periograf‡, Alveolgraf§), as a dense nonporous ceramic material, are available today for use in dentistry.

Although biocompatible and inert, these ceramics as a group are not ideal as synthetic bone materials (see Table 34–1). They are nonosteogenic, difficult to handle, cannot be molded in exact replicas, are difficult to shape, are not bacteriostatic, are cationic electrically charged, are hydrophobic, and are

*OsteoGen, Impladent, Ltd., Holliswood, N.Y., and G.B.D. Medical, Valley Stream, N.Y.
  †Calcitite, Calcitek Drug Co., San Diego, Calif.
  ‡Periograf, Sterling Drug Co., New York, N.Y.
  §Alveolgraf, Sterling Drug Co., New York, N.Y.

not microporous. Even when using hydroxylapatite as cones in alveolar ridges of humans for ridge maintenance, a 60% rate of failure and exposure of these cones was reported. The cones do not preserve the alveolar bone.[9]

Hydroxylapatite seems to act more like a filler than a bone stimulator. Six months after particulate hydroxylapatite replacement, one practicing dentist observed a "sand-like substance surrounded by dense connective tissue" (L. Linkow, D.D.S., written communication, 1987). Its greatest attribute seems to be its biocompatibility, allowing a noninflammatory *fibrous* healing. However, it should be noted that many successful hydroxylapatite procedures have been reported in the literature, using the material for ridge augmentation and in periodontal defect lesions,[28] even though hydroxylapatite has not been shown to regenerate a functional attachment apparatus or to possess osteoinductive properties.[33, 34]

In making ceramic hydroxylapatite porous,* one manufacturer improved its osteoconductive properties considerably.[35] But the end result is a material that is very brittle and difficult to use. Its use has been limited to periodontal lesions only. Some authors found technical problems in the use and handling of the material,[36] while others observed greater pocket depths with Interpore* as compared with clinical control areas.[37] LeGeros gave an extremely informative review of the field in 1988.[38]

DISCUSSION

Although there are strong indications that HTR polymer may be the ideal synthetic bone material that our profession has been seeking, the results of controlled human studies in the bone maintenance, ridge augmentation, and periodontal defect areas must continue to be submitted to the profession for peer review before a conclusion can be reached.

Can hydroxylapatite be improved for clinical use? If the material can be clinically controlled, mixed with other materials (collagen?), be made porous or moldable, elicit an osteogenic instead of a fibrous response, and be made less difficult to use,

*Interpore, Interpore, San Diego, Calif.

then hydroxylapatite would be indicated for increased use. It is proving useful in some clinical applications today, for example, as a chemical coating attached to subperiosteal and endosteal metal implants. Results still remain equivocal as Kent reported fibrous connective tissue around ceramic hydroxylapatite used alone or with hydroxylapatite-collagen blocks in a dog study.[39]

We are encouraged by the preliminary results of Linkow, Boyne (personal communication, 1988),

and Ashman,[40] who have utilized HTR polymer with various forms and sizes of metal implants (e.g., cylinders, blades, or subperiosteals). These dentists have placed implants into or on top of HTR polymer augmented ridges, used HTR polymer around osteotomy sites, around the neck of implants, and as an immediate tooth replacement (cylinder) in extraction sites, with outstanding results. In the case of the immediate tooth replacement, the HTR polymer cylinders were buried for 6 to 8 months. They were then

TABLE 34-2.

Uses and Applications of Synthetic Bone Materials in Dentistry

	Nonresorbable Microporous Polymers	Lactic Acid	Nonporous HA	Porous HA	TCP	Resorbable HA
1. Bone maintenance (post-extraction and post-implantation)						
a. Particulate (granular)						
Porous	***	0	0	0	0	***
Solid root shapes	0	0	0	0	0	0
b. Root forms						
Porous	***	0	0	0	0	***
Solid, as a coating on metal	0	0	***	0	0	*
c. Implant replica or placed with implants						
Porous	***	0	0	0	0	***
Solid	0	0	*	0	0	0
2. Ridge augmentation						
a. Particulate						
Porous	***	0	0	*	0	*
Solid	0	0	***	0	0	0
b. Ridge forms						
Porous	***	0	0	*	0	0
Solid	0	0	*	0	0	0
c. Immediate replication						
Porous	***	0	0	0	0	***
Solid	0	0	0	0	0	0
3. Periodontal defects						
a. Particulate						
Porous	***	0	0	**+	0	***
Solid	0	0	*	0	*	0
4. Maxillofacial reconstruction						
a. Particulate						
Porous	***	0	0	*	0	***
Solid	0	0	**	0	0	0
b. Ridge forms						
Porous	***	0	0	0	0	***
Solid	0	0	*	0	0	0
c. Immediate replication						
Porous	***	0	0	0	0	***
Solid	0	0	0	0	0	0

HA = hydroxylapatite; TCP = tricalcium phosphate; *** = best use; ** = routinely used; * = slightly used; 0 = unable to be used; + = porous HA disintegrates with too much pressure (packing).

placed in function with a crown. Only 2 years have elapsed with these implants in function, and results are excellent, although it is much too short a time for final judgments.

By recognizing the emergence of a new class of restorative material—synthetic bone—in the general practice of dentistry, the practitioner has taken a new step and is able to do an almost endless variety of new and exciting treatment procedures that were thought impossible only a few short years ago. Besides using synthetic bone with implants, the areas of single or multiple extraction bone maintenance,[4, 18, 19] periodontal defect lesions,[10] and restoring the atrophic mandible (ridge augmentation)[41] open a truly new and exciting extension, and with good scientific basis, for the practice of dentistry (Table 34–2).

SUMMARY AND CONCLUSIONS

A brief overview has been presented dealing with the clinical and philosophical uses of synthetic bone materials in dentistry. One material, HTR polymer, appears adaptable to many clinical situations. Other synthetic bone materials have been researched extremely well and all have a place in dentistry. But what is clear from the literature, as well as from clinical experience, is that all bone substitutes are not ideal. The ceramics as a group are difficult to use and are not osteogenic. Attempts to improve their acceptability have included forming a mixture (composite) with other materials (e.g., collagen, plaster of Paris) and making hydroxylapatite porous. In making hydroxylapatite porous, however, it becomes extremely brittle and weak with a very low compressive strength. As a group, the ceramics still have drawbacks. They are hydrophobic, not electrically charged, nonresistant to infection, not easily moldable into any shape or form, lack osteogenic potential, and are brittle in a microporous structure. We suggest that the nonresorbable, microporous polymeric materials will become the major synthetic bone substitute material in clinical practice. All of the materials reviewed are adaptable to some areas of dentistry and in a few years, synthetic bone will

be as common to everyday practice as bonding materials are today.

REFERENCES

1. Ashman A: The dramatic future of the polymers in dentistry. *NY J Dent* 1972; 42:331–341.
2. Ashman A: On implantable materials. *NY J Dent* 1974; 44(6):180–185.
3. Dragoo MR, Sullivan HC: A clinical and histologic evaluation of autogenous iliac bone grafts in humans. *J Periodontol* 1970; 41:566.
4. Schallhorn RC, Hiatt WH, Boyce W: Iliac transplants in periodontal therapy. *J Periodontol* 1970; 44:566-580.
5. Mellonig JT, Bowers GM, Bright RW, et al: Clinical evaluation of freeze dried bone allografts in periodontal defects. *J Periodontol* 1976; 47:125-131.
6. Urist MR, Strates BS: Bone formation in implants of partially and wholly demineralized bone matrix. *Clin Orthop* 1970; 71:271.
7. Hodosh M, Shklar G, Povar M: Current status of the polymer tooth implant concept. *Dent Clin North Am* 1970; 14:103–115.
8. Grenoble DE, Kim RL: Progress in the evaluation of a vitreous carbon endosteal implant. *Ariz State Dent J* 1973; 19:12.
9. Kwon H, el Deeb M, Morstad T, et al: Alveolar ridge maintenance with hydroxylapatite ceramic cones in humans. *J Oral Maxillofac Surg* 1986; 44:503–508.
10. Krejci CB, Bissada NF, Farah C, et al: Clinical evaluation of porous and nonporous hydroxylapatite in the treatment of human bony periodontal defects. *J Periodontol* 1987; 58:521–528.
11. Bowers GM, Vargo JW, Levy B, et al: Histologic observations following the placement of tricalcium phosphate implants in human intrabony defects. *J Periodontol* 1986; 57:286–287.
12. Rabalais ML Jr, Yukna RA, Mayer ET: Evaluation of durapatite ceramics as an alloplastic implant in periodontal defects I: Initial six months results. *J Periodontol* 1981; 52:680-689.
13. Leake D: Contouring split ribs for correction of severe mandibular atrophy. *J Oral Maxillofac Surg* 1976; 34:940.
14. Ashman A, Bruins P: Prevention of alveolar bone loss postextraction with HTR polymer grafting material. *J Oral Maxillofac Surg* 1985; 60:146–153.

15. Krejci CB, Farah CF: Osseous grafting in periodontol therapy, part I: Osseous graft materials. *Compendium* 1987; 8:722–724, 726, 728.

16. Ashman A, Bruins P: A new immediate hard tissue replacement (HTR) for bone in the oral cavity. *J Oral Implantol* 1982; 10:419–452.

17. Ashman A: Applications of HTR polymer in dentistry. *Compendium* 1988; 10(suppl):S330–S336.

18. Murray V: Clinical applications of HTR polymer in periodontal surgery. *Compendium* 1988; 10(suppl):S342–S347.

19. Norman BA: HTR polymer bone grafting material: A clinical survey of 647 cases. *Compendium* 1987; 8:832.

20. Kamen P: Attachment of oral fibroblasts to HTR polymer. *Compendium* 1988; 10(suppl):350–352.

21. Stahl S, unpublished data, Nov 1988.

22. Boyne PJ, Cranin AN, Leake D, et al: Preliminary reports. *Compendium* 1988; 10(suppl):S337–S341.

23. Masters DH: Bone and bone substitutes. *Can Dent Assoc J* 1988; 16:55–64.

24. Olson RAJ, Roberts RL, Osbon DB: A comparative study of polylactic acid, Gelfoam and Surgicel in healing extraction sites. *Oral Surg* 1982; 53:441–449.

25. Kaban LB, Glowacki J: Induced osteogenesis in the repair of experimental defects in rats. *Proc Am Inst Biol* 1980; 73:291–306.

26. Nirva S: Experimental studies of the implantation in HA in the medullary canal of rabbits. Presented at the First World Biomaterial Congress, Baden, Austria, May 1980.

27. Boyne PJ, Rothstein SS, Gumaer KI, et al: Long-term study of hydroxylapatite implants in canine alveolar bone. *J Oral Maxillofac Surg* 1984; 42:589–594.

28. Krejci CB, Farah CF, Bissada NF: Osseous grafting in periodontol therapy, part II: Non-osseous graft materials. *Compendium* 1987; 8:785–787,790,792–794.

29. Rabalais ML, Yukna RA, Mayer ET: Evaluation of durapatite ceramics as an alloplastic implant in periodontol osscous defects. *J Periodontol* 1981; 52:680–689.

30. Froum SJ, Kushner L, Scopp IW, et al: Human clinical and histologic responses to durapatite implants in intraosseous lesions. *J Periodontol* 1982; 53:719–725.

31. de Groot K, Geesink R, Klein CPAT, et al: Plasma sprayed coatings of hydroxylapatite. *J Biomed Mater Res* 1987; 21:1375–1381.

32. Golec TS: The use of hydroxylapatite to coat subperiostcal implants. *J Oral Implantol* 1983; 10:21–38.

33. Saphos S: The use of Periograf in periodontal defects. *J Periodontol* 1986; 57:7.

34. Ganeles J, Listgarten MA, Evian CI: Ultrastructure of durapatite–periodontal tissue interface in human intrabony defects. *J Periodontol* 1986; 57:133–140.

35. Piecuch JF, Fedorka NJ: Results of soft-tissue surgery over implanted replamineform hydroxylapatite (Interpore). *J Oral Maxillofac Surg* 1983; 41:801–806.

36. West TL: Coralline hydroxylapatite implants in canine and human periodontal defects. *Curr Clin Pract* 1985; 29:435–447.

37. Kenney EB, Lekovic V, Sa Ferreira JC, et al: Bone formation within porous hydroxylapatite implants in human periodontal defects. *J Periodontol* 1986; 57:76–83.

38. LeGeros RZ: Calcium phosphate materials in restorative dentistry: A review. *Adv Dent Res* 1988; 2:164–180.

39. Kent J: Bone response to hydroxylapatite and hydroxylapatite-collagen block implants in dogs. Presented at Osseous Integration Society Meeting, Louisiana State University, New Orleans, La, September 1988.

40. Ashman A: The HTR molded ridge for alveolar augmentation, an alternative to the subperiosteal implant, autogenous bone graft, or injectable bone grafting materials. *J Oral Implantol* 1986; 12:556–575.

Chapter 35

Use of Bone Augmentation or Substitute Material in Implantology

Wade B. Hammer, D.D.S.

The ability to restore satisfactory anatomic form to the deficient maxilla or mandible has long been the desire of the dental practitioner. The augmentation of deficient denture-bearing structures has historically led to the use of bone, metallic devices, numerous medical-grade polymers, and plaster of Paris. Recently, attention has turned to the use of sophisticated bioceramics. This chapter presents a brief review of the indications for bone substitute materials, the requirements for such materials, and a discussion of the current concepts of bone augmentation in dental implantology.

The loss of maxillary or mandibular bone height and contour, regardless of the cause in the particular patient, is very problematic for the dentist who must restore masticatory function with dental prosthetic devices. The lateral stability of full dentures is greatly influenced by the size and shape of the residual alveolar ridges. Even after the removal of one or several teeth the remaining ridge form is often less than desirable for the esthetic pontic design required in removable partial or fixed dental prostheses.

Alveolar ridge resorption is a continuous process, contributing to denture instability, especially the lower denture. Denture instability affects a large percentage of the more than 36 million edentulous people in the United States alone.[1] Upon the loss of teeth, particularly when the patient is rendered edentulous, changes in stress, which are usually due to denture pressure on the residual alveolar processes, result in remodeling of the endosteal trabeculae

bringing about overall dimensional decrease of the mandible or maxilla. Systemic factors such as osteopenia, osteomalacia, osteoporosis, hyperthyroidism, or hyperparathyroidism are believed to alter bone metabolism resulting in decreased mineralization and the eventual loss of height and form of the residual alveolar ridge.

The traumatic loss of bone results from sporting, industrial, or vehicular accidents, and from social encounters. Avoidable iatrogenic bone loss possibly has occurred when insufficient care has been exerted to avoid loss of alveolar bone and cortical plate during removal of teeth. The unnecessary elevation of large mucoperiosteal flaps during dentoalveolar surgery may also result in more rapid bone resorption.

Loss of bone contour and form resulting from surgical management of oral lesions is common. Defects resulting from surgical removal of malignant oral lesions often requires extensive bone and split-thickness skin grafting for reconstruction. Those defects, on the other hand, that result from operations to remove benign lesions, can often be corrected by bone grafting or by the implantation of a compatible material.

INDICATIONS FOR AUGMENTATION IMPLANTOLOGY

Defects and atrophy of the mandible and maxilla are crippling. Not only is denture-wearing ability and masticatory function jeopardized, but such patients are affected physiologically and psychologically. Regardless of the causes of the loss of bone, common procedures used to correct the anatomic defects relate to:

1. The augmentation of deficiencies in the labial contour of the maxilla or mandible
2. The augmentation of deficient maxillary and mandibular residual alveolar ridge
3. The prevention of alveolar bone loss
4. The reconstruction of discontinuity defects of the mandible[2]

BONE GRAFTING

For decades augmentation of the deficient mandible or maxilla has been performed using either autologous bone grafting or allogenic freeze-dried bone implantation or by a combination of these methods. Xenogenic bone implantation using animal bone has been attempted, but with unacceptable results. The use of autogenous bone grafting, whether the donor source be rib, iliac crest, or iliac marrow, initially seems successful. There remains the probability, however, that a skin graft vestibuloplasty is necessary and that a portion of the graft may subsequently be lost by resorption. When autogenous bone is used, the additional factors of hospitalization, procurement of the graft, cost, and the extensive nature of some bone grafting procedures limit the application of this method for a readily available bone augmentation procedure.[3, 4]

BIOMATERIALS

Owing to the problems with bone graft augmentation, the search continues for a superior alloplastic material, or one of synthetic, nonanimal, origin. In discussing the need for biomaterials research, Hall[5] has described the requirements for any alloplastic implantable device that is to be in contact with viable tissue. The following definitions have been offered for mutual acceptance by materials researchers and clinicians:

1. *Biocompatability*. A general term meaning capable of being implanted; causing no systemic toxic reaction, having no carcinogenic qualities, and having no local reaction that compromises function, causes pain, swelling, or necrosis in adjacent tissues.

2. *Tissue interfacing*. Being physically adjacent to viable tissue. When used without qualification, interfacing does not necessarily denote compatibility.

3. *Tissue compatability*. A specific term. Similar to the more general term "biocompatible," but relating to local tissue response.

4. *Nontoxic*. Nonpoisonous. That which causes no local tissue death and no systemic reaction due to degraded poisonous byproducts.

Considering these definitions, and clinical experience, any such biomaterial to be implantable for bone augmentation must be resistant to corrosion or resorption by body fluids, nonallergenic, capable of uniformly transferring functional forces, easily shaped or prepared for implantation, relatively inexpensive, and require relatively simple surgical procedures. Another desirable feature is that the biomaterial possess an interface surface into which viable tissue will proliferate, thus providing stability.

Numerous alloplastic materials have been used for augmentation of the maxilla and mandible. The various categories of biomaterials are discussed here with a major emphasis on the bioceramics.

Metallic Augmentation

Bone prostheses historically have been predominantly fashioned from biocompatible metals.[2] Such devices, except for more modern alloys, corrode in body fluids, produce inflammation, swelling, pain, and erosion of bone at stressed sites, or are experimentally carcinogenic.

As for augmentation of atrophic ridges, uncorroded smooth metallic prostheses do not attach to the adjacent tissues, remain unstable, and at the present time have proved unsatisfactory when used alone.

Extensive work and wide clinical use of metallic temporomandibular joint and other orthopedic prostheses that have porous ceramic coatings have proved more acceptable. The porous coating provides a surface to which interfacing surfaces may firmly attach. The bioceramics will be discussed subsequently in more detail.

Augmentation With Medical Polymers

Medical-grade organic polymers such as methyl methacrylate, polystyrene, polyethylene, polyurethanes, methylcellulose, polyvinyl alcohols, nylon, and silicone rubber substances are among the many polymeric compounds tested and used in the fabrication of prostheses.[2]

Presently, medical polymers are used for soft tissue implantation in essentially every organ system. Although there are many favorable features found with modern medical polymers, degradation and lack of compatibility between polymers and the physiologic environment present disadvantages for their clinical use. Degradation products such as carbon 14 have been found in the urine of rats after implantation of tagged polystyrene, polyethylene, and polymethylmethacrylate. Polyurethanes and polyvinyl alcohols have also been found to deteriorate and fragment.[6]

Certain high-grade silicone rubbers are the choice of materials for long-term soft tissue implantation in the human. These materials are not metabolized nor do they cause foreign body reactions as do the other polymers.[7] Boucher reported the successful use of Silastic to augment the deficient residual alveolar ridge.[8, 9] However, owing to the relatively low tensile strength of silicone rubber, the material hypothetically would have limited value in a load-bearing area such as an alveolar ridge undergoing masticatory function. Clinical use of injectable Silastic has resulted in breakdown of the material and dehiscense when pressure-loaded by the wearing of dentures. More recently, the injection of liquid silicone rubber has been limited because of the potential for material migration.

Ceramic Augmentation

Except for early reports of using inorganic substances such as plaster of Paris and epoxy-impregnated ceramic materials, the interest in bioceramics for internal prosthetic applications only became popular in the early 1970s.[10, 11]

Ceramics, substances made from various inorganic minerals, have been suggested as replacement for bone in reconstructive surgery. The compatibility of implanted ceramic pellets with the musculoskeletal system was reported by Hulbert et al. in 1970.[12] Calcium aluminate pellets with interconnecting pores of various sizes, from 44 to 75 μm to 150 to 200 μm, were placed within the femurs of adult dogs. The materials with pore size of less than 150 μm exhibited an ingrowth of fibrous connective tissue into the surface porosity. Specimens with pores greater than 150 μm had ingrowth of bone with well-formed haversian systems present as far as 2 mm inward from the surface. Soft tissue and bone filled the surface pores of the ceramic pellets, providing firm anchorage, thus greatly decreasing the problem of extrusion which often occurred with other alloplasts.[13]

Ceramic materials such as calcium aluminate and aluminum oxide were found to have a specific gravity, coefficient of friction, and strength comparable to bone.[14] These materials have proved nontoxic and nonantigenic by the use of laboratory tissue culture techniques and repeated intracutaneous and intraperitoneal injections.[15] Testing concluded that the undesirable aspects of porous ceramic materials, such as brittleness and lack of ductility, are of less biological importance after soft tissue or bone had filled the porous portions of the implanted material.

Powdered marble and alumina were the raw materials used to produce a calcium aluminate ceramic structure with an intricate network of interconnecting pores communicating with the sample surface. Pore size was produced by the inclusion of controlled-sized particles of calcium carbonate within the slurry prior to placement in the firing kiln.

Calcium aluminate ceramic segments with pore sizes of 150 to 200 μm were implanted to augment deficient residual mandibular ridges in dogs.[16] The implants were placed through either a tunneling procedure or through the development of a vestibular incision and full-thickness mucoperiosteal flap. Either procedure proved successful for alveolar ridge augmentation in the dogs. After a 1-year follow-up the implants were clinically, radiographically, and histologically compatible with the oral soft and hard tissues. Bone proliferation occurred at a distance of 1 to 2 mm into the surface porosity. The conclusion was that ceramic segments have potential value for augmentation of deficient alveolar ridges. This animal study, however, did not include pressure loading of the ceramic segments with dentures for masticatory function, as the dogs were maintained by a soft diet.

A study utilizing similar, but individually designed, calcium aluminate implants for mandibular ridge augmentation in human subjects was reported in 1974.[17] Of six patients who underwent augmentation of deficient mandibular ridges with the ceramic implants, three functioned with dentures for up to 3 years. However, owing to dehiscence, traumatic avulsion, or chronic infection, all the solid implants eventually were removed.

In 1976, implants fabricated from porous aluminum oxide and high-density polyethylene sponge blocks were studied in dog models. Neither of these materials proved successful in the laboratory phase because of brittleness, roughness, difficulty in implant preparation, and unacceptable bone resorption.[18] Research on the use of ceramics in solid block form for ridge augmentation came to a standstill.

The materials previously discussed have a continued popularity in orthopedic and cardiovascular research. Tibial plateau, segmental bone, and cardiac valve replacement research continues with solid preformed implants of calcium aluminate, aluminum oxide, and other inorganic ceramic materials.

Calcium Phosphate Bioceramics

Recently, interest in the calcium phosphate systems has intensified, particularly with those biomaterials composed of either nonbiodegradable hydroxylapatite $[Ca_{10}(PO_4)_6(OH)_2]$ or the biodegradable tricalcium phosphate $[Ca_3(PO_4)_2]$.[19] These biomaterials have chemical formulations similar to vertebrate bone and teeth. Dense calcium phosphate bioceramics are processed by using high-pressure compaction of calcium phosphate powder at a high sintering temperature to form a shaped block or other form. Porosity is produced with a minimum pore size of 100 μm. The porosity is accomplished by the inclusion of particles of naphthalene which evaporates during sintering.[20]

A unique property of the calcium phosphate implants is their ability to bond to bone. Extensive experiment and clinical research has proved these materials to be the most biocompatible known,[19] although their physical characteristics may limit their application as hard tissue substitutes.

Dense calcium phosphate, particularly hydroxylapatite, is used in many forms by oral and maxillofacial surgeons and dental implantologists. Block form, either porous or nonporous, and the particulate porous form of hydroxylapatite is by far the most commonly utilized biomaterial in dentistry and oral reconstructive surgery today.

The use of both block and particulate forms of hydroxylapatite are used for the establishment of stability in segmental maxillary and mandibular surgery.[21, 22] Hydroxylapatite placed in cystic defects, osteotomy sites, or in facial contour defects has proved satisfactory when used alone or in conjunction with autologous bone.

The use of particulate hydroxylapatite for alveolar ridge augmentation was reported by Kent et al. in 1982 after an extensive multi-institutional study.[23] The material when used alone or in combination with equal volumes of autologous bone marrow and a subperiosteal tunneling procedure serves as a suitable bone substitute for ridge augmentation. These studies indicated that after 6 years of denture wearing on augmented ridges, only 10% to 15% of the surgically acquired ridge height was lost over time. The conclusion was that this loss was due to compression of the material. In 1986 Kent et al. estimated that 20,000 patients had received such ridge augmentations in the United States alone. A classification and treatment of alveolar ridge deficiency as proposed by Kent et al.[23] is provided in Table 35–1.

Procedure for Hydroxylapatite Augmentation.—Today, the commonly used procedure for mandibular and maxillary ridge augmentation is the implantation of commercially available hydroxylapatite particles. Standard local anesthesia procedures are performed to provide anesthesia and hemostasis. An effort is made to prevent ballooning of the mucosa and periosteum since such an occurrence can produce undesirable extension of the pocket or tunnel where the hydroxylapatite is to be inserted.

For the mandibular augmentation procedure, an incision is made bilaterally and anterior to the mental foramina at the canine tooth site. These first inci-

TABLE 35–1.

Classification and Treatment of Alveolar Ridge Deficiency

Class I
  Alveolar ridge is adequate in height but inadequate in width, usually with lateral deficiencies on undercut areas. Patients received hydroxylapatite (HA) alone: 2–4 g for each anteroposterior area and 6–8 g for the total ridge.
Class II
  Alveolar ridge is deficient in both height and width and presents a knife-edge appearance. Patients received HA alone: 3–5 g for each anterposterior area and 8–10 g for the total ridge.
Class III
  Alveolar ridge has been resorbed to the level of the basilar bone producing a concave form in the posterior areas of the mandible and a sharp bony ridge form with bulbous mobile soft tissue in the maxilla. Patients received HA alone: 8–12 g or combined with autogenous iliac cancellous bone (1 g HA to 1 cc of bone).
Class IV
  There is resorption of the basilar bone producing a pencil-thin flat mandible or maxilla. Patients received HA: 10–15 g mixed with autogenous bone in a 1:1 ratio. Patients unable to permit harvesting of iliac bone may have HA alone to increase ridge heights modestly. HA combined with bone is recommended for larger augmentation and to strengthen the mandible.

Modified from Kent JN, Quinn JH, Zide MF, et al: *J Am Dent Assoc* 1982; 105:993–1004.

sions are made only through mucosa and extend from the attached gingival margin inferiorly into the vestibule, or approximately 1.5 to 2.0 cm. By blunt dissection, the mental foramina and neurovascular bundles are located, but extensive isolation of these structures is avoided. Using a periosteal elevator, a submucosal tunnel is elevated along the crest of the ridge posterior to the retromolar pad. These supraperiosteal tunnels are carefully controlled to avoid the neurovascular structures, lingual extension, and the forming of a pocket larger than the diameter of the plastic syringe that will be used to inject the hydroxylapatite. Through the incisions and below the roof of the mucosal tunnel, the periosteum is incised along the crest of the bony ridge and reflected buccally and slightly lingually. The removal of a strip of periosteum will allow contact of the injected hydroxylapatite with bone. The previously loaded syringes are moistened with normal saline and inserted into the tunnels. The hydroxylapatite is gently extruded from the syringe and finger-molded into the tunnels. When the tunnels, which can also extend into the anterior aspects of the mandible, are filled, the particles are firmly packed with an instrument such as mouth mirror handle. After finger-molding the augmented ridge again, the incisions are sutured with a

nonresorbable material. When the ceramic material is combined with bone marrow, a similar procedure is used.

Maxillary ridge augmentation is accomplished in a similar manner through bilateral incisions placed in the canine tooth sites. Care must be taken to avoid overextension of the tunneling to the labial aspect. The tunnel must be placed on the crest of the ridge if possible. The deficient maxillary ridge is often associated with fibrous and mobile redundant tissue. Such fibrous tissue can be removed through the incisions to form space for injection of the particulate material. Again, for satisfactory stability, the implanted material must be placed on bone rather than periosteum.

The use of postsurgical splints for stabilization is widely advocated; however, the previously designed splints must be supported by regions of the mandible or maxilla that are not augmented. Otherwise the splint will compress the implanted material. The mandibular splint is soft-lined and secured in place with circummandibular wiring or nylon sutures. Maxillary splints are likewise soft-lined to adapt to the newly acquired ridge form but are fixed into place with palatal or perialveolar screws, or pins. Needless to say, any such augmentation procedure should be planned conjointly with the dentist who is to design and fabricate the patient's dentures. The areas of desired augmentation are waxed onto a study cast. The splint is then designed to contact the nonaugmented ridge in at least the retromolar and the anterior labial areas. Maxillary splints are more stable since the entire palate serves as a rest to prevent compression of the ceramic particles. Patients are maintained on antibiotic coverage and a soft diet for 7 to 10 days when splints are removed. Four to 6 weeks' healing time should allow for stabilization of the ridge prior to the making of impressions for dentures.

Complications

Problems with the procedure include wound dehiscence, short-term infection, neuropathies, and a less-than-desirable ridge form. Experience has shown that dehiscence is minimal and will usually granulate over with maintenance of daily irrigation and adequate oral hygiene. Infection is rare and has usually been found to be secondary to splints. Pressure points, extended flanges, and circummandibular wires or sutures have been responsible for such complications. Careful attention to acrylic splint design, soft-lining procedures, and adherence to sterile procedures will prevent many such complications.

Altered sensation in the chin and inferior lip are unfortunately quite common following augmentation of the mandibular ridge and are caused by the manipulation of the mental neurovascular structures. Thus, the patient should be well informed of this potential hazard. It is again stressed that careful but minimal manipulation of these structures during surgery is critical. Every attempt should be made to avoid trauma to or placement of hydroxylapatite over the mental foramina or nerves. Unless the nerve fibers have been transected or compressed, the remission of hypoesthesia, paresthesia, or anesthesia has an acceptable prognosis.

Compression of the particulate ceramic mass and migration of the implanted material are common problems. When the surgically created tunnels are overextended the material dislodges or migrates buccally or lingually, often creating undesirable irregularities. Often additional surgical procedures are nec-

essary to reduce these irregularities to a more desirable ridge form. When the patient is to receive a previously planned split-thickness skin graft vestibuloplasty, the ceramic-fibrous irregularities are contoured simultaneously. Many patients, however, do not require the skin graft vestibuloplasty, but do require an alveoplasty of their augmented ridge.

Recently, alterations of the augmentation procedure to assist in retention of the desired ridge form have been reported. A multicenter report by Mehlisch et al.[24] describes the use of a material composed of purified fibrillar collagen and particulate hydroxylapatite for 99 ridge augmentations. They report a significant increase in retention of desired ridge form and superior handling characteristics of the material. Lew et al.[25] report the use of an intraoral alveolar ridge soft tissue expander. An inflatable device is inserted by way of the tunnel procedure. Approximately 2 weeks later, after the formation of a fibrous capsule around the expander, it is removed and particulate hydroxylapatite is inserted into the tunnel. An advantage is that a subsequent vestibuloplasty is probably not necessary.[25]

The use of collagen tubes for controlling the migration of particulate hydroxylapatite has been described by Shen and Gongloff in animals.[26] Gongloff has since used commercially available collagen tubes for particulate hydroxylapatite ridge augmentation in 20 patients.[27] Three segments of the sausagelike implants were inserted for each patient, leaving the sites above the mental foramina unenhanced. The conclusion was that the ceramic material is well stabilized. Lambert[28] has designed a two-piece surgical splint to eliminate the migration of hydroxylapatite particles.

The complications of ridge augmentation with the use of particulate ceramics are minimal, considering its the proven biocompatibility and stability. Diligent and continuous research is solving these minor drawbacks for a system which is proving to be revolutionary to dental prosthetics and the search for bone substitutes.

Solid Block Hydroxylapatite

Blocks of hydroxylapatite have been used successfully in orthognathic surgery as a material to maintain stability or to serve as spacer blocks,[21] and ceramic cones have been used in fresh extraction sites to prevent loss of alveolar ridge height and width. Both animal research[29] and human trials[30] concluded that preservation of alveolar bone is not significantly improved by the insertion of either cone-shaped or particulate hydroxylapatite into fresh extraction sites.

The use of porous ceramic blocks or anatomically shaped forms for augmentation of atrophic mandibular ridges has shown varied success. Experimentally, such procedures were satisfactory in animals[16] but a failure in humans[17] when solid porous calcium aluminate was implanted. Porous blocks of hydroxylapatite gave promising animal results. However, Hupp and McKenna,[31] in 1988, concluded that the use of blocks of porous hydroxylapatite to augment atrophic mandibular ridges was unsatisfactory because of numerous complications. They reported dehiscence, exposure of the implant, chronic pain, infection, and overall patient displeasure with removal of 37 of the original 45 implanted blocks. Time of removal ranged from 3 weeks to 35 months and only 2 of 11 patients continued to wear dentures over implanted blocks.[31]

Thus solid blocks of ceramic materials have had their trials and have been found unsatisfactory. When one considers the physiologic stress placed on the thin mucoperiosteum which overlies such implants, it is not difficult to expect dehiscence and exposure of the material. The wearing of dentures over such implants overtaxes the functional ability of this friable tissue. Even when such tissue is replaced by skin the prognosis is presently dismal.

Other Uses of Ceramic Materials

The literature is abundant with reports of the use of inorganic ceramic materials or substitutes for bone or for bone augmentation. The implantation of particulate hydroxylapatite for the correction of deficient facial contours has been reported. Hydroxylapatite, in combination with microfibrillar degradable collagen, was used for augmentation of the zygomatic eminence in 11 patients, resulting in a stable and esthetically satisfactory procedure when used as an adjunct to Le Fort I osteotomy procedures.[32]

Hydroxylapatite and autologous cancellous marrow from the ileum were used to augment the posterior mandibular ridge simultaneously with an interposed bone grafting procedure in the symphyseal area anterior to the mental foramina.[33] Enhanced denture-wearing ability was reported in 22 (81.5%) of 27 patients treated.

A biodegradable material, polyglycolic acid combined with proteolipid, has been used experimentally to successfully repair mandibular defects in dogs.[34] This method could serve as an alternative to more commonly used autogenous and allogenic bone substances for reconstruction following loss of mandibular form or continuity.

COMBINATION OF IMPLANT SYSTEMS

The systems of alloplastic implants that are available today are myriad. It was only a matter of time before researchers and clinicians began to find indications for the combination of these systems for management of their patients' oral problems. The placement of endosseous implants into reconstructed mandibles following bone grafting is commonly employed with success. Grafts are commonly performed using a combination of titanium mesh and cancellous bone marrow. After an 8- to 10-month graft consolidation period, an endosseous implant system can be employed. These combined procedures allow for the oral rehabilitation of patients who have lost segments or continuity of their mandible or maxilla as a result of trauma, infection, removal of a neoplasm, or other disease process.

Cranin et al.[35] have described the augmentation of the severely atrophied mandible in 15 patients by the placement of a bone marrow or bone marrow and hydroxylapatite–filled titanium mesh tray on the inferior mandibular border followed 6 months later by the construction and placement of a titanium subperiosteal implant. This method not only strengthens the mandible but also adds facial length, improves labial posture, and allows the implant to be placed on unaugmented solid basilar bone.[35] Dobson and Smith[36] describe the removal of an odontogenic myxoma by partial mandibular resection and reconstruction using a corticocancellous iliac bone graft.

The patient functioned with a removable partial denture for several years, then successfully underwent the placement of Noblepharma osseointegrated implants.[36]

The severely atrophic maxilla has also been reconstructed with iliac bone grafting and tissue-integrated prostheses. Keller et al.[37] report successfully reconstructing the atrophic maxilla in patients by sandwiching grafted bone between the downfractured maxilla and the maxillary sinuses following Le Fort I osteotomy, or by onlay grafting. The segments were stabilized, allowed to heal, and threaded titanium endosteal implants were placed in the newly fashioned maxillary ridge. Another method is to place the implants at the time of initial surgery. Both methods show that with careful selection, bone grafting in conjunction with a tissue-integrated prosthesis can provide superior functional and esthetic results.

The restoration of masticatory function aided by the use of aluminum oxide endosseous implants following microsurgically revascularized iliac crest grafts to the mandible or maxilla was described by Riediger.[38] Thirty-eight such devices were successfully placed in 13 secondarily and 15 primarily reconstructed mandibles and 5 maxillae, following reconstructions for various malignant tumors. Fifteen patients received irradiation therapy prior to or following their osteomyocutaneous groin flap reconstructions. All 38 implants were stable after undergoing masticatory functional stress from 3 to 30 months.

Small developed the titanium alloy mandibular staple bone plate and reported on an 8-year study with this implant device.[39] Although the mandibular staple is inserted into the inferior mandibular cortical bone through an extraoral incision, it is possible to think that this system could be used in conjunction with the grafted or hydroxylapatite-augmented mandibular ridge. The indication for such a combination might be the patient with a concave, grossly atrophic posterior mandibular ridge, and a less atrophic anterior ridge. The staple implant would be totally supported by bone while the deficient posterior ridges could be simultaneously augmented by the implantation of hydroxylapatite.

The long-term successful use of endosteal dental implants for placement in hydroxylapatite-aug-

mented ridges has not been reported. Experience has shown that the successful placement of endosseous implants requires the formation of precise, surgically created sites within the host bone. Since it is rare that bone proliferates beyond 1 to 2 mm into the fibrous tissue particulate hydroxylapatite mass, the ability to perform precise drill holes or grooves for such implants is not predictable. The continued compressibility of such augmented ridges likewise seemingly would lead to failure of implanted devices.

Work has, however, been initiated to study the direct bonding of dense, nonresorbable, nonporous hydroxylapatite onto implantable devices. Block et al.[40] report use of a 50 to 75-μm thickness of hydroxylapatite on machine-smooth pure titanium implants. Histologic evidence indicated that there was a bonding of the coated implants to bone that is defined as *biointegration*. This term applies to a mechanically significant biochemical bonding of living bone to the surface of the implant which is independent of any mechanical interlocking mechanism and which can be identified by electron microscopy. Stability occurs at a much faster rate in the coated implants when compared with the noncoated specimens. Conclusions were that the coated implants had superior bonding, had earlier biointegration, improved adjacent lamellar bone patterns, and maintained crestal bone around the devices.

DISCUSSION

The restoration of anatomic form and function to the maxilla and mandible is definitely not a new problem. Writers for many decades have described attempts to substitute bones and teeth from lower animal forms, from cadaveric implants, or from allogenic transplants. Except for the implantation of freeze-dried bone from human cadavers, the use of allogenic bone has usually resulted in failure. The use of autogenous bone grafting for augmentation or reconstructing the mandible or maxilla has been extremely successful, however.

For over 20 years, first Vitallium, and now more commonly titanium alloy mesh trays, have been used in combination with autogenous cancellous marrow for reconstruction of mandibular defects. Many combat veterans of the Vietnam conflict received such combination graft-implant systems for reconstruction of facial or skeletal bone defects.

With careful patient selection, meticulous planning, utilization of the proper implant system, be it subperiosteal, staple, or endosseous, the disappointments previously encountered are becoming less frequent. Many patients today benefit from the results of sound research relating to reconstructive oral surgery, bone grafting, the use of alloplastic bone substitutes, and the implantation of biocompatible devices.

The various titanium alloys used in orthopedics and oral and maxillofacial surgery in the form of mesh trays, joint prostheses, bone plates, and pins or screws have provided a vast armamentarium for bone reconstruction.

Likewise, the use of ceramic hydroxylapatite has evolved as a promising and compatible biomaterial for augmentation of mandibular and maxillary defects and deficiencies. As stated earlier, it is imperative that dentists who provide denture prostheses have a major role in the planning of such surgery. The fact that an augmented ridge requires additional care and more frequent denture relining must also be understood by the prosthodontist. Slowly changing ridge form, occasional dehiscences, the formation of hyperkeratosis, growth of hair following a skin graft vestibuloplasty, and altered sensation in the ridge and chin must be understood. The patient certainly must fully understand the details of such procedures, the alternatives, and the expectations of success and possible complications. Patients should expect such information and should be presented with a detailed operative permit. The American Association of Oral and Maxillofacial Surgeons urges its members to use such permits. Underwriters of liability insurance for this specialty also require such documentation for all patients.

Hopefully, the days of clinical trials of unresearched and unproven methods for implantology are past. The moratorium placed by the American Dental Association in the early 1970s on the use of "implants" served its purpose. There has since been a vast upsurge of investigative research to determine biologically sound principles and materials for dental implantology as we know it today. With study, the implantation of nonviable materials in sites that are less than surgically sterile can continue to be successful, as reported in recent years. Although commercial endeavors and our centers of higher learning have been responsible for a significant portion of the research regarding implantology, the clinician must continue to use his judgment and knowledge to differentiate sound research. Through thorough understanding and adherence to solid biological, surgical, ethical, and professional principles, the concept of bone augmentation implantology will be made acceptable. Otherwise, the concept could become merely a passing fad.

REFERENCES

1. *Bureau of Economic and Research Statistics: Prosthodontic Care: Number and Type of Denture Wearers, 1975*. Chicago, American Dental Association, 1976.
2. Topazian RG, Hammer WB, Talbert CD, et al: The use of ceramics in augmentation and replacement of portions of the mandible, in Hall CW (ed): *Bioceramics—Engineering in Medicine*. New York, Wiley Interscience, 1972, pp 311–332.
3. Boyne PJ: Restoration of alveolar ridges by intramandibular transposition osseous grafting. *J Oral Surg* 1968; 26:569–576.
4. Yeager JE, Boyne PJ: Use of bone homografts and autogenous marrow in restoration of edentulous alveolar ridges. *J Oral Surg* 1969; 27:185–189.
5. Hall CW: The need for biomaterials research, in Hall CW (ed): *Bioceramics—Engineering in Medicine*. New York, Wiley Interscience, 1972, pp 1–4.
6. Oppenheimer BS, Oppenheimer ET, Danishefsky I, et al: Further studies of polymers as carcinogenic agents in animals. *Cancer Res* 1955; 15:333–340.
7. Braley S: Medical uses of silicone rubber. *Ind Res* July 1966, pp 66–70.
8. Boucher LJ: Injected Silastic for tissue protection. *J Prosthet Dent* 1965; 15:73–82.
9. Boucher LJ: Injected Silastic in ridge extension procedures. *J Prosthet Dent* 1964; 14:460.
10. Davis H, Nystrom G: Plugging of bone cavities with Rivanol-Plaster porridge. *Acta Chir Scand* 1928; 63:296.
11. Smith L: Ceramic-plastic material as a bone substitute. *Arch Surg* 1963; 87:653.
12. Hulbert SF, Klawitter JJ, Talbert CD, et al: A histologic study of ceramic-bone compatibility (abstracted). *J Dent Res* 1970; 49:67.
13. Klawitter JJ, Talbert CD, Hulbert SF, et al: Artificial

bones, in Hulbert SF, Young FA (eds): *Use of Ceramics in Surgical Implants.* New York, Gordon & Breach Science Publishers, 1969, pp 95–114.

14. Klawitter JJ, Hulbert SF, Talbert CD, et al: Materials of construction for bone gap bridges, in *Orthopaedic Surgery Papers of the Duke University Medical Center and Affiliated Hospitals,* January 1969.

15. Autin J: Test reports from materials and toxicity laboratories. Knoxville, Colleges of Dentistry and Pharmacology, University of Tennessee, June 10, 1970.

16. Hammer WB, Topazian RG, McKinney RV Jr, et al: Alveolar ridge augmentation with ceramics. *J Dent Res* 1973; 52:356–361.

17. Hammer WB, Topazian RG, Lundquist DO, et al: Augmentation of human mandibular alveolar ridges with ceramics (abstracted). *J Dent Res* 1974; 53(special issue):88.

18. Hammer WB, Klawitter JJ: Porous aluminum oxide and high density polyethylene sponge for augmentation of the edentulous mandible (abstracted). *J Dent Res* 1976; 55(special issue):B243.

19. Jarcho M: Calcium phosphate ceramics as hard tissue prosthetics. *Clin Orthop* 1981; 157:259–278.

20. Klawitter JJ, Hulbert SF: Application of porous ceramics for the attachment of load bearing orthopedic applications. *J Biomed Mater Res* 1971; 161.

21. Kent J, Block M, Zide MF, et al: Hydroxylapatite blocks for increased stability in orthognathic surgery (abstracted). *J Dent Res* 1985; 64(special issue):215.

22. Kent JN, Zide MF, Kay JF, et al: Hydroxylapatite blocks and particles as bone graft substitutes in orthognathic and reconstructive surgery. *J Oral Maxillofac Surg* 1986; 44:597–605.

23. Kent JN, Quinn JH, Zide MF, et al: Correction of alveolar ridge deficiencies with nonresorbable hydroxylapatite. *J Am Dent Assoc* 1982; 105:993–1004.

24. Mehlisch DR, Taylor TD, Leibold DG, et al: Evaluation of collagen/hydroxylapatite for augmenting deficient alveolar ridges: A preliminary report. *J Oral Maxillofac Surg* 1987; 45:408–413.

25. Lew D, Clark R, Shahbazian T: Use of a soft tissue expander in alveolar ridge augmentation: A preliminary report. *J Oral Maxillofac Surg* 1986; 45:408–413.

26. Shen K, Gongloff RK: Collagen tube containers: An effective means of controlling particulate hydroxylapatite implants. *J Prosthet Dent* 1986; 56:65–70.

27. Gongloff RK: Use of collagen tube contained implants of particulate hydroxylapatite for ridge augmentation. *J Oral Maxillofac Surg* 1988; 46:641–647.

28. Lambert PM: A two-piece surgical splint to facilitate hydroxylapatite augmentation of the mandibular alveolar ridge. *J Oral Maxillofac Surg* 1986; 44:329–331.

29. Block MS, Kent JN: A comparison of particulate and solid root forms of hydroxylapatite in dog extraction sites. *J Oral Maxillofac Surg* 1986; 44:89–93.

30. Hak JK, El Deeb M, Morstad T, et al: Alveolar ridge maintenance with hydroxylapatite ceramic cones in humans. *J Oral Maxillofac Surg* 1986; 44:503–508.

31. Hupp JR, McKenna SJ: Use of porous hydroxylapatite blocks for augmentation of atrophic mandibles. *J Oral Maxillofac Surg* 1988; 46:538–545.

32. Waite PD, Matukas VJ: Zygomatic augmentation with hydroxylapatite. A preliminary report. *J Oral Maxillofac Surg* 1986; 44:349–352.

33. Stoelinga PJW, Blijdorp PA, Ross RR, et al: Augmentation of the atrophic mandible with interposed bone grafts and particulate hydroxylapatite. *J Oral Maxillofac Surg* 1986; 44:353–360.

34. Holliger JO, Schmitz JP: Restoration of bone discontinuities in dogs using a biodegradable implant. *J Oral Maxillofac Surg* 1987; 45:594–600.

35. Cranin AN, Sher J, Shpuntoff R: Reconstruction of the edentulous mandible with a lower border graft and subperiosteal implant. *J Oral Maxillofac Surg* 1988; 46:264–268.

36. Dodson TB, Smith RA: Mandibular reconstruction with autogenous and alloplastic materials following resection of an odontogenic myxoma. *Int J Oral Maxillofac Implants* 1987; 2:227–229.

37. Keller EE, Van Roebel, Desjardins RP, et al: Prosthetic surgical reconstruction of the severely resorbed maxilla with iliac bone grafting and tissue integrated prostheses. *Int J Oral Maxillofac Implants* 1987; 2:155–165.

38. Riediger D: Restoration of masticatory function by microsurgically revascularized iliac crest bone grafts using enosseous implants. *Plast Reconstr Surg* 1988; 81:861–878.

39. Small IA: Survey of experiences with the mandibular staple bone plate. *J Oral Surg* 1978; 36:604.

40. Block MS, Kent JN, Kay JF: Evaluation of hydroxylapatite-coated titanium dental implants in dogs. *J Oral Maxillofac Surg* 1987; 45:601–607.

Chapter 36

The Necessity for Controlled Clinical Implant Trials

Ralph V. McKinney, Jr., D.D.S., Ph.D.

The practitioner in private practice develops a personal practice basis for the selection and use of dental implants. These personal concerns can be summed up in a number of questions the practitioner wants to know about dental implants. For example, Is a given implant safe to use? How does an implant function biologically, particularly the implant I am interested in? Is the implant I'm interested in clinically successful? How can I select the correct implant to match the patient with a certain diagnostic situation? Can I predict the outcome for this implant? What type prosthetic restoration should I use for this particular implant? What type hygiene maintenance program do I prescribe for my patients with these implants? All these practitioner-oriented questions can and must be answered with knowledge based on adequate clinically controlled implant trials. This sort of information about implants cannot be developed from engineering designs that are then taken directly to the human mouth. Clinical trials, animal followed by human, are necessary for the generation of scientific implant data.[1]

One of the major reasons that implantologists in the past have received a poor reception from the rest of the dental profession has been this lack of adequate scientific information about the implant before it was made available to the profession at large.[2] Not only has there been a lack of clinical trial information but information on the tissue interface phenomena as well.[3]

How has this been allowed to happen? Dental implant materials are limited to a few—surgical stainless steel, chrome-cobalt-molybdenum alloy, aluminum oxide ceramics, the bioactive ceramics, pure titanium, and titanium alloy. All these materials have been tested toxicologically and approved for use in the human body.[4] How, then, have dentists been able to utilize dental implants in their practice setting without formal approval for the device?

Implant manufacturers are able to market their new implant designs and concepts without clinical trials or premarket approval under an amendment to the Federal Food and Cosmetic Act known as the Medical Device Amendment or commonly referred to as the 510 (k) amendment.[5] Under this amendment, which was passed by Congress in 1976, the new implant devices can be determined as "equivalent" if the device corresponds to a pre-1976 marketed implant. All endosteal implants qualify under this regulation. This is not an approval or a determination by the Food and Drug Administration (FDA) whether the new device is safe or effective. The FDA can still take the device off the market if adverse comments are received in the literature or through correspondence.

For American Dental Association (ADA) approval, the ADA has never provided any blanket approval for dental implants. Instead, in 1973, the ADA classified dental implants as in the "new technique phase" and suggested "continuing scientific review."[6] In 1980 the ADA's Council on Dental Materials, Instruments, and Equipment stated that implants are in need of continuing scientific review and are not recommended for routine clinical practice, but further stated that in selected cases in which the relative merits of benefits and risk are carefully evaluated and fully discussed with the patient, the endosseous implant may be used. The council further stated that responsibility for selection of patients and providing information for informed consent rested with the dentist.[6]

In 1981 the ADA issued guidelines for an acceptance program for dental implants. Now a manufacturer may apply for provisional or full acceptance based on strict criteria established by the Council on Dental Materials, Instruments, and Equipment.[7] (See Table 36–1 for summary of criteria.)

As mentioned, the FDA has allowed the manufacture and clinical use of dental implants under the Medical Device Amendment of 1976 which placed endosseous implants under general FDA control, as is imposed by law for all medical devices. This meant that dental implants were not subject to mandatory performance standards nor have they been subject to the FDA requirement for premarket approval (PMA).[5] This is now changing and the FDA is considering the establishment of premarket approval for new dental implants, effective September 1992 (B. Sands, FDA, personal communication, June 1990). A recent hearing was conducted by the Dental Products Panel of the FDA concerning new evaluation standards for premarket approval of dental implants.[8] Following this the FDA publicly announced in December 1989 that premarket approval was going to be required and the public had until May 1990 to respond and submit petitions for change(s) in this proposal. A summary of the FDA premarket approval clinical trial requirements is shown in Table 36–2.

Thus scientific knowledge about dental implants requires thorough evaluation of the implant to include physical properties, cytotoxicity, microbiological, and inflammation and mutagenic studies, and then clinical animal trials followed by well-con-

---

TABLE 36–1.

American Dental Association Council on Dental Materials, Instruments, and Equipment Acceptance Program for Endosteal Dental Implants

1. Establishment of negative levels of cytotoxcity, mutagenicity, inflammation, and other tissue pathologic factors as delineated in *American National Standard/American Dental Association Document No. 41.*[9]
2. Two independent clinical studies with a sample size of 50 patients evaluated periodically by two or more evaluators for a period of 3 years for *provisional acceptance*. Quantitation of clinical criteria must be carried out.
3. For *acceptance* the above clinical study must be evaluated periodically for a period of 5 years.
4. Physical properties and interface characteristics of the implant must be described.
5. Recommended operative techniques and anatomic considerations must be described and supported by clinical trial data.

TABLE 36–2.

Food and Drug Administration Premarket Approval Program for Acceptance of Dental Implants

1. Establishment of efficacy of the dental implant through appropriate biomaterial testing and animal testing for cytotoxicity, inflammation, mutagenic factors, and description of interface phenomena
2. Two independent clinical studies with a sample size of 100 patients periodically evaluated by two or more evaluators for 2 years for *provisional* premarket approval.
3. For *full* premarket approval the above clinical studies must be carried out for 5 years.

trolled human clinical trials.[7, 9] Only then can an implant be fully approved for wide clinical use in the hands of appropriately trained dentists. It would seem that all dentists would want assurance of this degree of biological tissue acceptance before beginning general clinical use of the implant.

The presence on the market of inadequately tested implants not only puts questionable devices on the market but also confuses the practitioner as to the type of implant to select for treatment. Advertising makes all implant selections sound highly compatible and successful. If the profession and implant manufacturers continue this type of blind endeavor, it will only bring heightened federal regulation concerning this treatment modality.

There are currently a number of well-controlled and scientifically established clinical trials being conducted in the United States,[10-13] Sweden,[14] and Canada[15] in which the clinical presentation of a particular implant system is measured in quantifiable clinical terms. These types of experimental and validation trials provide a rationale for selection and use of a particular implant system. Only in this way will the cause and professional acceptance of implants move forward in the future.[16, 17]

CONCLUSION

Dental implantology is an exciting treatment concept that relies on the diagnostic, surgical, prosthetic, and restorative-periodontal skills of the practitioner. The use of dental implants is now widespread throughout the profession and they are employed by generalist and specialist alike. One has only to look in the local telephone directory to see the dental advertisements for dental implants to realize how far this treatment modality has come in the past decade. There are still many areas of concern about the biological reaction of tissues to dental implants and only through adequate testing and clinical trials can we develop the answers that will result in a highly acceptable and predictable treatment device that the practitioner can select for restoration of the human dental structures.

REFERENCES

1. McKinney RV Jr, Steflik DE, Koth DL, et al: The scientific basis for dental implant therapy. *J Dent Educ* 1988; 52:696–705.
2. James RA: Dental implants—moving into the mainstream. *J Calif Dent Assoc* 1984; 6:22–25.
3. Misch CE, Judy KWM: Oral implantology: Speciality status. *Mo Dent J* 1985; 6:23–24.
4. Lemons JE: Dental implant interfaces as influenced by biomaterial and biomechanical properties, in McKinney RV Jr, Lemons JE (eds): *The Dental Implant: Clinical and Biological Response of Oral Tissues.* Littleton, Mass, PSG Publishing Co, Inc, 1985, pp 143–157.
5. Federal Food, Drug and Cosmetic Act as amended by the Medical Device Amendment, 510 (k), May 1976.
6. Wozniak WT: Dental implants and ADA acceptance. *J Am Dent Assoc* 1986; 113:879.
7. Council on Dental Materials, Instruments and Equipment. Expansion of the acceptance program for dental materials, instruments and equipment: Endosseous implants. *J Am Dent Assoc* 1981; 102:350.
8. Food and Drug Administration: Dental Product Panel hearing. Rockville, Md, US Department of Health and Human Services, Public Health Service, December 16, 1988.
9. Council on Dental Materials, Instruments and Equipment: *American National Standard/American Dental Association Document No. 41 for Recommended Standard Practices for the Biological Evaluation of Dental Materials.* Chicago, American Dental Association, ANSI/ADA document No. 41, 1982.
10. Koth DL, McKinney RV Jr, Steflik DE, et al: Clinical and statistical analyses of human clinical trials with the single crystal alumina oxide endosteal dental implant: Five year results. *J Prosthet Dent* 1988; 60:226–234.
11. Schnitman P, Rubenstein J, Jeffcoat M, et al: Three year survival results: Blade implant vs cantilever clinical trials. *J Dent Res* 1988; 67(special issue):347.
12. Kapur KK: Veterans Administration Cooperative Dental Implant Study: Comparisons between fixed partial dentures supported by Blade-Vent implants and removable partial dentures. II: Comparisons of success rates and periodontal health between two treatment modalities. *J Prosthet Dent* 1989; 62:685–703.

13. Smithloff M, Flitz ME: The use of blade implants in a selected population of partially edeutulous adults, a 15 year report. *J Periodontol* 1987; 58:589–593.

14. Albrektsson T, Dahl E, Enbom L, et al: Osseointegrated oral implants. A Swedish multicenter study of 8139 consecutively inserted Nobelpharma implants. *J Periodontol* 1988; 59:287–296.

15. Zarb GA, Symington JM: Osseointegrated dental implants: Preliminary report on a replication study. *J Prosthet Dent* 1983; 50:271–276.

16. Laney WR: On behalf of valid research (editorial). *Int J Oral Maxillofac Implants* 1990; 5:99–100.

17. McKinney RV Jr: Implantology into the next decade: The three I index (editorial). *Implantologist* 1990; 6:7–8.

Chapter 37

Implant Clinical Trials: Design and Statistical Management

David E. Steflik, M.A., Ed.D.
Harry C. Davis, Ph.D.

To clinically evaluate the efficacy of specific dental implant systems it is imperative to design appropriate clinical trials that set objective criteria which can be compared and tested. Inherent to this design and development process is the selection of an appropriate statistical protocol for analysis. This selection is most often based upon the investigator's familiarity with specific statistical protocols and the type of study to be evaluated.

Dental implant studies can usually be divided into two categories: prospective and retrospective studies. Clinical criteria, and thereby the statistical analysis of clinical behavior, can be preset (within limits) for prospective studies. However, retrospective studies usually restrict the type of analyses that can be performed. Statistical protocols to analyze implant studies can generally be divided into the two broad categories of descriptive and inferential statistics. As their names imply, descriptive statistics describe available data and inferential statistics make inferences from the sample that is being assessed to the general population.

This chapter is divided into three general sections. First, an overview of pertinent statistical methods is described. Second, a selective review of the oral implantology literature describes how dental researchers are utilizing statistical protocols in evaluating implant serviceability. Third, a summary of the incorporation of scientific method into statistically sound clinical implant trials is presented.

STATISTICAL METHODS

Why should statistics be utilized in clinical offices and research institutions? Guilford and Fruchter[1] have presented six advantages of statistical thinking and operations in research which can be modified for the purposes of this chapter.

First, statistics permit the most exact kind of description. As an adjunct to clinical diagnostic procedure and intuition, statistics allow a quantification of patient progress in an accurate and reproducible sense.

Second, statistics force the investigator to be definite and exact in procedures and thinking.

Third, statistics enable the investigator to summarize results in meaningful and convenient forms. Even though observations appear meaningless at the time, recording of these data is necessary. Before we can see the forest and the trees, order must be given to data. Statistics provide an important bridge to bring order out of chaos—for focusing in on one's results.

Fourth, statistics enable the investigator to draw general conclusions. Statistics allow the investigator to not only generate conclusions from the data using accepted rules, but also tell how much confidence to have in those conclusions.

Fifth, statistics enable the investigator to predict potential outcomes, within acceptable or discrete margins of error. In other words, by using statistics it may be possible to predict the serviceability of patients' implants.

Sixth, statistics enable us to analyze some of the causal factors underlying complex and often bewildering events. Why do some implants succeed and others fail? By examining evaluation data over time, generalization of implant serviceability or demise may become apparent. Even though the data may look unimportant in its raw sense, when graphed or analyzed and compared with what is expected, causal relationships can become expressed.

Therefore, statistics are critical to evaluate implant behavior in patients. An examination of specific statistical measures is now indicated, and begins with an overview of *descriptive statistics*.

Measures of *central tendency* provide the investigator, or clinician, the midpoint of a series of observations. For most situations *means* and *medians* are the statistics of choice. The mean $(\overline{X})$, or the sum of measurements divided by the number of measurements, can give a value which would be adequate for assessing how one patient does against the mean of all the patients. The mean is also the basis for most subsequent statistical analyses. The *median*, however, is perhaps better for assessing patient performance to overall central tendency. The median is defined as that point on the scale of measurements above which are exactly one half of the cases and below which are the other half.[1] The reader should be aware that, in general, this is defined as a point and not as a score or a particular measurement. The median allows for the elimination of variability due to individual patients with unusually high or low values which would artificially inflate or deflate the arithmetic mean.

Once the value is obtained that provides the measure of central tendency for a group of observations, it is necessary to examine how far values vary from that central tendency measurement. Statistics used to document the degree of dispersion from that value are *measures of variability*. The literature most commonly utilizes the *standard deviation* (SD) as the variance for such measurements. Guilford and Fruchter suggest that the standard deviation is the most commonly used indicator of the degree of dispersion and is the most dependable estimate of variability in the population from which the sample came.[1] The standard deviation is the square root of the arithmetic mean of the average squared deviations of the measurements from the mean.[2] Approximately two thirds (68.26% in a normal distribution) of the measurements should fall between 1 SD below and 1 SD above the mean. In most cases 3 SD above and below the mean will include all the observations. The term obtained when we have the mean of the squared deviations of the measurements from the mean is known as the variance of the distribution.

In contrast to the previous statistics describing variability, *coefficients of correlation* tells the individual to what extent two things are related or to what extent variations in one go with variations in the other. Values can vary from $+1$, which means perfect positive correlation, through 0, which means complete independence, through -1, which means a perfect negative correlation. Correlation coefficients are especially applicable to implantology evaluation to follow progress over time or to examine evaluation parameters relative to one another. The statistic of choice is usually the Pearson product-moment coefficient of correlation (r). Many other correlation coefficients (e.g., Spearman's rho(p), point biserial, phi) are variations of the Pearson correlation.

The sets of statistics discussed to this point represent descriptive statistics—those describing data at specific times. *Inferential statistics* are those statistics which suggest that the descriptive analysis can be projected to test hypotheses and make inferences. What the investigator attempts to accomplish with inferential statistics is estimation of inferences to the entire population. In other words, How near the truth are the statistical answers we've come up with? To answer this question the statistician has numerous tools at his disposal.

The first tool to examine the relative correctness of a given statistic is the standard error of the mean (SEM), usually represented in the literature as some mean $\pm$ SEM. The standard error of the mean can be defined as the standard deviation of the distribution of sample means for a given sample size.[1, 2] This statistic is often critical for the reader to have as it provides him with an estimate of how much confidence should be placed in a statistic.

When analyzing research data, whether they be basic research data or applied clinical research data, the investigator often needs to evaluate whether the experimental variable differs significantly from control variables. Further, an implantologist may require data as to whether implant behavior differs between implant types or from the behavior of control natural dentition. To examine the significance of differences, the statistician's tools include the *t*-test, the chi-squared (χ^2) test, and the *F* ratio in the analysis of variance.

Student's *t* test is generally used to compare two means. These means are usually based on data obtained from two different groups of subjects although they may be obtained from the same group at two different time points. For example, the investigator may compare a gingival evaluation index such as the crevicular fluid volume prior to implantation and 3 months' post-implantation. Or, the investigator could compare the fluid volume between control natural teeth and the implant at one time period.

When more than two means are being compared the analysis of variance is frequently used. When the means are computed from the same subjects at different time periods, the *repeated measures analysis of variance* is used to examine trends over time. This statistic permits the investigator to analyze patterns of a treatment variable over time. This is particularly important when the investigator has data points at large numbers of evaluation time periods.

Other forms of the analysis of variance (usually abbreviated as ANOVA) can also be used when more than one factor is present. For example, a two-way ANOVA might be used to compare implant patients with control patients by side of jaw for the crevicular fluid volume index.

Regression analysis[3] is often used when the researcher has several measures of a more or less continuous nature which are possible predictors of some continuous outcome measure. For example, regression analysis might be used to see if the age of the patient, the patient's systolic blood pressure, and overall health status are important determinants of the patient's crevicular fluid volume. In other words, are these three "predictors" related to the primary dependent variable of crevicular fluid volume? Given a specific value for the three independent variables (the predictors), we can get an expected value of the dependent variable. More commonly, this statistical technique can be used to determine if the three are significantly related to the outcome measure. Are these continuous predictors capable of predicting a continuous outcome?

Although the majority of interpreted statistical techniques make some assumptions about a hypothetical population's true values (known as a parameter), another class of inferential statistics does not make such assumptions. This class is known as *nonparametric statistics* and includes the χ^2 *test*, *Friedman's two-way* ANOVA, and life table analysis.

Life table analyses[3] are often used for data that have different starting times (for example, dates of implantation in a clinical practice) and in which some patients may be considered as having a specific end point. For example, a study of implants would have patients that have had implants for varying amounts of time. Some patients would have reached an end point (loss of implant). Others would be considered "censored," that is, there are no data on these patients after a given amount of time since implant insertion. Censored patients are most frequently those who still have their implants but the time since implantation is not the maximum time period. Other censored cases include patients who still had their implants when they were lost to follow-up (for example, those who have died or moved from the area of study). Two methods used to estimate survival time are the *Kaplan-Meier* technique[4] and the *actuarial life table method (Cutler-Ederer)*.[5] Other statistics are available for comparing survival curves.

A further, and important, nonparametric statistic is the χ^2 test of association. This statistic is commonly used to see if two variables are related in terms of frequency of occurrence. For example, the χ^2 test could be used to test if, in a group of implant patients, a crevicular fluid volume rate above 10 is related to implant failure.

Once a decision is made as to which statistic is used to test the hypothesis under investigation, the next item to consider is the decision making process for accepting or rejecting present *null hypotheses* and the subsequent *research hypotheses*. The null hypothesis can be defined as the statistical hypothesis which states essentially that there is no relationship between the variables of the problem.[2] The research hypothesis can be defined as the prediction derived from the theory under test. These terms are derived from the Neyman-Pearson null hypothesis model which developed from the logic of David Hume, R.A. Fisher, W.S. Gosset, and others. As an example, if we take clinical evaluation data for a sample of patients implanted with two different implant types, the null hypothesis would be that there is no difference between the clinical evaluation data for crevicular fluid volume for either type of implant. We might also express this as, "There is no relationship between implant type and mean crevicular fluid volume," although this is a less common form of the null hypothesis when looking at differences between groups. We must now consider the degree of error we are willing to risk to make our decisions. The two general categories of statistical errors are Type I error and Type II error. Type I error suggests that we are rejecting the null hypothesis when, in fact, it is correct. Type II error suggests that we are failing to reject the null hypothesis when, in fact, it is false. Table 37–1 reflects the decision making process and the type of error inherent in the decision making process.[1, 2]

As is apparent, Type I error suggests that there are differences when there are none. The probability of an investigator making a Type I error is designated as the alpha level of acceptable error. Type II error says that there are no differences when, in fact, some do exist. The probability of an investigator making a type II error is characterized by beta. Therefore, if the investigator sets an alpha level of 0.05, he specifies that he accepts the chance that any statistical significance that is found may be due to random chance in 5 out of 100 cases. In drug research, the investigator might not want to say there are no differences when in fact there may be a harmful side effect. Therefore, the investigator would specify a more stringent level of Type II error, therefore setting a beta level of 0.01 or lower. In experimental implant trials, the investigator may want to set a more stringent (lower) alpha level to diminish the possibility of Type I error. The investigator would not want to conclude that one implant treatment is different from a second implant treatment without satisfactory statistical support.

Sample size is also a major consideration for hypothesis testing. Generally, with all other concerns being equal (i.e., experimental control, homogeneity of subjects, reliability of measurement), the larger the sample size, the more likely you are to reject the null hypothesis when the null hypothesis is incorrect. There are numerous formulas for the estimation of needed sample size based upon alpha and beta probability, and the reader may desire to examine these.[1] Such objective analysis can help answer the proverbial question, "How large a sample do I really need?"

Finally, two last concepts should be considered. These are the concepts of the power & robustness of specific statistics. The power of a statistic is its ability to correctly reject a false null hypothesis. The statistic is correctly disclosing that there are differences when in fact there are differences. The robustness of a statistic is the capability of the statistic to violate an assumption underlying the statistic and still disclose truthful conclusions (D.A. Payne, personal communication, January 1981). The power and robustness of certain statistics are referred to in the literature and the reader of implant dentistry research should be aware of these concepts.

TABLE 37–1.

Decision Making*

	Decision	
	Do Not Reject H_0	Reject H_0
H_0 true	Correct	Type I error
H_0 false	Type II error	Correct

*David A. Payne, personal communication, January 1981.
H_0 = null hypothesis.

STATISTICAL REPORTING OF CONTEMPORARY IMPLANT STUDIES

When an investigator reviews the contemporary oral implantology research literature that is specifically related to clinical research trials, the preponderance of reporting methodologies are restricted to descriptive analysis of results. This is not surprising considering the fact that the investigator primarily desires to concentrate on implant success or failure, or the number of implants placed.[6-9]

However, the sophistication of the definition of success or failure is restricted to individual trials. Often, this definition is related only to having the individual implant "in function," with no attempt made to include objective data supporting this subjective analysis.[10-12]

Descriptive statistical analysis of clinical evaluation data usually is restricted to intrastudy measures of central tendency, for example, to examine the means of control sites to implanted sites. These data also report the central values of a group of implant treatments within that study, or the changes in the parameters for time points of a study.[13-15]

Even as simple descriptive statistics can provide extremely important information, simple inferential statistics can provide estimates of prolonged serviceability. Lemons[16] has been involved in dental implant retrieval analyses and retrospectively estimates survival using life table analyses, particularly the Kaplan-Meier survival curves. James also suggests the validity of this statistical tool (R.A. James, personal communication, April 1988).

Specific standards to evaluate implant serviceability are increasingly becoming mandated. As early as 1977 Cranin and colleagues[17] attempted to utilize a subjective radiographic interpretive index to substantiate implant serviceability. However, standardization of radiographs has always been a critical problem in implantology research. As Friedland stated, "certainly there is a lack of standardization between the authors with regard to the criteria used . . . also there was no attempt at standardization."[18] To standardize radiographs requires sophisticated radiographic techniques and the desire on the part of investigators to continue this protocol for long-term follow-up. Radiographic indices are useful

for success criteria, but these data should for the most part be viewed as subjective rather than objective criteria. This is particularly important when the reader examines radiographic evidence of bone changes due to implantations.[6] These are often important data and need to be reported, but the statistical analysis of these data may be tenuous.[19]

The use of specific and objective clinical evaluation criteria has been shown to be useful in interpreting implant success and failure. The most common indices are mobility and gingival health interpretations. Mobility and gingival recession or pocket formation have been used since 1978 by Gettleman and associates.[20] They used correlation coefficients and a linear regression analysis to analyze these objective data. The analysis of gingival evaluation data by descriptive statistics (means, standard deviation) was also reported by Cox and Zarb.[21] They suggested, however, that conventional soft tissue health indices may not be reliable monitors of implant efficacy. Deporter et al.[22] have developed a protocol for the standardization of serial radiographs to develop a bone implant score (BIS). This sophisticated protocol is useful when examining implant serviceability and assessing peri-implant bone height. Further, they were able to perform correlational statistics between gingival evaluation data and the BIS, finding that the BIS was strongly correlated with pocket depth and attachment level. In fact, the data were objectively sound to perform analysis of covariance statistical analysis. Criteria for success were also set forth by Albrektsson et al.[23] in their follow-up report of a Swedish multicenter study of Nobelpharma implants. These criteria again included immobility, peri-implant radiolucency, bone loss, and patient subjective symptoms. Such criteria were not subjected to any statistical analysis. In studies of mandibular staple implants, Kent et al.[24] and Small and Misiek[25] examined gingival criteria, mobility, and bone loss for their reporting of cumulative success rates (with associated standard errors). These conclusions of successful implant behavior were based upon these clinical evaluation criteria.

Steflik and associates have attempted to analyze the validity of both using and statistically analyzing quantifiable clinical evaluation parameters in implant clinical trials. The use of a gingival bleeding index (based on the work of Loe and Silness[28]), a plaque accumulation index (based on the work of Silness and Loe[27] and of Ramjford[28]), a mobility index (based on the work of Wasserman et al.[29]), and a crevicular fluid volume index (based on the work of Golub and Kleinberg[30] and of Garnick et al.[31]) was tested in an animal model[32] and validated for use in human clinical trials.[33] The obtained clinical evaluation data were shown to be suitable for both descriptive statistical analysis as well as for inferential statistical analysis using both parametric and nonparametric statistical protocols. These analyses included descriptive statistics, Pearson product-moment coefficients of correlation, repeated measures ANOVA, and the Friedman's two-way ANOVA. These objective indices were then used to set specific criteria for documenting implant success or failure for descriptive longitudinal reporting.[34, 35]

Similar criteria were used by Brose and associates during 8-year studies of alumina implants in baboons and humans. They developed their criteria in experimental animal studies[36] and subjected the data to descriptive statistical analysis. After these animal studies they utilized evaluation criteria of mobility, pocket depth, appositional bone height, and gingival bleeding to set standards for clinical serviceability of the implants. During their 31-patient study[37] a least squares curve was utilized as the statistical protocol to show patterns over time.

INCORPORATION OF THE SCIENTIFIC METHOD INTO STATISTICALLY SOUND CLINICAL IMPLANT TRIALS

This chapter has attempted to introduce the reader to various statistical protocols found in the reports of clinical implant evaluation trials. Descriptive reporting of these data provide important clinical observations. However, the dental scientific community is increasingly mandating that these descriptive data be further analyzed by more sophisticated statistical methodologies. Further, clinical implant evaluation studies will necessarily be required to set foundational planning criteria to make maximum utilization of human clinical evaluation data. In other words, clinical implant trials will have to be evaluated by the same sound scientific method as is required with conventional experimental investigations.

Speaking before the panel of the 1988 National Institutes of Health (NIH) consensus conference on dental implants, Kapur[38] suggested requirements for such clinical trials. These requirements were taken from the Veterans Administration cooperative study designed to determine whether endosteal blade-supported fixed partial dentures offered an acceptable substitute for mandibular unilateral or bilateral distal base extension removable partial dentures. Kapur suggested that "proper clinical trials must evaluate the relative efficacy of the new treatment modalities prior to their acceptance as a substitute for conventional approaches.[38] Schnitman et al.[39, 40] have accomplished just that in their blade implant randomized clinical trials. Their carefully controlled study examined the efficacy of blade-supported bridges as compared to equivalent cantilever bridges. The results at 4 years concluded that survival rates were similar for implants and cantilevers, but that patients preferred the implant-supported prostheses for function and comfort. Schnitman et al. utilized objective clinical evaluation criteria amenable to statistical analyses to support their conclusions based, partly, on life table analysis.

Kapur[38] proposed that the scientific approach to investigation be better brought to implant trials. Kapur proposed that the trials consist of the following seven steps[38]:

1. Delineation of study hypotheses
2. Determination of sample size
3. Definition of patient selection criteria
4. Definition of treatment procedures
5. Identification of outcome variables
6. Standardization of data collection
7. Development of a coordinated plan for statistical analysis

Since, other things being equal, statistical significance depends on the size of the sample being investigated, Kapur correctly implied that a small difference of little clinical value can be statistically significant, and concurrently, a large difference with clinical significance can appear statistically insignificant if there was a small sample in the study. He stated, "Therefore, researchers should provide full statistical information including sample estimates, confidence intervals, test statistics, p values, and sample size."[38] The importance of such experimental design was also discussed by Antczak-Bouckoms and Chalmers[41] and by Pocock and associates[42] as they examined statistical problems in the reporting of clinical trial data.

Therefore, after proper planning, the clinical evaluation study should commence with patient selection criteria. With this procedure, a proper patient sample can be obtained to ensure that clinically significant conclusions can be obtained. Objective clinical evaluation criteria must be set to ensure that a reliable test for clinical success or failure is available. These objective clinical parameters or indices must be capable of being subjected to statistical analysis. These objective criteria can be used in conjunction with more subjective criteria to develop a clinical evaluation protocol.

Once this prospective evaluation study begins, clinical evaluation data must be collected prior to treatment, at treatment, and at all subsequent evaluation time periods. Evaluation time periods should be at specified intervals. Descriptive statistics can be computed at individual time periods, and with these descriptive statistics (primarily means, medians, or frequencies) more sophisticated parametric or nonparametric inferential statistics can be calculated. Therefore we can start with the charting of individual patient data to evaluate how the individual patient is progressing by documenting any changes in implant behavior. This can be accomplished by simple charting procedures. Subsequently, samples can be compared. By performing simple descriptive statistics for the entire patient sample, means of central tendency can be obtained. These can provide the foundation point to compare the variability of individual patients from the mean or median of that clinical evaluation index. Therefore, we can analyze individual patients with respect to the "expected" norm of the group.

To analyze the patterns of the entire sample, the investigator can use the sample means at longitudinal evaluation time points. With these means various ANOVA protocols can be incorporated. By utilizing

the available data of when specific implants failed or were lost to the study, life table analyses, specifically the Kaplan-Meier, can be utilized to define prospective implant survival.

Therefore, with normal preplanning of the research process, and incorporating the traditional scientific process into clinical evaluation studies, the efficacy of various implant modalities may be more objectively analyzed. This must incorporate valid and reliable statistical protocols. Such protocols are nothing new, but need to be considered in the sphere of oral implantology. Oral implantology is one of the most rapidly growing spheres of discipline in dentistry and in 1990 a myriad of implant systems exist, some without any foundational experimental studies or rudimentary clinical efficacy trials. The decade of the 1990s will likely see the emergence of governmental agencies beginning to regulate corporate implant concerns. In fact, the Food and Drug Administration (FDA) and the American Dental Association (ADA) are mandating such objective trials as presented at the 1989 American Association of Dental Research annual meeting.[43] The future of implant dentistry systems will likely depend on reproducible clinical implant trials based on sound statistical methodology.

REFERENCES

1. Guilford JP, Fruchter B: *Fundamental Statistics in Psychology and Education.* New York, McGraw-Hill Book Co, 1978.
2. Bledsoe JC: *Essentials of Educational Research.* Athens, Ga, Optima House, 1972.
3. Lawless JE: *Statistical Models and Methods For Lifetable Data.* New York, John Wiley & Sons, 1982.
4. Kaplan EL, Meier P: Nonparametric estimation from incomplete observations. *J Am Stat Assoc* 1958; 53:457–481.
5. Cutler SJ, Ederer F: Maximum utilization of the life table method in analyzing survival. *J Chron Dis* 1958; 8:699–713.
6. Adell R, Lekholm U, Rockler B, et al: A 15-year study of osseointegrated implants in the treatment of the edentulous jaw. *Int J Oral Surg* 1981; 10:387–416.
7. Adell R: Clinical results of osseointegrated implants

supporting fixed prostheses in edentulous jaws. *J Prosthet Dent* 1983; 50:251–254.

8. Smithloff J, Fritz ME: The use of blade implants in a selected population of partially edentulous adults. *J Periodontol* 1987; 58:589–593.

9. Brånemark P-I, Adell R, Albrektsson T, et al: An experimental and clinical study of osseointegrated implants penetrating the nasal cavity and maxillary sinus. *J Oral Maxillofac Surg* 1984; 42:497–505.

10. Kirsch A, Mentag PJ: The IMZ endosseous two phase implant system: A complete oral reabilitation treatment concept. *J Oral Implantol* 1986; 12:576–589.

11. Linkow LI: Statistical analysis of 173 implant patients. *J Oral Implantol* 1974; 4:540–562.

12. Niznick GA: Implant prosthodontics: A team approach. *J Oral Implantol* 1985; 12:45–67.

13. Kenney EB, Lekovic V, Han T, et al: The use of a porous hydroxylapatite implant in periodontal defects. *J Periodontol* 1985; 56:82–88.

14. Adell R, Lekholm U, Rockler B, et al: Marginal tissue reactions at osseointegrated titanium fixtures. *Int J Oral Maxillofac Surg* 1986; 15:39–52.

15. Ericsson I, Lekholm U, Brånemark P-I, et al: A clinical evaluation of fixed-bridge restorations supported by the combination of teeth and osseointegrated titanium implants. *J Clin Periodontol* 1986; 13:307–312.

16. Lemons JE: Dental implant retrieval analyses. *J Dent Educ* 1988; 52:748–756.

17. Cranin AN, Rabkin MF, Garfinkle L: A statistical evaluation of 952 endosteal implants in humans. *J Am Dent Assoc* 1977; 94:315–320.

18. Friedland B: The clinical evaluation of dental implants—A review of the literature, with emphasis on the radiographic aspects. *J Oral Implantol* 1987; 13:101–111.

19. James RA, Altman AF, Clem DC, et al: A critical review of the "osseointegrated" literature. *Int J Oral Implantol* 1986; 3:35–41.

20. Gettleman L, Schnitman PA, Kalis P, et al: Clinical evaluation criteria of tooth implant success. *J Oral Implantol* 1978; 8:12–27.

21. Cox JF, Zarb GA: The longitudinal clinical efficacy of osseointegrated dental implants: A 3-year report. *Int J Oral Maxillofac Implants* 1987; 2:91–100.

22. Deporter DA, Friedland B, Watson PA, et al: A clinical and radiographic assessment of a porous-surfaced titanium alloy implant system in dogs. *J Dent Res* 1986; 65:1071–1077.

23. Albrektsson T, Dahl E, Enbom L, et al: Osseointegrated oral implants: A Swedish multicenter study of 8139 consecutively inserted Nobelpharma implants. *J Periodontol* 1988; 59:287–296.

24. Kent JN, Misiek DJ, Silverman H, et al: A multi-center retrospective review of the mandibular staple bone plate. *J Oral Maxillofac Surg* 1984; 42:421–428.

25. Small IA, Misiek D: A sixteen-year evaluation of the mandibular staple bone plate. *J Oral Maxillofac Surg* 1986; 44:60–66.

26. Loe H, Silness J: Periodontal disease in pregnancy. I. Prevalence and severity. *Acta Odontol Scand* 1963; 21:533–551.

27. Silness J, Loe H: Periodontal disease in pregnancy: II. Correlation between oral hygiene and periodontal condition. *Acta Odontol Scand* 1964; 22:121.

28. Ramfjord SP: Indices for prevalence and incidence of periodontal disease. *J Periodontol* 1959; 31:51.

29. Wasserman BH, Geiger AM, Turgeon LR: Relationship of occlusion and periodontal disease. Part VIII—Mobility. *J Periodontol* 1973; 44:572.

30. Golub LM, Kleinberg I: Gingival crevicular fluid: A new diagnostic aid in managing the periodontal patient. *Oral Sci Rev* 1976; 8:49–61.

31. Garnick JJ, Pearson R, Harrell D: The evaluation of the Periotron. *J Periodontol* 1979; 50:424–426.

32. Steflik DE, McKinney RV, Koth DL: A statistical analysis of the clinical response to the single-crystal sapphire endosseous dental implant in dog jaws. *J Dent Res* 1983; 62:1212–1215.

33. Steflik DE, Koth DL, McKinney RV: Human clinical trials with the single crystal sapphire endosteal dental implant: Three year results, statistical analysis, and validation of an evaluation protocol. *J Oral Implantol* 1987; 8:39–53.

34. Koth DL, Steflik DE, McKinney RV, et al: A clinical and statistical analysis of human clinical trials with the single crystal alumina oxide endosteal dental implant: Five year results. *J Prosthet Dent* 1988; 60:226–234.

35. McKinney RV, Koth DL, Steflik DE, et al: Statistical analysis of a nine year endosseous ceramic implant study. *J Dent Res* 1990; 69(special issue):267.

36. Brose MO, Rieger MR, Downses RJ, et al: Eight-year study of alumina tooth implants in baboons. *J Oral Implantol* 1987; 13:409–425.

37. Brose MO, Rieger MR, Avers RJ, et al: Eight year analysis of alumina dental root implants in human subjects. *J Oral Implantol* 1988; 14:9–22.

38. Kapur KK: Requirements for clinical trials. *J Dent Educ* 1988, 52:760–764.

39. Schnitman PA, Rubenstein JE, Jeffcoat MK, et al: Implant prostheses: Blade vs. cantilever—Clinical trial. *J Oral Implantol* 1986; 12:449–459.

40. Schnitman PA, Rubenstein JE, Whorle PS, et al: Implants for partial edentulism. *J Dent Educ* 1988; 52:725.

41. Antczak-Bouckoms A, Chalmers TC: The importance of design and analysis in clinical trials. *J Oral Implantol* 1988; 14:36–42.

42. Pocock SJ, Hughes MD, Lee RJ: Statistical problems in the reporting of clinical trials. *N Engl J Med* 1987; 317:426–432.

43. Implantology Research Group and Dental Materials Group of The American Association for Dental Research. Safe and effective implants—Criteria for pre-market approval (abstracted). Symposium VIII, American Association For Dental Research Annual Meeting, San Francisco, March 18, 1989. *J Dent Res* 1989; 68(special issue):62.

Chapter 38

Future Projections for Implantology

Ralph V. McKinney, Jr., D.D.S., Ph.D.

Modern implantology has progressed rapidly into all aspects of dental practice within the past 10 years.

Following ancient attempts at dental implantations, the original introduction of this type of treatment modality within the United States was most likely conceived by Edwin Greenfield and R.E. Payne at the turn of the 20th century (see Chapter 2). Although Greenfield reported his innovative design of a submerged two-stage porous rooted implant device to the profession both in the dental literature and orally at the National Dental Association meeting,[1] there was not a lot of enthusiasm for his implant technique and so the innovative implant ideas lay dormant for many years. Undoubtedly, World War I and the Great Depression further contributed to this lack of interest in dental implants. The Strock brothers, Alvin and Robert, both dentists in Boston, were the ones to renew and rejuvenate interest in the field of implantology by conducting animal and human scientific investigative studies. The Strock brothers inserted a screw-type root form implant made of castable metal in the jaws of dogs and studied the results clinically and histologically.[2] In addition, they treated patients with their endosteal implant system, developing quite a following for their innovative concepts.

If one had to cite a focal point of stimulation for the development of modern dental implantology in the United States, one would most certainly have to recognize the major role that the Strocks played in developing *sound scientific data* for presentation to the dental community. Again, international war intervened and set aside the use of these unique reconstruction techniques for the dental apparatus. Following World War II though, interest started again and we began to see a widespread application of implant protocols throughout the world. The details of this development are outlined in Chapter 2.

Although some dentists began to practice implantology as a bona fide part of their practice, a lack of enthusiasm on the part of other practitioners, and a lack of support for dentists wanting to conduct scientific investigations, led to the alienation between the professional dental community and implantologists for many years. Only through a great deal of dedicated work and personal effort were these implant dentists able to challenge the preconceived notions of the profession about dental implants and their service for patients.[3]

A number of factors occurring at approximately the same time heightened the interest in dental implants in the decade of the 1980s. Our society began changing with a larger group of older and retired Americans who had a higher dental IQ. These people had experienced good dental care all their lives and they expected the same in their late years. And they had the funds, or insurance coverage, to pay for the treatment. This was occurring at about the time that a decline in the caries rate was being recognized, and dentists perceived a business problem. Further, the first National Institutes of Health (NIH)–Harvard sponsored conference on dental implants was published in 1978,[4] and this was followed by publication in the scientific literature of the Swedish human clinical trials.[5] Professional and lay interest was aroused, and suddenly dental implants were a much discussed subject, both by the profession and by the public. In the short span of 10 years dental implants had gone from a type of treatment considered as charlatan in nature by many professionals to a treatment option in high demand by the public and by dentists as they scrambled to attend postdoctoral courses and seminars on the various implant systems.[6]

We are now in the last decade of the 20th century and we must examine the future directions of dental implantology.

A key to continued growth and success in this treatment field is the development of sound educational programs in implantology. Since the large segment of dental practitioners engaged in or starting implant practice are already graduate dentists, the educational programs must be organized along sound postdoctoral continuing education channels. This type of information and learning cannot be adequately assimilated in short weekend programs. The complex nature of the material requires a commitment on the part of the practitioner to attend a multiple-session program, 3 to 4 days a month, 9 months to 1 year in length, to acquire a knowledge about the entire field, from basic material properties to interface phenomena to treatment concepts. This type of instruction is best conducted in dental schools and institutes and these units of the dental profession must take the lead in developing academic programs so that the graduate dentist can become well-schooled in implant principles. The sessions must include some type of laboratory and clinical hands-on experience so the dentist becomes familiar with the intricacies of implant practice. There is no substitute for experiencing the sweaty feeling that occurs when a pilot or cannon drill suddenly drops into the soft trabecular bone of the jaw interior when not anticipated or planned in the treatment approach. Experience and education must go hand in hand if implant longevity is to succeed.

The other part of an implant educational program that needs to be developed and initiated is predoctoral and graduate student and resident programs.[7] Dental students must be given some beginning exposure to the field so they can make sound

decisions about postdoctoral implant education; and residents must have a competent program of instruction that includes actual clinical treatment and follow-up. Three of the dental specialities now require experience in implantology as part of their resident training requirements: oral and maxillofacial surgery, periodontics, and prosthodontics. All of these implant instruction programs are best developed and directed by those persons who are the professional educators in the profession.[7] They can utilize the services of the experienced implant clinician as a presenter in various parts of the course.

Clearly, instruction is the future for implantology. Experienced implantologists must expand their knowledge base while the beginning implant therapist develops the skills and background that will make him or her a successful implant practitioner.

The other major future direction for implantology is investigation. Implant science must develop a bigger and broader base of inquiry into implant function and success. We can no longer rely on empiric experiences of individual practitioners or the advertising hyperbole of implant manufacturers. Reputable investigative studies led by dental scientists skilled in the investigative process must head this effort. This is starting to occur now. But the research process must be championed by the profession. This is a critical direction in which the speciality of implantology must expand in the next decade. And the individual dentist must be an advocate for this type of scientific effort. He must encourage his dental school alma mater and various federal agencies such as the National Institute of Dental Research to fund scientific implant studies and encourage agencies like the Food and Drug Administration to establish scientific requirements and premarket standards for implants prior to their availability to the entire profession (see Chapter 36). The general dentist and the specialist must contribute to the investigative process themselves. They need to keep accurate records on the implants they place, and report this information at dental study groups, implant organizations, and dental society meetings. They need to participate in implant registry and retrieval programs that are being made available to the profession. When an implant fails, they should not sweep this fact under the carpet, but submit the specimen for analysis to an implant retrieval service.* Only in this manner will knowledge about the biological tissue reaction be shared with the profession.

Investigation is a key ingredient to the growth of the implant field. Sound, well-conceived basic materials, and biological tissue interface and clinical studies must be conducted for the continued future growth of implant dentistry.

CONCLUSION

As implantology moves into the final decade of this century a number of challenges are clearly projected as the future direction of implant practice and service. The major challenges are education in implantology and in depth research in implantology using the scientific process. The door is just ajar now so dentists must become advocates of implantology for the profession and strongly support educational requirements and sound research data about implant systems. Only then will the implant knowledge base grow and a better and more reliable service be provided to our patients.

Implantology has become an exciting and dynamic force within dentistry during the past decade; from a less-than-well-accepted treatment option it has mushroomed into the current hottest issue in dentistry. Implantology provides many new and exciting ways to help dental patients achieve function and social well-being, and provide a certain amount of personal professional satisfaction to the dentist himself.

*American Academy of Implant Dentistry Research Foundation–Medical College of Georgia Implant Retrieval Service, School of Dentistry, Augusta, Ga, established March 1990.

The future is bright for implantology and as we move into the next decade and a new century, the dental professionals need to become advocates of the treatment protocol and support increased education and investigation with enthusiasm.[8]

REFERENCES

1. Greenfield EJ: Implantation of artificial roots for crown and bridge work. *Dent Rev* 1914; 28:1–7.
2. Strock AE: Experimental work on a method for the replacement of missing teeth by direct implantation of a metal support into the alveolus. *Am J Orthodont Oral Surg* 1939; 25:467–472.
3. James RA: Dental implants—moving into the mainstream. *J Calif Dent Assoc* 1984; 6:22–25.
4. Schnitman PA, Schulman LB (eds): *Dental Implants: Benefit and Risk. An NIH-Harvard Consensus Development Conference*. Bethesda, Md, US Department of Health and Human Services Publication No. (NIH)81-1531, 1980.
5. Adell R, Lekholm U, Rockler B, et al: A 15-year study of osseointegrated implants in the treatment of the edentulous jaw. *Int J Oral Surg* 1981; 10:387–416.
6. Balkin BE: Implant dentistry: Historical overview with current perspective. *J Dent Educ* 1988; 52:683–685.
7. Steflik DE, Gowgiel JM, James RA, et al: Oral implantology instruction in dental schools. *J Oral Implantol* 1989; 15:6–16.
8. McKinney RV Jr: Implantology into the next decade: The three I index (editorial). *Implantologist* 1990; 6:7–8.

Index

A

Abutment head(s)
  bending adjustments to, in
      plate/blade implant
      insertion, 98–99
  one-stage and two-stage, adjusting
      of, for interocclusal
      clearance, 91–92
  preparation of gingival tissue
      around, in plate/blade
      implant insertion, 100–101
Age, pharmacologic considerations
      on, 82
Alloys for endosteal implants, 28
Alpha aluminum oxide for Bioceram
      implant systems, 219–221,
      222
Aluminum oxide single crystal
      material for Bioceram
      implant systems, 219–221,
      222
Alveolar bone breakdown around
      implant failures,
      physiology of, 149
Amorphous component of bone, 54
Ancient era of implantology, 8–9
Anesthesia, local, for plate/blade
      implant insertion, 92
Antimicrobial agents, topical, in
      plaque control for implant
      patient, 407
Antimicrobial therapy of wound
      infections, 84–85
Apical arteries in bone, 59
Armamentarium
  for Flexi-Cup implant system,
      180, 181
  for Flexiroot implant system, 258
  hygiene, with implant, 112–113
  for oral hygiene by implant
      patient, 402–405,
      406–407

for Oratronics plate/blade implant
      system, 131–133, 134,
      135
for Startanius blade implants,
      156–157, 158, 159
Arteries, nutrient, in bone, 58
Attachment complex, implant-tissue,
      49
A-type design for Bioceram
      implants, 216, 217
Augmentation of bone in
      implantology, 438–446
  biomaterials for, 439–444
  with calcium phosphate
      bioceramics, 441–443
  ceramic, 440–441, 444
  with combination of implant
      systems, 444–445
  complications of, 443
  discussion of, 445–446
  indications for, 438–439
  with medical polymers, 440
  metallic, 439–440
  with solid block hydroxylapatite,
      443–444

B

Bar attachments in overdentures,
      379–380
Biblades as reentry implants, 150
Bioceram implant systems, 215–229
  A-type design for, 216, 217
  ceramic material in, 219–221
  discussion on, 229
  E-type design for, 215, 216
  implant in, 215–219
  instrumentarium for, 223–224
  patient considerations for, 222
  porous root design for, 216, 218
  prosthodontic considerations for,
      228–229
  site selection for, 222

S-type design for, 215, 216
surgical procedure for, 224–228
Type II-Two Stage Design for,
      217, 219
Biochemical interactions,
      implant-to-tissue interfaces
      and, 34
Biointegration vs. osseointegration,
      111–112
Biological properties of tissues, 30,
      32
Biological seal, tissue-implant, role
      of, 46–49
Biological tissues
  in body-implant interactions,
      37–38
  response of, to implants, 37–50
    peri-implant bone, 41–45
    peri-implant connective tissue,
      45–46
    peri-implant gingival, 38–41,
      42
Biomaterials
  in body-implant interactions, 37
  for endosteal implants, 28–30, 31
    implant-to-tissue interfaces and,
      33–34
    mechanical properties of, 30,
      31
Biomechanical considerations,
      implant-to-tissue interfaces
      and, 34–35
Biomechanics
  in body-implant interactions, 37
  of endosteal implants, 30, 32–33
    research on, 33
Blade form endosteal implants, 30,
      32
Blade form series of Stryker implant
      system, 203–214 (see also
      Stryker precision dental
      implant system, blade form
      series in)

Blade implants in Omni system, 171–172
Blade-Vent implant(s), 139–154 (*see also* Ultimatics Blade-Vent implant system)
  choosing implant site for, 143
  insertion of, 145–146, 145–148
    healing after, 146
    implant selection and bone for, 146–148
    making osteotomy groove for, 145–146
    postoperative considerations for, 146
    seating in, 146
  modification of, 143, 145
  principles of design for, 143
  rationale for, 143
  sterilization of, 145
  treatment of, during insertion, 145
Blood
  diseases of, in patient evaluation, 73
  supply of, to bone, 58–59
Blood vessels in hemostasis, 78
Body-implant interactions, sphere of, 37–38
Body serviceability in body-implant interactions, 38
Bone
  augmentation of, in implantology, 438–446 (*see also* Augmentation of bone in implantology)
  biology of, basic, in implantology, 52–62
  blood supply to, 58–59
  bundle, 56
  compact, 56
    remodeling of, 57–58
  fine-fibered, 57
  formation of, 53–54
    hormones and, 60
    vitamins and, 59
  fractured and damaged, healing of, 60–61
  grafting of, 439
  haversian, 57
  healing of, 77
  immature, 56
  lamellar, 57
  mature, 56, 57
  membranes of, 54–55
  osteonal, 57
  repair of, 56
    hormones and, 60

  vitamins and, 59–60
  response of
    to endosteal implant placement, 61
    peri-implant, 41–45
  synthetic, in implantology, 427–436 (*see also* Synthetic bone)
  trabecular, 56
  woven, 56
Bone tissue, 52
  histologic classification of, 56–57
  morphologic classification of, 55–56
  types of, 55–57
Brånemark single-tooth abutment in Nobelpharma implant system, 313
Bundle bone, 56

C

Calcification in bone formation, 54
Calcium aluminate for augmentation of bone, 440–441
Calcium phosphate bioceramics for augmentation of bone, 441–443
Calculus removal from implant surfaces, 407–408
Callus in bone healing, 61
Canaliculus in bone formation, 54
Canal(s)
  haversian, in remodeling of compact bone, 57
  Volkmann's, in bone, 58
Carbons for endosteal implants, 28–29
Cardiovascular disease in patient evaluation, 71
Cartilage, Meckel's, 52
Casts, study, in patient evaluation, 70
Cells
  mesenchymal, in bone formation, 53
  osteogenic, in bone formation, 53
  osteoprogenitor, in bone formation, 53
Cellular components of wound healing, 76–77
Cement line in remodeling of compact bone, 58
Central fossa-ridge crest relationships for Oratronics plate/blade implant system, 135–136

Central tendency, measures of, in clinical implant trials, 453
Centrifugal circulation of blood
  in bone, 58
  in mandible, 59
Centripetal circulation of blood in mandible under abnormal conditions, 59
Ceramic and nonceramic derivatives as synthetic bone, 433–434
Ceramics
  for augmentation of bone, 440–441, 444
  for Bioceram implant systems, 219–221
  for endosteal implants, 28–29
Chemical interactions, implant-to-tissue interfaces and, 34
Chemical mediators in wound healing, 77
Clinical evaluation tools for implant performance, 388–394
  controls in, 393
  gingival bleeding index as, 389, 390
  minimal standards for clinical serviceability and, 393
  mobility index as, 391–392
  patient comfort index as, 393
  peridontal probe index as, 390
  plaque and calculus index as, 390–391
  practical criteria for, 388–389
  purpose of, 389
  radiographic index as, 392
  sulcular fluid volume index as, 390, 391
Clinical implant trials
  contemporary, statistical reporting of, 456–457
  controlled, necessity for, 448–450
  design of, 452–458
  statistically sound, incorporation of scientific method into, 457–458
  statistical methods for, 452–455
Clinical observation in diagnosis of failing implant, 422–423
Co-abutment(s), natural, serving as support under same prosthesis as implants, preparing and temporizing, 89
Coagulation in hemostasis, 78–80

Cobalt alloy for endosteal implants, 28
Coefficients of correlation in clinical implant trials, 453
Collagen in wound healing, 76
Compact bone, 56
  remodeling of, 57–58
Composites for endosteal implants, 29
Connective tissue response, peri-implant, 45–46
Contamination, avoiding, in plate/blade implant surgery, 88
Controlled clinical implant trials, necessity for, 448–450
Core-Vent implant in Core-Vent implant system, 315, 317
  indications for, 319
  surgical protocol for, 320, 321
Core-Vent implant system, 315–330
  Bio-Vent implant in, 317, 318
  complete edentulous prosthodontic options with, 325–326, 327
  discussion of, 328–329
  for fixed-detachable prosthetics, 324–325
  for fixed prosthetics, 323–324
  healing with, 323
  Micro-Vent implant in, 315–316, 317
  partially edentulous prosthodontic options with, 326–328
  patient evaluation for, 318–319
  prosthetic applications of, 323–328
  Screw-Vent implant in, 315, 317
  SUB-Vent implant in, 317–318
  surgical procedures for, 319–323
  Swede-Vent implant in, 316–317
Coronal screws in Steri-Oss implant system, 357–358
Corrugated reentry devices, 150, 151
Culturing in diagnosis of failing implant, 424
Cutting cone in remodeling of compact bone, 57

D

Dental implants (*see* Implant)
Dermatologic diseases in patient evaluation, 73
Descriptive statistics in clinical implant trials, 453

E

Edentulous patient, prosthetic rehabilitation with Flexiroot implant system for, 263
Education
  patient, on oral hygiene with implant, 405, 407
  postgraduate, in practice management, 412
Embryologic development of jaws, 52–53
Endocrine system diseases in patient evaluation, 72–73
Endosseous implant, two-stage, 5
Endosteal area, periodontal considerations for, 107–109
Endosteal implant, 5
  biomaterials for, 28–30, 31
    overview of, 27–28
  biomechanics of, 30, 32–33
    overview of, 27–28
  patient with (*see* Patient)
  placement of, bone response to, 61
Endosteal implants
  stage I, history of, 12
  stage II, history of, 13
Endosteal implant system(s), 117–371
  Bioceram, 215–229 (*see also* Bioceram implant system)
  Core-Vent, 315–330 (*see also* Core-Vent implant system)
  Flexi-Cup three-dimensional blade implant devices, 174–186 (*see also* Flexi-Cup three-dimensional blade implant devices)
  Flexiroot, 255–265 (*see also* Flexiroot implant system)
  IMZ-interpore osteointegrated, 331–347 (*see also* Intramobile cylinder (IMZ)-interpore osteointegrated implant system)
  Integral, 362–371 (*see also* Integral implant system)
  ITI, 240–254 (*see also* ITI implant system)
  Nobelpharma, 293–314 (*see also* Nobelpharma implant system)
  Omnii, 163–173 (*see also* Omnii implant system)
  plate/blade oratronics, 119–138 (*see also* Plate/blade oratronics implant system)
  Startanius, 156–162 (*see also* Startanius implant system)
  Steri-Oss, 349–361 (*see also* Steri-Oss implant system)
  Stryker precision, 188–214 (*see also* Stryker precision dental implant system)
  Titanodont, 231–239 (*see also* Titanodont implant system)
  Ultimatics Blade-Vent, 139–154 (*see also* Ultimatics Blade-Vent implant system)
  Vent-Plant osseointegrated compatible, 266–291 (*see also* Vent-Plant osseointegrated compatible implant system)
Endosteal plexus in bone, 58
Endosteum, 55
  in bone formation, 54
Endothelium in hemostasis, 78
Erosion tunnel in remodeling of compact bone, 57
E-type design for Bioceram implants, 215, 216
External oblique blade-vent implants, 151–152
Extraction sites, new, implanting, in plate/blade implant insertion, 100

F

Failing implant, clinical management of, 422–426
  bacteriologic considerations in, 425
  diagnosis in, 422–424
  discussion of, 425–426
  prosthesis evaluation in, 425
  treatment intervention in, 424–425
Fibro-osseous integration vs. osseointegration, 109–110
Fibro-osseous retention, definition of, 107
Fibrous component of bone, 54

Figure-of-8 reentry implants,
150–151
Fine-fibered bone, 57
Flexi-Cup three-dimensional blade
implant devices, 174–186
armamentarium for, 180, 181
discussion on, 185–186
implant in, 174, 175
selection of, 176–180
patient evaluation for, 174–176
prosthetic considerations for,
184–185
surgical procedure for, 180–183
Flexiroot implant system, 255–265
concept of, 255
discussion of, 264
implant in, 255–258
indications for, 258–259
instrumentation for, 258
prosthetic rehabilitation with,
261–264
in fully edentulous patient, 263
in overdenture procedure,
263–264
surgical procedures for, 259–261
in vivo fluorochrome stain-test
implant-bone biopsy
technique in evaluation of,
264–265
Force distribution with Blade-Vent
implant, 148–149
Force transfer in biomechanics of
endosteal implants, 30
Foundational period of implantology
of, 10–11
Frame implants in Omni system,
172, 173

G

Gastrointestinal diseases in patient
evaluation, 72
Genetic factors, pharmacologic
considerations on, 82–83
Gingival bleeding index, 389, 390
Gingival plastic surgery in
plate/blade implant
insertion, 100
Gingival response, peri-implant,
38–41, 42
Gingival tissue preparation around
abutment head in
plate/blade implant
insertion, 100–101

Globulin, cold-soluble, in wound
healing, 76
Glucocorticoids, bone formation and
repair and, 60
Glucose-6-phosphate dehydrogenase
(G6PD) deficiency,
pharmacologic
considerations on, 82
Grafting, bone, 439
Ground substance in wound healing,
76

H

Hard tissue replacement (HTR)
polymer as synthetic bone,
430–433
Haversian bone, 57
Haversian canal
in bone formation, 54
in remodeling of compact bone,
57
Haversian system in remodeling of
compact bone, 57
Head height adjustment for
interocclusal clearance in
plate/blade implant
insertion, 99
Healing following Blade-Vent
implant insertion, 146
Healing time and sequencing
one-stage and two-stage
systems for plate/blade
implant insertion, 103–104
Hemostasis, 78–81
Histologic classification of bone
tissue, 55–56
History of implantology, 8–16
ancient era in, 8–9
contemporary oral implantology
in, 14–15
dawn of modern era in, 12–13
foundational period in, 10–11
medieval period in, 9–10
premodern era in, 11–12
professional status in, 15
Hollow-cylinder implants, 246–254
(*see also* ITI implant
systems, hollow-cylinder
implants in)
Home car after plate/blade implant
insertion, 103
Horizontal basket reentry implants,
151

Hormone effects on bone formation
and repair, 60
Host tissue reaction, 19–23
handling implant in, 22–23
material properties in, 19–22
Host vs implant, functional
biocompatibility of, 23–24
Hydroxylapatite
for augmentation of bone,
441–443
solid blocks of, for augmentation
of bone, 443–444
as synthetic bone, 433–434
Hydroxylapatite crystals in bone
formation, 54
Hygiene, oral, protocol for,
400–408 (*see also* Oral
hygiene protocol for
implant patients)
Hygiene instrumentation with
implant, 112–113

I

Immature bone, 56
Implant(s)
biological tissue response to,
37–50 (*see also* Biological
tissue response to implants)
demographics and economics of,
6–7
design and function of,
biomechanics and, 30,
32–33
endosseous, two-stage, 5
endosteal, 5 (*see also* Endosteal
implant)
failing, clinical management of,
422–426 (*see also* Failing
implant, clinical
management of)
handling of, host tissue reaction
and, 22–23
management of, clinical
considerations of,
373–463
performance of, clinical evaluation
tools for, 388–394
plate/blade, surgery for, 88–104
(*see also* Plate/blade
implant(s), surgery for)
reentry, 149–152
safety of, host tissue reaction and,
19–22
science of (*see* Implantology)

Implant(s) *(cont.)*
  sinus-lift, 152–153
  subperiosteal, 4–5
  and tissues, interfaces between, 33–35
  vs host, functional biocompatibility of, 23–24
Implantology
  background of, 3
  bone biology in, basic, 52–62
  clinical considerations for, 19–24
    host tissue reaction in, 19–23
    host vs implant in, 23–24
  contemporary, history of, 14–15
  current treatment concepts and progress in, 4–5
  four B's of, 37–38
  future projections for, 461–463
  history of, 8–16 *(see also* History of implantology of*)*
  overview and progress of, 3
  science and developing of, 4
Implant-tissue attachment complex, 49
Implant-tissue interface, biological and clinical mechanisms operative at, research into, 5–6
Incision
  for plate/blade implant insertion, 92–93
  trimming edges of, for plate/blade implant insertion, 94
Infection(s), wound, 83–86
  antimicrobial therapy of, 84–85
  microbiology of, 83–84
  pharmacologic considerations on, 83–86
Inferential statistics in clinical implant trials, 453–454
Insertion visit for plate/blade implants, 92–103
  adjusting head height for interocclusal clearance in, 99
  bending adjustments to abutment head in, 98–99
  cleansing ridge crest in, 94
  final closure in, 101–102
  final seating in, 99–100
  gingival plastic surgery in, 100
  implanting new extraction site in, 100
  incision in, 92–93
  local anesthesia in, 92

locating implant receptor site in, 94
  preliminary bending adjustments to implant body in, 96–97
  preliminary seating of implant in, 97–98
  preoperative and postoperative medication in, 92
  preparation of gingival tissue around abutment head in, 100–101
  preparing receptor site in, 95–96
  temporization and function during healing in, 102–103
  tissue reflection in, 93–94
  trimming edges of incision in, 94
Instrumentation *(see* Armamentarium)
Instruments, titanium, for Oratronics plate/blade implant system, 132
Integral implant system, 362–371
  bone preparation for, 366–367
  closure in, 369
  discussion of, 369–370
  implant in, 362, 363
  implant placement in, 368–369
  instrumentation for, 364–365, 366
  patient consideration for, 362–364
  patient selection for, 362–364
  postoperative care for, 369
  surgical procedure for, 366–369
Intercellular space in bone, 53
International Team of Implantologists (ITI) implant system, 240–254 *(see also* ITI implant systems)
Interocclusal clearance
  adjusting head height for plate/blade implant insertion for, 99
  adjusting one-stage and two-stage abutment heads for, 91–92
Intraalveolar arteries in bone, 59
Intramobile cylinder (IMZ)-interpore osteointegrated implant system, 331–347
  with additional abutment, 334
  bilateral free-end reconstruction with, 334
  clinical indications for, 333–335
  coronal fixation screw in, 344

fixed restorative design for, 344–345
  frame waxing for, 344
  for fully edentulous arch, 335
  impression making for, 343
  insertion of final prosthesis with, 345–347
  laboratory intramobile element in, 344
  pouring impression for, 344
  presurgical evaluation for, 335–336
  prosthetic phase in, 341–344
  for single tooth replacement, 333
  two-stage implantation procedure for, 338–341
    stage I in, 338–341
    stage II in, 341
  unilateral free-end reconstruction with, 333, 334
  for wide edentulous span, 334
Intraosseous vessels in bone, 59
In vivo fluorochrome stain-test implant-bone biopsy technique in evaluation of Flexiroot implant system, 264–265
ITI implant systems, 240–254
  hollow-cylinder implants in, 246–254
    discussion on, 253–254
    placement procedures for, 247
    prosthetic technique for, 251, 253
    surgical indications for, 247
    surgical procedure for
      F implant, 247–250
      H implant, 250–251, 252
      K implant, 250
  implants in, 240–242
  Titanium plasma-sprayed screw in, 240–246
    indications for, 242–243
    patient considerations on, 242–245
    prosthetic technique for, 245–246
    surgical procedures for, when used as overdenture, 243–245

J

Jaws, embryologic development of, 52–53

K

Kidney diseases
in patient evaluation, 72
pharmacologic considerations on,
81–82

L

Laboratory tests in patient
evaluation, 73
Lacuna in bone formation, 54
Lamellar bone, 57
Laminin in transmucosal seal
formation, 48
Landmarks, clearing, adjusting
implant for, 90–91
Life table analysis in clinical implant
trials, 454
Liver disease, pharmacologic
considerations on, 82

M

Magnetic attachments in Steri-Oss
implant system, 360
Magnets in overdentures, 380–381
Malignant disease in patient
evaluation, 73
Marketing in practice management,
411–412, 413–414
external, 414–415
internal, 415–419
vs. external, 414–419
Marrow, red and yellow, 56
Material properties, host tissue
reaction and, 19–22
Matrix, organic, 54
Mature bone, 56, 57
Maxilla, circulation of blood in, 59
Meckel's cartilage, 52
Mediators, chemical, in wound
healing, 77
Medical evaluation in patient
evaluation, 71–73
Medication, preoperative and
postoperative, in
plate/blade implant
insertion, 92
Medieval period of implantology,
9–10
Medullary cavity, 56
Medullary plexus in bone, 58
Membranes of bone, 54–55
Mesenchymal cells in bone
formation, 53

Mesial and distal abutment head
location with Oratronics
plate/blade implant system,
128
Metallic augmentation of bone,
439–440
Metallurgy and interface texture with
Oratronics plate/blade
implant system, 125–126,
127
Metals for endosteal implants, 28
Metal transfer, avoiding, in
plate/blade implant
surgery, 88
Microbiology of wound infections,
83–84
Micro-Vent implant in Core-Vent
implant system, 315–316,
317
indications for, 318, 319
surgical protocol for, 322, 323
Mineralization in bone formation, 54
Mineralization phase in bone
formation, 54
Mobility index, 391–392
Modern era of implantology, dawn
of, 12–13
Morphologic classification of bone
tissue, 55–56
Mucous membrane diseases in
patient evaluation, 73

N

Nervous system diseases in patient
evaluation, 72
Nobelpharma implant system,
293–314
abutment connection in, 302–303,
304
implant insertion in, 294–302
in mandible, 294–299
in maxilla, 299–302
instrument preparation for,
293–294
laboratory procedures for,
310–311
patient placement for, 312–313
patient selection for, 293–294
prosthodontic procedure for,
303–310
after abutment connection, 305
early care in, 303–305
final impression procedure in,
305–307
interim prosthesis in, 303–305

maxillomandibular relationship
records in, 307–308
patient try-in in, 308–310
trial setup of teeth in, 308–310
single tooth abutment for,
313–314
surgical procedure for, 294–303
Nonparametric statistics in clinical
implant trials, 454–455
Nutrient arteries in bone, 58

O

Omnii implant system, 163–173
background of, 163
blade implants in, 171–172
frame implants in, 172, 173
root form implants in, 163–165,
166–169
sinus implants in, 165–166,
170–171
Oral hygiene protocol for implant
patients, 400–408
armamentarium for, 402–405,
406–407
maintenance care in, 408
pathogenesis of "peri-implantitis"
and, 400–401
patient instruction in, 405, 407
plaque regulation by patient in,
402–407
removing calculus from dental
implant surfaces in,
407–408
topical antimicrobial agents in,
407
Oratronics Generation Ten Blade
Implant System, 119, 121
Oratronics Osteo-Loc Plate Form
Implant, 119, 122–123
Oratronics Standard Blade Implant
System, 119, 120
Organic matrix, 54
O ring attachments in Steri-Oss
implant system, 360
Osseointegration, 42
definition of, 108–109
two-stage endosseous implant and,
5
of Vent-Plant implants, 276, 286
vs biointegration, 111–112
vs. fibro-osseous integration,
109–110
Ossification, definition of, 53
Osteoblasts in bone formation, 53,
54

Osteocalcin in bone, 54
Osteoclasia, definition of, 54
Osteoclasts
  in bone formation, 54
  in remodeling of compact bone, 57
Osteocytes in bone formation, 54
Osteogenesis, definition of, 53
Osteogenic cells in bone formation, 53
Osteoid formation phase in bone formation, 54
Osteoid in bone formation, 54
Osteo-Loc Plate Form Implants
  mesial and distal abutment head location for, 128–131
  serial placement of, 131
Osteolysis, definition of, 54
Osteomalacia, 59
Osteonal bone, 57
Osteonectin in bone, 54
Osteon in remodeling of compact bone, 57–58
Osteoprogenitor cells in bone formation, 53
Osteotomy groove, making of, for Blade-Vent implant, insertion of, 145–146
Overdenture procedure, prosthetic rehabilitation with Flexiroot implant system for, 263–264
Overdentures, implant prosthodontics in, 379–381, 382

P

Parallelism with Oratronics plate/blade implant system, 128
Parallel pins in Integral implant system, 365
  surgical procedure using, 368
Parathyroid hormone (PTH), bone formation and repair and, 60
Patient
  clinical examination of, 64–67
  dental evaluation of, 63
  dental history of, 63–64
  instruction of, on oral hygiene with implant, 405, 407
  medical evaluation of, 71–73
  photographs of, 71
  radiographs of, 67–70
  selection of, 63

study casts of, 70
Patient comfort index, 393
Peri-implant bone response, 41–45
Peri-implant connective tissue response, 45–46
Peri-implant gingival response, 38–41
Perimucosal area, periodontal considerations for, 105–107, 108, 109
Periodontal considerations for implantology, 105–114
  discussion on, 113–114
  in endosteal area, 107–109
  fibro-osseous integration vs. osseointegration as, 109–110
  hygiene instrumentation as, 112–113
  osseointegration vs. biointegration as, 111–112
  in perimucosal area, 105–107, 108, 109
  in transgingival area, 105–107, 108, 109
Periodontal plexus in bone, 59
Periodontal probe index, 390
Periosteal plexus in bone, 59
Periosteum, 55
  in bone formation, 54
Perivascular cells in remodeling of compact bone, 57
Personality in practice management, 413
Pharmacologic considerations in implant surgery, 81–83
Philosophy of life, practice management and, 419
Photographs in patient evaluation, 71
Physiologic loads in biomechanics of endosteal implants, 30
Pilot drill in Integral implant system, 364
  surgical procedure using, 367
Plaque, regulation of, by implant patient, 402–407
Plaque and calculus index, 390–391
Plate/blade implant(s)
  adjusting, to clear landmarks, 90–91
  body of, preliminary bending adjustments to, in plate/blade implant insertion, 96–97
  final seating of, in plate/blade implant insertion, 99–100

form selector for, for final model selection, use of, 90
one-stage system for
  insertion of
    final closure in, 101–102
    preparation of gingival tissue around abutment head in, 100–101, 102
    temporization and function during healing in, 102–103
    vs. two-stage system, 88–89
  preliminary seating of, in plate/blade implant insertion, 97–98
  proper, selection of, 89–92
  receptor site for, locating, in plate/blade implant insertion, 94
  single- vs. double-headed, selection of, 90
  surgery for, 88–104
    avoiding metal transfer and contamination in, 88
    exposure of two-stage implant after healing in, 104
    healing time in, sequencing one-stage and two-stage systems and, 103–104
    insertion visit in, 92–103 (*see also* Insertion visit for plate/blade implants)
    preinsertion visit in, 88–89
    selecting proper implant in, 89–92
  two-stage system for
    insertion of
      final closure in, 102
      preparation of gingival tissue around abutment heads in, 101
      temporization and function during healing in, 103
    variations in, 89
Plate/blade Oratronics implant system, 119–154
  armamentarium for, 131–133, 134, 135
  central fossa-ridge crest relationships in, 135–136
  discussion of, 137–138
  finishing lines in, 137
  implants for, 119–123
    Oratronics Generation Ten Blade Implant System, 119, 121

Oratronics Osteo-Loc Plate Form Implant System, 119, 122–123
Oratronics Standard Blade Implant System, 119, 120
materials for, 137
metallurgy and interface texture with, 125–126, 127
occlusion with, 137
one-stage sequencing with, 126
prosthetic procedures with, 133, 135–137
prosthodontic considerations on, 135–137
prosthodontic fulfillment with, 128–131
ridge-lapping implant abutments in, 136–137
two-stage sequencing with, 126, 128
Platelets in hemostasis, 78
Polymer derivatives as synthetic bone, 429–433
Polymers
for endosteal implants, 29
medical, for augmentation of bone, 440
Porous root design for Bioceram implants, 216, 218
Porphyria, pharmacologic considerations on, 82–83
Practice management, 411–421
discussion of, 421
happiness in, 419–421
marketing in, 411–412, 413–414
external, 414–415
internal, 415–419
vs. external, 414–419
personality and, 413
postgraduate education and, 412
role model and, 412
Prebone, 54
Premodern era of implantology of, 11–12
Professional status of implantology, history of, 15
Prosthesis(es)
fixed, implant prosthodontics in, 378–379
fixed-removable, implant prosthodontics in, 381–384
Prosthetic attachments, Steri-Oss, 351–352
Prosthetic considerations
for Blade-Vent implant, 148–149
for Flexi-Cup implant system, 184–185
Prosthetic laboratory relationships for endosteal implants, 395–399
dental laboratory education on, 399
dental laboratory's obligations for, 398
dentist's obligations for, 397–398
diagnostic wax-up of, 396–397
written work authorization for, 398
Prosthetic procedure for Oratronics plate/blade implant system, 133, 135–137
Prosthetic reconstruction with Steri-Oss implant system, 357–360
Prosthetic rehabilitation with Flexiroot implant system, 261–264
Prosthetics
fixed, Core-Vent implant system for, 323–324
fixed-detachable, Core-Vent implant system for, 324–325
Prosthodontic fulfillment with Oratronics plate/blade implant system, 128–131
Prosthodontic options for Core-Vent implant system
complete edentulous, 325–326, 327
partially edentulous, 326–328
Prosthodontics, implant
applications of, 377–384
diagnostic evaluation and, 376–377
discussion of, 384–385
in fixed prostheses, 378–379
in fixed-removal prosthesis, 381–384
functional considerations in, 375–376
in overdentures, 379–381, 382
practical, 375–385
in single tooth replacement, 377–378
treatment planning and, 376–377
Proteoglycans in wound healing, 76

R

Radiographic findings in diagnosis of failing implant, 423–424
Radiographic index, 392
Radiographic measurement template in patient evaluation, 68–70
Radiographs in patient evaluation, 67–70
Receptor site
locating, in plate/blade implant insertion, 94
preparing, in plate/blade implant insertion, 94–96
Red marrow, 56
Reentry implants, 149–152
Regression analysis in clinical implant trials, 454
Rehabilitation, prosthetic, with Flexiroot implant system, 261–264
Remodeling of compact bone, 57–58
Repair bone, 56
Repeated measures analysis of variance in clinical implant trials, 454
Respiratory system diseases in patient evaluation, 71–72
Retention, fibro-osseous, definition of, 107
Rickets, 59
Ridge crest cleansing in plate/blade implant insertion, 94
Ridge-lapping implant abutments, 136–137
Root form endosteal implants, 30, 32
Root form implants in Omni system, 163–165, 166–169
Root form series of Stryker implant system, 188–201 (*see also* Stryker precision dental implant system, root form series of)
Rosette bur in Integral implant system, 364
surgical procedure using, 367

S

Safety, implant, host tissue reaction and, 19–22
Scientific method, incorporation of, into statistically sound clinical implant trials, 457–458
Screw-Vent implant in Core-Vent implant system, 315, 317
indications for, 319

Screw-Vent implant in Core-Vent
        implant system *(cont.)*
    surgical protocol for, 321, 322
Scurvy, 59
Semisubmerged system for
        plate/blade implants
    exposure of two-stage implant
        after healing in, 104
    vs. submerged system, 88–89
Sequential multiple analyzer (SMA
    P/60, SMA 6/60), 73
Sex, pharmacologic considerations
    on, 82
Shiner magnet in Steri-Oss implant
    system, 360
Shock-absorbing element, implant
    system with, 331–347 *(see
    also* Intramobile cylinder
    (IMZ)-interpore
    osteointegrated implant
    system)
Sinus implants in Omni system,
    165–166, 170–171
Sinus-lift implants, 152–153
Skin diseases in patient evaluation, 73
Snakelike reentry devices, 150
Spade drills in Integral implant
        system, 364–365
    surgical procedure using,
        367–368
Stainless steel, surgical, for
    endosteal implants, 28
Standard deviation (SD) in clinical
    implant trials, 453
Startanius blade implants, 156, 157
    surgical procedures for, 158–161
Startanius implant system, 156–173
    discussion on, 162
    implants in, 156, 157, 158
    instrumentation for, 156–157,
        158, 159
    surgical procedures for, 158–162
Startanius Star Vent implants, 156,
        158
    surgical procedures for, 161–162
Statistical methods for clinical
    implant trials, 452–453
Steri-Oss implant system, 349–361
    discussion of, 360–361
    implant exposure in, 356–357
    implant placement in, 352–356
    implants in, 349–350
    patient preparation for, 353
    patient selection for, 352
    postoperative management with,
        356

prosthetic attachments for,
    351–352
prosthetic reconstruction in,
    357–360
surgical preparation for, 352
surgical procedure for, 353–354
surgical system for, 350–351
treatment planning for, 352
Stryker precision dental implant
        system, 188–214
    blade component surgical
        procedure for, 207–210
    blade form series in, 203–214
        head options for, 213–214
        patient considerations for,
            204–205, 206
        patient selection for, 204–205,
            206
        placement of head component
            in, 210–213
        preoperative procedures for,
            205–207
        rationale for use of, 214
    root form series in, 188–201
        implant head options for,
            199–201
        patient considerations for,
            191–192
        patient selection for, 191–192
        placement of head component
            for, 198–199, 200
        preoperative procedures for,
            192, 193
        root component surgical
            procedure for, 193–198
Study casts in patient evaluation, 70
S-type design for Bioceram
    implants, 215, 216
Submerged system for plate/blade
        implants
    exposure of two-stage implant
        after healing in, 104
    vs. semisubmerged system,
        88–89
Subperiosteal implants, 4–5
    history of, 12–13
SUB-Vent implant in Core-Vent
        implant system, 317–318
    indications for, 319
    surgical protocol for, 322–323
Sulcular fluid volume index, 390, 391
Sulcus depth index, 390
Surface conditions, implant-to-tissue
    interfaces and, 33–34
Surgical principles, 75–86
    hemostasis as, 78–81

pharmacologic considerations as,
    81–83
for plate/blade implants, 88–104
wound healing as, 75–78
wound infections as, 83–86
Suture removal after plate/blade
    implant insertion, 103
Synthetic bone
    ceramic and nonceramic
        derivatives as, 433–434
    discussion of, 434–436
    hard tissue replacement (HTR)
        polymer as, 430–433
    hydroxylapatite as, 433–434
    in implantology, 427–436
    material(s) for
        available, 429–434
        comparisons of, 428
        ideal, 427
    polymer derivatives as
        nonresorbable and porous,
            429–433
        resorbable and nonporous, 433
    in prevention of bone loss, 427,
        429
    in restoration of bone loss, 427,
        429
    uses and applications of, 435

T

Telescoping abutments in Steri-Oss
    implant system, 358, 359
Thyroid hormone, bone formation
    and repair and, 60
Tissue(s)
    biological, in body-implant
        interactions, 37–38
    biological properties of, 30, 32
    bone, 52 *(see also* Bone tissue)
    and implant, interfaces between,
        biomechanics and, 33–35
    reflection of, for plate/blade
        implant insertion, 93–94
Tissue-implant biological seal, role
    of, 46–49
Titanium for endosteal implants, 28
Titanium instruments for Oratronics
    plate/blade implant system,
    132
Titanium plasma-sprayed screw (TPS
    Screw) implant, 240–246
    (see also ITI implant
    systems, Titanium
    plasma-sprayed screw in)

Titanodont implant system, 231–239
  development of, 231–232
  discussion of, 238
  healed, buried, exposure of,
    236–237
  Miter System 2000 for, 238–239
  placement technique for, 232–234
  sterile surgical technique for, 232
  subcortical blade implants for,
    238–239
  surgical placement of, 234–235
  suturing site for, 235–236
  treatment crown coverage in, 237,
    328
Tooth, single, replacement of,
    implant prosthodontics in,
    377–378
Trabecular bone, 56
Transgingival area, periodontal
    considerations for,
    105–107, 108, 109
Transmucosal seal, formation of,
    after implant surgery, 48
Try-in guide in Integral implant
    system, 365
  surgical procedure using, 368
Tunnel, erosion, in remodeling of
    compact bone, 57

U

UCLA abutment system in
    Nobelpharma implant
    system, 313–314
Ultimatics Blade-Vent implant
    system, 139–154
  background on, 139

Blade-Vent implant insertion in,
    145–148 (*see also*
    Blade-Vent implant,
    insertion of)
Blade-Vent implant modification
    for, 143, 145
failures of, physiology of alveolar
    bone breakdown around,
    149
force distribution with, 148–149
implant in, 139–143, 144
implant site selection in, 143
patient considerations on, 143,
    145
principles of, 140–142
prosthetic considerations for,
    148–149
reentry implants in, 149–152
sinus-lift implants in, 152–153
sterilization for, 145
treatment of blades during
    insertion in, 145
Urinary tract diseases in patient
    evaluation, 72

V

Variability, measures of, in clinical
    implant trials, 453
Vent-Plant osseointegrated
    compatible implant system,
    266–291
  current designs in, 268–269
    suggested clinical uses of,
    270–276
  cylindrical-type implants in,
    clinical verification of, 270

discussion on, 284, 285, 286–291
implant clinical selection in,
    276–277
patient considerations on, 267,
    270
prosthetic considerations for, 278,
    279–284
screw design implant in
    clinical verification of, 270
    original, 266–267
surfaces of implant in, 277
Vitamins, effects of, on bone
    formation and repair,
    59–60
Volkmann's canals in bone, 58

W

Weight, pharmacologic
    considerations on, 82
Wound healing, postsurgical, 75–78
Wound infections
  antimicrobial therapy of, 84–85
  microbiology of, 83–84
  pharmacologic considerations on,
    83–86
Woven bone, 56

X

X^2 test of association in clinical
    implant trials, 454–455

Y

Yellow marrow, 56